First International Congress on Cataract Surgery

Documententa Ophthalmologica
Proceedings Series volume 21

Editor H. E. Henkes

Dr. W. Junk bv Publishers The Hague-Boston-London 1979

First International Congress on Cataract Surgery Florence, 1978

Edited by J. Francois,
E. Maumenee & I. Esente

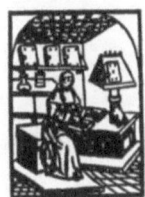

Dr. W. Junk bv Publishers The Hague-Boston-London 1979

Cover design: Max Velthuijs

ISBN-13:978-94-009-9615-1   e-ISBN-13:978-94-009-9613-7
DOI: 10.1007/978-94-009-9613-7

CONTENTS

Docum. Ophthal. Proc. Series, Vol. 21

SOCIAL ASPECTS OF THE CATARACT

R.T. VYAS

(Bombay, India)

Indeed, it is a rare privilege for a lay person such as myself to be invited to speak before an august and renowned organisation such as yours. May I at the outset express my sincere gratitude and thanks of my own and on behalf of the Royal Commonwealth Society for the Blind for this unique honour done to me.

You the experts have gathered together today to discuss for the first time at International level the 'cataract surgery'. This branch of Ophthalmic surgery has been practised since time immemorial. Cataract surgery and its technique has reference in the ancient Indian Science of Medicine called 'AYUR VEDA' which dates back 5,000 years. While you sit here and deliberate over new techniques of cataract surgery, there are millions of people in the developing countries of the world who are condemned to lives of perpetual darkness. Cataract for the developed countries of the world and their citizens really speaking is no problem at all. The onset of cataract for the citizens of the developing world relegates them to a life of utter dependence, destitution, and degradation. In India alone according to the statistics provided by the Indian Council of Medical Research five million men and woman today are totally blind because of operable cataract. According to the same organisation in the year 1978, 1.8 million eyes will go blind and would need cataract surgery. What holds good for India is equally true and perhaps more depressing for other countries in the Indian sub-continent and parts of the developing world.

Cataract is responsible for 55% of the total cases of blindness in India. Thus it is by far the most dominant factor in causing blindness. The situation is further aggravated by the fact that for the whole of India with a population of over 700 million, we have only approximately 3,500 ophthalmic surgeons. For Bangladesh which has an estimated number of 1 million blind people in a population of 80 million, the number of ophthalmic surgeons is only 25 or thereabout. Most of the Ophthalmic surgeons reside in the towns and cities, while bulk of the population of these countries lives in rural areas. This again makes it impossible for an average villager to receive ophthalmic aid for the restoration of his sight.

In Europe and other parts of the developed world, cataract sets in on or after an average age of 60 years. In India the average age at which cataract sets in is 45 years or thereabout. As is well known in the developing

1

countries of the World, there is no old age or disability pension. Thus when a person becomes blind, he is thrown out of employment, has no means of supporting himself and his family which results in gradual starvation and death.

MAGNITUDE OF THE PROBLEM

It is a contradiction of our age that while the mechanism does exist to cure cataract blindness, it is far too inadequate to meet the colossal nature of the problem. While large cities and towns have facilities, and that too, to a limited extent, the vast majority of the people sit helplessly waiting for the day of deliverance from their miserable existence through death. People just do not go blind in numbers. On paper they are cold statistics but in actual life, they are individuals. Are we going to allow them to pass their days in darkness and destitution?

In the Indian sub-continent, 80% of its 850 million people live in the rural areas pursuing traditional agricultural pursuits. When they go blind at an average age of 45 years which according to European standards is almost the 'Youth', you can imagine what will be their predicament. Let us take the example of Shankar. He lives in a small village of Kathor on the bank of the river 'Tapi'; 47 year old Shankar has a wife and 4 young children to maintain. He would leave his home early in the morning much before sunrise to work on a farm. Throughout the day, he would be working under the blazing sun and as the sun set, he would return home with his daily wage of 50 cents. With this money his wife would pay for the purchase of the food and cook the evening meal and possibly a little extra to be used the following morning for Shankar to take with him to his farm. The family of six was without an income for almost two years when Shankar could no longer work because of 'cataract'. His wife did some chores for the neighbours and earned a little income to keep the family of six alive. Shankar resigned himself to the will of God thinking that he was destined to be blind.

EYE CAMPS

One day news came to the village that eye doctors were camping in the near-by village to provide free treatment. A Rotary Club with the help of the Royal Commonwealth Society for the Blind had organised an eye camp. By word of mouth, by beating the drum and through posters people having eye trouble were notified to go to the eye camp.

A school building was converted into a temporary Eye Hospital. Desks and tables were removed; rooms washed and beds laid for the operated patients. The Rotarians worked as volunteers, patients queued up in the school compound for registration. Some came walking from miles away, some used the bullock cart, while some came by buses praying that they would get back their sight. An unassuming quiet looking gentleman in simple clothes examined the patients, in an improvised dark room. He was Dr. R.R. Doshi. It was Shankar who was sitting before Dr. Doshi, blind due to bilateral cataract. Shankar was admitted to the eye camp and operated in one eye. On the seventh day when the bandages were finally removed, Shankar saw the light for the first time after two years. His joys knew no bounds. Throughout the duration of the camp in which over 260 people were operated for cataract in three days time, free food was provided to the patients and their relatives.

Each year, the Royal Commonwealth Society for the Blind in 22 States of India, in Bangladesh and in Pakistan supports over 1,500 rural eye camps. For the year ended 31st December, 1977, eye camps supported by the Royal Commonwealth Society for the Blind in co-operation with Lions Clubs, Rotary Clubs and other Organisations examined the eyes of 668,826 Indian villagers and restored sight to 85,176 cataract blind men and woman.

EYES OF INDIA CAMPAIGN

Since 1970, when the Royal Commonwealth Society for the Blind launched the eyes of India campaign, the eyes of over a million people were examined and treated and sight of more than 4,00,000 totally blind people restored.

India has about 12,000 ophthalmic beds in its hospitals which are mainly in towns and cities. Its 3,500 ophthalmic surgeons are based in towns and cities. Eye camps are the only means which can help to restore sight to cataract blind people.

STRATEGY

The Government of India have evolved a national programme for the Control of Blindness and Visual impairment. Under this programme mobile ophthalmic units will eventually cover the rural areas of India and base hospitals in the rural areas will be set up to provide ophthalmic treatment. Till this becomes fully operative, eye camps will have to continue to play an effective role.

SUPPORT OF THE OPHTHALMOLOGISTS

Ever since Sir John Wilson, President of the International Agency for the Prevention of Blindness and Director, Royal Commonwealth Society for the Blind, addressed the Indian Ophthalmic Society in 1973, the ophthalmic surgeons are coming forward in large numbers to give their free services in the rural eye camps. Careful scrutiny of eye camps statistics have given very encouraging results. The rate of success at an eye camp is as high as 94%. Bearing in mind that these eye camps are held in improvised hospital-like accomodation, these statistics are indeed very heartening.

100 CATARACT OPERATIONS IN A DAY

At an eye camp, the day begins before sunrise, and by the time sun sets, one eye surgeon does as many as 100 cataract operations. Yes, 100 cataract operations, which will be unbelievable for most ophthalmologists, in the developed countries.

Cataract to a European or to an American is a minor inconvenience which lasts only for a short duration till he is able to have himself operated. Cataract to an Asian villager, is a crippling, handicapping, and devastating situation which only terminates with his death. The civilized Society has assured right to life to all citizens. It should be equally our endeavour to ensure right to see. To make millions of cataract blind people see again and not remain blind till they die, we may have to think of new strategy — a strategy involving the use of trained para-medical personnels to be sent to the villages to operate on cataract. Perhaps, this is too bold a statement. But extraordinary situations require extraordinary remedies. Let us hope this view of Sir John Wilson may be translated into action not in too distant a future. May I in conclusion thank you once again for inviting me to tell you that millions of people in the developing world go blind due to cataract and die blind for want of a simple operation. Let us all resolve today that while we discuss the most modern methods in cataract surgery, we also think of those who do not have access to even the traditional and simplest methods.

CATARACT, A MAJOR CAUSE OF UNNECESSARY BLINDNESS

M.L. TARIZZO

(Geneva, Switzerland)

Accepting the definition of blindness given in the 1977 edition of the International Classification of Diseases — categories 3, 4 and 5 of visual impairment, corresponding to a visual acuity with best possible correction of less than 3/60, or 20/400, or a visual field no greater than $10°$ — it has been estimated recently that there are today approximately 40 million blind persons in the world, and that 80 per cent of this blindness is in the developing countries.

The World Health Organization is now developing a global programme for the prevention of blindness or — as we like to put it — for the eradication of the intolerable burden of unnecessary blindness. Among the categorical priorities identified, cataract has been recognized as being by far the main cause of curable blindness. As I said in my short introduction in Italian, I am therefore particularly happy to be here today and to have this opportunity of bringing to your attention the extent of this problem in other parts of the world. The timing is especially appropriate, as only three weeks ago I participated in a meeting on the strategy for restoring sight to the curable blind, organized in New Delhi by the WHO Regional Office for South-East Asia, meeting attended by representatives from 7 countries of that region — Bangladesh, Burma, India, Indonesia, Nepal, Sri Lanka and Thailand — as well as by representatives of other international and non-governmental organizations. According to the data presented at that meeting, in all these 7 countries cataract is considered not only as the main cause of curable blindness, but of blindness in general. In India alone, with a total population estimated at 630 million, or almost 1/6 of the world population, the rate of blindness is estimated at 1.5 per cent of the total population, this accounting for about 1/4 of the world's blind. Of this estimated 10 million blind, 55 per cent, or 5.5 million are blind because of cataract; similar figures apply to most of the countries of that region, which has an estimated total population of almost 1 000 million.

Although these figures are estimates, extrapolated from partial data, they fit with the overall pattern in other countries, where blindness rates range from a few hundred to a few thousand per 100 000 population, i.e. from a few tenths to about 1 or 2 per cent, reaching higher values where infections and deficiency diseases still take a high toll in mortality and morbidity, the latter including eye diseases and blindness as well.

Apart from the magnitude of the problem, senile cataract in India and in other countries of that region appears to have an earlier onset than in other parts of the world, its incidence becoming significant already in the 40 to 50 age group. Various hypotheses have been put forward to explain this, including those involving environmental or genetic factors, but the most plausible seems to be that which links senile cataract to the aging process and to life expectancy. Observations made in India over the past 20 years suggest that, in parallel to an increase in life expectancy from approximately 28 to 40–45 years, there has been a shift in the age of onset of cataract. It has also been recently reported that in Nepal there is a difference in age of onset among different populations, cataract apparently starting earlier at about 35 years of age in the Terai, the low altitude belt along the border with India, while in the so-called hills, that is the high altitude zone above 2 500 m., the age of onset is usually around 60 years.

A number of other observations in different countries point to other differences, without indentifying the underlying factors and there is an obvious need for more information on the epidemiology of cataract and on the factors favouring its development.

Apart from its purely medical aspects, the problem posed by cataract is a complex one, with implications in all spheres of life. It becomes even more important in developing countries where its early incidence adds to its social and economic impact, and to the burden it represents for the affected persons and for the community.

The solution of the problem is for the moment essentially one of delivery of services. Existing knowledge and methods could restore sight to millions, if they were applied. In countries of South-East Asia, and to a certain extent in some African countries, one approach which has been followed is that of mobile units and of eye camps, i.e. setting up of temporary facilities for cataract surgery and to a lesser extent for providing the necessary attention for other eye conditions, thus bringing to rural populations the resources otherwise limited to the eye hospitals and eye clinics of the major towns. But even this approach is not adequate to cope with the needs. In India alone, which has a relatively high number of ophthalmologists, in comparison to other countries, 3 800 or 1 per 170 000, there is still a considerable backlog of cases. It is estimated that the number of cases of cataract increases in India by 10 per cent every year. Approximately 500 000 operations are performed yearly there and this barely copes with the annual increase, without reducing the backlog. Current plans call for an increase of the number of cataract operations to about 1 million per year, together with the strengthening of eye services and of eye care at all levels to cope with other existing eye problems.

I stressed in the introduction that some of the figures I have quoted might not be accurate, but they give an idea of the order of magnitude of the problem. Activities which are already under way or which are planned will provide additional information which will further facilitate the development of an effective approach to this problem. Among them is the setting up of a pilot project to test the feasibility and to determine the cost of eliminating the backlog of curable blindness caused by cataract in a well-defined geographical area of South-East Asia.

I hope this short presentation might have helped in giving a wider perspective to the problem which is the theme of this Congress. I also hope that in the course of your discussions you will keep present in your mind that beyond the refinements of techniques, beyond the technical breakthroughs, there are millions and millions of needlessly blind and that they will be the ultimate beneficiaries of progress in this field.

Author's address:
W.H.O.
1211 Geneva 27
Switzerland

Docum. Ophthal. Proc. Series, Vol. 21

BIOCHEMISTRY OF CATARACT

A.J. BRON

(Oxford, England)

When considering the biochemical causes of cataract, attention may be directed (1) to those types of change in lens morphology which may be designated an opacity, and (2) those biochemical derangements responsible for them.

INCREASED LIGHT SCATTERING-LENS OPACITIES

The normal lens is not as transparent as the cornea, it yellows with age, and absorbs a considerable amount of visible blue light. With aging also, there is increasing glare sensation (Wolf, 1960, Wolf & Gardiner 1965) associated with increased backscattering from the lens. There is also an increasing incidence of lens opacities in the 'normal' population with aging e.g. about 65% of people in the age group 50–59, 83% in the group from 60–69, 91% in the group 70–79 and 100% for those over 80 years (Cinotti & Patti 1968).

Any structure which interferes with the optical homogenity of the lens, producing a discontinuity of refractive index over a zone of sufficient size, will produce increased light scattering, i.e. a lens opacity. Opacities may therefore include:

1. Accumulation of fluid in or between the lens fibre (Miller & Benedek 1973)

2. Disordered fibres and complexes formed from lens fibre membranes (Dilley et. al. 1974).

3. Aggregates of lens proteins into groups with large average molecular weight, and a refractive index differing from that of the average refractive index of the lens (Benedek 1971).

4. Other structures such as capsular deposits of calcium orthophosphate (van Heyningen 1972), sub-capsular connective tissue, and deposits such as calcium oxalate (Goldberg, 1967, Bron & Habgood 1976) may also create lens opacities.

Combinations of such lens opacities may be found in the same cataract.

LENS ANATOMY AND PHYSIOLOGY

In the adult lens, there is an anterior monolayer of cells, the lens epithelium, and a concentric arrangement of spindle-shaped lens fibres posterior to this.

9

The epithelium is responsible for secreting the collagenous capsule of the lens, and for generating new lens fibres by pre-equatorial cell division. The outer, cortical lens fibres are nucleated, and contain those organelles essential for the intermediary metabolism of the lens such as mitochondria, rough endoplasmic reticulum, ribosomes and Golgi apparatus.

ATP is generated in the lens and supplies energy for active cation transport and synthesis of nucleic acid, enzymes, and structural lipids and proteins (e.g. cell membrane components and the lens crystallins). (van Heyningen 1969).

1. Respiration

Anaerobic respiration (glycolysis) is the cheif source of enery (in the form of A.T.P.) for the lens, and takes place chiefly in lens fibres. Aerobic respiration takes place almost exclusively in the lens epithelium and is responsible for a small percentage of the glucose utilised by the lens (Kuck 1975). Amino acids and fatty acids are the chief substrates for oxidation in the mitrochondria of the lens epithelium and in some species this process is responsible for between 20–30% of the energy produced (Kuck 1975, Trayhurn & van Heyningen 1972).

2. The cation pump of the lens

The main cation pump of the lens resides in the lens epithelium. Kinsey described the lens as a pump-leak system, in which the level of cations is regulated by a balance between active transport of cation, and passive diffusion (Kinsey 1965, Kinoshita 1974).

Sodium is actively extruded from the lens by the epithelium, and diffuses into the lens across its posterior surface. Potassium is transported into the lens at the epithelium and diffuses out posteriorly.

The enzyme involved in the cation pump is $NA^+K^+ - ATP$ ase, which is located chiefly in the lens epithelium. The enzyme possesses a reactive $-SH$ group thought to be involved in binding ATP to the enzyme. It is thought that the tripeptide, glutathione, whose concentration is highest in the epithelium, may protect the reactive group and hence the enzyme, from oxidation (Giblin et al. 1976).

LENS MEMBRANES

The lens fibre membrane is made up chemically of cholesterol, cholesterolester, fatty acids, glycerides, phospholipids lipoproteins and carbohydrate (Broekhuyse 1973). 70% of total phospholipid is sphingomyelin Obara et. al 1976. Lens crystallin, in particular alpha cyrstallin, is in some way closely associated with fibre membranes (Bracchi et. al. 1971, Spector & Rothchild 1973).

LENS CRYSTALLINS

The crystallins are the specific water-soluble proteins of the lens and are responsible for over 30% of the wet weight of the lens. They are termed alpha, beta and gamma and differ according to their molecular weight, chemistry and configuration.

The alpha crystallins are of the highest molecular weight, next the beta crystallins, with the gamma crystallin of lowest molecular weight. The alpha and beta crystallins exist as aggregates while gamma crystallins exist as a series of related monomers. Alpha crystallin is present throughout the lens cells, in both epithelium and fibres, while gamma and beta are found in the lens fibres only, excluding the earliest elongating fibres. (McAveroy 1978).

LENS ASCORBATE AND GLUTATHIONE

Ascorbic acid is actively secreted by the ciliary body and its concentration in human aqueous greatly exceeds that in the plasma. Ascorbic acid is thought to enter the lens from the aqueous by diffusion, and is a normal lens constituent.

Glutathione is an —SH containing tripeptide whose highest concentration is in the epithelium, next the lens cortex, and least in the nucleus.

Both these substances are reducing agents, probably performing a protective function in the lens against oxidation. The glutathione concentration is reduced in many forms of cataract, excluding that due to diquat.

ANIMAL MODELS OF CATARACT FORMATION

Certain biochemical mechanisms of cataractogenesis in animal models may be relevant to cataract formation in man (Fig. 1).

Experimental models of cataract formation

Mechanism	Cataract
1. Inhibition of Cation Pump	Nakano mouse
2. Increased lens permeability	Anticholinesterase
3. Osmotic Swelling	Hyperglycaemic
4. Disturbed glycolysis	2 deoxyglucose
5. Disturbed aerobic respiration	2.4 DNP
6. Drug induced lipidosis	Chloroquine
7. Protein denaturation	D.M.S.O.
8. Free-radicle formation	Chlorpromazine

1. Inhibition of the cation pump

In the Nakano cataract strain of mouse, a pinhead lens opacity develops at three weeks of life, which is associated with a sudden increase of lens sodium and water. This increases as the cataract matures. Radioactive studies (^{86}Rb and ^{22}Na) have shown a defective transport of potassuim inwards and of sodium extrusion in the presence of normal permeability in the early stage. At 13 days there is a 50% inhibition of $Na^+ K^+$ ATP ase. Inhibition appears to be due to the presence of a heat-labile inactivator (Kinoshita 1974, Iwata & Kinoshita 1971). Ouabain in a concentration of $10^{-4}M$ inhibits 90% of (rabbit) $Na^+ K^+ -$ ATP ase activity with a resulting rise in water and a loss of potassium.

2. Increased lens permeability

In-vitro studies of anticholinesterases demacarium bromide and phospholine iodide (Michon and Kinoshita 1966) and of surface active agents (Cotlier and Apple 1973), have demonstrated an increase in lens permeability which is regarded as a possible basis of experimental cataract with these agents. Other factors may be involved with the anticholinesterases.

3. Osmotic swelling – sugar cataracts

A rise in aqueous sugar levels initially induces lens fibre swelling by osmotic means, and later results in a rise in lens fibre permeability resulting in disruption of the fibre.

The cataractogenic sugars, xylose, galactose and glucose entering the rat lens, are converted into their respective sugar alchols in the presence of the enzyme aldose reductase.

These alcohols accumulate within the lens fibre which is poorly permeable to them. The hypertonicity it creates is corrected immediately by an influx of water (Kinoshita et. al. 1963, van Heyningen 1959, 1962, 1969).

Initially the activity of the cation pump compensates for the increased water content of the fibre. This results in extra-cellular vacuole formation. Eventually, fibre membrane permeability breaks down and both water and electrolyte content of the fibre increases. At the stage of dense nuclear cataract, there is loss of free amino acids and the sugar alcohol itself, associated with disruption of the fibre. (Sakuragawa et. al. 1975).

Other early changes include a fall in glycolysis, a marked fall in gluta-thione, and a small fall in ATP, which could itself be important to cation pump function. (Sippel 1966, van Heyningen 1963).

4. Disturbed glycolysis

Glucose enters the glycolytic pathway through the action of the pacemaker enzyme, hexokinase, which is involved in the formation of glucose 6-phosphate. This enzyme is competitively inhibited by the glucose analogue 2 deoxyglucose. This compound is capable of inducing cataract in vitro in the same way as a low glucose concentration, presumably acting by reduced production of ATP, affecting the cation pump, and reduced pentose shunt activity (which provides ribose –5-phosphate for ribonucleo-tides and coenzymes, and NADPH coenzyme needed for fatty acid synthesis and maintainance of reduced glutahtione) (Chylak 1975, van Heyningen 1977). Chylak (1977) believes that the cataract associated with neonatal hypoglycaemia is caused through such a mechanism, and that a secondary loss of hexokinase activity occurs due to the thermolability of this enzyme at body temperature in the absence of glucose.

5. Disturbed aerobic metabolism

2.4. Dinitrophenol (DNP) uncouples oxidative phosphorylation from the respiratory chain and prevents the generation of ATP by aerobic respiration.

Cataract has been produced in ducklings and chickens by feeding with D.N.P. but not in mature rabbits. This species difference appears to be related to the ability of D.N.P. to enter the aqueous in different species (Gehring & Buerge 1969), and in the immature rabbit whose blood aqueous barrier is more permeable than the adult, cataract is also produced by ingestion.

Since lenses may be maintained clear in vitro in the presence of glucose but the absence of oxygen, it is not certain that the action of DNP is due to its inhibition of aerobic metabolism, but this appears likely. It may be relevant that the initial location of the lens opacity in this condition is anterior subepithelial while the major location of aerobic metabolism is in the epithelium.

6. Drug induced phospholipidosis

Lullman et. al. (1975) have advanced the hypothesis that certain cationic amphiphilic drugs (having both hydrophilic and hydrophobic moieties) are capable of inducing a generalised phospholipidosis, which may include the lens, by binding firmly with cell phospholipids. The complexes so-formed are poorly digestible by lysomal acid lipases, accumulate within lysosomes as membranous lamellar and crystalloid inclusions. The amphiphilic compound chloroquine produces cataracts in rats and such lamellar inclusions are found within the opacities. This mechanism may also be relevant to the formation of lens opacities due to Triparanol and phenothiazine (chlorpromazine).

7. Protein Denaturation

Oral administration of dimethyl sulphoxide (DMSO) in dogs and rabbits produces a curious change in the lens nucleus after some months, in the absence of lens opacity (Rubin and Mathis 1966). This is associated with a marked refractive change in the lens. The excised nucleus is harder than normal (Wood et. al. 1967) and there is a marked increase of insoluble lens protein at the expense of soluble (mostly gamma crystallin) (van Heyningen & Harding 1972). It is suggested that DMSO or its metabolic products may react with −SH groups to encourage denaturation.

8. Free-radicle formation

This is discussed under phenothiazine cataract.

THE BIOCHEMISTRY OF SELECTED FORMS OF HUMAN CATARACT

Figure 2 lists those cataracts in man in which the biochemical mechanisms have been identified or may be inferred.

13

SELECTED FORMS OF CATARACT IN MAN

1. Inherited and other endocrine and metabolic causes

   A. Fabry's disease
      Mannosidosis
      G-6-PD deficiency
      Cholestanolosis

   B. Diabetes mellitus
      Galactosaemia
      Galactokinase deficiency
      Wilsons disease

   C. Hypocalcaemia
      Hypoglycaemia
      Hypoxia

2. Drugs and toxic agents

   Anticholinesterases
   Corticosteroids
   Chloroquine
   Naphthalene
   Phenothiazines
   Triparanol

3. Senile cataract

Inherited Cataracts

A: In Fabry's disease and Mannosidosis there is a genetically determined deficiency in lysosomal acid hydrolases resulting in the intra-lysosomal storage of macromolecular substances. Cataract is encountered in each disorder and may be presumed to result from an intra-lenticular enzyme defect, thought this has yet to be demonstrated.

Fabry's disease

In this sex-linked disorder, there is a deficiency of the enzyme alpha-galacto-sidase which results in the tissue accumulation of the glycolipid ceramide trihexoside due to the failure to cleave the terminal galactose moiety.

A typical spoke-like cataract is found not only in the affected male, but also in a proportion of the female hetrozygotes (Spaeth & Frost 1965). Also anterior wedge-shaped opacities, anterior sutural opacities and sub capsular opacities are described (Franceschetti 1974, Karr 1959, Dempsey et. al. 1965, Bronner et. al. 1970). In the lens both the epithelium and cortex may show inclusions on histological examination (Franceschetti 1976).

Mannosidosis

This is an autosomal recessive disorder resulting from deficient activity of acidic alpha-mannosidase A and B (Caroll et. al. 1972 and Norden et. al.

14

1973). There is an accumulation of mannose-rich glycopeptides, glyco-proteins and oligosaccharides in the tissues and body fluids of affected individuals. The disorder shows some phenotypic resemblance to Hurlers syndrome and there are two clinical subtypes, a severe form (Type 1) and a mild form. Lens opacities have been noted in both forms, and appear to be posterior cortical (arranged in a wheel or spoke pattern) in Type I, and scattered dot-like opacities in the entire lens in Type II (in one case an anterior plaque-like opacity is recorded). (Arbisser et. al. 1976 Murphree et. al. 1976. Letson & Desnick 1978). Residual mannosidase enzyme appears to be more stable in milder forms of mannosidosis.

Glucose 6-Phosphate Dehydrogenase deficiency

Cataract has occasionally been observed in this disorder (Kinoshita 1964). The enzyme deficiency is know to affect the lens, (Zinkham 1961) as well as the red cell. The enzyme is essential for the pentose shunt pathway.

B. DIABETES MELLITUS

The mechanism of sugar cataract has been outlined in an earlier section. In diabetes there is an increase in lens sorbitol leading to the fibre swelling described. Such an accumulation is thought to occur in nerve and vascular cells also and may contribute to the important neuropathic and vascular complications in human diabetics (Gabbay 1973).

Recent studies have shown the ability of certain relatively non-toxic flavonoid compounds, such as quercetin, to inhibit the activity of lens aldose reductase in vitro and in vivo (Varma et. al. 1975) and to reduce both the production of sugar alcohol within the lens fibre, and also the consequent osmotic swelling. It has been possible both to delay the onset of swelling, and to reduce the incidence of galactose-induced cataract in the rat.

Galactosaemia and Galactokinase deficiency

The conversion of galactose in the tissues into glucose-1-phosphate requires two basic steps. In the first step, galactose-1-phosphate is formed in the presence of galactokinase, and in the second step, galactose-1-phosphate is converted to glucose-1-phosphate in the presence of galactose-1-phosphate uridyl transferase.

Galactosaemia results from a deficiency of the transferase; there is an accumulation of galactose, with high concentrations in blood and urine, hepatosplenomegaly, failure to thrive, mental retardation and cataract. The lens opacity develops in the first weeks of life. (Wilson et. al. 1976, Sidbury 1969).

The cataract in its early stages has an oil droplet appearance in the red reflex but eventually may become total. Its occurence may be prevented by dietary means. In galactokinase deficiency there is galactosuria and no mental defect. The onset of lens opacity is in the juvenile age group

(Gitzelman 1967) and the lens opacity may not be severe. Recently Beutler et. al. have suggested that heterozygotes for galactokinase deficiency may be at increased risk for cataract. (1973).

Wilson's disease

Wilson's disease is an autosomal recessive disorder in which there is a deficiency of the enzyme caeruloplasmin. Free copper levels are raised in the blood while total copper levels are reduced. A polychromatic anterior and posterior, capsular cataract (sunflower cataract) occurs rarely and is reversible on treatment with penicillamine (Walshe 1976, Cairns et. al. 1969). In the copper cataract of chalcosis, copper is deposited in the epithelium (causing degeneration), and within the capsule itself. (Hanna 1975)

OTHER ENDOCRINE AND METABOLIC CAUSES

Hypocalcaemia

Hypocalcaemia occurs in man in association with hypoparathyroidism, pseudohypoparathyroidism, rickets and idiopathic hypocalcaemis of infancy (Brooks 1975). Lens opacities may occur in as many as 50% of post-parathyroidectomy patients with hypo-parathyroidism (Ireland et. al. 1968).

Rarely the embryonal or foetal nucleus is involved. In the infant or child, the cataract is generally lamellar. In the adult, hypocalcaemia produces anterior and posterior punctate subcapsular opacities and eventually a total cataract (Bellows 1944 Haft 1953).

In animal lenses, calcium deficiency induces a reversible increase in permeability, leading to a decrease in the K^+ / Na^+ ratio within the lens (Harris and Gehrsitz 1951), (Thoft & Kinoshita 1965) without a decrease in sodium pump activity. It is presumed that this is the cause of cataract.

Hypoglycaemia

An association has been observed between neonatal or infantile cataract and hypoglycaemia of the idiopathic, ketotic or neonatal type (Brooks 1975). The majority are in males and are associated with prematurity, low birth weight, and complicated pregnancy (Scheie 1964, McKinna 1966, O'Connor et. al. 1967, de Loore & van Gelderen 1967, Fraser & Friedman 1967, Hull 1969, Wilson 1969, Gabilan & Chaussain 1969, Merin & Crawford 1971).

The cataracts are often bilateral but not necessarily of simultaneous onset. The onset is usually after birth and the opacities are usually made up of concentric lamellar changes. In some eyes the changes are posterior subcapsular.

Occasionally, lens opacities may be seen in adult diabetics in whom the blood sugar is rapidly being reduced by insulin therapy.

The mechanism of hypoglycaemic cataract has been outlined (supra).

Hypoxia

Cataracts have been produced in rats and other animals raised in a low concentration of atmospheric oxygen (Bellows and Nelson 1944). Hypoxia lowers the epithelial mitotic rate in rats while air restores it (Pirie & van Heyningen 1960). It has been suggested that opacities may result from the direct action of hypoxia, to high levels of lactic acid in the aqueous, or to osmotic factors (van Heyningen 1969) but it is of note that the lens can survive in vitro in the absence of oxygen, as long as glucose is supplied.

It is not certain whether hypoxia is a factor in neonatal cataract.

2. DRUGS AND TOXIC AGENTS

Antocholinesterases

Antocholinesterases such as phospholine iodide produce a dose related anterior subcapsular cataract whose incidence is cited as between 33—62% after six or more months of treatment (Axelsson 1969 Axelsson & Holmeberg 1966, de Roetth 1966, Schaffer & Hetherington 1966).

Laties has demonstrated localisation of D.F.P. at the anterior lens surface (1969), while de Roetth (1966) demonstrated reduced lens anticholinesterase activity with such agents. It has been suggested that cholinesterase may have a role in ion transport. Michol & Kinoshita (1968) demonstrated a depression of oxidative metabolism in the lens which differed with different miotics and the role of this in cataract formation is unclear. However, they demonstrated an increased permeability and altered sodium and potassuin content which may be the initiating factor in cataractogenesis.

Corticosteroids

The ability of long-term cortico steroid therapy to induce posterior subcapsular cataract in a dose-related fashion, is well established. Spaeth and von Sallmann (1966) suggest that a dose of prednisone or its equivalent of 10 mg a day is safe to a total dose of 3.5 gm.

Cultured lenses lose potassium and gain sodium and water when incubated with prednisone and a number of glucocorticoids prevent the cooled lens from re-establishing its cation levels on rewarming. It appears that steroids increase the permeability of the lens to cations (Harris 1966 Becker & Cotlier 1965).

Paterson (1971) suggests that the posterior location of the lens opacity may be best explained by assuming that a generalised increased permeability of the lens may be offset anteriorly by the activity of the cation pump.

Chloroquine

The mechanism of experimental chloroquine cataract has been discussed. In some reports of chloroquine toxicity in man, the occurence of tiny flake-like posterior subcapsular lens opacities have been recorded in 20—40% of patients (Francois & Maudgal 1965, Hermann & Sourdille 1963, Hobbs, Sorsby & Freedman 1959, Whisnant et. al. 1961, Young & Brosnan 1963). They do not appear to progress or affect vision.

2.4. DNP

The mechanism of DNP cataract has been discussed. The agent was found to be cataractogenic after it was introduced as a slimming agent in the 1930's. The cataracts begin in the anterior cortex and progress to involve the posterior cortex and the whole of the lens. Onset was several months after the start of therapy (Grant 1974).

Naphthalene

Cataract has been induced in man after ingestion or exposure to the toxic vapour (Paterson 1971). The mechanism of cataract has been elucidated by the studies of van Heyningen & Pirie 1967, and Rees & Pirie 1967.

Naphthalene is oxidised in the liver, through a precursor to naphthalene diol (1,2-hydro 1,2-dihydroxy naphthalene). This is further metabolised in the eye to form 1,2 dihydroxynaphthalene in the aqueous humour and the lens. This is thought to autoxidize to 1,2 naphthaquinone, a highly reactive substance thought to react with ascorbic acid, glutathione, enzymes, amino acids and lens proteins in the eye.

Naphthaquinone causes the catalytic oxidation of ascorbic acid with the formation of dehydroascorbic acid and hydrogen peroxide. Aqueous ascorbic acid and probably oxygen levels, fall.

(Quinone formation is unlikely to be a general mechanism of cataractogenesis resulting from the ingestion of potential precursors, since the lens does not contain polyphenol oxidase capable of participating in enzymic-oxidation (van Heyningen 1976)).

Chlorpromazine

Chlorpromazine is a dimethylamino substituted phenothiazine capable of causing an anterior capsular and subcapsular lens opacity when used in chronic high dosage, say 500 mg daily for three years or more. The opacities are coloured light brown.

Apart from the mechanism noted earlier, of drug induced lipidosis, it has been suggested that chlorpromazine may increase lens permeability (Michon & Lambert 1968); the effects are not necessarily mutually exclusive.

Chlorpromazine is a powerful photosensitizing agent. The molecule is capable of absorbing light energy, with the loss of an electron, to produce a highly reactive free radical. The absorbed energy may be transferred to tissue constituents as part of a damaging photochemical reaction. It has been suggested that the lens opacity, which is located in the pupillary zone of the lens may be the result of such a photosensitization reaction. The brown opacities might be a metabolite of chlorpromazine itself, or the product of a photochemically denatured protein (Howard et. al. 1969).

Triparanol Cataract

Triparanol was introduced in the 1950's as a hypocholesterolaemic agent. It blocks the enzymic reduction of 2.4 dehydrocholesterol to cholesterol. It

18

was found to induce posterior subcapsular cataracts and was withdrawn in 1961 (Kirby 1967).

In experimental cataract there is an accumulation of a sudanophilic material, which has been surmised to contain desmosterol in addition to other lipids (von Sallman et. al. 1963). The possibility that a drug induced lenticular lipidosis might occur has already been discussed.

Harris & Gruber (1969) found evidence of increased lens permeability in experimental triparanol cataract.

SENILE CATARACT

Excellent reviews of the biochemical changes in senile cataract are given by Barber (1973) and Harding & Dilley (1976).

Both clinical and biochemical considerations indicate that senile cataracts exist as two subgroups which may co-exist. These are cortical and nuclear cataract. The mechanisms responsible for loss of transparency appear to be different.

In cortical cataracts there are significantly lower wet weights and total protein contents than in normal lenses. (Maraini & Mangili 1973, van Heyningen 1976). An increase in interdigitation has been observed between fibres in the aging lens and in human senile cataract (Kobayashi & Susuki 1975). In cortical cataracts of various kinds there is evidence of fibre breakdown leading to the formation of complex membrane figures and myeloid bodies (membranous lamellar bodies) (Dilley, Bron & Habgood 1976, Bron & Habgood 1976). There is also evidence for the presence of crystallins in the aqueous in cortical cataract (Sandberg 1976).

Van Heyningen (1976) has suggested that loss of protein from the lens could result from the action of a neutral proteinase, present in highest concentration in lens cortex and closely associated with alpha crystallin. This enzyme is active against all the major crystallins though alpha crystallin is its preferred substrate, and is able to split the lens proteins into short peptides. Recently Dr. van Heyningen has identified the presence of free peptides in cataractous lenses and suggests that once fibre membranes begin to disrupt and become leaky, the products of digestion may diffuse from the lens. The absence of feedback inhibition would accelerate the process of digestion. Proteolysis is increased in the presence of calcium, and calcium levels are increased in cortical cataract, in both cortex and nucleus. It may be that Morgagian cataract, in which the cortex may become completely liquified and absorbed, may represent an extreme example of cortical proteolysis (Bron & Habgood 1976).

A particularly high level of capsular calcium is found in Morgagnian cataract, which may explain the development of calcium orthophosphate plaques in this form of cataract. Duncan (1976) and Duncan & van Heyningen (1976) have shown that there is strong binding of calcium in cataract to the water insoluble fraction of the lens.

In nuclear cataract there is less evidence of protein loss and the characteristic feature of senile nuclear cataract appears to be the brown discolouration and aggregation of proteins mainly in the nucleus of the lens (Dilley &

19

Pirie 1974). It is likely that light scattering by large protein aggregates and light absorbtion by coloured proteins both contribute to loss of lens transparency.

With aging there is a conformational change in the crystallins, which is shown in many kinds of cataract, and the change is greater in the nucleus than in the cortex (Harding 1972). The proteins of the nucleus are the oldest of the crystallins and there is no evidence of turnover in the adult lens (Dilley & van Heyningen 1969, Pirie 1973). The conformational change in nuclear cataract explains the increased reactivity of the lens protein thiols, the formation of disulphide-bonded aggregates (Harding 1972, 1973) and formation of urea-insoluble protein after extraction of crystallins in air. Truscott & Augusteyn (1977) suggest that in nuclear cataract there is true protein intramolecular disulphide bond formation responsible for the production of a cross linked yellow protein. Harding (1972 a and b) has suggested that this urea insolubility is a preparative artifact due to oxidation of exposed −SH groups of denatured proteins. This is an important area of disagreement which requires resolution.

There is also evidence for denaturation of a proportion of the nuclear proteins into a brown, high molecular weight component which is covalently cross-linked and fluorescent. The cross-links include non-disulphide covalent bonds, and this insoluble fraction contains some non-protein material (Dilley & Pirie 1974). It will be of future interest to know whether the material contains membrane components.

REFERENCES

Arbisser, A.I., Murphree, A.L., Garcia, C.A. & Howell, R.R.: Ocular findings in mannosidosis. *Amer. J. Ophthalnol.* 82, 465 (1976)

Axelsohn, U. Glaucoma miotic therapy and cataract. *Acta ophthal.* 47, *Suppl.* 102, 1969

Axelsohn, U. & Holmeberg, A. The frequency of cataract after miotic therapy. *Acta Ophthal.* 44, 421 (1966)

Barber, G.W.: Human cataractogenesis: a review *Exp. Eye Res.* 16, 85 (1973)

Becker, B. & Cotlier, E. The efflux of 86Rubiduim from the rabbit lens. *Invest. Ophthal.* 4, 117, (1965)

Bellows, J.G.: Cataract and anomalies of the lens. St. Louis, Missouri, Mosby 1944

Bellows, J.G. & Nelson, D.: Cataract produced by anoxia A.M.A. *Arch. Ophthal.* 31, 250 (1944)

Benedek, G.B. Theory of transparency of the eye. *Appl. Optics* 10, 459 (1971)

Beutler, E., Matsamoto, F. Kuhl, W. et. al.: Galactokinase deficiency as a cause of cataracts. *N. Engl. J. Med.* 288, 1203, (1973)

Bracchi, P.G., Carta, F. Fasella, P. & Maraini, G.: Selective binding of aged α-crystallin to lens fiber ghosts. *Exp. Eye Res.* 12, 151 (1971)

Broekhuyse, R.M.: The Human Lens- in Relation to Cataract, Ciba Foundation Symposium 19 (new series) Amsterdam, 1973 Elsevier Publishing Co. p. 135

Bron, A.J. & Habgood, J.O. Morgagnian Cataract, *Trans. Ophth. Soc. U.K.* 96 265, (1976)

Bronner, A., Payeur, G. & Mossart, J.M., et. al. A propos d'un cas de glycolipidose de Fabry. *Bull. Soc. Ophtalmol. Fr.* 70 710 (1970)

Brooks, M.H.: Lenticular abnormalities in endocrine dysfunction. In, Cataract and abnormalities of the lens J.G. Bellows (ed) New York, Grune & Stratton Inc. (1975) p. 285

Cairns, J.E. Parry Williams, H. & Walshe, J.M.: 'Sunflower Cataract' in Wilsons Disease. Br. Med. J. 3 95 (1969)

Caroll, M., Dance, N., Masson, P.K., Robinson, D. & Winchester, B.G. Human mannosidosis — the enzyme defect. *Biochem. Biophys. Res. Comm.* 49, 579, 1972.

Chylak, L.T. Mechanism of hypoglycaemic cataract formation in the rat lens. I The role of hexokinase instability. *Invest. Ophthalmol.* 14, 746, (1975)

Cinotti & Patti (1968) cited by Miller, D. and Benedek G. In, Intra ocular light scattering: Springfield, Thomas (1973) p. 62

Cotlier, E. & Apple, D.: Cataracts induced by the polypeptide antibiotic polymyxi B sulfate. *Exp. Eye Res.* 16, 69 (1973)

Dempsey, H. Hartley & M.W. Caroll, J. et. al.: Fabrys disease *Ann. Intern.* 63, 1059 (1965)

de Loore, I & van Gelderen H.H.: Liver glycogenosis and cataracts in a mentally deficient child

de Roetth, A. Jr. Lens opacities in glaucoma patients on phospholine iodide therapy. *Amer. J. Ophthal.* 62, 619, 1966;

Dilley, K.J., Bron A.J. & Habgood J.O.: Anterior polar and posterior subcapsular cataract in a patient with retinities pigmentosa. *Exp. Eye Res.* 22, 155 (1976)

Dilley, K.J. & Pirie, A.: Changes to the human lens nucleus in cataract. *Exp. Eye Res.* 19, 59 (1974)

Dilley, K.J. & van Heyningen, R. Some aspects of human lens metabolism, glycosis and protein synthesis. *Docum. Ophthal.* 8, 171, (1976)

Duncan, G.: The concentration and state of calcium in the lens Biology of the epithelial lens cells. *Inserm.* 60, 19, (1976)

Duncan, G. & van Heyningen, R.: Differences in the calcium binding capacity of normal and cataractous lenses. Documenta Ophthalmologica Proceedings Series 8, 229 (1976)

Franceschetti, A.Th.: Fabry Disease: Ocular Manifestations In The Eye and Inborn Errors of Metabolism., Birth defects: Original Article series XII No. 3 p. 195 Eds. D. Bergsma, A.J. Bron, E. Cotlier. Pub. Alan Liss. New York (1976)

Francois, J. & Maudgal, M. Experimental chloroquine retinopathy. *Ophthalmologica* 148, 442 (1964)

Fraser, G.R. & Friedman A.I.: The Causes of Blindness in Childhood, Baltimore, Johns Hopkins Press (1967)

Gabbay, K.H.: The sorbitol pathway and the complications of diabetes, *N. Eng. J. Med.* 288, 831, (1973)

Gabilan, J.C. & Chaussain, J.L.: L'Association hypoglycemie idiopathique et cataracts chez l'enfant. *Arch. Fr Pediatr.* 26, 633, (1969).

Gehring, P.J. & Buerge, J.F. The distribution of 2,4 dinitrophenol relative to its cataractogenic activity in ducklings and rabbits. *Toxic Appl. Pharmacol.* 15, 574, 1969

Giblin, F.J., Chakrapani, B. & Reddy, V.N. Glutathione and lens epithelial function. *Invest. Ophthalmol.* 15, 381, 1976

Gitzelman, R.: Hereditary galactokinase deficiency: A newly recognised cause of juvenile cataracts. *Pediatr. Res.* 1, 14 1967

Goldberg, M.F. Cytologic diagnosis of phacolytic glaucoma utilising millipore filtration of the aqueous. *Brit. J. Ophthalmol.* 51. 847, (1967)

Grant, W.M. Toxicology of the Eye. 2nd Edition Springfield: Thomas (1974)

Haft, A.S. Idiopathic hypoparathyroidism and cataract. Report of four cases. *Arch Ophthalmol.* 50, 455, 1953

Hanna, C.: Chalcosis of the lens p. 279 In, Cataract and abnormalities of the lens. J.G. Bellows, New York, Grune and Stratton Inc. (1975)

Harding, J.J. The nature and origin of the urea-insoluble protein of human lens *Exp. Eye Res.* 13, 33, (1972 a)

Harding, J.J. Conformational changes in human lens proteins in cataract. *Biochem. J.* 129, 97 (1972 b)

Harding, J.J. Disulphide cross-linked protein of high molecular weight in human cataractous lens. *Exp. Eye Res.* 17, 377 (1973)

Harding, J.J. & Dilley K.J.: Structural Proteins of the Mammalian Lens: A review with

Emphasis on Changes in Development, Aging and Cataract. *Exp. Eye Res.* 22, 1, (1976)

Harris, J.E. The temperature-reversible cation shift of the lens *Invest. Ophthal.* 4, 709, (1965)

Harris, J.E. & Gehrsitz, L.O.: Significance of changes in potassium and sodium content of the lens. *Amer. J. Ophthalmol.* 34, 131, 1951

Harris, J.E. & Gruber, L. The reversal of triparanol induced cataracts in the rat. *Docum. Ophthal.* 26, 324, (1969)

Hermann, P. & Sourdille, P.: Ocular lesions produced by a synthetic antimalarial drug. *Ann. Oculist (Paris)* 196, 1004, 1963.

Hobbs, H. Eadie, S. & Somerville, F. Ocular lesions after treatment with chloroquine, *Brit J. Ophthal.* 45, 284, 1961

Howard, R.O., McDonald, C.J. Dunn, B. & Creasey, W.A. Experimental chlorpromazine cataracts. *Invest. Ophthal.* 8, 413, (1969)

Hull, D.: Cataracts associated with metabolic disorders in infancy. *Proc. Soc. Med.* 62, 694, 1969.

Ireland, A.W., Hornebrook, J.W., Neale, F.C. & Posen, S: The crystalline lens in chronic surgical hypoparathyroidism. *Arch. Int. Med.* 122 408 (1968)

Iwata, S. & Kinoshita, J.H. Mechanism of development of hereditary cataract in mice. *Invest. Ophthal.* 10, 504, (1971)

Karr, W.J. Fabrys disease. *Am. J Med.* 27, 829, (1959)

Kinoshita, J.H. Selected topics in ophthalmic biochemistry. *Arch. Ophthal.* 72, 554, (1964)

Kinoshita, J.H. Mechanisms initiating cataract formation *Invest. Ophthal.* 13, 713, (1974)

Kinoshita, J.H., Futterman, S., Satoh, K. & Merola, L.O. Factors affecting the formation of sugar alcohols in ocular lens. *Biochim. biophys. Acta.* 74 340 (1963)

Kinsey, J.H. Cataracts in galactosaemia. *Invest. Ophthal.* 4, 786 (1965)

Kirkby, T.J.: Cataracts produced by triparanol. (MER-29) *Trans. Amer. Ophthal. Soc.* 65 493, (1976)

Kobayashi, Y. & Susuki, T.: The aging lens: Ulltrastructural changes in cataracts, In Cataract and abnormalities of the lens J.G. Bellows (ed) New York, Grune and Stratton Inc (1975) p. 313

Kuck, J.F.R. Jr. The Metabolism of the Lens. p. 97. In, Cataract and abnormalities of the Lens J.G. Bellows, New York, Grune and Stratton, 1975

Laties, A.M. Localisation in cornea and lens of topically applied irreversible cholinesterase inhibitors. *Amer. J. Ophthal.* 68, 848, (1969)

Letson, R.D. & Desnick, R.J. Lenticular opacities in Mannosidosis. *Amer. J. Ophthal.* 85, 218, (1978)

Lullman, H. Lullman-Rauch, R. & Wasserman, O. Drug induced Phospholipidosis. *Critical Reviews in Toxicology* 4, 185, (1975)

Maraini, G. & Mangili, R. Characteristics of alpha-crystallin in human senile cataract. *Exp. Eye Res.* 16, 123, (1973)

McAvoy J.W., Cell division, cell elongation and distribution of α-, β- and γ-crystallins in the rat lens. *J. Embryol. exp. Morph.* 44, 149, (1978)

McKinna, A.J. Neonatal hypoglycaemia. *Can. J. Ophthalmol.* 1, 56, (1966)

Merin, S. & Crawford, J.S.: Hypoglycaemia and infantile cataract. *Arch. Ophthalmol.* 86, 495, (1971)

Michon, J. & Kinoshita, J.H.: Experimental miotic cataract. II Permeability, cation transport and intermediary metabolism. *Arch. Ophthal.* 79, 611, (1968)

Michon, J. & Lambert, B.W. The effects of chlorpromazine on the lens. Presented at Meeting of the Association for Research in Ophthalmology, Florida, April 1968

Miller, D. & Benedek, G. In Intraocular Light Scattering. Springfield, Thomas (1973)

Murphree, A.L. Beaudet, A.L. Palmer E.A. & Nichols B.L. Jr. Cataract in Mannosidosis, In Birth Defects: Original Article Series Vol. XII No. 3 p. 319 (1976), Alan Liss, New York

Norden, N.E., Ockermann, P.A. & Szabo, L.: Urinary mannose in mannosidosis. *J. Pediatr.* 82 686, (1973)

22

Obara, Y. Cotlier, E., Kim, J.O. Lueck, K. & Tao, R. Sphingomyelin species stored in human senile cataract *Invest. Ophth.* 15, 966, (1976)

O'Connor, C.F., Crawford, J.D., Cohen J.M., De Vivo, D.C., Cogan D.G. & Crigler J.F. Jr., Hypoglycemia in infancy. *Clin. Pediatr.* 6, 94 (1967)

Paterso, C.A.: Effects of Drugs on the lens. In, International Ophthalmology Clinics Vol II, No. 2 p 63, Little, Brown & Co. Boston (1971)

Pirie, A.: Chairman's introduction. The human lens in relation to cataract. Ciba Foundation Symposium 19, 1–3, Elsevier, Amsterdam.

Pirie, A. & van Heyningen, R.: Comparison between the effects of cysteine and of anoxia on the rate of mitosis in lens epithelium. *Nature, Lond.* 187, 947 (1960)

Rees, J.R. & Pirie, A. Possible reactons of 1,2 naphthaquinone in the eye. *Biochem. J.* 102, 853 (1967)

Rubin, L.F. & Mattis, P.A.: Dimethyl Sulphoxide: Lens changes in dogs during oral administration. *Science* 153, 83, (1966)

Trayhurn, P. & van Heyningen, R.: Neutral Proteinase Activity in the Human Lens. *Exp. Eye Res.* 22, 251, (1976)

Sakuragawa, M. Kuwabara, T., Kinoshita, J.H. & Fukui, H.N. Swelling of the lens fibers. *Exp. Eye Res.* 21, 381, 1975

Sandberg, H.O.,: The alpha-crystallin content of aqueous humour in cortical, nuclear and complicated cataracts. *Exp. Eye Res.* 22, 75 (1976)

Shaffer, R.N. & Hetherington, J. Jr.: Anticholinesterase drugs and cataracts. *Amer. J. Ophthal.* 62, 613, (1966)

Scheie, H.G. Rubenstein, R.A. & Albert, D.M. Congenital glaucoma and other ocular abnormalities with idiopathic infantile hypoglycemia. *J. Pediatr. Ophthalmol.* 1, 45 (1964)

Sidbury, J.B. Investigations and speculations on the pathogenesis of galactosemia, in Hsia D.Y.Y. (ed) Galactosemia, Springfield, Illinois, Thomas, (1969) p. 14

Sippel, T.O. Energy metabolism in the lens during development of galactose cataract in rats. *Invest. Ophthal.* 5, 576, (1966)

Spaeth, G.L. & Frost, P.: Fabry's disease. Its ocular manifestations. *Arch. Ophthalmol.* 74, 760 (1965)

Spaeth, G. & von Sallmann, L. Corticosteroids and cataracts. *Int. Ophthal. Clin.* 6, 915, (1966)

Spector, A. & Rothschild, C. The effect of calcium upon the reaggregation of bovine alpha crystallin. *Invest. Ophthalmol.* 12, 225 (1973)

Thoft, R.A. & Kinoshita, J.H. The effect of calcium on rat lens permeability. *Invest. Ophthal.* 4, 122, (1965)

Truscott & Augusteyn, R.C. Oxidative changes in human lens proteins during senile nuclear cataract formation. *Biochim Biophys Acta* 492, 43 (1977)

van Heyningen, R. Formation of polyols by the lens of the rat with 'sugar'cartaract.

van Heyningen, R. The sorbitol pathway in the lens. *Exp. Eye Res.* 1, 396, 1962

van Heyningen, R. Changes in weight and adenosine triphosphate content in the lens of the xyolse-fed rat. *Exp. Eye Res.* 2, 362, (1963)

van Heyningen, R. The lens: Metabolism and cataract. In H. Davson (Ed.). The Eye (2nd ed) London Academic 1969

van Heyningen, R. The human lens. I. A comparison of cataracts extracted in Oxford (England) and Shikapur (W. Pakistan) *Exp. Eye Res.* 13, 136 (1972)

van Heyningen, R. Experimental studies on cataract. Proctor Lecture. *Exp. Eye Res.* 15, 685, (1976)

van Heyningen, R. The biochemistry of the lens, – selected topics. In, Scientific Foundations of Ophthalmology E.S. Perkins and D.W. Hill (eds.) London, Heinemann 1977 p. 44

van Heyningen, R. & Harding. J.J.: Some changes in the lens of the dimethyl sylphoxide – fed rabbit. *Exp. Eye Res.* 14, 91, (1972)

van Heyningen, R. & Pirie, A.: The metabolism of naphthalene and its toxic effect on the eye. *Biochem.. J.* 102, 842, (1967)

Varma S.D., Mikuni, V.I. & Kinoshita, J.H.: Flavonoids as Inhibitors of Lens Aldose Reductase. *Science* 188, 1215 (1975)

von Sallmann L, Grimes P. & Collins E. Triparanol induced cataract in rats. *Arch. Ophthal.* 70, 522, 1963

Walshe, J.M.: The Eye in Wilsons Disease. In The Eye and Inborn Erros of Metabolism. Birth Defects: Original Article Series XII No. 3 1976 New York, Liss (1976) p. 187

Whisnant, J. Espinosa, R. Kierland, R. & Lambert, E. Chloroquine neuromyopathy. *Proc. Staff. Meet. Mayo Clin.* 38, 501, (1963)

Wilson, W.A., Donnell, G.N. & Bergren, W.R. The dietary prophyllaxis of cataracts in patients with galactosaemia. In, The Eye and Inborn errors of Metabolism. Birth defects: Original Article Series XII No. 3 New York, Liss, (1976) p. 313.

Wolf, E. Glare and age. *Arch. Ophthal.* 64, 502, (1960)

Wolf, E. & Gardiner, J.S.: Studies on the scatter of light in the dioptric media of the eye as a basis for visual glare. *Arch. Ophthalmol.* 74, 338, (1965)

Wood, D.C., Sweet, D. Van Dolah, J., Smith J.C. & Contaxis, I. A study of DMSO and steroids in rabbit eyes. Ann. *N.Y. Acad. Sci.* 141, 346 (1967)

Young, P. & Brosnan, D. III Simple tests for the early detection of retinopathy due to chloroquine and hydroxychloroquine *Amer. Rheum. Ass.* Dec. 1963.

Zinkham, W.H. A deficiency of glucose-6-phosphate dehydrogenase activity in lens from individuals with primaquire sensitive erythrocytes. Bull Johns Hopkins Hosp. 109, 206. 1961.

Author's address:
University of Oxford
Nuffield Laboratory of Ophthalmology
Walton Street
Oxford OX2 6AW
England

GENETICS OF CATARACTS

I.H. MAUMENEE

(Baltimore, Maryland U.S.A.)

I am not going to give an extensive classification of cataracts, and I refer for that to the excellent work by Nicholas Brown (1976). I would like to discuss some specific genetic problems based on observations of lens pathology.

Most of us senesce while keeping our sight, with sometimes the exception of interference from some haze due to nuclear sclerosis. However, we all see families in which cataracts occur in consecutive generations as presenile or senile cataracts. Their mode of inheritance seems at times compatible with autosomal dominant inheritance with delayed onset. However, other modes of inheritance cannot be excluded with certainty.

Why do we know so little about a possible genetic basis of this most common of all eye diseases? There are some obvious reasons. Patients who are now in their 50's or 60's usually know vaguely whether their parents had ocular problems, and of what type; but they usually do not know why their grandparents went blind, the exact reason why they were operated upon, and certainly not what type of cataract they had. Another problem lies in the phenotypic overlap between various types of cataracts as they mature and come to the attention of the ophthalmologist. Also, the segregation frequencies — as aspected under autosomal dominant, autosomal recessive with high gene frequency, and polygenic inheritance — are not all that different (Barrai & Cann, 1965; Neel, 1967). Nor is it known what influence environment has, and so it is again difficult to differentiate between familial disease due to a common genetic background and that due to a shared environment. Thus, any disease with delayed age of onset and with probable heterogeneity but phenotypic overlap is not very amenable to genetic studies; and all these results will be open to much critisism such as the studies of open-angle glaucoma or diabetes have encountered. Thus, large numbers of families are needed for us to come possibly to a conclusion about the inheritance pattern or patterns of presenile and/or senile nuclear lenticular sclerosis, and posterior subcapsular or other types of cataracts.

The situation is much clearer for congenital cataracts not associated with other ocular or systemic pathology. Several clinical types — which breed

Supported in part by Grant No. 5 RO1 EYO1773 from the National Eye Institute Bethesda, Maryland, U.S.A.

true, although they may show a variable amount of severity — are recognized: anterior and posterior polar, nuclear, zonular pulverulent, nuclear pulverulent, etc. The vast majority of them are inherited as autosomal dominant diseases. Autosomal recessive and X-linked inheritance are also recognized, although both are considerably rarer.

Why should most cataracts, congenital or senile, be inherited as autosomal dominant diseases? Nicholas Brown (1978) recognises three basic mechanisms for the formation of lens fiber opacities: 1) previously clear lens fibers become opaque; 2) newly-formed fibers may be opaque at the time of their formation; 3) granular material may be laid down in the subcapsular region in a lens which has lost the ability to produce properly formed fibers. What happens in autosomal dominant diseases? The old statement that one gene produces one polypeptide (or protein) still holds. In the lens and the cornea the autosomal **dominant** dystrophies are the more common types, and both tissues are made up of highly organized structural proteins. In case of a mixture of products of a normal and an abnormal gene, slight abnormalities can lead to interference with the physical properties of the lens and hence to a cataract. Neither the actual sequence nor the number of amino acids in the lens fibers or in the proteins of the lens capsule are known, but most polypeptide chains are composed of some 100 to 200 amino acids, each coded for by three bases, for each of which three different base substitutions can occur. Thus, the number of different possible mutation is very large, and these are likely to become clinically manifest, although phenotypic differences are not to be expected for all the different mutational events. It seems clear that much more research on cataracts is needed before the mutational event and the phenotypic appearance can be correlated, as has been done for mutations of the human hemoglobin chains. By 1976, 102 mutations were recognized for the α-chain and 166 for the β-chain (McKusick, 1976).

How can the blinding disorder of cataract reach as high an incidence as 5 million new cases in India a year? Are such figures evidence against a genetic basis for this disease? Any gene frequency in a given population depends upon mutation rate and selection with selection being the reciprocal of fitness. There is no reason to assume that presenile and senile cataracts give rise to a measurable reduction in fitness in Western countries, since their onset occurs after the end of a patient's reproductive age and leads to little interference with a patient's earning capacity. However, in countries such as India where the mean age of blindness from cataracts is 45 years (Vyas, personal communication) and surgery is not readily available, there may be an effect on the suvivorship of the later-born children. However, cataracts have a high incidence in India and therefore a large non-genetic componet for presenile and senile cataract formation cannot be excluded. It would be very interesting to examine a group of Indians living in a different country under improved socio-economic conditions, to evaluate the respective effects of environment and genes on this condition.

The majority of cases of congenital cataracts arise as new dominant mutations in view of the strong selective disadvantage of those affected. If there were only one recessive and one dominant type of cataract, and each type equally severe, one could expect twice as many patients suffering from autosomal dominant cataracts as from autosomal recessive ones ($\mu_r = q^2 c$ for autosomal recessive diseases and $\mu_d = \frac{1}{2}$ q c for autosomal dominant diseases; thus, if the mutation rates and selection coefficients are equal, twice as many autosomal dominant as autosomal recessive cases will occur.) However, many more autosomal dominant types and cases of cataracts are reported, pointing towards the existence of more heterogeneity of autosomal dominant cataracts than of recessive types.

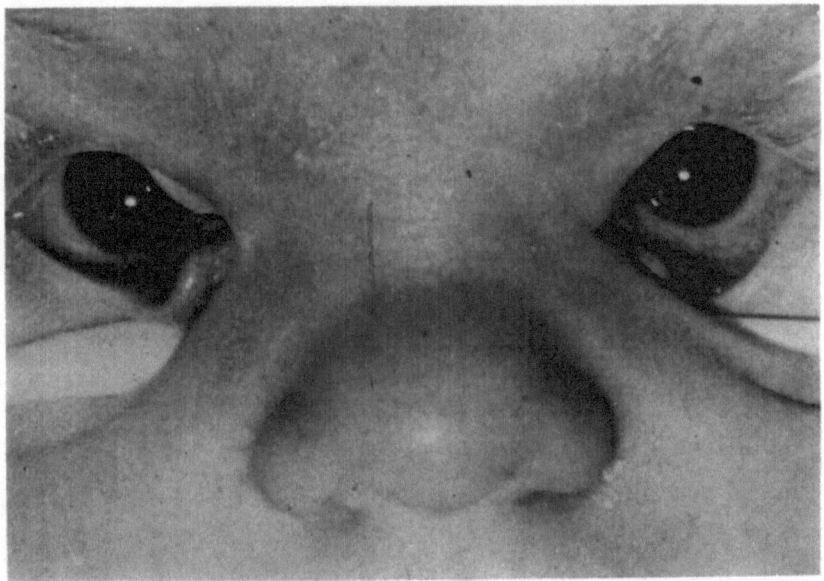

Fig. 1. Congenital cataracts in a 10-day-old infant, son of carrier mother depicted in Figure 2.

In X-linked congenital cataracts a special situation arises. Affected boys usually have complete cataracts, microcornea and probably microphthalmos (Fig. 1). The surgical results are usually poor. Carrier mothers have reduced corneal diameters and y-sutural opacities not interfering with vision, and are usually unaware of their carrier state (Figs. 2 and 3). To what extent should the ophthalmologist investigate such families and inform carrier females of their respective risks? Are ophtalmologists obliged to, and will they be liable if they do not? In this family (Fig. 4) about one-half of the 11 sisters in generation III are expected to be carriers, with the probability of multiple affected boys in the following generation; but inversely the other one-half are expected to be normal and not at risk of having affected sons. In these cases, unnecessary anxiety can possible be relieved by counseling. Medical geneticists have been very much concerned with the ethical and legal

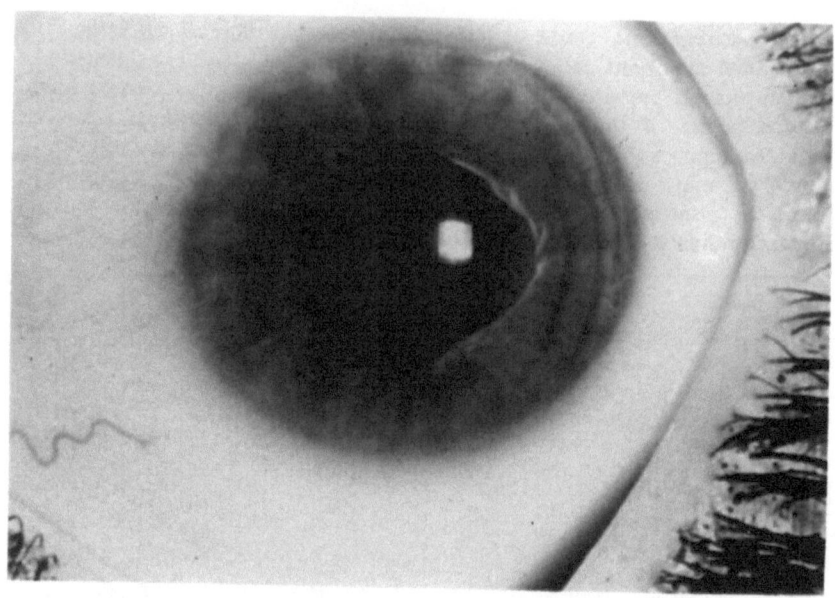

Fig. 2. Carrier state of X-linked cataract as evidenced by reduced corneal diameter (8.5 mm OU) and here faintly visible y-sutural opacity.

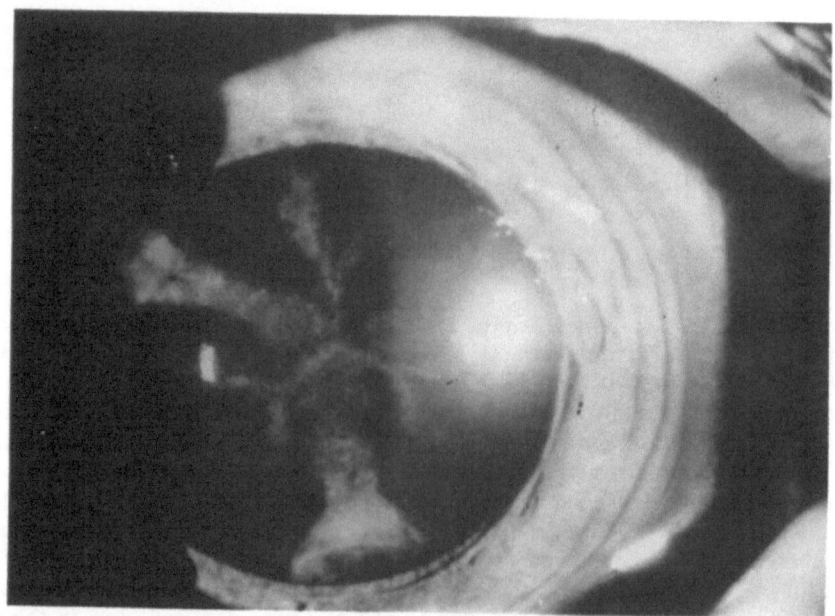

Fig. 3. y-sutural opacities in a more severely affected carrier female, member of the family depicted in Figure 4.

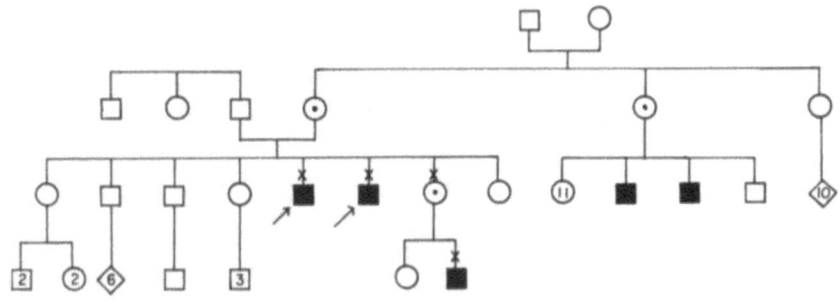

■ X-LINKED CATARACTS

⊙ OBLIGATORY CARRIER

Fig. 4. X-linked inheritance of cataracts over three generations with at least 15 unexamined possible carrier females at risk of having affected sons.

problems of such situations, but no accepted guidelines have been arrived at for such situations.

Thus, very specific problems for the study of hereditary cataracts exist – encompassing the fields of population genetics, biochemical genetics, and genetics and the law. All of this makes the field of ophthalmic genetics an exciting one for the use of the eye as a test tube and focal point in development of genetic methodology.

REFERENCES

Barrai, I. & Cann, H.M.: Segregation of juvenile diabetes mellitus. *J. Med. Genet.* 2:8–11, 1965.
Brown, N.: Cataract and diseases of the lens. In, Medical Ophthalmology; F. Clifford Rose, Editor, The C. V. Mosby Company, St. Louis, 1976, pp. 495–517.
McKusick, V.A.: Mendelian Inheritance in Man. Johns Hopkins University Press, Baltimore, 1976, pp. 51–52.
Neel, J.V.: Current concepts of the genetic basis of diabetes mellitus and the biological significance of the diabetic predisposition. Excerpta Medica Intern. Congress Series No. 172S; 1967. pp. 68–78.
Vyas, (N.I.): Personal communication.

Author's address:
The Wilmer Institute
John's Hopkins Hospital
601 N. Broadway
Baltimore, Md 21205
USA

Docum. Ophthal. Proc. Series, Vol. 21

IATROGENIC CATARACTS

F. D'ERMO & P. STEINDLER

(Padova, Italy)

Substances which have been shown to be cataractogenic are commonly used in therapy, and this use is becoming more and more frequent. It is necessary to distinguish between drugs which affect the transparency of the crystalline lens through a simple depository action, and those which cause metabolic alterations of the lens.

Silver salts, apart from producing the more frequent corneal and conjunctival argyrosis, can cause a greenish sheen behind the anterior lens capsule (argyrolentis), although this does not impair the vision (Bryk 1956, Larsen 1927). Similar changes can be caused by mercuric salts when mercuric eye ointments are applied (Fisher 1947) and by gold salts when administered parenterally (Roberts & Wolter 1956).

However, lesions caused by drugs which affect the metabolism of the crystalline lens, are much more important and frequent. These drugs have been listed under the following headings: hydrocarbons, antimitotics, enzymatic inhibitors, ferrothiazine derivatives, corticosteroids, miotics, contraceptive oestroprogesterone hormones.

HYDROCARBONS

Dinitrophenol: First marketed many years ago as a slimming aid after Gibbs & Reichert (1891) had demonstrated that the drug could increase the metabolic rate, this therapy was widely used, especially in the United States, until it was found to cause progressive opacity of the lens (Horner 1941). The onset of the cataract varied greatly, from the beginning of the therapy (generally not before several months) and often continued, even after suspension of the treatment. The pathogenesis of this cataract is unknow, and it has been proved impossible to reproduce it in animals (Duke Elder, 1972).

Paradiclorobenzene: a trinitrophenol derivative used as an insecticide and insect repellent. The cataract which develops in humans exposed to inhalation of the substance is sometimes preceded by a toxic hepatitis (Duke Elder 1972).

Antimitotic drugs: Many of these drugs have been shown to cause cataracts in animals. The nitrogen mustards, melamintriethylene (TEM) (Conklin et al 1963) 2, 3, 5, TRIS (Ethylene-Imino) benzoquinoline (Trenimon), cause a unilateral cataract in the mouse 30-40 days after intracarotid injec-

31

tion (Apponi et al. 1964). Ericson (1964) has shown a clouding of the rat lens following intravitreous injection of nitrogen mustard, Cyclophosphamide (Endoxan) and Methrotrexate.

During this treatment in man, ocular changes of various types, especially inflammatory (Iridocyclitis, uveitis, choroiditis, etc.) have been described.

Of course it is difficult to distinguish the toxic effects of the drug, from those of the disease to be treated, when patients have generalised neoplasia.

ENZYMATIC INHIBITORS

Triparanol. Triparanol is used as an antiarteriosclerotic drug because it inhibits the enzymatic reduction of cholesterol from dehydrocholesterol.

This drug, after prolonged use, has caused in man not only cataract, but also cutaneous changes, hair-loss and icthyosis (Kirby 1962).

The ocular lesions have also been reproduced in the rat (Salman 1963).

Clomiphene (Clomid). This substance is structurally similar to triparanol and is used to induce ovulation in sterile women, particularly in the case of the Stein-Leventhal syndrome. It too causes cataract (Walsh & Hoyt 1969).

PHENOTHIAZINE DERIVATIVES

Greiner & Berry (1964) were the first to pay attention to ocular complications arising from long term therapy involving Largactyl administered in high doses (500-1.500 mg a day). They observed a peculiar skin pigmentation in 70 patients, all women. In 12 cases corneal and lenticular opacities appeared. Later, numerous reports of corneal and lens toxicity were published (Baron 1968; De Long 1968; Francesconi 1968; Moschini 1968).

The first changes consist of fine pinpoint anterior subcapsular opacities in the pupillary area, well seen with the slit lamp. At first, the opacity is round in appearence, but soon because of the sutures, it becomes star-like. Initially the granules are pale, but they gradually darken.

The cataract incidence is influenced by both the total dosage and duration of the therapy. Doses of under 0,5 Kg. do not usually give rise to lenticular deposits. They become frequent when the doses is above 1 Kg. The incidence rises to 90 % of cases treated when the dose is approx. 2,5 Kg.

CORTICOSTEROIDS

a) General treatment. It has been observed in a significant number of cases, that corticosteroids administered for long periods cause the development of posterior subcapsular opacities of the lens. It seems that the process is related both to duration and dosage of therapy. According to Duke Elder, patients treated with prednisolone doses below 10 mg per day do not develop a cataract while the cataract appears in 75% of patients treated with doses of above 15 mg/day for over a year. However, doubts concerning the direct responsibility of cortisones in the cataractous process have been expressed (Moro 1965).

Most of the patients who undergo prolonged corticosteroid therapy and have developed a cataract, are already suffering from rheumatoid arthritis. So it is possible that opacification may be due, at least in part, to the rheumatic disease, Gordon and coll. (1961) have observed an unusual percentage of posterior cataracts in patients under the age of 50 suffering from rheumatoid arthritis who have not undergone cortisone treatment.

b) Local treatment. The onset of cataracts after local instillation of cortisone has been observed by numerous authors (Valerio 1963; Neuschuler 1966; Quaranta 1967, etc.).

The process starts as a pulverulent opacity, discoid at the posterior polar level, immediately subcapsular. This opacity tends to advance, reaching the intermediate strata and the anterior cortex.

If the treatment is interrupted, at least in the initial cases, the cataract may regress partially (Streiff 1964) yet in other instances, it progresses. Well known (though here only mentioned) is the cataract + glaucoma link with cortisone (Frendsen 1964).

The pathogenesis of this type of cataract is not yet well known. Harris (1962) claims that corticosteroids affect the permeability of the lens to cations and that their action is similar to that of galactose and triparanol. Pecori Giraldi et al. (1973) have observed a significant diminution of the ascorbic acid in the lens of rabbits undergoing prolonged instillation of 9-fluoro-16 methylprednisolone.

MIOTICS

The prolonged use of miotics of the anticholinesterase group (DFP, Echotiophate, Decamerium bromide, Diethyl-P-Nitrophenyl phosphate, Mintacol) used in glaucoma therapy, can cause opacity of the lens. The toxicity of these drugs was first observed by Kreibig (1954), but it has since been confirmed by numerous observations (Shaffer 1966; Harrison 1960; Nordmann 1965, Levene 1968).

The lens alterations consist of anterior subcapsular vacuoles, posterior subcapsular and nuclear opacities. The visual damage is initially very slight, but may become more noticeable after the second year of treatment. The alteration presents a significant degree of reversibility when treatment is suspended.

The pathogenesis of the lens opacification remains to be clarified. Experiments 'in vitro' and 'in vivo' evidence a change of lens permeability to cations of rabbits treated with Phospholine Iodide (Secchi 1971).

Such toxic effect may be partially inhibited, both 'in vivo' or 'in vitro', by the administration of Taurine (Secchi 1974).

Other studies carried out 'in vitro' have failed to evidence such damage in the permeability to cations after incubation of lenses in Pilocarpine or Aceclidine, which in this case, would be the least harmful.

All the authors agree with the claim that the lenticular opacity caused by anticholinesterases appears exclusively when these drugs are used for glaucoma therapy. With the exception of one case, (Harrison 1960) the anterior subcapsular vacuoles were not observed in children treated with anticholinesterases to correct the accomodative esotropia.

CATARACTS CAUSED BY ORAL OESTROPROGESTINIC CONTRACEPTIVES

In 1968 Kogan reported the case of a young woman who developed acute myopia after taking an antiovulatory preparation for 4 months. This myopia normalized when she interrupted treatment. The author thought this might be due to a lens swelling induced by the hormone.

The first two cases of cataract which appeared following prolonged oral contraceptive treatment were described by Davidson (1971) as occurring in two women of 21 and 25 who had taken the oestroprogestional drugs for approx. 2 years.

Other authors reported the development of lens opacities in patients who used contraceptives habitually (Goddé-Jolly 1972; Varga 1973; Offret 1974). Trux et al. carried out a systematic study of 120 patients 22 to 40 years old who had been taking oestroprogestional drugs habitually for 7-8 months. In 7 cases posterior cortical opacities of the lens were observed, which did not progress after suspension of the treatment. Cataracts caused by oral contraceptives have the following characteristics (Volpi 1977).

a. Most cases were between 20 and 30 years old; b. The average duration of administration is 1 year for the onset of opacities, 2 years for the onset of cataract; c. The cataract usually occurs in both eyes as posterior subcapsular, even if at different stages.

The features of the cataract caused by oestroprogestinases are similar to those caused by corticosteroids. This would suggest a similar pathogenesis for the two forms.

The basal structure, steroidal, is common to the two types of drugs.

The hypothesis of a relationship between the taking of progestinics and the development of cataract is supported by other researches. Lamber (1968) evidenced an increase of 30% in the permeability to cations after exposure of the lens to progesterone in concentrations of 10^{-4} M for 48 hours. The effect was dependent on and directly correlated to duration of exposure.

Not all authors agree in establishing a relationship between cataracts and oestroprogestines. Drill et al. (1975) in a long term study of monkeys and dogs given high doses of 2 types of contraceptives ('Ovulen' and 'Eno E') failed to find a significant cataractogenic potential of the two drugs.

In humans, Conel & Kelman (1969) showed no statistically significant difference between cataract development in women taking oral contraceptives and in the control group.

At present, our knowledge does not permit a definite conclusion. All the studies, in fact, have been conducted on groups which are too small to allow statistically significant conclusions.

The relationship between contraceptive treatment and opacification of the lens deserves further research especially when we consider the increasing use and social importance of these drugs.

SUMMARY

Numerous drugs administered either generally or locally have shown a cataractogenic action.

From a pathogenic point of view a distinction must be made between drugs which modify the transparency of the lens due to accumulation (mercuric, silver, gold salts, etc.) from those influencing its metabolism.

Among the latter, Triparanol, antimitotic drugs, various phenothiazinic derivates, corticosteroids and certain miotics cause the most significatn damage.

It is necessary to indicate the most frequent reports which evidence a relationship between a prolonged oestroprogestinic therapy and alterations of the lens transparency.

The authors also indicate pathogenic mechanisms which probably cause iatrogenic cataracts.

REFERENCES

Apponi G., Rinaldi E. & De Simone S. Cataratta monolaterale dopo iniezione endocarotidea di 2-3-5 Trisetilenimmino 1-4 benzochinone (Trenimon Bayer). *Ann. Ottal.* 90, *224*, 1964.

Baron J.B., Morel P., Rivollan Y. & Soulairac A.: Incidences ophtalmologiques du traitement prolongé par la chloropromazine associée ou non à des troubles cutanés. *Agressiologie*, 9, (2) *293*, 1968.

Bryk E.: Generalized argyrosis with involvement of lenses. *Klin. Oczna* 26, *217*, 1956.

Conel E.B. & Kelman C.D.: Ophthalmologic findings with oral contraceptives. *Obstet. Gynec.* 31, *456*, 1968.

Conklin, Upton & Christenberry & Mc.Donald: Citato da Duke-Elder. *Radiat. Res.* 19, *156*, 1963.

Davidson S.I.: Reported adversa effects of oral contraceptives on the eye. *Trans. Ophthal. Soc. U.K.* 91, *561*, 1971.

De Long S.L.: Incidence and significance of chloropromazine-induced eye changes. *Dis. Nerv. Syst.* 29 (3), Suppl. 19, 1968.

Drill V.A., Martin D.P., Gollway P.L. & Hart E.R.: Ocular effect of oral contraceptives. II. Studies in the rhesus monkey. *Fertil. Steril.* 16, 9, *914*, 1975.

Drill V.A., Rao S.K., Mc.Connell R.G. & Souri E.N.: Ocular effects of oral contraceptives. I studies in the dog. *Fertil. Steril.* 26, (9), *908*, 1975.

Fischer F.P. Mercuriosis du cristallin. *Ann. Ocul.* 180, *508*, 1947.

Francesconi G., Di Tizio A. & Cameo D.: Alterazioni oculari e cutanee in pazienti sottoposti a terapia di lunga durata con farmaci neurolettici. *Ann. Ottal.* 94 (7), *835*, 1968.

Frandsen E.: Glaucoma and posterior subcapsular cataract following topical Prednisolone (Ultracortenol) therapy. *Acta Ophthal.* 42. *108*, 1964.

Fricson L., Karlberg B. & Rosengren B.H.O.: Trials of intravitreal injection of chemotherapeutic agents in rabbits. *Acta Ophthal.* 42, *721*, 1964.

Gibbs, Reichert: Riferito da Duke-Elder in System of Ophthal. vol. XIV part II p. 1291. *Am. Chem. J.*, 13, *289*, 1891.

Godde-Jolly M., Ruellan Y.M., Bremme C. & Theron H.P.: Trois observations de cataracte survenue chez des femmes prénent le même contraceptif par voie orale. S'agit-il d'une coincidence? *Bull. Soc. Ophtal. de France* 72, *441*, 1972.

Gordon D.M., Camerer W.H. & Freyberg R.H.: Examination for posterior capsular cataracts. J.A.M.A. 175, 127, 1961.

Greiner & Berry: Riferito da Duke-Elder in System of Ophthal. vol. XIV part II, p. 1295. *Canad. Med. Ass. J.*: 90, *663*, 1964.

Lambert P.W.: The effects of progestins and estrogens on the permeability of the lens. *Arch. Ophtal.* 4, *957*, 1965.

Larsen B.: Ueber Argyrosis Corneae bei Hollensteinarbeitern. *Albrecht v. Graefes Arch. klin. exp. Ophtahl.* 118, *145*, 1927.

Levene R.Z.: Echothiopate Iodide and lens changes. Symposium on Ocular Therapy, Vol. 4. I. H. Leopold. The C.V. Mosby Co., Saint Louis, 1968.

Moschini G.B., Cancrini L., Bietti C. & Gastona: Tossicologia nei trattamenti protratti con farmaci neurolettici. *Riv. Psichiatr.* 3, *674*, 1968.

Harris J.E., Gruber L.: The electrolyte and water balance of the lens. *Exp. Eye Res.* 1, *372*, 1962.

Harrison R.: Bilateral lens opacities associated with use of Di-Isopropyl Fluorophosphate eyedrops. *Am. J. Ophthal.* 50, *153*, 1960.

Horner: Riferito da Duke-Elder in System of Ophthalmology. Vol. XIV part II, p. 1252. *Trans. Am. Ophthal. Soc.* 39, *405*, 1941.

Kirby T.J., Achor R.W.P., Perry H.O. & Winkelmann R.K.: Cataract formation after Triparanol therapy. *Arch. Ophthal.* 68, 486, 1962.

Kogan J.: Miopia aguta cristaliniana por anovulatorios. *Arch. Oft. B. Aires* 43, 1, 1968.

Kreibig W.: Zur operativen Behandlung des akuten Glaukomanfalles. *Klin. Mbl. Augenheilk.* 125, 39, 1954.

Neuschuler R.: Ulteriore contributo casistico alle cataratte da uso locale di cortisonici: cataratta totale in età infantile. *Boll. Ocul.* 45, 48, 1966.

Nordmann J. & Gerhardt J.P.: A propos de la cataracte par miotiques. *Bull. Soc. Ophtal. Fr.* 69, 649, 1969.

Offret G., Haut J., Limon S & Clay C.: Pilules contraceptives et cataracte. *Bull. Soc. Ophtal. Fr.* 74, 1119, 1974.

Roberts W.H. & Wolter J.R.: Ocular crysiasis. *Arch. Ophthal.* 56, 48, 1956.

Salmann L., Ivon J., Grimes P. & Collins F.: Triparanol induced cataract in rats. *Arch. Ophthal.* 70, 522, 1963.

Secchi A.G., Levi Minzi S., Segato T. & Steindler P.: Ricerche sperimentali sull'azione di un inibitore delle colinesterasi (Phospholine Iodide) sulla permeabilità del cristallino ai cationi. *Ann. Ottal. Clin. Ocul.* 97, 9, 1971.

Secchi A.G., Fregona I. & Mancini B.: Azione normalizzante della Taurina nella alterazione della permeabilità del cristallino. indotta da 'Phospholine Iodide'. Atti del LVI Congr. S.O.I., Roma, 1975.

Shaffer R.N. & Hetherington J.R.: Anticholinesterase drug and cataract. *Am. J. Ophthal.* 62, *619*, 1966.

Streiff E.B.: Evolution de l'opacité cristallinienne par cortisone locale. *Ophthalmologica* 147, *143*, 1964.

Trux E., Varga M. & Follma B.: Complications oculaires au cours du traitement contraceptif par voie orale. *Bull. Soc. Fr. Ophtal.* 87, *310*, 1975.

Varga M.: Ophthalmologische Komplikationen nach oraler Kontrazeption. *Klin. Mbl. Augenheilk.* 162, *621*, 1973.

Walsh F.B. & Hoyt W.F.: Clinical Neuro-Ophthalmology. 3rd Edit. Williams & Wilkins, Baltimore, 1969 p. 2687.

Author's address:
Institute of Ophthalmology of the
University of Padova
Padova
Italy

Docum. Ophthal. Proc. Series, Vol. 21

CATARACT EPIDEMIOLOGY:
PUBLIC HEALTH IMPLICATIONS AND
RESEARCH NEEDS

B. NIZETIC

(Copenhagen, Denmark)

It is largely recognized today that the picture and understanding of a disease process cannot be complete without the description or the thorough study of its behaviour in the population.

Epidemiological studies of cataract are therefore aiming to provide us with reliable data on

a. its frequency and distribution in a given population (descriptive epidemiology),

b. determinants of the noted distribution (analytic epidemiology).

The third and not less important aspect of the epidemiological studies is to give us guidance in the planning and provision of eye-health services and particularly in the evaluation of medical eye care.

The data on which epidemiological studies rest are dependent, for their validity, upon certainty and consistency of diagnostic criteria and upon completeness of ascertainment. As far as cataract is concerned, these data derive from three sources: statistics of blindness registration, population surveys, and surgical statistics.

From a statistical point of view each of these sources presents some pitfalls which have been analyzed elsewhere, and I will, however, consider only a few which are relevant from a public health point of view.

Of all eye diseases, 'cataract' registration figures are likely to be most misleading due to a variety of reasons:

The first is the one resulting from the confusion that exists in the literature between 'cataract' and lens opacities.

Many people visually impaired by cataract are not registered because they are thought to be awaiting surgical treatment.

According to Sorsby, the availability of this treatment is the single major factor explaining the drop in registered cases between 1949 and 1968 (83:100.000 to less than 50:1.000.000 among the 70plus age group).

Very many people with bilateral cataract are not visually impaired (if WHO classification is applied), and the slow progression toward their visual impairment must affect the ageing person's perception of his own visual ability.

This is why Wyatt in a relatively recent (1973) survey found that 89 per cent of 154 people with lens opacities could not be counted as visually impaired.

To reduce further the reliability of figures on cataract registration it would seem likely from Brenner and Knox's observations that most of the elderly in the community with cataracts who were suffering severe visual impairment at the time of examination, had some other systemic disease making operation inadvisable, or had a dual eye pathology such as macular degeneration.

A range of 22 per cent (Sorsby 1966) to 33 per cent (Mann 1966) of blindness registration attributable to senile cataract is probably the expression of some of the difficulties just mentioned.

As far as second source of epidemiological data is concerned, it is regretable that extremely few population surveys of cataract have been made, in the sense of studies of random samples of the general population rather than of patients presenting themselves for ophthalmological examination.

These studies (considering opacities of all types) have revealed a steady increase with age (McGuiness 1967; Fisher 1948), but here again the lack of well defined denominator population makes the results questionable.

Data from surgical statistics related to cataract extraction have the advantage of dealing with events in which occurrence can certainly be determined, but the interpretation of data is difficult in view of many imponderable factors. According to Caird who has carefully analyzed this problem, cataract extractions should be studied only in a clearly defined population. Definitions of various types of cataract are another prerequisite. Before definite inferences about the frequency of cataract in these population groups can be made, it is necessary to consider the relation between cataract extraction and lens opacities in the population as a whole, and efforts should be deployed to standardize for the population under study and probably the visual indications for cataract extraction.

This having been said about the validity of our present knowledge on cataract epidemiology, a few figures representing estimations rather than findings, should illustrate the public health dimension of the problem.

At least 300 000 – 400 000 new visually disabling cataracts occur yearly in the United States, and 5–10 million world-wide, according to Sommer.

Venkataswamy estimates that nearly 17 million people are blind due to cataract at any one time in the world. This estimate is based also on the fact that, according to the same author, not even 20 per cent of blind afflicted with cataract is being operated upon, for restoration of sight.

In India nearly 5 per cent of the population (30 million people) suffers from cataract and more than 1 per cent is economically blind from the same cause.

In Kenya it is estimated that nearly 1.7 per cent of the population is blind and 44 per cent of this blindness is attributable to cataract. It is estimated that similar figures are applicable to most of the African countries.

Venkataswamy estimates the total number of blind from cataract to be nearly 7.5 million.

Belforts Junior attributes 31.3 per cent of all registered blindness to cataract in Brazil.

Finally, complications of modern surgical techniques alone probably result in at least 7000 irreversibly blind eyes annually in the United States, and a potential 100 000 to 200 000 world-wide, according to Sommers.

Age distribution of cataract differs considerably from region to region. In India and some other developing countries, 70 per cent of cataract blindness occurs below the age of 60, while in the United States, 70 per cent of the people with cataract are 65 years of age, or older.

Socio-economic impact of this situation is enormous for both medically affluent and developing countries.

The former face problems related to spiralling costs of hospitalization, and the latter face those related to unemployment and loss in productivity.

About 10 years ago a study was made in India on the economic impact of blindness due to cataract. This study was done on 440 patients operated for cataract in one of the eye-camps in Tamil Nadu. These people were blind for varying periods and they had ceased working as farmers or shop keepers. The average duration of unemployment due to blindness was found to be six months. The average monthly earning of a man was $10 a month and a woman $8. The average earning loss was about $55 per person at the time of surgery; in developing countries, however, few people receive surgery at all, and seldom at an early stage. In addition to personal income loss there is family economic loss, since family members are responsible for the care of these blind people. If the present cost entailed a loss of $100 per person per year, for 17 million people in the world who are blind due to cataract, the economic loss would be more than 1.7 billion dollars per year even by the Indian economic standard. The real economic loss on a world-wide scale is impossible to estimate, but must be much greater than this conservative figure. In one district of Tamil Nadu there were at least 60 000 people blind from cataract, many of whom were farmers or farm workers whose visual disability rendered them unfit for work.

On a very long range it is to be hoped that basic research coupled with carefully conducted clinical-epidemiological studies will bring us the necessary knowledge on etio-pathogenesis of cataract and clues for successful prevention.

I would like to mention just one of the fields in which more basic and clinico-epidemiological research is possibly needed, particularly in industrialized countries. To elucidate, if the steadily increasing use of microwaves so widely used in affluent countries for cooking, transmitting long-distance calls, bringing civilian airliners down for landings and monitoring the seas and skies for foreign military craft, really has any impact upon cataractogenesis.

Today, more concerted multidisciplinary research efforts seem mandatory to improve the treatment from a clinical point of view, to improve the efficiency and the effectiveness of eye-care services, due consideration being given to the health system of each respective country and its socio-economic stage of development.

As an example, I would mention the necessity of controlled clinical trials of such procedures as phacoemulsification and lens implantation before they are recommended on a mass scale. Furthermore, health service research should provide guidance to health authorities for reorganizing appropriately eye-care services, for reducing the duration of costly hospital stay, for considering possible extra-mural clinical and surgical activities.

The case of India which uses the so-called 'camp approach' is an example of an imaginative solution under given conditions which need not be adopted, but could be improved and adapted in many other areas of the world.

REFERENCES

Belforts, R. Jr.: A survey of cases of blindness. *Archivos Brasileiros de Ophtalmologia.* 35:1–28–33 (1972).

Caird, I.F.: Problems of cataract epidemiology with special reference to diabetes in the human lens. A Ciba Foundation Symposium Elsevier Excerpta Medica (1973).

Nizetic, B.: Public health ophthalmology. Chapter 29 of 'The theory and practice of public health', (Hobson W. Editor) Oxford University Press (1975).

Nizetic, B.: Introduction to epidemiology. Chapter 22 of Scientific Foundation of ophthalmology. (Perkins E.S. and Hill B.W. Eds) William Heinemann Medical Books, London (1977).

Sommer, A.: Cataract as an epidemiologic problem. *American Journal of Ophthalmology,* 83(3):334 – 9, (1977).

Venkataswamy, G.: Problems of blindness in India. National Society for Prevention of Blindness (1974).

Author's Address:
World Health Organization
Regional Office for Europe
8, Scherfigsvej
DK-2100 Copenhagen
Denmark

Docum. Ophthal. Proc. Series, Vol. 21

GENERAL AND OPHTHALMOLOGICAL PROBLEMS PRECEDING THE OPERATION

C. A. QUARANTA

(L'Aquila, Italy)

As regards general and pre-operative ophthalmological problems in cataract surgery, all of those factors which together condition individual indications of operability must be analyzed. The different clinical peculiarities of each individual patient must be attentively considered in order to obtain the best surgical and functional results. Within the individual clinical context, general and local, precise critical pre-operative evaluation of the indications, contraindications and potential complications is essential for the best preparation for the operation and the exact choice of the most appropriate surgical techniques. A precise general anamnesis is the first step to be taken in examination of the patient.

As a general rule, cataract operations are not extremely urgent. Therefore the surgeon has the necessary time for programming his decisions so that the operation can be performed under the best possible conditions, with the best prognostic expectations.

The final aim of cataract surgery is the restoration of the visual functions. Any operative risk, whether potentially linked to the patient's general condition, to local conditions, or to a psychological situation, must be carefully evaluated before the operation. To avoid as far as possible any complication springing from general or local conditions, the surgeon must intervene beforehand, either with therapeutical techniques or with surgical precautions, as the case requires. Each decision must be made individually, case by case.

Annual statistics tell us of high and truly praiseworthy percentages of success in the field of cataract surgery, success in both the anatomical and the functional sense. Present-day surgical and microsurgical technical possibilities have contributed to these results, as regards both intra- and extracapsular extractions, individually programmed in the pre-operative and peroperative stages, including the possible decision to perform intracamerular implantation.

The reduction in the incidence of per- and post-operative complications is fundamentally based on complete examination and precise evaluation of the general and ocular conditions of each individual patient. In present-day standardized surgical methodologies, both classic and more recent, the study of general and local pre-operative conditions has been essential in bringing about continual, progressive improvements and new knowledge necessary

41

for avoiding all those complications and failures linked to unrecognized or underestimated pre-disposing pathological factors.

The present discussion, rather than defining absolute or relative indications or contra-indications to cataract operation, will limit itself to a study, from a prophylactic point of view, of conditions pre-existent to the operation, which must be treated or given appropriate consideration when choosing surgical procedures in order to avoid more or less serious complications.

The greater possibilities of succes which are undoubtedly within our reach must not make us forget that even the most precise techniques and the most refined surgical methods cannot give us the results desired unless the operative indications are perfectly recognized. In this sense, pre-operative examination of each individual patient's condition is a basic element for obtaining the best functional and anatomical results. General and local pre-operative problems, appropriately detected and studied, give precise and objective direction as to criteria of operability. The patient's state must be assessed from all aspects, not only those strictly pertaining to the operation itself.

It must always be remenbered that although the cataract operation, considered comprehensively in its various stages, preóperative, peroperative and post-operative, usually has well-defined stages and a certain codification of post-operative therapies, any possible complication may lead to the necessity of special treatment, often urgent. The patient's general level of tolerance and individual contraindications must also be considered, on the basis of knowledge gained from preliminary examinations.

In the field of cataract surgery, too, interdisciplinary collaboration can assure a better safety margin and better functional and anatomical results, also as regards the patient's psychological situation and his trusting acceptance of surgical decisions. Since cataract operation is usually not urgent, any general therapy, even a rather long one, may be used to put the patient in the best general pre-operative condition.

Any possible risk must be a calculated risk. In these cases, all the necessary supplementary precautions must be taken. Careful, precise study of cardio-vascular and circulatory conditions, of renal function, of endocrine equilibrium, especially as regards a possible diabetic state, of blood dyscrazia, of the hemogenic state, of hepatic, gastro-enteric and respiratory functions, can give the surgeon the possibility of operating under the best general conditions.

The conditions of the respiratory system, states of emphysema or bronchitis or laryngo-tracheitis, all of those conditions, in short, which can influence respiratory function or give rise to attacks of coughing, must naturally be given due consideration, both causal and symptological, for proper medical therapy. Chronic or episodic disturbances of gastro-enteric and urinary functions, of any cause whatever, should be noted in the anamnestic stage for appropriate testing, to avoid incurring possible ocular damage from causes which are often banal and moreover easily preventable with proper treatment.

Special attention must be given to a preliminary study of possible allergic conditions or hyper-sensitive reactions to medicines. The patient must be carefully questioned about general and local therapies being followed at the time of the examination, or before, in order to define, if possible, the reasons for the prescribed treatment.

A study of anamnestic data and of the general conditions of the individual patient can be greated aided by the collaboration of his family doctor, when possible. This collaboration can provide more precise information on medical therapies used either in the past or at the present, on their efficacy and on the possibility of individual intolerance.

Interdisciplinary collaboration is especially useful on the clinical and scientific level and for surgical purposes in congenital and infantile cataracts. Before the operation, an aetiopathogenetic classification of the cataract should be made. Cataracts resulting from embryopathies, foetopathies and metabolic alterations and cataracts associated with more or less serious and complex general syndromes often involve special anaesthetic and surgical problems, including the question of the best age for operation. The best time for cataract operation in infants and children is a special problem involving comparative study of visual, anatomical and functional results and of the psychological development of the child within his environment. Sometimes in infancy the cataract operation must be programmed in time in relation to the subject's general condition and to the possible need for preventive medical therapies or surgical operations for other malformations.

Still on the subject of the influence of general conditions on operative and post-operative complications, it must be remembered that it is sometimes possible, through careful examination of the fundus oculi, to recognise all those elements having to do with the patient's vascular condition which are useful for determining the most appropriate precautionary, general and local therapeutic measures.

Arterial hypertension, pathological states of cardio-circulatory and renal functions and pathological vascular states can be elements giving rise to the most diverse complications. Detachment of the choroid and choroidal haemorrhages, and even expulsive hemorrhage, papillary and retinal oedemas, retino-vitreal hemorrhages, cystoid macular oedema, neuropathies and ischaemic retinopathies, can all originate from particular general and local conditions preceding the operation; therefore the need for well-oriented pre-operative therapy must always be given due value. The anamnestic data of the individual case, the data from preceding examinations, the eventuality of being able to examine the fundus oculi, even if only in the eye with a less-advanced cataract, can raise the question of the necessity of precautionary prophylactic treatment against detachtment of the retina.

Among ophthalmological problems to be considered specifically before operating, the conditions of the anterior segment of the eyeball and in particular the condition of the cornea must not be forgotten. Corneal edema can be a serious post-operative complication. The most diverse factors can enter into its pathogenesis, such as for example, induced toxic effects of corneal trauma during the operation, with consequent endothelial lesions and rupture of the descemet, cutting in the corneal area, vitreous in the anterior chamber with vitreo-corneal adherences, the type and location of corneal or sclero-corneal sutures. It is clear that a pre-existing corneal pathological state can in itself be a predisposing cause of the development of serious complications.

The Cornea Guttata and the endothelial dystrophies of Fuchs, although of sub-clinical importance, must be carefully examined, using the most modern instruments available such as the corneal specular biomicroscope, in order to limit as far as possible corneal complications of the oedematous type.

All of the possible triggering causes, whether of mechanical or toxic nature, must be prevented and avoided in the various stages of the operation. In cases where there is persistent oedema in the pre-operative state, the appropriateness of a combined operation for cataract extraction and corneal transplant should be investigated. The possibility of co-existence of a glaucomatous state should naturally be carefully evaluated in order to choose the best therapeutic decisions, medical or surgical, to be practiced during the operation or beforehand. Combined operations, with deep protected sclerectomy and cataract extraction are at present preferred by many surgeons.

Other local problems which must be attentively weighed before the operation are those connected with the condition of the adnexa of the eyeball. Of course any inflammatory process which is conjunctival, palpebral, or involving the lacrimal apparatus must be detected and treated, if necessary by recurring to microbiological examinations and studying the relative antibiograms. Dacryocystitis must be surgically treated, with successive microbiological examinations, above all when dacryo-rhinostomy operations have been performed.

Study of the numerous reports in the literature leads us to affirm that a careful approach, in the prophylactic sense, to the possible post-operative infections, immediate or late-appearing, can give highly significant results. Even though at present the incidence of post-operative inflammatory is statistically low, two cases in a thousand, with occasional highs of six-seven per thousand, the gravity of post-operative endophthalmitis is such that every precaution must be taken to prevent it.

It should be mentioned that the statistics for the years 1900-1946 report average percentages of endophthalmitis as twelve in a thousand, with highs of 30 per thousand. Of course the statistics reported in the literature dealing with this subject may be conditioned by various causes of error. If on the one hand we can consider post-operative non-septic reactions as inflammatory states, on the other hand we must consider the natural reluctance to publish cases of infection, which, moreover, are often quickly dominated by the proper therapy.

Post-operative infections are actually a rare occurrence nowadays, notwithstanding the fact that the possible sources of infection in the various stages of the operation are innumerable. In the pre-operative phase, the eyeball cannot be completely sterilized, and it is contiguous to numerous structures, such as the eyelids, the lacrimal ducts, the pharyngonasal and sinus cavities, which are also not completely sterilizable.

The ever-more refined methods of antisepsis and of asepsis now in use are certainly a determining element in the present-day low incidence of post-operative endophthalmitis. To this may be added the importance that should be given to the prophylactic use of general and local antibiotic treatments. Pre-operative general treatment must of course be limited to special cases, with general or local inflammatory processes requiring such therapy. It is obvious that in these conditions, it is best to postpone the operation until after the inflammatory process is cured. The utilization of local antibiotic prophylaxis before the operation is, instead, generally favoured. Recent statistics have shown how local pre-operative antibiotic prophylaxis leads to a reduction of the rate of post-operative infections by about 12 times, from 0.75% to 0.06%.

A short-term prophylactic therapy, of only a few days but with closely-spaced doses, seems preferable for avoiding alterations of the normal bacteric flora with the consequent appearance of mycetes and of pseudomonas. Local therapy makes use mostly of those antibiotics which are not usually used generally and which produce fewer allergic reactions: various combinations of neomycin, bacitracin, polymyxin B, chloramphenicol, erythromycin, kanamycin, gentamycin.

About 50% of post-operative infections are probably due to staphylococcus and about 25% to pseudomonas. It must be remenbered that conjunctival bacterial, viral and mycotic flora can be increased by prolonged treatment with cortisones. In these cases a preliminary cultural examination is prudent to determine specific pre-operative treatment for avoiding as far as possible serious post-operative complications.

In this discussion we have attempted to synthesize some of the main general and ophthalmological pre-operative problems in cataract surgery. In conclusion, it must be emphasized again how an exact pre-operative investigation of each single individual case, both on the general clinical and on the ocular level, can allow us to utilize better, with a surer critical sense, the most modern surgical techniques, further increasing the possilibities of their anatomical and functional success, to the greater benefit of our patients.

Author's address:
Instituto Universitario di Medicina e Chirurgia
Cattedra di Clinica Oculistica
L'Aquila
Italy

45

Docum. Ophthal. Proc. Series, Vol. 21

GUIDELINES OF HAEMORRHAGIC PROPHYLAXIS IN CATARACT SURGERY

M. PANDOLFI

(Malmö, Sweden)

HAEMOSTASIS AND CATARACT OPERATION. GENERAL REMARKS

Any full-thickness lesion of the wall of a blood vessel is followed by the escape of blood. The blood-loss is generally limited since the organism can provisionally plug the gap whereafter cellular proliferation gradually reconstitutes the vascular wall. Fig 1 summarizes the haemostatic process after trauma of a minor vessel.

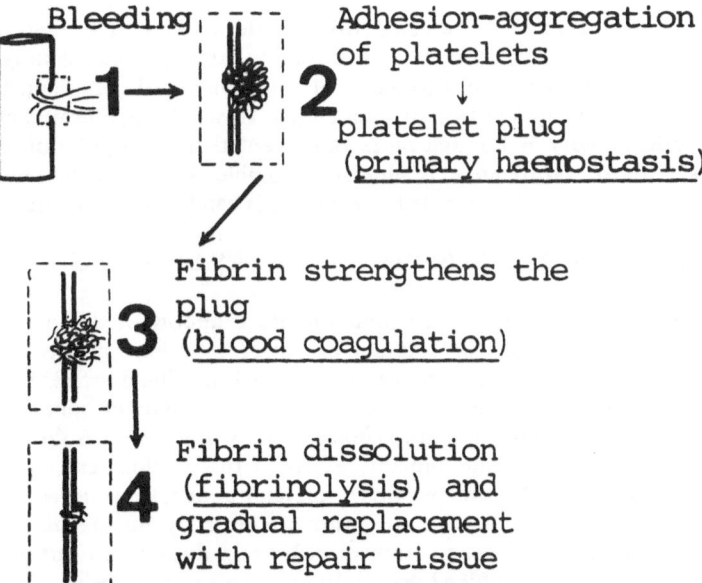

Fig. 1 Haemostatic process after the trauma of a small vessel. Bleeding through the vascular wound (1). Platelats adhere to the exposed subendothelial collagen and aggregate forming the haemostatic plug (primary haemostasis) which arrests the haemorrhage (2). Following the activation of the coagulation system fibrin strengthening the plug is formed (3). The obstructing clot is gradually dissolved by the fibrinolyctic system and replaced by repair tissue (4).

* Supported by grants from the University of Lund and the T. and E. Segerfalk's Fund for Medical Research.

In any operation involving vascular trauma bleeding is unavoidable; such a bleeding, however, has to be 'normal' since a persisting haemorrhage makes the operation difficult and may cause serious loss of blood. Cataract surgery is virtually never complicated by life-threatening haemorrhages. However, because of the optic function of the eye it is especially indicated to avoid intra- and postoperative haemorrhages involving this organ.

A patient with a haemostatic defect can be expected to bleed unusually freely at as well as after the operation. In patients with a depression of the clotting factors, such as of those occuring in haemophilia or treatment with anticoagulants even a small surgical trauma, such as tooth extraction, may be followed by profuse bleeding. The platelet count and platelet function seem to be less important than clotting factors for the haemostasis in medium and major operations, and it is often possible to perform such operations on patients with severe platetet disorders (i.e. splenectomy in thrombocytopenia) without serious complications. On the other hand platelets and other factors of the primary haemostasis are crucial in case of minute surgical trauma (operation for cataract, for example).

It follows that before an operation for cataract, care has to be taken to detect defects of haemostasis and especially those of the primary haemostasis.

As for fibrinolysis an increased fibrinolytic activity of the blood interferes with haemostasis in operation both by causing fibrinogenolysis and thereby inhibiting the reinforcement of the haemostatic plug and later by causing premature dissolution of such a plug. However, an elevated systemic fibrinolytic activity is a much more rare event than a coagulation disorder and its clinical significance is almost negligible. On the other hand, the importance of local fibrinolysis in haemostasis can hardly be overestimated.

RECOGNITION OF A BLEEDING TENDENCY BEFORE OPERATION

The presence of an undetected (and therefore uncorrected) haemorrhagic diathesis in a candidate for cataract operation may have disastrous consequences. Which are the tests necessary to check the haemostasis before the operation? Some ophthalmologists feel safe if the platelet count, coagulation time and bleeding time are normal. Others, on even less grounds, feel safe when coagulation time and the results of the suction tests are normal. It should be vigorously stressed that a platelet count, suction test, bleeding time and coagulation time within normal limits by no means exclude a mild or even moderate coagulation disorder and thereby do not guarantee that the patient will not bleed profusely at and after operation. Actually, to be completely sure that haemostasis in a given case is normal would require scores of other tests most of which are feasible only in specialized laboratories.

Fortunately, routine haemostatic tests may be corroborated by a simple and inexpensive means allowing operation without a significant rist of haemorrhage, i.e. a careful inquiry into the patient's bleeding history which, according to Nilsson (1976), is the best screening method. Since many haemorrhagic diatheses are hereditary, the patient should first be asked whether any member of his family bleeds readily. The patient should be asked whether he/she bruises readily, whether he/she bleeds profusely and for a long time after trivial traumata (shaving, cutting of the skin, biting of the tongue. Recurring spontaneous nasal bleeding is suspicious. Women should be asked about the amount of menstrual blood loss. Inquiry about previous operations is important. Extraction of a tooth is a sensitive test of haemostasis. At Nilsson (1976) stated, extraction of a wisdom tooth without indue loss of blood almost excludes a congenital bleeding disorder.

As a rule of thumb proneness to develop skin petechiae and to bleed from mucosae speak for a platelet disorder, while coagulation defects usually cause profuse bleeding and haematomas in the subcutaneous tissues, muscles and joints.

As for acquired disorders of haemostasis the examiner should mainly check that the patient is not receiving anticoagulants or drugs with a side effect on haemostasis such as aspirin, indomethacin and phenylbutazone which are known to impair the aggregation of platelets (Caen et al 1977). The danger of these drugs in ophtalmic surgery has already been pointed out (Newell 1972).

As for hyperfibrinolysis the patient's medical history is less important since hyperfibrinolytic states are almost exclusively acquired and generally short-lasting, the only exception being the few cases with a congenital defect of fibrinolytic inhibitors described by Hedner et al (1970). Liver cirrhosis is often accompanied by a sustained increase in the fibrinolytic activity of the blood (Fletcher et al 1964) and so is myeloma (Niléhn and Nilsson 1966).

In conclusion, a platelet count, estimation of the coagulation time and the bleeding time may be considered sufficient measures before cataract operation only if accompanied by an accurate bleeding history. [1] If the value of any of these tests is near to the upper normal limit the test should be repeated. Whenever a disorder of haemostasis is discovered or suspected, ocular surgery must be done under the supervision of a coagulation expert.

MAIN HAEMORRHAGIC DISORDERS AND THEIR MANAGEMENT AT CATARACT SURGERY

Congenital disorders. As an example of the frequency of hereditary haemorrhagic disorders in Sweden it might be mentioned that there is about one case of verified hereditary bleeding tendency per 5000 persons (Nilsson 1976). Table 1 classifies the patients with congenital bleeding disorders in Sweden. These disorders can be divided into 1) disorders of primary haemostasis and 2) disorders of coagulation.

---

1   If possible these tests should be complemented by the PTT (partial thromboplastin time) which is a sensitive method to detect defects of the first phase of blood coagulation (formation of blood prothrombinase).

Table I. Congenital bleeding disorders in Sweden (data from Nilsson 1976).

Bleeding disorder	Deficiency	No. of patients
Haemophilia A	Factor VIII	436
" B	" IX	121
" C	" XI	44
v Willebrand's disease	" VIII- v Willebrand	785
Platelets defects	Thrombocytopenia Thrombopathia	
	Thrombasthenia	225
Other defects	Factor V, VII,	
	Fibrinogen	36

1. *Disorders of primary haemostasis.* Such disorders may be due to a rare congenital thrombocytopenia and qualitative platelet defects as thrombasthenia, in which platelets are unable to form aggregates. Severe thrombasthenia cannot be missed since it gives bleeding symptoms from early childhood. On the other hand, a mild thrombasthenia can be overlooked.

For the management of these disorders at surgery see the treatment of the acquired platelet disorders.

2. *Disorders of coagulation.* In Sweden there is one patient haemophilia for every 20.000 inhabitants and one patient with von Willebrand's disease for every 16.000. Von Willebrand's disease is not a pure coagulation defect since it affects also primary haemostasis. Severe cases may hardly pass unnoticed because of the early onset and the gravity of the symptoms.

Moderate and mild forms may escape recognition especially if the bleeding history has been defective. Sandax et al (1961) and Rubenstein et al (1966) described cases of undiagnosed von Willebrand's disease which were operated upon for cataract and had postoperative intraocular bleeding that eventually led to the loss of vision.

When operated upon these patients should receive substitution therapy to raise the blood level of the missing factor before and after the operation Such therapy may consist of transfusions of fresh plasma, plasma cryoprecipate, plasma fractions selectively rich in the missing factor i.e. factor VIII in haemophilia A (Kabi fraction I-0) or factor IX in haemophilia B. For details of such a treatment see Nilsson (1974). The plasma level of the missing factor should be raised to 30-50 % of normal on the operation day and first post operative day. Lower levels (20-30 %) are sufficient for the following 6 days. Until fairly recently (1940) cataract extraction was not considered possible in patients with severe haemophilia because of the risk of uncontrollable orbital (following retrobulbar injection) and intraocular haemorrhages and textbooks advised couching or discission as alternatives. When an operation for cataract had to be done according to the conventional technique former authors warned against iridectomy (Van Lint 1939). As late as 1965 a special technique for cataract operation (no retrobulbar injection, corneal section etc.) in haemophiliacs was described by Poweleit. This author used this technique successfully at operation for cataract in a patient with a mild bleeding tendency without substitution therapy. However, whatever the surgical technique used, substitution therapy should always be given before any type of ocular surgery if the patient has even a mild disorder of coagulation. Thus transfusions of frozen plasma (Lakatos et al 1967), Kabi fraction I-0 (Osterlind & Nilsson 1968), and porcine factor VIII, (Strauss & Ramsell 1968) have been used with success in patients with haemophilia A operated for cataract. Cryoprecipitate from human plasma has been used for an operation for antiglaucomatous iridectomy by Richards & Spurling (1973).

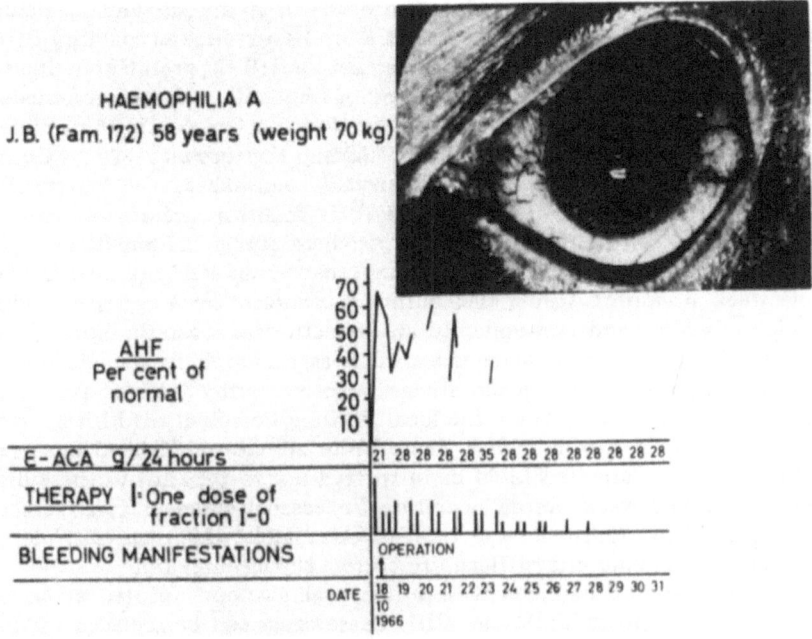

Fig. 2 Dosage of factor VIII in a patient with severe haemophilia A operated upon for cataract (from Osterlind and Nilsson, 1968). The patient was operated upon under protection of repeated infusions of factor VIII concentrate (fraction 1-0 Kabi). No bleeding complication occurred. The inset shows the eye 4 weeks after operation. Corrected visual acuity: 1.0.

Fig. 2 shows the factor VIII dosage and the plasma factor VIII levels as Osterlind and Nilsson's patient. The factor VIII level was kept between 70 and 30 % during the operation and the first 6 postoperative days. An antifibrinolytic drug (EACA) was also given. Lower values of factor VIII, i.e. 15 % or above, were sufficient to prevent haemorrhagic complications of a peripheral iridectomy in the case of Richards & Spurling (1973).

b. Acquired disorders. They are more common than the hereditary disorders. They can be devided into disorders of primary haemostasis, coagulation and fibrinolysis (Table 2).

51

Table 2. Acquired defects of haemostasis.

Defects of the primary haemostasis	Thrombocytopenia
	Thrombopathia (from drugs such as aspirin)
Defects of coagulation	Iatrogenic (heparin, dicoumarol)
	Vit-K deficiency
	Disseminated intravascular coagulation (D.I.C.)
	Circulating anticoagulants

1. *Disorders of primary haemostasis.* Acquired disorders of haemostasis because of impaired platelet function occur in uremia, myeloma, Waldenström's macroglobulinemia. In uremia there is a reduced capability of the platelets both to adhere and aggregate (Larsson 1971) presumably due to a toxic effect. In IgA myeloma and macroglobulinemia the macromolecules present in blood interfere with platelet function by coating the platelet membranes or the vascular surfaces (Vigliano & Horowitz 1967). Correction of uremia or blood dyscrasia usually normalizes the haemostasis.

An important group of disorders is that following treatment with certain drugs impairing platelet function such as aspirin, indomethacin, phenylbutazone etc. (Table 3). These drugs have a long effect (aspirin acts for one week or more). Under their influence platelets form aggregates which rapidly dissolve and consequently are defective haemostatic plugs. In patients with disorders of haemostasis such as haemophilia a single dose of aspirin can cause a joint haemorrhage. Also in healthy subjects aspirin can cause bleeding in sites where the local fibrinolytic activity is high as in the nasal mucosa (Petruson 1974). These drugs are contraindicated in surgery of the eyeball. Patients should be instructed not to take any of these drugs during the last week before operation. In case of emergency, surgery can be preceded by transfusions of fresh blood, platelet rich plasma or platelet concentrates in amounts sufficient to correct the bleeding time.
Bank blood should be avoided since it is generally poor in platelets as well as in coagulation factor V and VIII. These drugs can be replaced by analgesics (such as paracetamol) with no side effects on haemostasis.

2. *Disorders of coagulation.* Circulating antibodies with an inhibitory activity against coagulation factors (factor VIII, IX, XII as well as thromboplastin) may develop in different diseases, such as lupus erythematosus disseminatus, and haemophilia following substitution therapy and induce a tendency to bleeding.

The most common acquired coagulation disorders are those following

Table 3. Agents impairing the haemostatic action of platelets.

Inhibition of adhesion to the vessel wall	Dipyridamole
Inhibition of the release from platelets of procoagulant factors ('release reaction')	Aspirin R, phenylbutazone, oxyphenbutazone, indomethacin
Inhibitors of aggregation by ADP	Adenosine, ATP, AMP, prostaglandin E, furosemide.

therapy with anticoagulants, i.e. heparin and vitamin K antagonists mainly derivatives of dicoumarol.

Several reports have appeared on anticoagulation in relation to general surgery but not ophthalmic surgery. According to Storm (1958) and other authors (ref. in Wieberdink 1967), it is possible to operate on patients with pulmonary tumours and mitral stenosis under full anticoagulant treatment. However, most surgeons claim that full anticoagulation causes bleeding during and after operation. According to Nilsson (1974) patients under full dicoumarol therapy should not be operated upon; the prothrombin-proconvertin level examined by the P&P test should be allowed to rise above the therapeutic level (10 to 15%) to 30% . Postoperatively the prothrombin-proconvertin level should not be allowed to fall below 20% if bleeding is to be avoided.

As regards ocular surgery, in the absence of specific reports hereon, the cautious approach seems preferable. Thus before operation the dosage of anticoagulant should be modified to adjust the P&P levels to values over 30% .

An illustrative example of an operation on the eyeball follows. The patient, an 80-year-old man was to be operated upon for cataract extraction combined with trabeculectomy, but he had been receiving anticoagulant treatment with dicoumarol since 1969 because of deep venous thrombosis of the lower limbs, which relapsed as soon as the therapy was withdrawn. Before operation dicoumarol was withdrawn and the P&P level gradually rose from therapeutic levels to about 50% . However, the day before operation the patient manifested deep venous thrombosis of the left leg. The operation was postponed and anticoagulant treatment was resumed, first with heparin and then with small doses of dicoumarol. Two weeks later the patient was operated upon for cataract extraction combined with trabeculectomy according to Cairns.

The P&P level on the day of operation was 40% and no undue bleeding occurred. Dicoumarol was continued and its dose was increased to reach therapeutic levels 10 days after operation.

The postoperative course was uneventful. Six months later the patient was readmitted to hospital for the same operation on the other eye. This time dicoumarol was not withdrawn, but the dose was decreased and the patient was operated upon when the P&P level was around 30% . After the operation dicoumarol was increased and P&P reached a therapeutic level as soon as one week after operation. No bleeding complications were seen.

COMMENTS. HAEMOSTATIC AGENTS

The frequency of disorders of haemostasis and the serious consequences of haemorrhages in cataract surgery make it desirable that the eye surgeon has some basic knowledge on the mechanisms of haemostasis and their pathology. Only a precise diagnosis of a haemostatic defect may allow its proper treatment i.e. with specific haemostatics (Table 4). In absence of diagnosis the surgeon is obliged to recur to unspecific haemostatic substances (Table 4) whose effect is uncertain. As regards unspecific haemostatics these substances have the disadvantage of offering a pseudocover against haemorrhagic complications: with an unjustified sense of security the surgeon may neglect to study the haemostasis of the patient and abstain from treatment with specific haemostatics. On the other hand, with recognition of their limits some of these agents may be used according to the personal beliefs and clinical experience of the surgeon, especially since they have no side effects, but then only as a supplement to the specific haemostatic therapy.

Table 4. Tentative classification of the haemostatic agents.

I Haemostatics in eccessive surgical bleeding from any cause (unspecific, effect not proven), caused by:

a)	Congenital disorders of haemostasis	Substitution therapy (missing coagulation factor, platelet concentrate, fresh plasma)
b)	Acquired disorders	Specific drugs (Vit-K, protamine sulfate, fibrinolytic inhibitors i.e. EACA, AMCA, aprotinin)

II Haemostatic in 'normal' and excessive surgical bleeding from any cause (unspefic, effect not proven)

Oestrogens	Premarin R, Styptanon R
Ethamsilate	Dicynene R
Calcium dobesilate	Doxium R
Snake venoms	Botropase R, Reptilase R
Vitamins	K, 'p'
Miscellaneous	Clauden R, Tachostyptan R, Sango-stop

REFERENCES

Caen J., Cronberg S. & Kubisz P.: Platelets: Physiology and Pathalogy. Stratton, New York, 1977.

Fletcher A. Biedeman O., Moore D., Alkjaersig N., & Sherry S.: Abnormal plasminogen-plasmin system activity (fibrinolysis) in patients with hepatic cirrhosis: its causes and consequences. *J. Clin, Invest* 43: *681-689*, 1964.

Hedner U., Nilsson I. M. & Jacobsen C. D.: Demonstration of low content of fibrinolytic inhibitors in individuals with high fibrinolytic capacity. *Scand J. Clin. Lab. Invest.* 25: *329-336*, 1970.

Lakatos, L., Brenner E. & György T.: Kataraktoperationen bei Hämophilie A *Klin, Mbl. Augenheilk.* 151: *82-86* 1967.

Larsson S. O.: On coagulation and fibrinolysis in renal failure. *Scand. Haemat Suppl.* 15; 1971.

Newell E. W., Aspirin, bleeding and ophthalmic surgery. *Amer J. Ophthal.* 74: *559-560*, 1972.

Niléhn J.E. & Nilsson I.M.: Coagulation studies in different types of myeloma. *Acta Med. Scand Suppl.* 445: *194-199*, 1966.

Nilsson I. M.: Haemorrhagic and Thrombotic Diseases. K. Wiley & Sons. London 1974.

Nilsson I. M.: The problem of coagulopathies. In: Gastrointestinal Emergencies. Bárány F. and Torsoli A (eds) Pergamon Press. Oxford & New York 1976, pp. 129-147.

Oesterlind G. & Nilsson I. M.: Extraction of cataract in a patient with severe haemophilia *A. Acta Ophtal.* 42: *176-181*, 1968.

Petruson B.: Epistexis. A clinical study with special reference to fibrinolysis. *Acta Oto-Laryng Suppl. 317*, 1974.

Poweleit A.: A procedure for cataract extraction in the haemophiliac *Amer J. Ophtal. 59: 315-317,* 1965.

Richards R.D. & Spurling C.L.: Elective ocular surgery in haemophilia. *Arch. Ophtal.* 89: *167-168,* 1973.

Rubenstein R. A., Albert D. M. & Scheie H. G.: *Ocular complication of haemophilia. Arch. Ophthal.* 76: *230-232,* 1966.

Sandax E., Remigy A., Duprez A. & Ducret J.: Hémorrhagies post-operatoires révélatrices d'une maladie de Willebrand. *Bull. Soc. Ophthal. France* 5/6: *332-334,* 1961.

Storm O.: Anticoagulant protection in surgery. *Thrombos Diathes Haemorrh.* 2: *484-491,* 1958.

Strauss L. & Ramsell T. G.: Successful cataract extraction in a severe haemophilia. *Brit. J. Ophtal.* 52: *242-244,* 1968.

Van Lint: Extraction extracapsulaire de la cataracte. In: Traité d'Ophthalmologie (tome VII). Baillart P et al eds, Mason, Paris 1939, p 680.

Vigliano E. M. & Horowitz H. L.: Bleeding syndrome in patients with IgA myeloma: interaction of protein and connective tissue. *Blood* 29: *823-836,* 1967.

Wieberdink J.: Safe pre-operative anticoagulation. *Thorax* 22: *567-571,* 1967.

Author's address:
Univertsity of Lund
Department of Ophthalmology in Malmö
S-214 01 Malmö
Sweden.

Docum. Ophthal. Proc. Series, Vol. 21

GENERAL ANAESTHESIA IN CATARACT SURGERY

M. ARIANO & I. SALVONI

(Florence, Italy)

The use of the general aneasthesia in ophthalmology began very early in 1847. In that year Prett used ether as anesthetic for the extraction of a cataract. In 1850 Jungken used chloroform for the same purpose. Stoeber in 1860 and Welker in 1866 report the use of general anaesthesia by inhalation of ether fumes in eye operations. However, while the popularity of general anaesthesia in various branches of surgery was steadily increasing, in the ocular field an event occurred which seemed to decree its final abandonment: this was the discovery by Köller in 1884 of the corneo-conjuctival analgesic properties of cocaine solutions.

Thus general anaesthesia was almost totally abandoned, also due to the successive contributions brought to the technique of local anaesthesia by Van Lint in 1914 and O'Brien in 1927. This renunciation, with the exception of a few isolated cases (such as Davis who used general anaesthesia for some operations in 1931, Lyle & Fenton in 1934, Berro in 1936, Graves in 1937 and Saval in 1938) was to last until relatively recently. In 1935 the synthesis of the thiobarbiturates and their introduction into anaesthetic technique signalled the end of the oculist's ostracism of general anaesthesia.

In recent years, the use of general anaesthesia in ophthalmosurgery has constantly increased although it is still far from supplanting local and regional anaesthesia. However, the statistics reported by Atkinson in 1955, according to which 93.2% of oculists all over the world were still using local anaesthesia, are no longer up-to-date.

Even ophthalmic surgeons who accept general anaesthesia are not in perfect agreement as to its indications. Some believe that the use of general anaesthetic should be restricted to children under 14 years of age, to excessively fearful patients, to erethistics and to highly irresponsible subjects, while in adults it should be considered indispensable only for certain types of operation. According to others, it should be used indiscriminately in all eye operations.

All this is based on two main reasons: 1. almost all operations can be performed under local or regional aneasthesia due to the facility with which the eye is affected by local anaesthetics. 2. the 'quoad vitam' risk is frowned upon in ocular surgery, where no operation is of life-or-death importance to the patient.

In order to resolve the problem of the choice between local and general anaesthetic, the advantages and disadvantages of each type must be considered.

It should be mentioned incidentally that the supporters of local anaesthetic include surgeons who like to follow established habits and those who have had some bad experience with general anaesthesia (caused perhaps by an inexpert anaesthetist) and who consider it extremely risky. It must be said however that in eye surgery, good local anaesthesia is always better than bad general anaesthesia, and that general anaesthesia is enormously useful to the eye surgeon only when performed correctly.

The following advantages are attributed to **local anaesthesia**: 1. It allows the patient to get up more quickly: but this is confutable, since the patient who has been anaesthetized well can get up the day after the operation. 2. There is lesser incidence of nausea and vomiting, and better control of secretions with almost total absence of coughing: but it must be admitted that nausea and vomiting are present with the same frequency in general and in local anaesthesia and are caused above all by stimulation of vagal fibers, all the more so that general modern anaesthetics are very little emetogenic. Coughing can be prevented by the proper treatment and moreover, though it was highly dangerous when the surgical wound was not sutured at all, it has lost most of its danger now that the incision is sutured. 3. Alterations of 'organismic homoestasis' are abolished: but even this is arguable since emotional stimulus can modify humoural equilibrium even more than a good aneasthetic. 4. There is less danger of complications such as emboli, inhalation pneumonia, etc. (complications which, however, were typical of the epoch of ether and which are today irrelevant). 5. Less postoperative surveillance: actually the patient who has undergone ocular surgery needs constant care whether he has been operated under general or local anaesthetic, as his eyes are bandaged and he must keep his head as still as possible. The only difference lies in the fact that, upon awaking with both eyes bandaged, the patient may be disoriented and may go into a state of psycho-motor agitation, as often happens with elderly arteriosclerotics: on the one hand, this danger has diminished due to the fact that we tend more and more to bandage only the operated eye; on the other hand the danger may be averted by good post-operatory sedation. 6. The patient's collaboration can be obtained during the operation: however, most of the time this is useless as the patient is not able to perform exactly what is asked of him.

Beside these advantages of local anaesthesia, all of which are easily confutable, there exist real disadvantages which are represented by: 1. variations in intraocular tension which easily occur during the operation due to the patient's emotional state which leads him to breath irregularly, causing venous stasis in the cephalic region with repercussions on the choroidal vessels and a general rise in pressure which leads to stress on the vitreous; 2. technical difficulties (such as insufficient anaesthesia of the iris, appearance of retrobulbar hematomas, the rare possibility of traumatizing the optic nerve with the needle, intravasal retrobulbar injection of anaesthetic, etc.).

As regards **general anaesthetic**, its advantages may be summed up on four counts: 1. it is preferred by patients. 2. it lets the surgeon work with greater security, as the patient is unable to perform irresponsible acts. 3. it allows better control of intraocular tension. 4. it can reduce the loss of blood in long operations.

Complications of general anaesthesia may be divided into two categories: those involving the eye and those endangering the patient's life.

1. Complications involving the eye (which, however, can also occur with local anaesthetic): a. hemorrhage in the anterior chamber, b. vitreous loss, c. prolapse of iris, d. so-called expulsive hemorrhage.

2. Complications endangering the patient's life: a. cardiocirculatory collapse. which may be due to:

— anaesthetic factors (hypoxia from overdose of anaesthetic, from obstuction of the respiratory system, from hypoventilation, etc.).
— the presence of congenital malformations, very often found in children with congenital ocular malformations.
— surgical factors, such as the triggering of the oculocardiac reflex, which can be considered responsible for most of the incidents of mortality reported in the literature. This is rare in cataract surgery. It occurs above all in surgery for strabismus and for detached retina, where the ocular muscles are hooked and stretched directly. It can, however, occur even when compression is exerted on the eyeball, for example, in pre-operative massage.

The oculocardiac reflex manifests itself through the following phases: sinusal bradycardia, disturbance of cardiac rhythm and finally cardiac arrest. In 1960 Bellucci declared that 'there are no anaesthetic or medicinal techniques which can be used as absolutely sure preventive measures for protecting the heart during operations on ocular muscels, nor does it seem that regional anaesthesia is free from this danger'; the situation today is practically the same.

Correct procedure is based first of all on prevention by means of vagolytics and by constant checking of heart activity and on collaboration between the surgeon and the anaesthetist so as to suspend stimulations at the first sign of disturbance.

From a review of the negative and positive aspects of the two types of anaesthesia and considering the complications which can arise during ocular surgery, we must admit that general anaesthesia offers many advantages and does not introduce substantial negative effects. Of course it is obvious that, for the inadmissability of anaesthetic risk and for the dramatic consequences of any error in an eye operation, general anaesthesia is valid only when administered perfectly correctly.

Limiting the problem in discussion to cataract surgery alone, the concepts basic to good anaesthesia are four in number: 1. It is important that the level of arterial pressure remains constant, since any variation has repercussions on ocular circulation and may cause stress on the vitreous humour by the choroidal vessels, with pushing forward of the vitreous, extremely dangerous when the eye is open. 2. To facilitate venous drainage, two procedures are helpful: a. keep the patient's head raised higher than the rest of the body on the operating table. The utility of this manoeuvre has been documented recently (1977) by Frova & Musini. b. Ventilate the patient with negative expiratory pressure to reduce the mean intralung pressure, thus favouring the return of venous blood to the right side of the heart. 3. Good ventilation is protection against the highly dangerous occurrence of anoxia and of CO_2 accumulation; this is fundamental in maintaining uniformity of ocular tone. 4. For reduction of intraocular tension, the anaesthetist must choose medicines and techniques which are appropriate not only during anaesthesia, but also in the preparatory and post-operative phases. It should be remembered that a hypotensive effect is made on the eyeball by diuretics acting by osmosis, which, by dehydrating the tissues including the vitreous humour, lower ocular tension by reducing the volume of the vitreous humour itself. Mannitol and glycerol are usually used for this purpose. However, even when preparing the patient for the operation, pharmaceuticals influencing ocular tone should be used. The first step to be taken is that of sedation, as the role played by the emotional factor in increasing tone is well known.

Pre-anaesthesia presents the problem of whether to use atropine. In fact, the parasympatholytic effect of atropine seems to manifest itself in the eye too, determining (though in a much smaller measure, varying according to greater or lesser individual reactivity) those same modifications observed following instillation of this alkaloid into the conjuctival sac. However, the author's observations have led to the conclusion that the administration of intramuscular atropine does not bring about any severe rise in tension (never superior to 5 mm of Hg), not only in normotensive eyes but not even in eyes affected by various forms of glaucoma, as long as the latter are treated with the necessary general and local antiglaucomatous agents. Moreover, as mentioned above, atropinization is an indispensable step in the prevention and attenuation of the oculocardiac reflex.

As regards the effects of the most important anaesthetics on ocular tone, Guillaumat and collaborators (1971) maintain that, by choosing suitable anesthetics and adequate techniques, endobulbar tension can be reduced by 30 or 40%. Therefore it is necessary to discuss individually intravenous and inhalatory anaesthetics and other medicines used in anaesthesia.

Among the **intravenous anaesthetics** we find: 1. the thiobarbiturates, which produce a rapid and striking bulbar hypotonia in the first 15-20 minutes of anaesthesia, slowly returning to the original values afterward. 2. ketamine, which in the opinion of most writers produces ocular hypertonia, as observed also by the author (Ariano and Giovannoni, 1974); however, some writers have reported a slight reduction of tone. 3. Althesin is the most recent intravenous anaesthetic. The author's experience has confirmed what had already been reported by Fordham (1972), Deguerris (1976), and Longhi (1977) attributing to the effect of this anaesthetic a striking and constant lowering in ocular tone, caused, in the opinion of some writers (Longhi and collaborators) by a certain degree of depression of the neurogenous centres of regulation of ocular tone by means of an increased drainage of aqueous humour.

A few other intravenous anaesthetics, such as Viadril and Gamma OH may be omitted from this discussion. Their effects on ocular tone have been reported in the past, but they are by now to be considered obsolete.

We must now examine the **inhalatory anaesthetics**: 1. ether was the first anaesthetic used in eye surgery (Brett, 1847), and it was used for a cataract operation. Ether, however, certainly did not contribute to the spread of general anaesthesia in eye operations owing to the problems it caused in the post-operative period (vomiting, coughing, hiccupping, etc.); in fact, general anaesthetic only began to be used again after the Second World War when ether was supplanted by other more manageable and non-inflammable anaesthetics. Ether's effect on ocular tone is not advantageous for cataract surgery; on the more superficial levels, in fact, there is a rise in tension attributed at least partially to an increase in muscular tone: only in the deepest anaesthetic levels does the ocular tone tend to decrease. This last finding is not confirmed by Rubino & Esente (1947) who have found ocular tone slightly increased with hypnotic doses, and further increased with narcotic doses. 2. Chloroform causes moderate bulbar hypotension (Magora & Collins, 1961) but it is no longer used in general anaesthesia. 3. Cyclopropane has never been used in ocular work because it is inflammable. Its effect on ocular tone has been found to be inconstant (Bellucci and collaborators, 1960), sometimes causing increase, sometimes decrease. 4. Trichlorethylene is rarely used in general anaesthesia because of the disturbance it provokes in cardiac rhythm. Collet (1960) seemed to find in it a clearly hypotensive effect on the eyeball. More recently, however, Alabrak & Samuel (1975) may have found an increase in ocular tone with this anaesthetic. 5. Halothane has been recognized by Bellucci (1962) as the ideal anaesthetic for ocular surgery. Its rapid and pleasant action, its low toxic level, its gentle re-awakening without nervous agitation or vomiting, and its hypotensive effect on the eyeball all go to make this volatile anaesthetic the most widely-used in ophthalmic surgery. 6. Metoxifluorane is a very powerful anaesthetic, whose chief characteristic is that of assuring post-operative analgesia. It is not easily manageable since induction is rather slow and re-awakening time is prolonged. With this anaesthetic too, a considerable reduction in ocular tension can be obtained (Barbieri, 1964). 7. Ethrane is one of the more recent volatile anaesthetics. Its basic characteristics are quick induction and rapid re-awakening. Intraocular pressure is slightly reduced by this anaesthetic as has been demonstrated by Radtke & Waldmen (1975), by Bellucci and collaborators (1973) and by the author himself (1974).

A discussion of anaesthetic pharmaceuticals must include the **myolaxators**:

1. Dextrotubocurarine is unanimously judged to exert a marked bulbar hypotensive effect, largely due to its relaxing effect on the extrinsic muscular system of the eye and to reduction of venous pressure (Bellucci and collaborators 1960).

2. Succinylcoline, as has been well-documented, increases ocular tone, probably by means of fascicular contraction of the extrinsic muscles which precedes depolarization and by the effect of the increase in venous pressure determined by the fascicularization of the entire musculature of the area (Bellucci and collaborators 1960).

3. Decametonium causes an increase in ocular tone by a mechanism similar to that of succinylcoline (Greaves, 1958).

4. Pancuronium is one of the most recent muscle relaxors, very similar to dextrotubocurarine in the mechanism by which it acts and in its effect on ocular tone. It has been studied by Stankovic (1971), who attributes the lowering of intraocular pressure caused by this drug both to an increase in drainage of aqueous from the anterior chamber due to miosis, and to relaxation of the extra-ocular musculature.

For reducing vitreous hydration, various diurectics are used; the most widely employed are osmotic diuretics, mannitol in particular. Mannitol is considered one of the most active osmotic diuretics, practically free from toxicity and unpleasant side effects. Therapeutic doses used go from 1 to 3.50 g/Kg administered in 20% solution, in a length of time that goes from 30 to 120 minutes. The maximum hypotensive effect is reached from 30 to 60 minutes after beginning the perfusion.

The mechanism by which hypertonic mannitol solutions act is osmotic: bulbar hypotonia takes place due to a reduction in volume of the posterior segment, consequent both to the removal of aqueous hymour from the posterior chamber and to the dehydration of the vitreous humour. The percentual reduction of tension is greater in glaucomatous eyes with high initial tensive levels: in these cases the decreases reported vary from 40 to 80% with a prevalence of high percentages; in eyes with normal intraocular tension, the pressure drop percentage is more modest, from 20 to 70% with a prevalence of lower values.

It is obvious that the use of mannitol requires precautionary measures in severe hepatic insufficiency, in cardiac insufficiency and above all in the oligo-anuric syndromes; these, however, are conditions in which intraocular operations are not even to be considered. It may happen instead that patients affected by prostatomegaly are treated with this drug. In these patients, the abundant diuresis caused by mannitol makes necessary the fitting of a vesical catheter. This is a small precaution which can prevent serious disturbances.

Mannitol has shown itself to be highly useful in preparation for operation on eyes with special types of cataract, such as congenital cataracts, cataracts in myopics and those of a complicated type. In rare cases, in young people especially, when notwithstanding all precautions there is a forward thrust of the vitreous, associated with a more or less elevated arterial pressure, the use of 'controlled hypotension' has been suggested. With trimetaphone (Arfonad), which is very active and manageable, a peripheric vasodilation is provoked which, utilizing the anti-Trendelenburg position, permits emptying of the choroidal bed. However, controlled hypotension is extremely dangerous as it causes a reduction of the blood flow in the coronary, cerebral, renal, and hepatic regions.

According to Pintucci and collaborators (1977), a similar but more transitory effect can be provoked by the administration of small supplementary doses of sodium thiopentone during the operation.

This examination of the effects of anaesthetic drugs on ocular tone does not furnish results allowing precise rules to be established. In practice, it can be said that any anaesthetic may be utilized on the condition that it is administered by safe techniques and means. It is a general rule that the choice of anaesthesia must be made on the basis of various parameters, the first of them being the patient's condition.

Pre-operative evaluation of a patient is the synthesis of a thorough analysis of the various organs and systems involved in the operation; therefore a complete study of the condition of the subject who must undergo general anaesthetic is imperative.

The condition of the heart and its functions must be clinically and functionally examined before any operation. An electrocardiogram is absolutely necessary. The surgeon must be able to exclude the possibility of a cardiopathy; if such a cardiopathy should exist, he must be able to distinguish between vitium cordis, myocardic damage and coronary insufficiency: on the practical level it is important to know the state of efficiency of these cardioapthics, i.e., whether or not they are able to lead an active life without limitations.

For evaluating circulatory conditions, an examination of arterial pressure is neccessary, as we have already seen how its variations can influence ocular tone. Special attention must be given to the anaesthesia of hypertensives who have been following a therapy with hypotensives before the operation, as these patients are particularly fragile from the point of view of pressure. Noteworthy is the special attention to be given when hypotensive agents causing blockage of the central adrenergic system (rauwolphia alkaloids) or those blocking autonomous ganglia at the periphery have been used, keeping in mind that these may continue to act for 8-14 days.

Evaluation of the pulmonary function assumes obvious importance in cataract patients who, because of their age, are often affected by asthma, emphysema or bronchitis. In conditions of repose, these pathological situations might remain in a state of compensation; however, under the stress of the operation, respiratory insufficiency is probable.

Proper evaluation of these situations can be made by a series of clinical and laboratory examinations permitting us to classify the gravity of the risk and indicating the means of preventing it, if possible.

Since most anaesthetic agents involve the liver or the kidneys, knowledge of the **hepato-renal function** is particularly important for evaluation of anaesthetic risk. Moreover, knowledge of the glomerular and of the tubular functions would be of great importance in preventing post-operative hydro-electrolytic disturbances; it would be necessary before every operation to study both the hydroelectrolitic balance and the acid-basic state, which depend directly on the patient's metabolic state.

Among the activities of the **endocrine glands**, the greatest attention must be given to the adrenocortical and to the pancreas especially as regards the problem of the underestimated hyperglycemias, with hyperosmosis of the extra-cellular space and intra-cellular dehydration. This affects circulatory conditions and reduces cellular oxidation of glucose, with metabolic acidosis, loss of potassium and of phosphates, electrolytic deficiency and in the end, cardiac insufficiency.

As already noted, the accidental discovery of a diabetic state is not rare in patients requiring cataract surgery, and it is well known that a general anaesthetic and stress in general are important disturbing elements of glucidic homeostasis. Therefore it is imperative to postpone the operation until the hyperglycemia has been adequately controlled.

The **psychological behaviour** of the more elderly patients is a direct consequence of the blood supply of the brain and of the neuronal condition. In the anaesthetic field, great importance must be attributed to the cellular state of wear of the neurons, which leads to a reduction of synaptic and metabolic reactivity, as well as, of course, a diminishing of the cerebral circulation. This situation directly conditions the risk of the post-operative period. In fact, when the patient returns to consciousness with both eyes bandaged he may show a certain lack of orientation requiring special surveillances to avoid irrational action.

In pre-operative evaluation of the patient, it is necessary to analyse very carefully his state of reactivity to his surroundings, his state of alertness and capacity for self-control in order to pre-arrange suitable psycho-pharmacological treatment. This problem has no ideal solution, since the particular type of surgery discussed here involves a predominantly old population with degenerative disturbances against which even the most refined therepeutic means are often ineffective. In practice, in fact, pre-operative evaluation of a cataract patient may conclude with the prescription of suitable pharmacological therapies, but, and perhaps more often than not, it concludes only with an evaluation of risk: it is obvious that this risk must not exceed a certain limit.

CONCLUSIONS

To put into practice the theoretical presuppositions here stated, we must briefly discuss the duties generally assumed by the surgeon with a subject who must be operated for cataract.

Clinical examination is the first and most important approach to the patient. This examination must be as careful and painstaking as possible, since it serves as a guide for requests for laboratory and instrumental examinations, some of which are routine while others are indicated by the objective examination and the patient's case history. From evaluation of all of the data, including the patient's biological age, the surgeon can estimate the degree of operative risk, if necessary proposing the alternative of loco-regional anaesthesia.

As regards pre-operative infusion of 20% mannitol, its use should be limited to cases where it is truly indispensable, where it seems that bulbar hypotonia cannot be obtained by other means. The administration of mannitol, in fact, provokes a circulatory overload due to its calling into circulation of a quantity of liquid equal to four times the volume of that administered. Therefore it must be limited to those patients who have the power of establishing cardio-circulatory and renal compensation following the increase of the blood volume. In all other cases, one hour before the operation, always on condition that there are no contraindications of the metabolic order or having to do with acid-basic equilibrium, we utilize carbon diozide inhibitors as well as acting directly on the ocular tone with suitable anaesthesia techniques.

The basic limit which, in our experience, must be put to the use of general anaesthesia in cataract surgery is represented by the presence of serious disturbance of the respiratory system. In these cases, in fact, the success of the operation could be severely compromised by dyspnea, lung congestion, coughing, etc.

In conclusion, it should be emphasized once again that there is no single technique for anaesthesia in cataract surgery. Each anaesthetist must adopt, case by case, the technique in which he has the greatest experience and with which he has had the best results.

Author's address:
c/o Prof. Esente
Corso Italia
2 Firenze
Italy

NEUROLEPTANALGESIA IN OPHTHALMIC SURGERY

R. WITMER

(Zurich, Switzerland)

Neuroleptanalgesia has been introduced as a special form of general surgical anesthesia in 1959 by De Castro and Mundeleer. It consists essentially in a combination of a rapid but long acting sedative tranquilizer with potent antiemetic properties (Droperidol) with a short lasting narcotic analgesic (Fentanyl). Its analgetic effect is about 100 times that of morphine.

The combination of the two drugs is known in the U.S. as Innovan, in Europe as Thalamonal. Intramuscular administration of 1-2 ml of Thalamonal leads to a state of calmness without anxiousness or drowsiness after about 4 to 20 minutes. There is little reaction to pain, the patient remains quiet but is able to cooperate on command.

If general anesthesia is then performed, the patient will be given another dose of Droperidol (15-20 mg) and Fentanyl (0.3-0.7 mg) intravenously. He will then breathe nitrous oxide and oxygen in a relation of 75% to 25%, an intravenous injection of Succinylcholin (50 mg) is made and intubation is performed.

Later the patient remains under nitrous oxyde and oxygen, and pulse and blood pressure are being constantly watched.

As soon as pulse and blood pressure rise, another dose of Fentanyl 0.05-0.2 mg is given intravenously.

The main indication for general neuroleptanalgesia are elderly patients with cardiac disorders. Since Droperidol is a long acting drug, the duration of the surgical intervention should be at least 40-60 minutes. Most surgical interventions can be performed under neuroleptanalgesia, but for reasons to be mentioned later, it is not used in children.

Absolute contraindications for general neuroleptanalgesia are: ambulatory patients, interventions of less than 30 minutes, obstetrical operations because of the respiratory depressive action of the Fentanyl passing through the placenta, patients with asthma bronchiale and hypertensive patients. In children Fentanyl can cause bradycardia and hence a dangerous drop of blood pressure.

The main advantages of neuroleptanalgesia are: the very little toxicity of the drugs used, the protection of the neurovegetative system, and the fast postoperative recovery.

The disadvantages, however, have to be mentioned as well. They are due to the drop in systolic blood pressure about 30 minutes after the administration of Droperidol. Transient bradycardia may also occur as well as a marked shallowness of respiration, probably due to the action of Fentanyl. These side effects can be overcome easily if the patient is intubated and respiration artificially controlled.

Since the effect of the combination of Droperidol with Fentanyl leads to a state of calmness, analgesia and still good cooperation, this kind of treatment has been used by different authors (Wine, 1966, Tait & Tornetta, 1966, Klaus & Franicevic, 1966) as a premedication for ophthalmic surgery, combined with normal local anesthesia, but without intubation of the patient.

They claim to have rather good results, although Wine says that this kind of incomplete neuroleptanalgesia is not the final answer for sedation in cataract surgery. This is mostly due to the above mentioned side effects of bradycardia, drop of blood pressure, shallowness of respiration, which eventually call for the administration of an antidote (Nalorphin or Lorfan Ho-La Roche). In any case, our anesthetist does not recommend this kind of neuroleptanalgesic premedication without the presence of an anesthetist during the entire surgical procedure. He further thinks, that it should only be used by an experienced anesthetist and certainly not a young resident, which is often the case in teaching hospitals.

For these reasons we do not have any personal experience with this variation of neuroleptanalgesia in cataract surgery.

We do, however, often use neuroleptanalgesia with intubation and controlled respiration with nitrous oxide and oxygen in longer lasting operations (retinal detachment) and find it very convenient in old patients with cardiac disorders. But a normal cataract operation lasts not more than 40 minutes and does therefore not need the complete neuroleptanalgesia.

REFERENCES

De Castro, J. & Mundeleer, P.: Anesthésie sans barbituriques: La neuroleptanalgésie. *Anesth. et Analg.* 16, 1022 (1959).
Klaus, P. & N.F. Franicevic: Die Anwendung der Neuroleptanalgesie in der Ophthalmochirurgie. *Klin. Mbl. Augenhk.* 148, 707 (1966).
Tait, E.C. & Tornetta, F.J.: Neuroleptanalgesia as adjunct to local anesthesia in intraocular surgery. A preliminary report. *Amer. J. Ophth.* 59, 412 (1965).
Wine, N.A.: Sedation with neuroleptanalgesia in cataract surgery. *Amer. J. Ophth.* 61, 456 (1966).

Author's address:
Rämisstrasse 100
8091 Zurich
Switzerland

LOCAL ANAESTHESIA IN CATARACT SURGERY

R. WITMER

(Zurich, Switzerland)

Due to the progress in anesthesiology and the introduction of neuroleptanalgesia there are today almost no contraindications to general anesthesia.

Despite this fact local anesthesia keeps its indications in ophthalmic surgery. Different factors are important:

1. Physics and psyche of the patient
2. Type of surgical intervention
3. Technique of local anesthesia
4. Premedication
5. The relationship between the patient and the surgeon
6. Economic aspects
7. Complications

1. PHYSICAL AND PSYCHOLOGICAL STATUS OF THE PATIENT

General anesthesia may represent a high risk for patients with cardiovascular disturbances, angina pectoris, advanced arteriosclerosis and hypertension, or patients with liver diseases. If in such a case the ophthalmic surgeon insists on having a general anesthesia, he has to take full responsibility for any complication, which may occur. Most of us will choose local anesthesia in such circumstances.

Let me give you a few examples. Among 243 patients with retinal detachment or vitreous hemorrhages hospitalized for surgery 17 were operated under local anesthesia:

− in 2 patients intubation was impossible due to anatomical reasons,
− in 4 patients the duration of the operation was less than 30 minutes,
− in 11 patients the internist did not allow general anesthesia because of cardiovascular distrubances.

All 17 patients were operated without the slightest complication in local anesthesia.

The psychological attitude of the patient is very important. Some patients prefer general anesthesia because they are afraid of the operation. But the reverse may also happen, the patient may be afraid of general anesthesia, because he remembers the aftereffect of his latest general anesthesia.

Some patients may be very uncooperative, for instance small children or inmates,; they need general anesthesia even for minor surgery.

69

2. TYPE OF SURGICAL INTERVENTION

We prefer local anesthesia for
- cataract and
- glaucoma operation,
- lamellar and perforating keratoplasty,
- squint surgery in adults,
- minor lid and
- retinal surgery of short duration.

But in fact all eye surgery can be done under local anesthesia if necessary, even encircling procedures in retinal detachments or combined vitrectomies in diabetics (extraction of the lens and vitrectomy), enucleation or dacryocystorhinostomy.

3. TECHNIQUE OF LOCAL ANESTHESIA

It is simple and can be achieved in different ways.

We prefer the method of Van Lint for akinesia of the lids. It may produce a lid hematoma, which as a rule is no contraindication to surgery. Retrobulbar anesthesia is made through the lower lid deep into the muscle cone, using a 4.5 cm long needle. If correctly placed, this injection leads to very good akinesia of the globe, and to a lowering of intraocular pressure. It also blocks the oculocardiac reflex. For cataract, glaucoma and keratoplasty 2 cc of Lidocain with Adrenalin and Permease are sufficient, for squint and retinal surgery we inject 5 cc. An additional subconjunctival injection of not more than 1 cc is then made at the upper limbus. Retrobulbar hematoma occurs very infrequently. If severe, surgery has to be postponed.

In high myopes this retrobulbar injection has to be done with the utmost care to avoid perforation of a posterior staphyloma.

4. PREMEDICATION

As mentioned in my previous presentation, some people use a combination of Droperidol and Fentanyl as so-called neuroleptanalgesia. It is, however, dangerous because of the drop in systolic blood pressure and bradycardia. We therefore still prefer in younger patients a combination of Scopolamin, Dilaudid and Ephetonin (Scophedal). In elderly patients from 70-80 years we take a combination of phenergan and prazine, and in very old patients above 80 years Rohypnol.

I think that this is a field where personal experience of the surgeon is of greatest importance. Many different combinations are possible, and I am convinced, that within this audience no two surgeons use exactly the same drugs. I do not dare to say therefore, that our method is the best. But we are very statisfied with it.

5. THE RELATIONSHIP BETWEEN THE PATIENT AND THE SURGEON

The relationship between the patient and the surgeon is of utmost importance in local anesthesia. The patient must have confidence in his surgeon and the surgeon must be sure of himself. If one of the two is full of fear, then general anesthesia is preferable. The surgeon can then operate practically without the presence of the patient and mutual psychological difficulties are less likely to occur.

6. ECONOMICS

In our country economic criticism of the entire health system is very popular today. There is no doubt, that local anesthesia is much cheaper: we need less personnel, less drugs, less time.

7. COMPLICATIONS

There is no doubt either that complications are less frequent with local anesthesia. Cardiac arrest due to the oculocardiac reflex and hyperthermia do not occur. The only complication may be a hematoma, usualy without any further consequences.

REFERENCES

Van Lint: Paralysie palpébrale provoquée dans l'opération de la cataracte. *Ann. d'ocul.* 151, 420-424 (1914).
Witmer, R.: Lokalanaesthesie in der Ophthalmochirurgie. *Klin. Mbl. Augenhk.* 170, 329 (1977).

Author's address:
Rämisstrasse 100
8091 Zürich
Switzerland

Docum. Ophthal. Proc. Series, Vol. 21

STERILIZATION

F. HERVOUET

(Nantes, France)

It is now nearly two years since we, together with some American authors (R.K. Forster, for example) deplored the new outbreak of infections following opening of the eyeball, especially after cataract operation. This was a new fact in ophthalmology, which has led, after close investigation conducted with the aid of bateriologists, to the following conclusions:

— A dangerous operatory smear, i.e., one containing granulocytes and infracellular pyogenes can be responsible for an infection, but in reality it seems that this rarely occurs.

— Nine times out of ten, in fact, infection occurs because the patient has been operated in a polluted environment; in normal circumstances, this pollutions of the operating room is inevitable or almost so, when the operation is important and prolonged.

— Therefore, the author now operates in a sterile environment, which has had the radical effect of abolishing all infections.

1. THE MODERN OPERATING ROOM

Let us first of all examine all that which concerns the operating room in an endeavour to analyze the reasons why its pollution now begins more rapidly, much more rapidly, than in the past. The reason lies in the fact that modern operating rooms are equipped with material which is without doubt indispensable, but which is large in amount, larger and larger: we have seen the successive appearance of anaesthesists, cryotherapy, the microscope, the vitreotom, etc., etc., in addition to all the other things already present; moreover, the para-medical assistants required are more and more numerous.

Of course after every operation the room and the equipment are washed, sterilized with formol vapors and with the latest product seemed to be most efficacious; after disinfection, at least in some hospitals, a germicide is placed in the operating room, the emanations of which help to keep the operating area sterile. However, despite all aseptic precautions taken, the arrival of the surgical team quickly leads to pollution of the atmosphere; and the stirring of the air caused by movements in the room contributes to the development of a dangerous environment: Peremptory proof of this is that constant bacteriological testing of the air in the room (any surgeon may make the experiment) shows that the air becomes polluted (development of microbic colonies on Petri dishes) more and more as the morning goes on.

But this is not all. We have wondered if the **place itself** where the operating room is found, be it hospital or private clinic, does not play a role in the more or less rapid pollution of this atmosphere. It seemed probable, in fact, that a surgical complex located not far from contamination coming from the street, from traffic which is always more intense, would be more liable to engender inflammatory complications than one isolated on the outskirts of the city, or in any case far from heavy traffic.

2. THE STERILE OPHTHALMOLOGICAL COMPLEX

Neurosurgeons among others, plastic surgeons, orthopedic surgeons especially, have made observations identical to the foregoing, with the last years in England (at Wrightinston), a team of bone surgeons has had the idea of closing themselves within a sterile enclosure, kept sterile during the whole course of the operation, however long it may last.

The pinciple of this enclosure is to keep the patient and the surgeon and assistants closed within a compartment made of detachable plates of glass. Air conditioning feeds this transparent, almost hermetically closed room where is no recirculation of air, as fresh air is constantly thrown back. The surgeons wear loose gowns in a special material which hinders the transmission of particles carrying bacteria, constantly emanating from their bodies, from spreading in the atmosphere; a system of air cooling under the gown has been designed for maintenance of the most comfortable temperature, thus avoiding perspirations and fatigue; the masks are equipped with a system for removal of expired air by aspiration, which is achieved by means of a narrow flexible plastic tube connected to the exterior. The anesthetist remains outside of the 'ultra-sterile' complex. The surgical instruments are arranged on trays closed within cloth sacks; they are introduced as needed through the service door of the complex, without entering into contact with the air outside the enclosure where nurses, anaesthetists and spectators are present.

Upon first learning of the existence of this enclosure, we decided to put an end to our troubles by installing it in the Clinique Sourdille. This has been done, with a few modifications of the original model (Charnley Howorth): for ophthalmology, where the operating field is very small and where the risks of operative infection are less, it has been decided, after trials made by the constructors, (1) that the glass cage is not indispensable (which simplifies things remarkably), nor are the 'diving-suit gowns'.

The photograph shows the characteristics of the 'ophthalmological' enclosure. A square with sides measuring 3.50 m., it is attached to the ceiling. The conditioned air (adjustable temperature) is sucked in directly by the device which returns this air, completely sterilized; this 'falls' on everything within the enclosure, thus assuring safety.

Numerous bacteriological tests of the surrounding air have been made:

1. S.F.F.C. Midy, Division équipment, 62-64, Bd Arago, 75013 Paris.

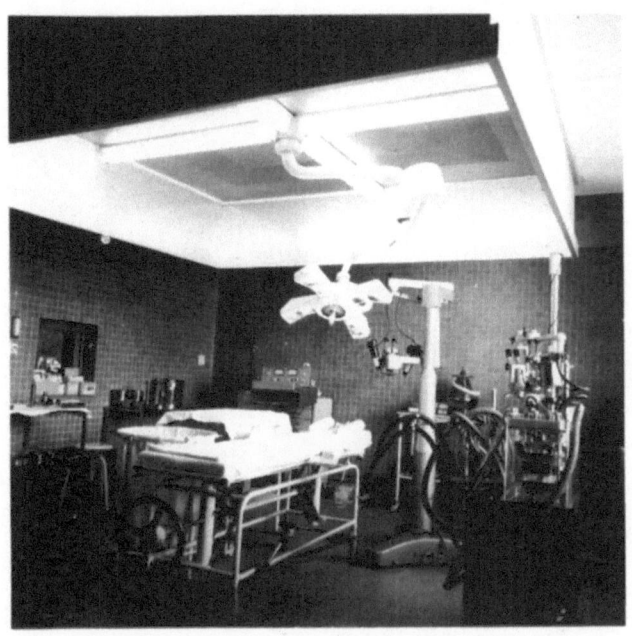

nothing enters, ever, even into the corridor (1 to 2 m.) outside of the cubicle and this is true no matter how long the operation lasts.

Not a single post-operative infection or initial infection has occurred for almost two years (for six years previously there were two cases per year on the average).

Further information regarding this sterile cubicle:

— Price: at present it costs about 40,000 dollars (work of transforming the operating room, equipment, lamps, air conditioners).

— Noise: the same noise, slightly amplified, as a standard air conditioner. This noise, however, as it is continuous, is not disturbing; it may even be considered desirable, as it isolates the cubicle from the outside world, cutting out the unusual noised inherent to every operating room.

Despite the obvious advantages outlined above, such a cubicle is not advisable, because of its high cost, for the surgeon who does not have a heavy operating schedule. One or two hours in the operating room, especially when the surgical team is limited to two or three persons, does not seem to present a risk for the patient. However, any hospital service of a certain importance should have a steriel enclosure: in the very special 'modern' circumstances in which we operate, it can be predicted that soon we cannot, we will not have the right to do without it.

Author's address:
16, Boulevard Gabriel-Guist 'Hau
44000 Nantes
France

Docum. Ophthal. Proc. Series, Vol. 21

INSTRUMENTS

A. VANNINI, G.M. GASTALDI, M. FAGIANO

(Torino, Italy)

Our paper is meant to be a concise review of the present state of surgical instruments overlooking those topics for which individual and detailed treatment is specifically provided.

Over the past decade we have witnessed a progressive and constant development of the instruments used in cataract surgery. It is superfluous to recall how such development has been imposed and guided by the progressive and invariable use of the operating microscope which has acquired an extremely prominent role, even if it was only used by some forerunners up to a few years ago.

The percentage of those who routinely use the microscope in cataract surgery, be it for the whole operation, for some of its phases, or, at least, in some particular cases, is very high.

The answers to a questionnaire we formulated and proposed to more than three hundred ophthalmologists show that only 28% of the respondents never use the microscope, as opposed to 55% who use it routinely, 8% who use it systematically, but only for certain phases of the operation, and 9% who use it only in particular cases.

In general, the advantage (Table 1) deriving from the use of the microscope that has been pointed out is a less traumatic surgery, thanks to the better accuracy the microscope allows for. In particular, greater precision in the making of the cut out and of the sutures, and the possible reduction and quantification of post-operative astigmatism.

The only two drawbacks that have been pointed out are a reduction of the usable field of observation and a lengthening of the operating time.

According to a majority of the respondents, the microscope is to be exclusively used in the case of congenital, complex, and secondary cataracts.

We shall start discussing the instruments by briefly describing an ideal microscope, which, also according to the opinions generally expressed by our Colleagues, must feature:
— a stable suspension system, preferably attached to the ceiling;
— a cold light coaxial lighting system, integrated by lateral lighting (including the slit), both with light intensity controllable by the operator;

ADVANTAGES INDICATED IN THE USE OF THE
MICROSCOPE IN CATARACT SURGERY

— Less traumatic surgery
— More reliable
— More accurate
— Better control of unusual situations
— Better apposition of surgical wound edges
— Less residual astigmatism
— Better cutting precision
— Non-perforating sutures

MAIN DEFECTS

— Lenthening of operating times
· Reduction of field of vision

ABSOLUTE INDICATIONS

— Complicated cataracts
— Secondary cataracts
— Congenital cataracts

— one or, better, two optical shunts for the surgeon's aides and for the recording systems;
— focussing, lateral and tilting movements, and magnifying lens zooming must be under the operator's direct control;
— possibility of sterilizins the microscope's whole body.

Some manufacturers are now approaching this ideal microscope, after going through a various phase evolution (Fig.1).

Even so there is a number of ophthalmologists who satisfactorily use magnifying glasses or loupes (Fig. 2).

The use of a microscope entails such variations in focus depths and in usable field of observation as to make necessary certain parallel variations in all surgical instruments.

The criteria for the making of surgical instruments have thus had to conform to the spread of microsurgery. In fact, modern microsurgical techniques require the use of smaller and smaller instruments, with thiver and thiver ends and different angles. The relationship established between the instrument and the pathway of the rays produced by the optical system used to visualise the operation is of fundamental importance. The operator's hand must not interfere with the instrument vision, as to allow for a constant visual control of the instrument operating tip (Fig. 3).

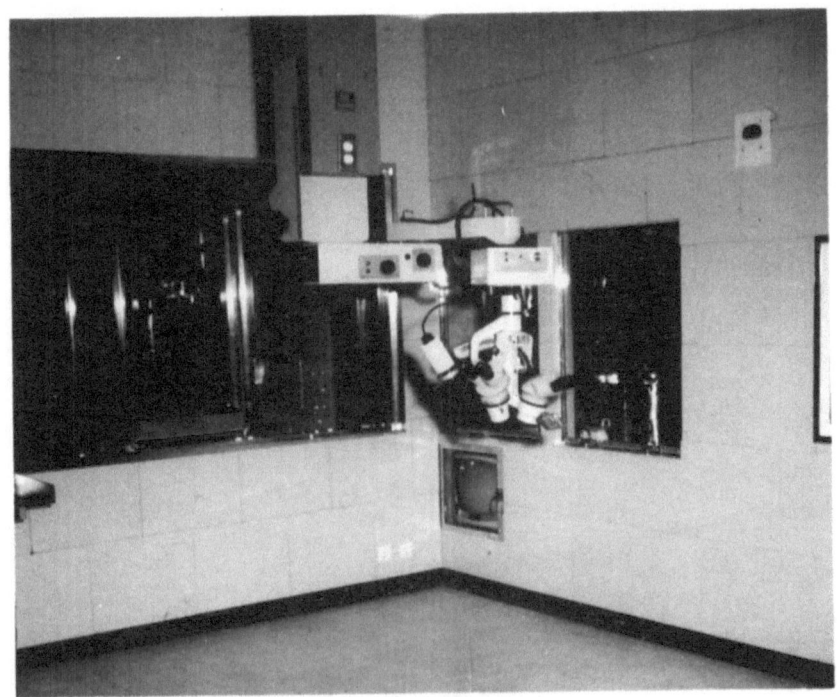

Fig. 1. Modern microscope for ophthalmic microsurgery

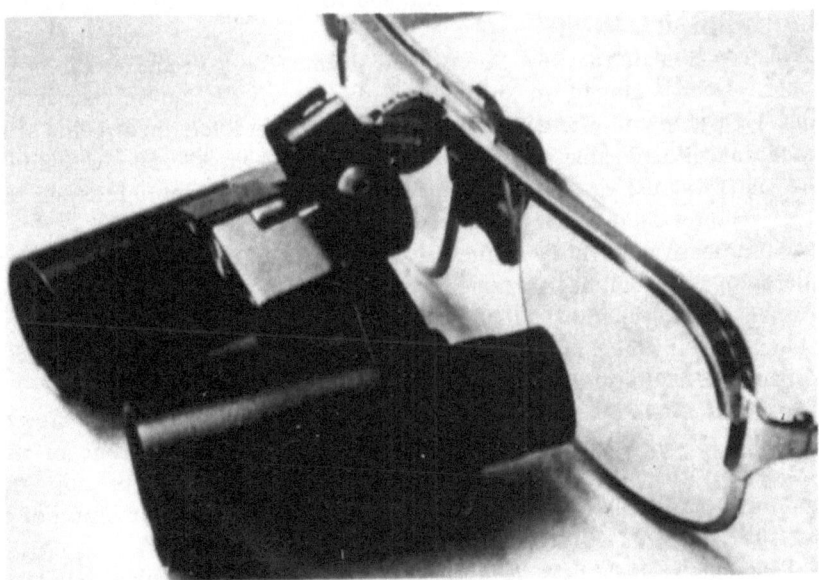

Fig. 2. Magnifying glasses (Jaeger)

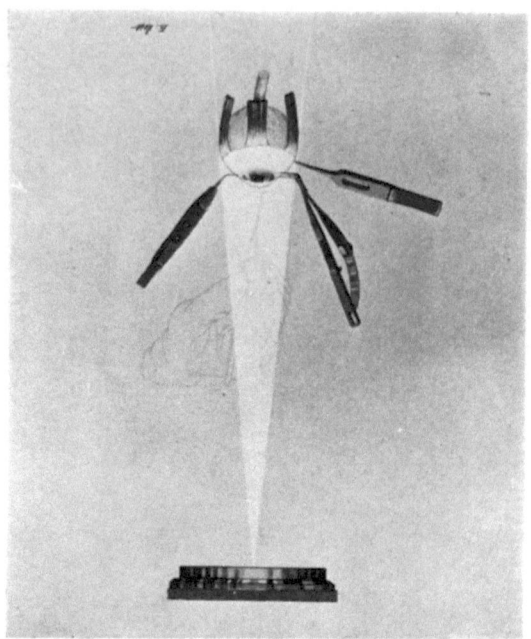

Fig. 3. See text for explanation

It is necessary for the forceps to grip in a non-traumatic way; for the cutter not to deform the structures; and for the needle-holder to be light, but sturdy and safe.

The creation of the new line of instruments (Fig. 4) requires the use of special steels, alloyed in different percentages with chromium, carbon, nickel, sulphur, tungsten, in order to have the characteristic of being at the same time inoxidizable, tempered, flexible, hard. One also has to underline the increasing use of titanium, which, being lighter and more resistent than steel, represents the metal of tomorrow's instruments.

Anti-reflectiveness is fundamental when one works with a coaxial light microscope. Titanium instruments' characteristic of absolute anti-reflectiveness is even superior to that of dull finished steel (Fig. 5).

Let us now examine in a more analytical fashion some of the micro-surgical instruments at our disposal.

As far as numerous and different available incision instruments are concerned, the characteristics one has to keep in mind at the time of their choice are: the quality and the durability of the edge; the pressure they require to make the cut; the visibility they permit; and the precision of the cut.

  — Diamond scalpels have in absolute terms the sharpest edge, but at the detriment of their thinness; they require minimum pressure for cutting,

80

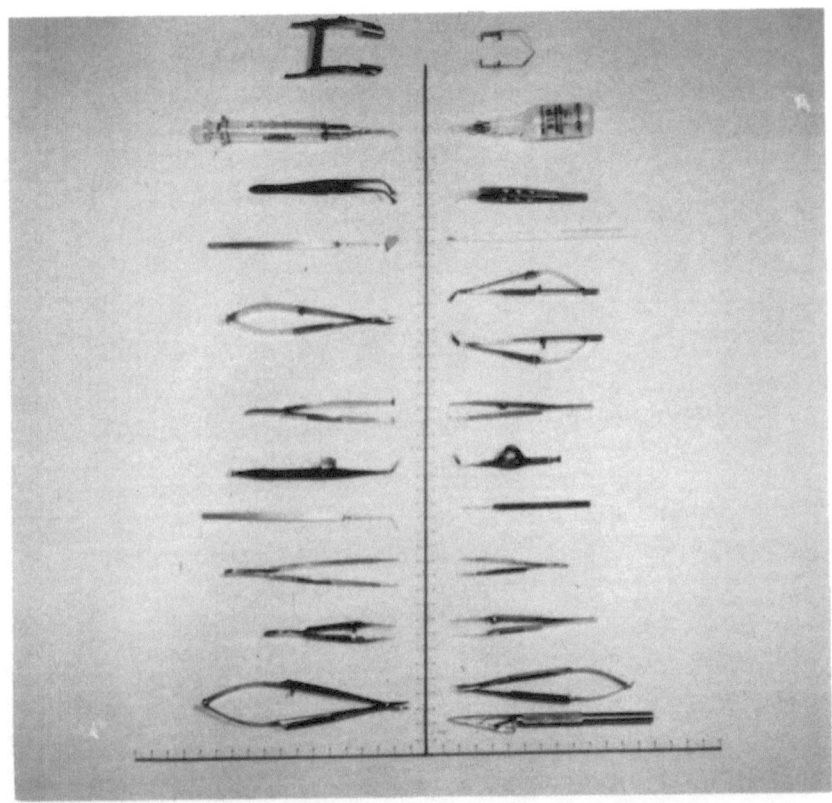

Fig. 4. Old (left) and actual (right) set of instruments for cataract surgery

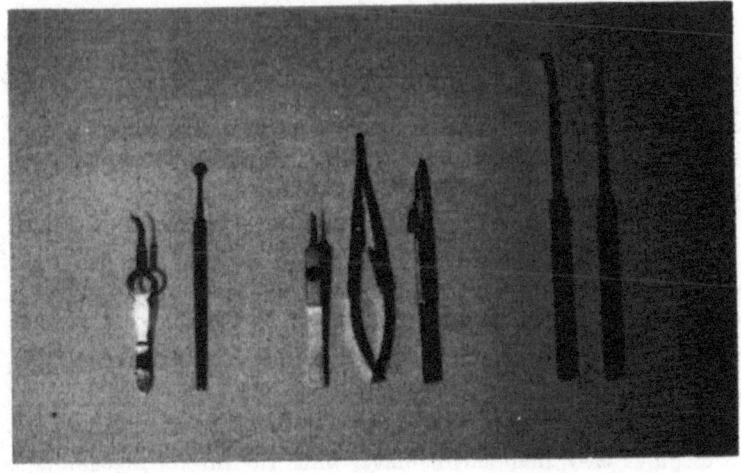

Fig. 5. From left to right: shine steel, dull finished steel and titatium instruments

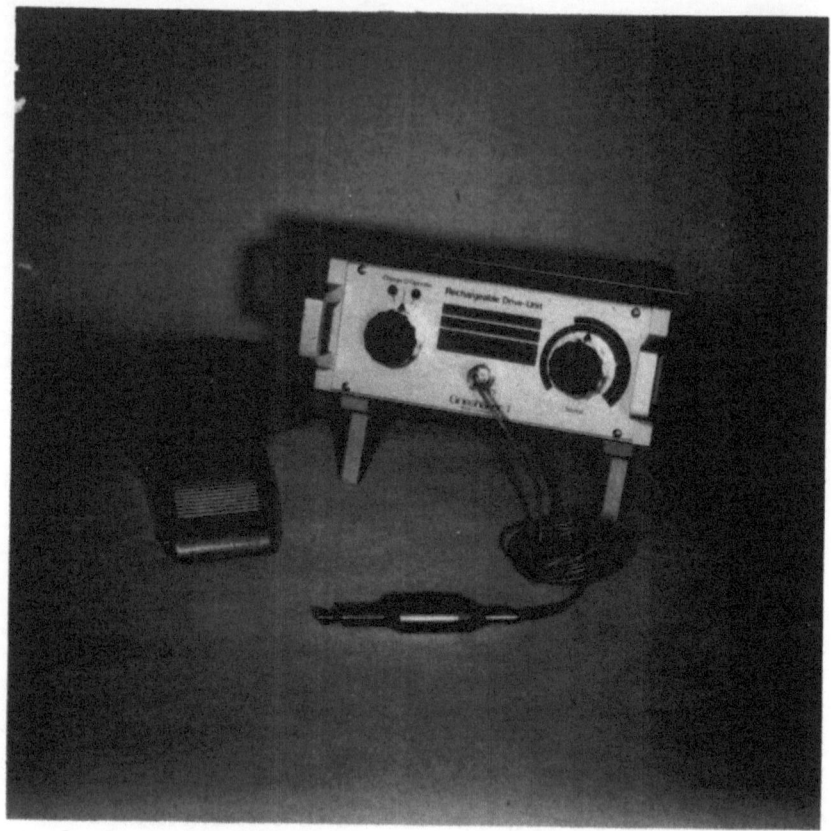

Fig. 6. Melbourne oscillotome

but are expensive and delicate. An interesting application of the diamond tip is done in Pintucci's compass keratotome.
– Some types of disposable blades (Beaver, Medical Workshop) are, in terms of easiness in cutting, only slightly inferior to diamond ones, without having any of the latters' defects. These blades no doubt appear to be much superior in quality than the traditional fragments of Gillette blades.
– A recent innovation in the use of various cutting instruments is linked to the introduction of the Melbourne oscillotome, by Grieshaber (Fig. 6).

This instrument, owing to an electric mechanism which by giving adjustable frequency scillations, allows for a very good control of the incision planes, and a shortening of operating times, while requiring a minimal pressure. The instrument displays easy manoeuverability, while the interchangeability of the blades allows the individual operator to personalize the instrument according to his needs.

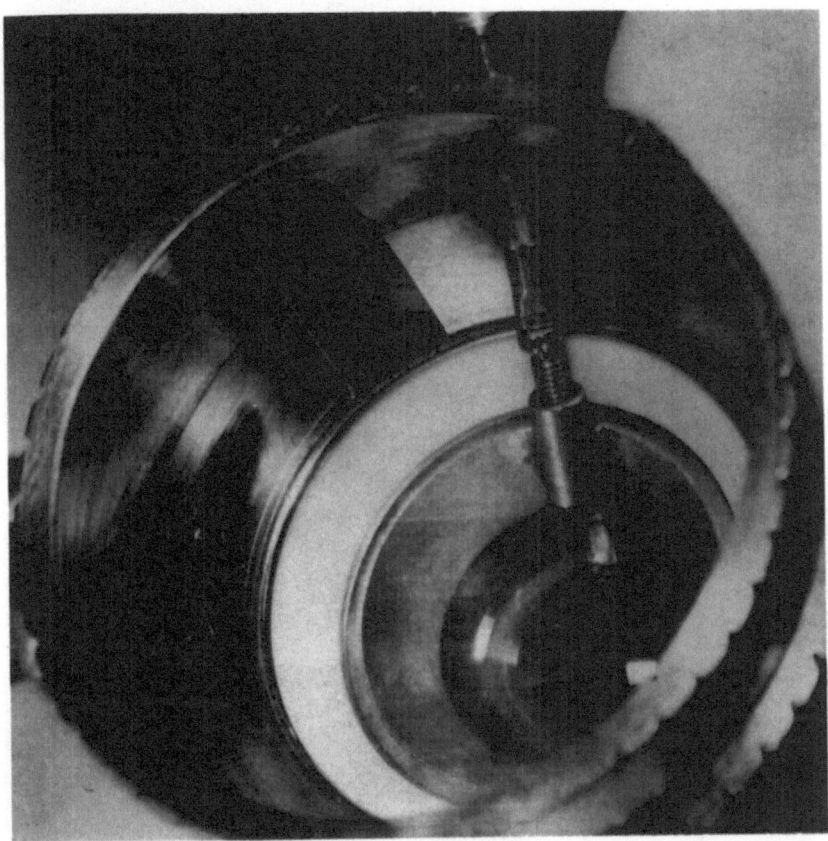

Fig. 7. Contact corneal cutter

A new corneal cutter coupled with a contact lens, which permits one to make an incision in a progressive and circular way, has also been designed at the Univertity of Melbourne, Ophthalmology Department. This instrument, conceived for use in keratoplasty, is also usable in cataract surgery (Fig. 7).

It is not appropriate to enter in detail the discussion of needle-holders, forceps, scissors, on whose constructional generalities, at any rate, we have already reported and of which we have shown some slides. in fact the choice of those instruments is ultimately up to the individual operator's personal experience. On the other hand, a different approach would force us to substitute for catalogues.

The following have at least to be mentioned:

— the Hoskin line forceps, which in our experience have proven to be among the least traumatic;

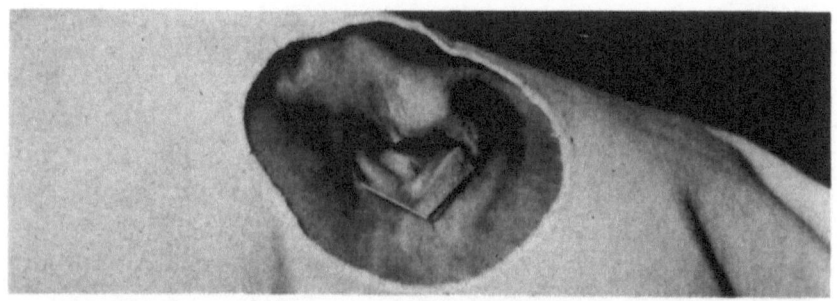

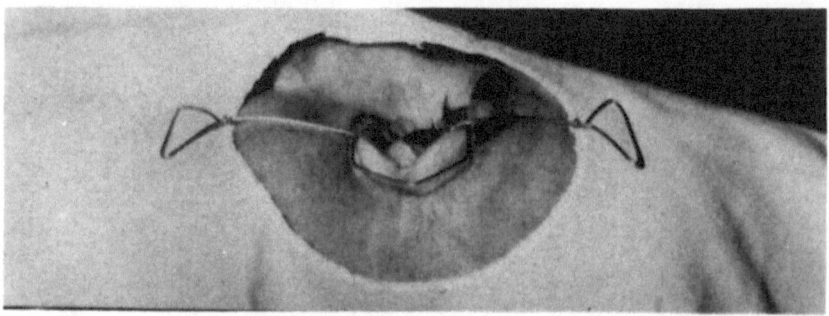

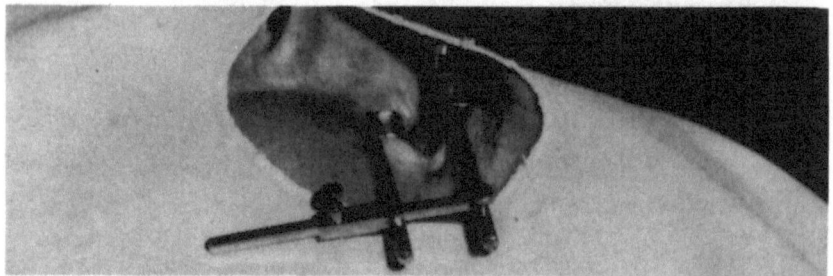

Fig. 8. See text for explanation

— the Bonn forceps, regularly mentioned by the respondents to our questionnaire;
— the thread tightening forceps and the forceps used for embedding single
filament sutures' knots.

As far as blepharostats are concerned, we point out a change made by
Dr. De Angelis to Barraquer's 'colibri' blepharostat. This extremely simple
change gives the instrument the characteristics of bone supported blepharostats, which lift the eye-lids while avoiding any ocular pressure increase. (Fig. 8)

Cataract extraction is by now carried out by most operators by means of
a cryogenic apparatus. The constructional principles by which cryo-extrac-

tors are presently inspired, are basically four. In fact the following stand out:
— cryo-probes containing the refrigerating element and working by an immersion of the element itself;
— cryo-probes cooled by a substance's phase change;
— cryo-probes exploiting the Peltier effect;
— cryo-probes based on the Joule-Thompson effect.

All modern apparatus presently employed in cataracts surgery utilize the Joule-Thompson effect. Owing to such an effect, a suitable gas, by expanding, cools the point to the desired temperature. Such a gas can be either carbon dioxide or nitrogen protoxide.

We shall limit ourselves to the consideration of a cryo-extractor's ideal characteristics, which, in short are:

1— The cryode must be applicable at room temperature, that is to say not previously cooled.

2— The cooling of the cryode must be instantaneous.

3— The thermal isolation of the cryode must be such as to reduce the danger of adhesions of the adjecent tissues.

4— The cryode must be designed in such a way as to be manageable and light.

5— Operational safety is another essential factor; not only must a cryode work in an predictable way but also in a safe one.

6— Cryode defrosting must take place at the operator's will very readly.

7— One must be able to sterilize the cryode easily and rapidly.

As far as expendable supplies are concerned, they depend on individual preferences even more than surgical instruments.

The following are worth mentioning: small self-adhesive sterile sheets, which fix the operating area in a stable way; various kinds of absorbent cellulose tampons: disposable containers for detergent liquids as opposed to the more common silicon tanks; filters for liquids to be introduced into the anterior chamber.

Author's address:
Via Juvarra 19
10122 Torino
Italy

MICROSURGERY NOW AND IN THE FUTURE

R.C. TROUTMAN

(New York, U.S.A.)

At a recent multidisciplinary International Microsurgery Symposium held in New York and sponsored by Ethicon, it was evident that microsurgery today is being employed in almost every surgical specialty. In addition to our sister specialty, otolaryngology, the specialties of plastic surgery, urologic surgery, neurosurgery, peripheral vascular surgery, gynecologic surgery, cardiac surgery, orthopedic surgery, and even general surgery were represented there.

The enthusiasm and frustrations of the pioneering surgeons representing the various specialties recalled my early attempts to introduce microsurgery to ophthalmologists. As was I two decades ago, several of these surgeons are among a small minority of their specialty now advocating the use of microsurgical instrumentation and techniques. In the more highly developed microsurgical specialties, such as ophthalmology and otolaryngology, most new techniques presented were at least partially, if not wholly, dependent upon microsurgery for their development and proper execution. Much of the hazard and morbidity of preexisting techniques had been reduced to more acceptable levels through the use of microscopic techniques. This trend was particularly striking in neurosurgery wherein Mallis reported that the mortality from surgery of aneurisms of the circle of Willis had been reduced by 80%. The gynecology representative reported reversal of female sterilization by recanalizing severed or tied fallopian tubes in 80% of cases. This feat was equalled by the urology surgeon who recanalized the vas deferens in males. Since the irreversibility of these sterilization procedures has been a major impediment to primary acceptance of sterilization, these accomplishments have tremendous import in the overall implementation of world population control.

The plastic, peripheral nerve, and vascular surgeons demonstrated their ability to replace and to restore function to severed digits and even to an entire limb.

The instruments presented were ingenious and may have some application to our own field. The surgical microscopes, compared to ours, seemed somewhat unsophisticated, lacking essentials such as motorized zoom magnification and focusing. Semiautomatic servo controls now beginning to appear on some ophthalmic microscopes have not even been considered.

As we had experienced in ophthalmology, microsurgical instrumentation in the other surgical specialties showed an evolutionary development with the refining and miniaturization of the working tips of standard instruments, along with the redesigning of the handles to prevent the obstruction of the limited field of view at higher magnifications. In contradistinction to ophthalmology, few specialties had yet adopted motorized instruments or made use of automated or computerized control units. Most instrumentation was manually actuated or controlled and dependent on the surgeon's tactile and visual senses.

At the conclusion of the meeting, each specialty representative speculated on the future of microsurgery within his or her specialty. It was concluded that as microsurgery had expanded to include almost every surgical specialty, in the future it would be practiced in all fields with increasing frequency by increasing numbers of surgical specialists.

In the last two decades, ophthalmic microsurgery, at first advocated by only a few of us, has become the standard of ophthalmic surgical practice. It seems hardly possible that when Harms, Mackensen, and I formed the Microsurgery Study Group just 12 years ago, we had great difficulty to assemble, for that inaugural meeting, 30 ophthalmic microsurgeons from around the world. In that same year, Harms and Mackensen published their pioneering book 'Ocular Surgery Under the Microscope'. This work served as an impetus to advance microsurgery in Europe. The publication of the English translation in 1967, complimented by my several publications, fortified the trend in the Americas. A symposium on ophthalmic microsurgery was held at the American Academy of Ophthalmology and Otolaryngology in 1968. The majority of the speakers at this symposium were members of the original Microsurgery Study Group.

In 1957, the Barraquers, Harms, Mackensen, and I had initiated an extensive redesign of instrumentation, and I had introduced the first zoom microscope. Our first and most logical application of ophthalmic microsurgery was to the surgery of the anterior segment, in particular, to corneal surgery. Monofilament nylon suture was introduced by Harms & Mackensen in 1962. This radically different suture material, coupled with the new zoom microscopes and microsurgical instrumentation, so improved our techniques as to cause a quiet revolution in anterior segment surgery, in particular, in penetrating keratoplasty.

Recently, after reviewing a series of my penetrating keratoplasty cases in an attempt to establish the immunologic basis for graft reaction, Henle reported to me that my patients' homografts remained clear even when marked immunologic sensitivity could be demonstrated preoperatively. This was in contradistinction to his findings some years earlier when he surveyed a group of patients of several prominent corneal surgeons who used macroscopic techniques and silk sutures for keratoplasty.

Nevertheless, ophthalmic surgeons the world over resisted the use of the microscope for the surgery of cataracts until 1967, when Kelman reintroduced extracapsular surgery by phacoemulsification. To use this technique, the surgeon was told he had to be able to use the microscope. Subsequently, some 3,000 American ophthalmologists were introduced to microsurgery when they took Kelman's course. Though most of these ophthalmic surgeons did not adopt phacoemulsification as their cataract procedure of choice, they did acquire an interest in anterior segment microsurgery. The qualitative improvement in technique, together with reduced wound complications and postoperative morbidity, was so striking that most of them continued to use the microscope for intracapsular cataract surgery. Since 1975, an added impetus to use microsurgery has been the increasing use of alloplastic lens substitutes. Even more recently, a new interest in preserving the viability of the corneal endothelium by refining the performance of the cataract operation has added further to the ranks of ophthalmic microsurgeons.

As a corollary to the increased accuracy and reproducibility of the cataract incision and closure through the use of microsurgery, the new subspecialty of refractive surgery of the cornea is now developing.

Thirteen years ago, I began my work on surgery to correct corneal astigmatism. These techniques are applicable not only in keratoplasty as originally conceived but also in cataract surgery. Within the same time frame, José Barraquer has continued his work to perfect his lamellar refractive keratoplasty techniques, keratomileusis for aphakia or myopia and keratophakia. Both of these techniques of corneal refractive surgery are dependent totally on microsurgery.

Out of a necessity for better identification and quantification of optical errors during refractive surgery and to monitor their correction, I developed the surgical keratometer. Refinements of my original instrument are now attracting wide interest in the United States.

Coreoplasty and suturing of the iris, severely condemned ten years ago, is now performed commonly, especially since the reintroduction of alloplastic lens substitues with iris supported lens fixation.

Only six years ago, Machemer and Douvas in the United States and Kloti in Switzerland introduced new instrumentation to perform microsurgery within the posterior segment. The ability to excise surgically the diseased or compromised vitreous was a direct result of the improved visualization of the posterior segment through the surgical microscope equipped with coaxial illumination. Patients with severe vitreous pathology obstructing or otherwise affecting retinal function, formerly condemned to blindness, are now being rehabilitated successfully. As importantly, the morbidity of operative and postoperative vitreous complications of anterior segment surgery has been reduced markedly by machine vitrectomy.

Microsurgery has been employed in surgery of the lacrimal apparatus, surgery of the lid margins, and, occasionally, in surgery of orbital and periorbital structures. In the majority of cases, extraocular muscle surgery is performed macroscopically. However, microsurgery has been advocated in secondary or complicated cases as reported by Veronneau, and in denervation and extirpation of the inferior oblique, as reported by Gonzalez.

What of the future of microsurgery? In my opinion, we are now reaching the practical limit of usefulness of our present microscopes and manual instrumentation.

Many ophthalmic surgical microscopes in use today are of a design more than 20 years old and were made originally for industrial use. Often, the useful magnification is limited because of poorly designed support systems and the necessity for manual or foot control of the most basic functions prevents precise orientation. Modifications and additions to these old microscopes often have made them even more ungainly and difficult to manipulate than they were in their original state. I foresee a new generation of exclusively ophthalmic surgical microscopes utilizing new computer-generated optical designs, integrally incorporated mechanical systems, and servo- and computer-controlled basic functions.

Manual microsurgical instruments also have reached a practical limit of performance. New instruments will have to be increasingly electromechanically, servo, or computer controlled so as to provide finer and exactly reproducible surgical manipulations. Such accuracy is essential to obtain maximal results from refractive corneal surgery. As refractive corneal surgery is refined, the use of alloplastic lens substitutes for aphakic correction will become obsolete.

New methods of cataract surgery will be developed as the role of the posterior capsule in causing or preventing postoperative complications is clarified by ongoing prospective clinical studies. It is the opinion of this author that to create extensive intraocular scarring by an extracapsular extraction and then to incorporate in it an alloplastic lens substitute is the height of surgical physiologic folly. Total removal of the lens and the adjacent, often pathologic vitreous body, by a pars plana approach, currently being evaluated by Girard, may eliminate the wound complications of the present intracapsular method, and prevent the postoperative intraocular scarring of extracapsular techniques. Postoperative aphakic correction can be performed at the primary procedure by the keratomileusis or keratophakia technique of José Barraquer.

I foresee an increasing use of vitrectomy during primary intracapsular cataract surgery and secondarily in the management of wound, iris, and retinal complications caused by degenerating or diseased uveal tissue and vitreous.

There is the probability that, through application of nerve and vessel anastimosis techniques used currently by neurosurgeons and microvascular surgeons, we will soon develop surgical techniques to alleviate orbital and ocular vascular disease and selectively to alter or to reestablish innervation of extraocular muscles.

What man (or woman) can imagine in ophthalmic surgery, can be accomplished by microsurgery!

90

Docum. Ophthal. Proc. Series, Vol. 21

RECENT ADVANCES IN MICROSURGICAL CUTTING TECHNIQUE

J. DRAEGER

(Bremen, B.R.D.)

Suturing was the first procedure in ophthalmic microsurgery, which was improved by use of a microscope. But no doubt also incision means a delicate, in many cases even dangerous manouver too. This also is true for cataract surgery. Of course it seems in possible to replace the classical Graefe knife by any means of motorized or remote controlled instrument. With this technique too much depends on the skill and the experience of the surgeon himsel, comparably little depends on the design of the instrument.

Any attempt to improve our cataract incision technique by a novel typ of instrument means the complete change of our surgical approach.

G. Crock was the first to build a motorized knife, which was practically applicable.

With a relatively high frequency the blade oscillates.

This additional motion of the cutting edge multiplies the distance covered per time by the blade. The faster the blade is moved, the less pressure is transmitted to the tissue. Following this principle cutting could be facilitated especially in very soft tissues with little resistance to the cutting edge. Of course this relation also can be utilized for cataract surgery: On the one hand less pressure is need to penetrate the corneoscleral region on the other hand no longer the surgeon has to perform the cutting manually. He just has to control the motorized incision through the microscope.

In the beginning we also applied the oscillating blade to perform cataract incision (Fig. 1).

The actual penetration of the tissue was facilitated, but the transmission of the vibration to the tissue surface – even using higher frequencies – was disturbing the precise observation.

Raising the cutting speed of a blades edge also can be achieved by continuous motion in one direction, if rotating blades are used: This principle 100 years ago was applied by v. Hippel for his motorized corneal trephine.

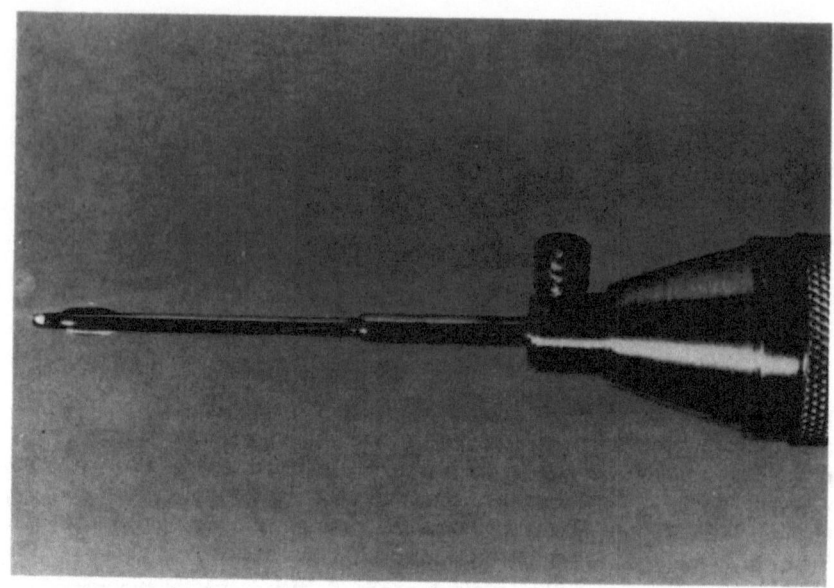

Fig. 1. Oscillating knife, electric knife (Draeger).

This principle of continuous cutting motion has become the basis of modern rotor instruments used for years in clinical practise. (Fig. 2)

The higher the speed of the cutting edge, the less cutting pressure is needed. This of course is also advantageous for cataract incision. (Fig. 3)

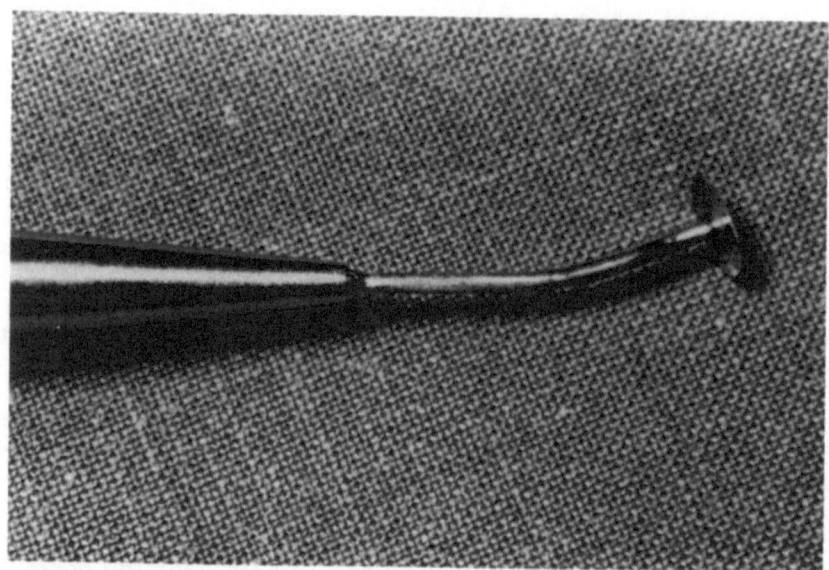

Fig. 2. Rotating blade.

92

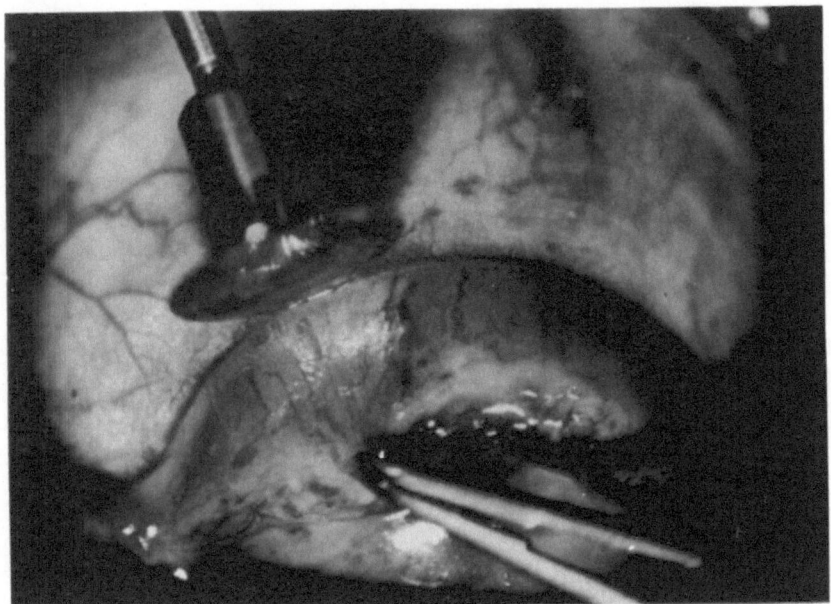

Fig. 3. Rotating blade before cataract incision.

Increasing the cutting speed per 10 times means decreasing cutting pressure to a tenth.

The transmitted pressure was measured by means of an electrical precision balance, the scale of which carried the embedded globe. In the same time the intraocular tension was controlled.

Using the new rotor knife only one p cutting pressure is needed compared with 37,7 p applied by using even the sharpest razor blade. Due to the adhesion at the flanks of the blade an opposite force reduces the pressure needed almost to zero. (Fig. 4)

Guards of different diameter allow precise depth control. For further increase of speed, for even higher reliability and safety recently we changed to air motors.

A small turbine, rotating at 30.000 rpm provides a higher torque – about 5 times as much as an electric motor of the same size.

This new motor also is remote controlled from the chair of the microsurgical unit, the pressure can be read at the panel. (Fig. 5).

By reduction of the pressure torque and number of revolutions can be altered.

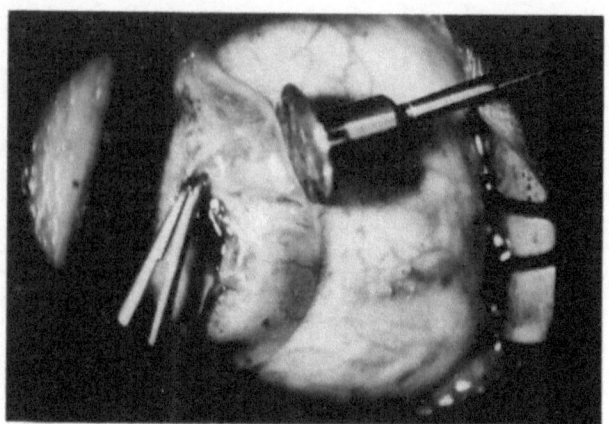

Fig. 4. Pressure components using the rotor blade.

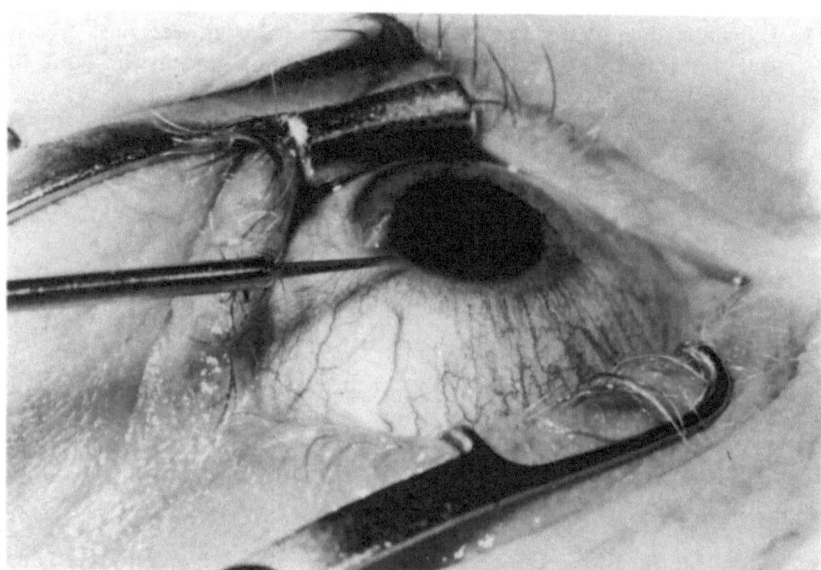

Fig. 5. Panel of the microsurgical unit, pressure gauge.

Using this new drive the rotating blades are even more handsome and useful in cataract surgery, especially to guarantee precise and smooth incisions.

REFERENCES

Draeger, J. & R. Hackelbusch, Experimentelle Untersuchungen und klinische Erfahrungen mit neuen Rotorinstrumenten. *Ophthalmologica* (Basel) 164 (1972), 273–283.
Draeger, J. Ein halbautomatisches elektrisches Keratom für die lamelläre Keratoplastik. *Klin. Mbl. Augenheilk,* 167 (1975) 353–359.

Author's address:
Augenklinik Zentralkrankenhaus
St. Jürgenstrasse
D-28 Bremen
F.R.G.

Docum. Ophthal. Proc. Series, Vol. 21

LENS SURGERY IN THE LAST DECADES

DEMETRIO PITA-SALORIO, MANUEL DEO VALERA &
RAMON BERNIELL TROTTA

(Barcelona, Spain)

Cataract surgery constitutes a central subject of ophthalmology. All the problems that it states are of great concern to all ophthalmologists. From our point of view, this generalized interest is based upon two circumstances. On the one hand, as lens opacity appears with a regularly high frequency in a clinic, every ophthalmologist, specialized or general, has a daily contact with the problem. On the other hand, the wide range of pathogenic and physiopathologic features that are related to this subject obliges the specialized ophthalmologist to intervene and take part in its discussion, whatever specific branch he is exclusively or prevailingly dedicated to. All of which indicates that this great item in ophthalmology should be focussed on in a multidisciplinary rather than a partial way, if a complete and accurate comprehension of it is required.

When looking at (the) 'Lens surgery in the last decades' we find out that many are the aspects which are related to this subject. Historical, conceptual, biological, sociological, technical problems, etc.; all of them conditioning decisively all scientific aspects. We will try, therefore, to give a global view of the problem, in front of such a diversified collection of aspects, without attending to concrete details to which other reports of this Symposium will certainly refer.

The beginning of cataract surgery's modern history takes place around the first half of the 18th century, being at the same time cause and consequence of a much more transcendental event: the birth of surgery as a speciality within modern scientific medicine.

In fact, the predominating idea in the scientific world of the second half of the 18th century is the 'rationalization of knowledge', understanding 'reason' as the supreme faculty that allows man to bring sense and order to his surrounding reality. In medicine, this rationalization of knowledge reaches into three fundamental orders. And so we can see how in clinical medicine the heritage of Hermann Boherbare and Thomas Sydenhan advances the development of nosography. Giving birth to Modern Pathologic Anatomy, Moraqui's works establish that specific abnormalities correspond to every disease. And in the area of therapeutics the essential change involves surgery, which becomes a science. With the basis of data and knowledge, that the fundamental sciences offer him (anatomy & physiology) the surgeon will build up his technique. Thus surgery appears as a rational discipline, the concept of regulated operations takes form and the surgeon is no more a skilful empiric but a rigorous scientist. And then from scientific surgery specialisation is born, for science and specialization are very closely attached, as the need of an 'exclusive dedication' to ophthalmologic work becomes clear, given the embarrassment that a 'rational surgery' of ocular diseases supposes.

In this way, cataract surgery is but a clear expression of the foresaid. And so, thanks to Daviel traditional couching of the lens is followed by a more rational method: extraction. Thereby a fundamental idea is introduced, and the same time an important technical advance is achieved, which is the 'penetration of the surgeon to the inside of the ocular globus'. The idea had already been conceived by other surgeons, as J. L. Petit (1696-1762), eminent surgeon at that time and one of the pioneers of the rationalization of surgery, the same as John Conrad Freytag, Johann Heinrich Freytag, Stephan Blarkaart (1659-1702), Ch. Saint Yves (1667-1736), and A. Maitre Jean (1650-1730) fundamentally. All the same, Jaques Daviel was the one who could accomplish succesfully the operation.

Since Daviel's work, it has all been a continuous perfection, still going on nowadays. And all the development and the improvements attained in cataract surgery have been tightly related to and conditioned by the achievements that surgery, as a scientific and technical discipline has obtained.

Daviel was followed by Pierre Pammard (1728-1793), who was the first to operate on a supine patient, and who also introduced a number of technical variants in order to attain a greater 'immobilization' of the eye and the patient. They were both continued by Guillaume Pellier de Quengsy (1752-1835), who performed the incision on the upper part of the cornea. About that time William Cheselden introduces the iridectomy, but this practice was not a part of cataract surgery until Jaeger, and later on Von Graefe, introduced it. The technical innovations of Georg Heurmann (1723-1768), Pierre Guérin (1740-1827), J. Virgilius Casaamata, and Joseph Barth (1745-1818), follow them. Barth is of crucial importance, for he was the first professor of the newly formed chair of Vienna, a centre that was to contribute in a fundamental way to the teaching of ophthalmology all over Europe.

In the first half of the 19th century, the task of technical perfection was to be of great importance. To be recognised, in that sense, was the work of Friederich Jaeger (1784-1871), who focussed his efforts on a standardization of techniques, especially of iridectomy. Also to be cited are Himly (1772-1832), who introduced the use of 'atropine' to help extraction, George Critchett (1817-1882), the first one to employ the Blepharostat and to practice the lineal incision, Pierre Demours, Victor Stoeber (1803-1871), Julius Sichel (1802-1868), Louis Auguste Desmarres (1810-1882), and Joseph Beer (1763-1821), successor of Barth in the chair of Vienna.

In the second half of the century, important innovations and changes of high significance take place. It is in this period when ophthalmology reaches its full age, for it begins to understand and treat the diseases of the eye with the orientations of modern scientific medicine. And all this accompanied by contributions as decisive as that of Hermann von Helmholtz, who introduces the ophthalmoscope, and those of Frans Cornelis Douders en Albracht von Graefe.

The technical improvement concerning surgery is of relevant importance, as the great enemies of surgical intervention begin to be dominated: pain with the help of anaesthesia, infection by means of antisepsis and asepsis.

Horace Wells (1815-1848) marked the beginning of anaesthesia when introducing laughing gas in dental operations, but it is Karl Köller who made the definitive contribution with the introduction in ocular surgery of anaesthesia by means of cocaine. Thanks to the recognition of antisepsis in ocular surgery by Alfred Carl Graefe (1830-1899), the works of Lister (1827-1912) were going to operate a decisive penetration with regard to the surgery of the eye. E. Fuchs and von Arlt would be the ones to undertake the application of Pasteur and Koch's eminent work.

As the concept and 'philosophy' of cataract surgery became clearly established, everything would be oriented from now on to the perfection and creation of more accurate methods of performing the operation.

We can systematize this second great stage of cataract surgery in the following way:

METHODS OF CATARACT EXTRACTION

a. Discission

Though it had already been recognized by Paul Barbette in 1672, as well as by W. Read (1706), Maître Jean (1711), Percival Pott (1713-1783), John Cunningham Sanders (1811), pioneer of the anterior approach, and Benjamin Travers (1814), this method was largely perfected by Dor (1892), Schwmitz (1903), Elschnig (1908), Blaskovic & Kreiker (1939), Offret (1949), Kirby (1950), Kuhnt (1959), and many others.

b. Extraction with forceps

The idea was first used by Albert Terson (1870) and was widely followed by Landsberg (1878), Kalt (1861-1941), Stanculenu (1847-1917), Knapp (1915), Torok (1915), Elshnig (1863-1939), Sinclair (1925), Nevertheless the universal use of this method is due to two illustrious spanish surgeons: Hermenegildo Arruga (1886-1972) and Ramon Castroviejo.

c. Suction

Proposed in former times by Galeazzo (1533) as well as Borri (1669), Pachili (1838), Blanchet (1847), Langer (1848), Teale (1863), Stoewer (1902), and Hullen (1910). Nevertheless, the fundamental contribution because of its orginality, usefulness and revolutionary value, is that of Ignacio Barraquer, who introduced the erysiphake, a method of continuous and controlled aspiration. The ventouses of Perez Llorca and of Arruga would be development of this method.

d. Cryoextraction

Undoubtedly, much later than all the preceding methods. In 1933, Bietti had already pointed out the possibility of using it, although it appears in Ophthalmology in 1960 introduced by Kewawicz. From that time on, a series of papers saw the light in several countries, the most important of which we cite here: Kellman (1963), Bellows (1954), Girard (1965), Amoils (1965), Haik (1965), Conway (1965), Grave (1966), Osher (1967), Levy (1967), Boke (1965), Mackevicus (1964), Paton (1965), Zanen (1965), Mawas (1966), and so on. Casanovas School of Barcelona, Sanchez Salorio's of Santiago de Compostela and Perez Llorca's School of Madrid, introduced it in Spain.

METHODS OF ZONULAR RUPTURE

Altough Di Lucca in 1866 and Andrew in 1883 were the introducers of the mechanic rupture, the most important contribution was that of Joaquin Barraquer, in 1957, when he brought zonulolysis by alpha-chymotrypsin into use.

ANAESTHESIA

We have already seen how anaesthesia began with the discovery of the anaesthetic properties of cocaine in 1884 by Karl Köller. In 1902 Willstater synthesized it. In 1889 Einhorn introduced the use of procaine and novocaine for local anaesthesia. Elshign and Arruga generalized the retrobulbar injection of novocaine.

Circa 1919 and 1920, Villard, Rochat & Lint introduced the akinesis of the orbicular muscle. Years later (1949) Atkinson introduced the adding of hyaluronidase.

INCISION

Conjunctival Incision

Corneal incision was introduced by Daviel in 1745. The contribution of Graefe's knife meant an important advance. Jaeger and Lancaster also contributed to obtain it.

But in 1951, Dunnington & Regan made evident the superiority of the sclerocorneal incision.

Finally, sclerocorneal incisions were performed and described by Castro-viejo and Troutmann and Barraquer (J.I.), who practiced them with 'pike' and scissors.

SUTURE

Suture was first employed by Williams, in 1865, who sutured the cornea. This practice was abandoned, retaining the use of the suture of the conjunctival flap.

Later on, Kalt (1894), Suarez de Mendoza (1888), advised this practice, and after them Verhoeff, Chandler and Gomez Marquez.

The most characteristic aspects of cataract surgery being now analyzed, let us study, by way of practical synthesis, the different standing problems of nowadays.

ANAESTHESIA

At the present time, there exists a clash between two different currents of opinion: those who support local anaesthesia and those who prefer general anaesthesia. In the first case, akinesis and a previous sedation are absolutely necessary. We are, in general terms, more inclined towards the second policy.

INCISION

Conjunctival Incision

We are not going to discuss the different possibilities. We will simply state that the possible options are:
— Base on the fornix.
— Base on the limbus.

Corneal and/or scleral incision

The following options can be named:
— Corneal incision.
  — Classical bevel.
  — Inverted bevel.
— Sclerocorneal Incision.
  — From within
  — From without
— Scleral incision.
  — Incision on four planes.
Though some surgeons still use the corneal incision, nowadays the sclerocorneal incision is more widespread, especially the ab externo form. We prefer the latter with limbus based flap.

IRIDECTOMY

The are possibilities are:
— Iridectomy
  — Peripheric
  — Sectorial

- Idiotomy
  - peripheral
  - radial
- Iridodialysis.

Although all of them can be indicated, today the peripheral iridectomy is the most systematically used.

ZONULAR RUPTURE

- Mechanical.
- Enzymatic.

Their use is equally popular. We prefer the enzymatic, for its efficience and innocuousness.

EXTRACTION

- Expression.
- Erysiphake.
- Forceps.
- Cryoextraction.
- Phacoemulsification.

SUTURE

The actual discussion involves those who prefer absorbable sutures and those who prefer non-absorbable ones.

It can be said that we have assisted in the last decades in a progressive perfecting of the techniques of cataract surgery. The introduction of the operation microscope, the increasingly thinner sutures, the much more sophisticated instrumentation, the osmohvpotensors, the enzymatic zonulolysis, etc., have helped this branch of surgery to be safer and more attainable to our ophthalmologist appretice pupils.

Authors' address:
Department of Ophthalmology
Ophthalmology Clinic
University of Barcelona
Barcelona
Spain

Docum. Ophthal. Proc. Series, Vol. 21

INTRACAPSULAR LENS EXTRACTION

JOAQUIN BARRAQUER

(Barcelona, Spain)

DEEP GENERAL ANAESTHESIA

Induction with intravenous thiopental (Pentothal) sodium and momentary muscular relaxation with succinylcholine to facilitate tracheal intubation. After tracheal intubation, anaesthesia is continued with another general anaesthetic agent.

Halothane (Fluothane) offers considerable advantages over ether. It is non-inflammable, the anesthesia can be deepened rapidly, and the recovery is uneventful. Postoperative vomiting is minimal. Halothane produces moderate hypotension. Epinephirine should not be used because halothane increase cardiac sensitivity to epinephrine and may cause cardiac arrest.

GENERAL AKINESIA

The drug of choice is curare (d-tubocurarine chloride), which has a highly specific blocking action at the myoneural junctions of skeletal muscle. It also has a nicotine-like effect on autonomic ganglia. The muscles innervated by the cranial nerves are expecially sensitive to curare. This is a particular advantage in ophthalmic surgery.

Succinylcholine, on the other hand, appears to cause a contracture of the extraocular muscles instead of relaxation. It should only be used for intubation.

The fundamental advantage of careful general aneasthesia and akinesia is the complete relaxation of the patient with excellent ocular hypotony. It is not necessary to count upon the collaboration of the patient and the surgical manoeuvres are carried out more easely than under local anaesthesia. It is essential, however, that the anaesthesiologist should be familair with the problems of ocular surgery and the ideal would be to have a full time anaesthesiologist for ocular surgery.

INCISION

Total extraction of the lens requires an ample incision into the anterior chamber to facilitate the delivery of the lens and to minimize the trauma to

103

the corneal endothelium and the iris during the extraction. A small incision may lead to capsule rupture and vitreous loss.

The size, form, and consistency of the lens must be taken into consideration in determining the length of the incision. For extracting the lens by the sliding manoeuvre the incision may be somewhat smaller.

A large corneoscleral incision with a conjunctival flap allowing a two-plane closure is considered of choice (Fig. 1). It may be performed with a Graefe knife, with keratome and scissors or with the new axially oscillating knife (Barraquer-Grieshaber) (11.000 oscillations per minute).

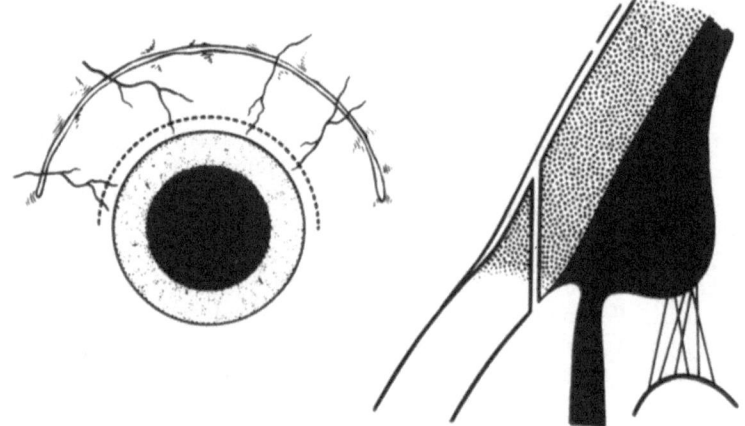

Fig. 1. Two-plane incision, sclerocorneal with limbus-based flap.

PERIPHERAL IRIDECTOMY

Before sutures were used to close the cataract incision, iridectomy was found to reduce considerably the incidence of iris prolapse. Although multiple well-placed corneoscleral sutures now provide tha major security against iris prolapse, the establishment of a peripheral communication between the posterior and the anterior chamber in the area of the incision is still indicated. This measure is a safeguard against the sequelae of pupillary block and, in addition, reduces the incidence of iris prolapse.

In the normal eye there is no peripheral communication between the chambers. In the aphakic eye, however, such communication is desirable. Without it, a wound leak would cause the aqueous in the posterior chamber to push the iris toward the incision (Fig. 2 a). This would lead to the formation of anterior synechiae, iris incarceration, or iris prolpase (Fig. 2 b). The natural communication between the posterior and anterior chambers, the pupil, may not suffice to prevent these complications from occurring. A wound leak creates an unequal pressure gradient between the two chambers in the corresponding area. The aqueous humor follows the path of least resistance, and, because of the flaccidity of the iris, it tends to push the

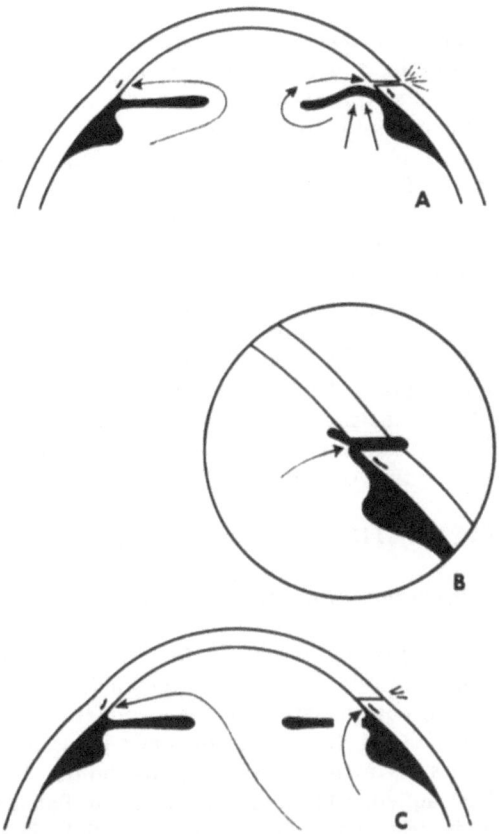

Fig. 2. The postoperative dynamics of the aqueous humor. a. Without iridectomy a wound leak would cause the iris to be pushed toward the incision by the aqueous in the posterior chamber. b. This can lead to iris prolapse. c. A peripheral iridectomy opening may prevent prolapse or anterior synechiae by providing free passage for the aqueous humor.

iris in this area toward the incision. In the presence of a wound leak this may happen in spite of an unobstructed pupil. Displacement of the iris will not occur if a peripheral communication, through which the aqueous humour can pass freely, has been established between the chambers (Fig. 2. c.).

Postoperatively the pupil may be blocked by the vitreous, especially if the hyaloid is intact, In the absence of a patent iridectomy opening the iris will bulge forward. The resulting angle closure leads to increased tension, which may be followed by wound rupture and iris prolapse.

A moderate amount of air injected into the anterior chamber may block the flow of aqueous in the absence of a patent peripheral iridectomy opening.

With an effectively closed wound and an unobstructed pupil, an iridectomy opening may seem superfluous. Although it is true that good results may be obtained without iridectomy, it still would be a grave mistake to perform a simple extraction, since the occurrence of wound leak and pupillary block cannot be predicted.

The fundamental purpose of iris surgery is thus related to the postoperative dynamics of the aqueous humor. In addition, sector iridectomy or radial iridotomy may serve to facilitate the delivery of the lens, to prevent rupture of the sphincter, or to provide an improved optical aperture. Extensive synechiae are dealt with before the lens is extracted. Certain surgical complications require additional iris surgery.

For peripheral iridectomy the iris is stroked toward the pupil with a marten hair brush. The brush keeps the incision open and exposes the base of the iris, which is grasped with the colibri forceps (Fig. 3). The iris is gently pulled into the incision, and a small fragment is excised with a single snip of the Wecker-Barraquer scissors (Fig. 4). A regular peripheral iridectomy opening is thus obtained.

APPLICATION OF ALPHA-CHYMOTRYPSIN

a. Preparation of the alpha-chymotrypsin solution

The selectivity of alpha-chymotrypsin for the zonule is related to the strength of the concentration used and the limiting of the duration of action. The optimum concentration of the enzyme solution for zonulolysis is 1:5.000 or 1:10.000. A fresh solution must be used since the enzyme, once disolved, loses its activity within a few hours. The most adequate diluent is artificial aqueous humour (P.E.V.A.) or Balanced Salt Solution (Alcon) which is less cytotoxic than a physiologic sodium chloride

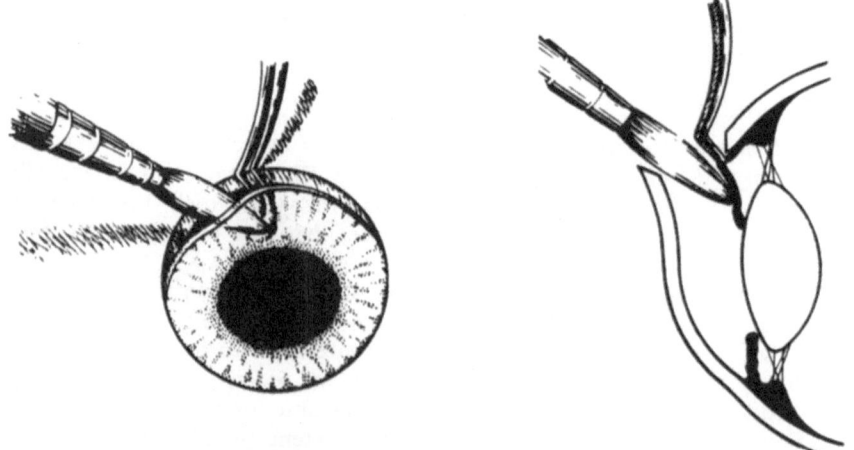

Fig. 3. For peripheral iridectomy the base of the iris is exposed with a marten hair brush. The iris is grasped with a colibri forceps.

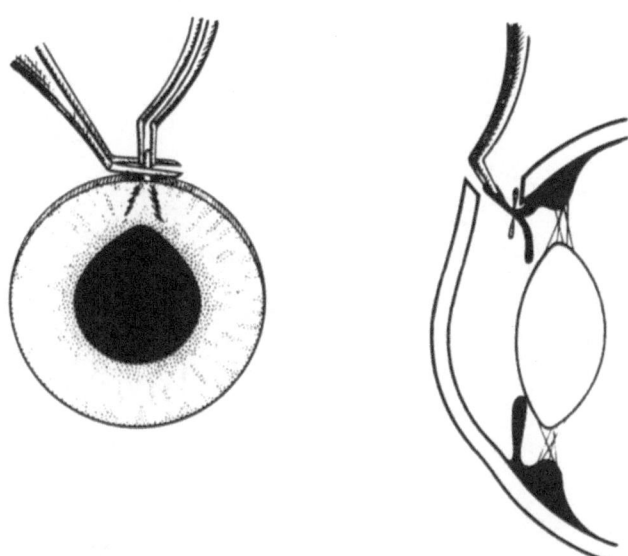

Fig. 4. Peripheral iridectomy with the de Wecker-Barraquer scissors.

solution. The activity of the enzyme depends on the temperature. The optimum temperature is $37°C$, but it is more practical to use the solution at room temperature.

The syringe and cannula must be sterilized by heat, since traces of alcohol or detergents inactivate the enzyme. External sterilization of the alpha-chymotrypsin vials should be avoided, because the enzyme may be inactivated by the accidental penetration of some of the sterilizing agent into the vial. The stopper is wiped with alcohol and dried with sterile gauze.

Application of the alpha-chymotrypsin solution

The anterior chamber must be free of blood, which may have entered at the incision or following the iridectomy. Blood is expelled by irrigation with artificial aqueous humor. Adherent clots are removed with a marten hair brush.

The introduction of the enzyme solution into the posterior chamber must be carried out precisely. The syringe is held in one hand, and the base of the attached cannula is steadied with a forceps held in the other hand (Fig. 5). The lens is slightly depressed with the smooth tip of the cannula to avoid trauma to the iris and dispersion of pigment. The danger of luxating the lens is minimal since this manoeuvre requires less pressure than grasping the lens with a capsule forceps. Only 0.5 cc. of the enzyme solution is slowly injected. For uniform zonulolysis the solution is injected in each quadrant. Contact of the cannula with the corneal endothelium, which may produce striate keratopathy, is prevented by having the assistant raise the cornea slighty.

107

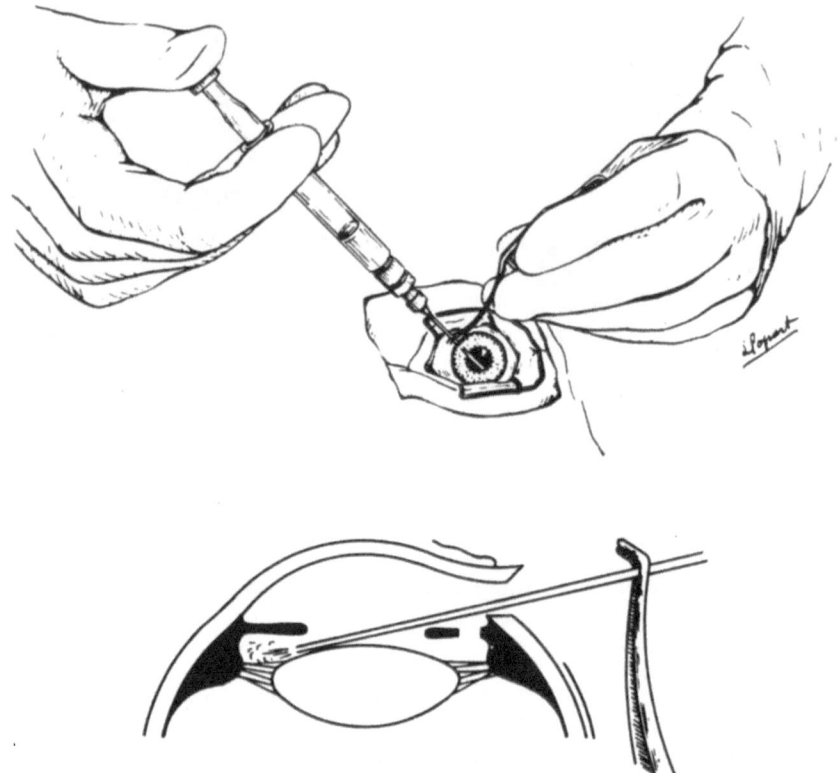

Fig.5. The technique of introducing alpha-chymotrypsin into the posterior chamber. The cannula is steadied with a forceps.

IRRIGATION OF THE INCISION AND THE ANTERIOR CHAMBER

Immediately after the injection of the enzyme solution, the incision is irrigated with artificial aqueous humor to prevent prolonged contact of the wound edges with the enzyme (Fig. 6).

Two minutes after the injection of the enzyme solution has been started, the anterior chamber is irrigated with artifical aqueous humor for the removal of any remaining enzyme (Fig. 7). The duration of action of the enzyme is varied according to the case and the degree of zonuloysis desired. The lens may be seen to come forward and to assume a spherical shape as zonulolysis becomes complete (Fig. 8). However, these signs are often masked by hypotony.

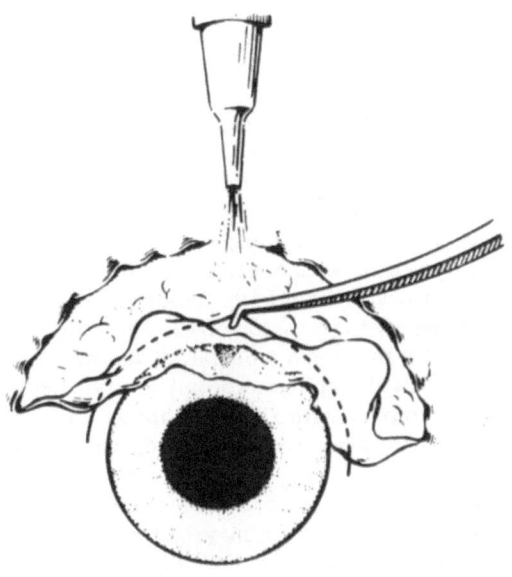

Fig. 6. Irrigation of the incision with artificial aqueous humor. The anterior chamber is kept closed.

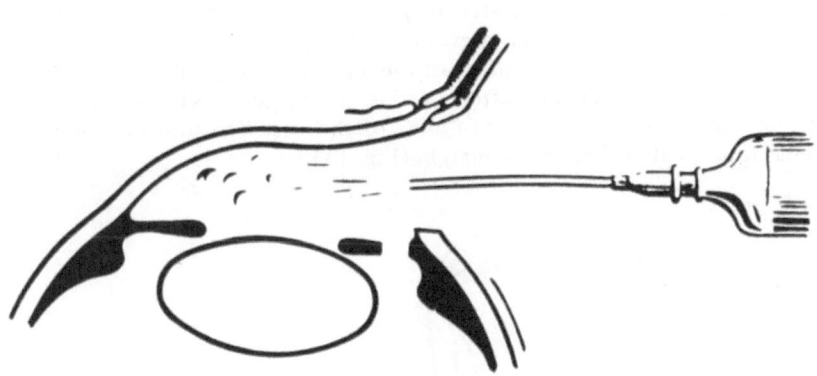

Fig. 7. Elimination of alpha-chymotrypsin from the anterior chamber.

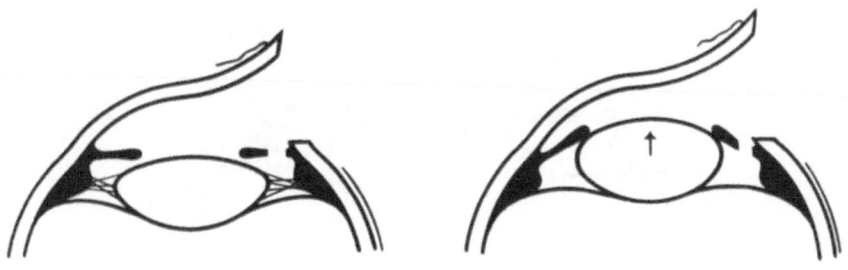

Fig. 8. Signs of zonulolysis. The lens comes forward and assumes a spherical shape.

INTRACAPSULAR EXTRACTION

a. Enzymatic phakoerysis with tumbling manoeuvre and 'open sky' technique

1. To prevent contact between the corneal endothelium and the erysiphake, it is advisable to use the open sky technique. In this technique the incision is opened widely by raising the cornea with the colibri forceps. The anterior lens capsule is dried with a marten hair brush, and the erysiphake is applied eccentrically toward the inferior border of the lens, so that the rim of the cup comes close to the equator of the lens (Fig. 9). The erysiphake passes without difficulty through a moderately dilated pupil, unless the iris is rigid. When the iris is rigid a sphincterotomy is indicated. When the entire rim of the cup is in contact with the lens capsule and free of the iris, the vacuum is started. It is not necessary to depress the lens to establish good contact.

The vacuum pressure should be about 30 cm. Hg for the average lens. In young patients the vacuum pressure may be raised to 45 or 50 cm. Hg to increase the contraction of the lens. For intumescent cataracts a vacuum pressure of 5 or 10 cm.Hg is used.

The vacuum grasps the anterior lens capsule, which partially prolapses into the cup of the erysiphake. The equatorial diameter of the lens is thus reduced (Fig. 10), which facilitates the passage of the lens through the pupil and the incision. This also facilitates the tumbling maneuver.

2. To ensure a firm engagement of the lens by the erysiphake it is necessary to pause a few seconds after starting the vacuum. The erysiphake is raised and tilted to initiate the tumbling of the lens. The inferior border of the lens appears at the pupillary margin (Fig. 11).

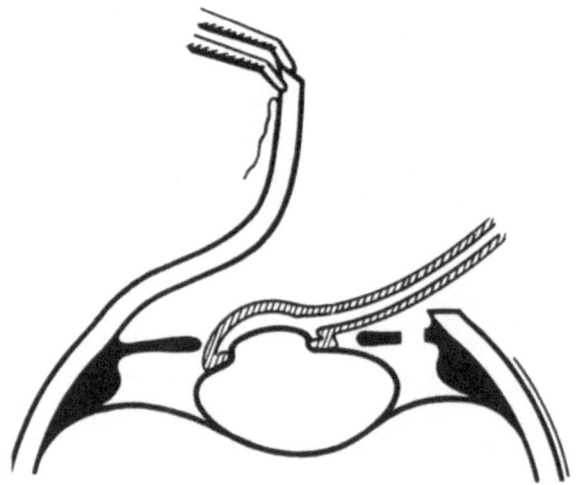

Fig. 9. Application of the erysiphake with the 'open sky' technique.

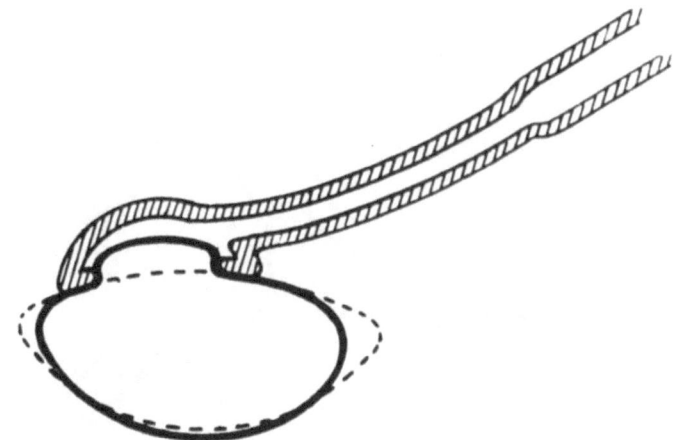

Fig. 10. Reduction of the equatorial diameter of the lens by the erysiphake.

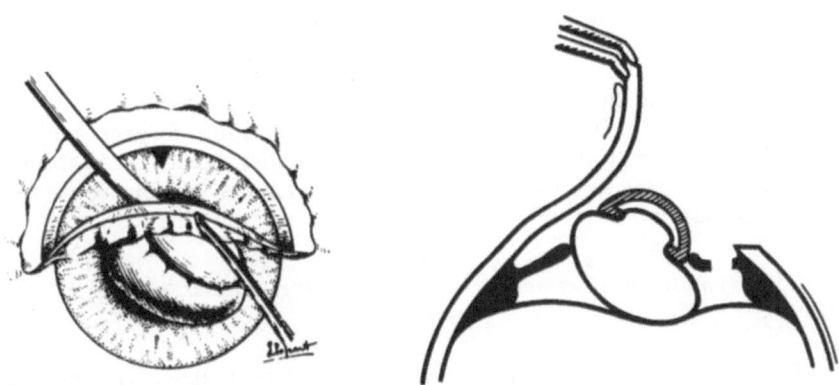

Fig. 11. Beginning of the tumbling manoeuvre. The inferior border of the lens enters the anterior chamber.

3. The tumbling of the lens is continued by raising and tilting the crysiphake and moving it superiorly at the same time. As the hyaloid is visualized, its position and relation to the lens are noted. With good hypotony tumbling of the lens 100 to 120° is sufficient.

To facilitate the tumbling manoeuvre the handle of the erysiphake is rotated between the fingers. The hand is steadied on the forehead of the patient or against his temple, avoiding pressure on the globe at the external canthus. The vacuum tube must be flexible and not impede the rotation of the erysiphake. A twisted tube may interfere with the rotation or cut off the vacuum.

4. The superior border of the lens is made to leave the anterior chamber last. The open sky technique permits the lens to be raised enough to prevent the superior border from damaging the hyaloid (Fig. 12). Usually the iris is

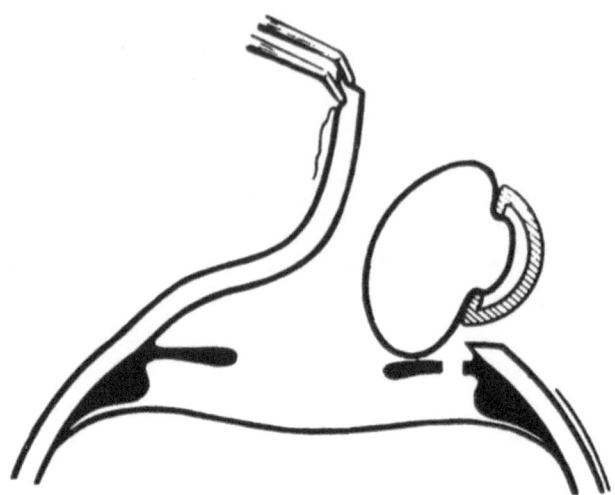

Fig. 12. Termination of the tumbling manoeuvre. The lens touches neither the hyaloid nor the corneal endothelium.

not drawn up, and the pupil remains perfectly round and central.

5. The incision is kept wide open with the colibri forcpes. and the position of the iris root and the pupil is noted under direct visualization. If necessary, a marten hair brush is used to replace the iris. The incision is then closed and sutured.

Enzymatic cryoextraction with sliding maneuver and 'open sky' technique

1. The pupil should be dilated widely for the sliding maneuver. The open sky technique is used. The anterior lens capsule is dried with a marten hair brush.

2. The iris is retracted toward the 12 o'clock meridian with a fine forceps or an iris reatractor.

3. The cryoprobe is placed on the anterior lens capsule, sufficiently separated from the iris and the corneal enothelium to avoid the freezing extending to these structures.

4. With a foot control the gas (CO_2) is opened to freeze the tip of the probe. After 2 or 3 seconds good adhesion between the tip of the probe and the lens capsule and cortex is obtained.

5. When an ice ball of ½ mm. around the tip has formed, the adhesion is considered adequate and the probe is raised. The superior border of the lens appears at the pupillary margin, and the lens is delivered by sliding horizontally through the incision.

The traction on the iris which was exerted to separate it toward the 12 o'clock meridian is released as soon as the border of the lens appears in the anterior chamber.

112

Immediately after the extraction of the lens a solution of 1 per cent acetylcholine in artificial aqueous humor is instilled to constrict the pupil. When the open sky technique is used, acetylcholine is instilled directly on the iris the moment the extraction of the lens is completed. Usually direct manipulations are not required for obtaining a round and central pupil. A simple but effective manoeuvre is to massage the cornea gently with the lens while the lens is still attached to the erysiphake. After tying the first suture the anterior chamber is irrigated with 1 per cent acetylcholine to constrict the pupil maximally.* The irrigation must be done gently; a forceful jet of fluid may traumatize the iris and rupture the hyaloid. It may even perforate the iris, especially when the iris is atrophic. The cannula should not be allowed to touch the iris or the corneal endothelium, nor should it be allowed to pass the pupillary border (Fig. 13). To prevent accidents, a cannula with a side opening may be used; the stream is directed toward the corneal endothelium.

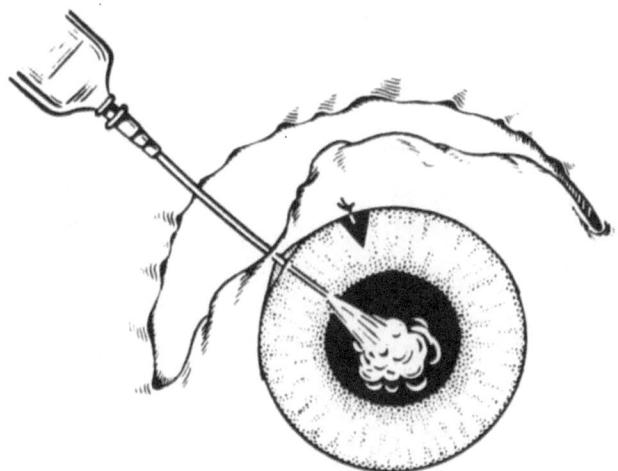

Fig. 13. Irrigation of the anterior chamber with acetylcholine. The cannula should not be allowed to pass the pupillary border.

SUTURE

Corneoscleral sutures must be placed accurately in order to promote early and firm healing with minimum astigmatism. The sutures should be able to withstand the intraocular pressure, and they should be well tolerated.

The sutures are placed edge-to-edge and radially. They are passed through the middle third of the corneoscleral thickness, and a bite of 0.5 mm. is

* Lyophilyzed acetylcholine should be used, freshly disolved in Balanced Salt Solution (Alcon) to avoid toxic effects on the corneal endothelium.

taken at each side of the incision (Fig. 14). All sutures should be tied to the same degree of tension, sufficient to keep the wound edges in good apposition.

The number of sutures used must be in direct proportion to the length of the incision and in inverse proportion to the diameter of the suture material.

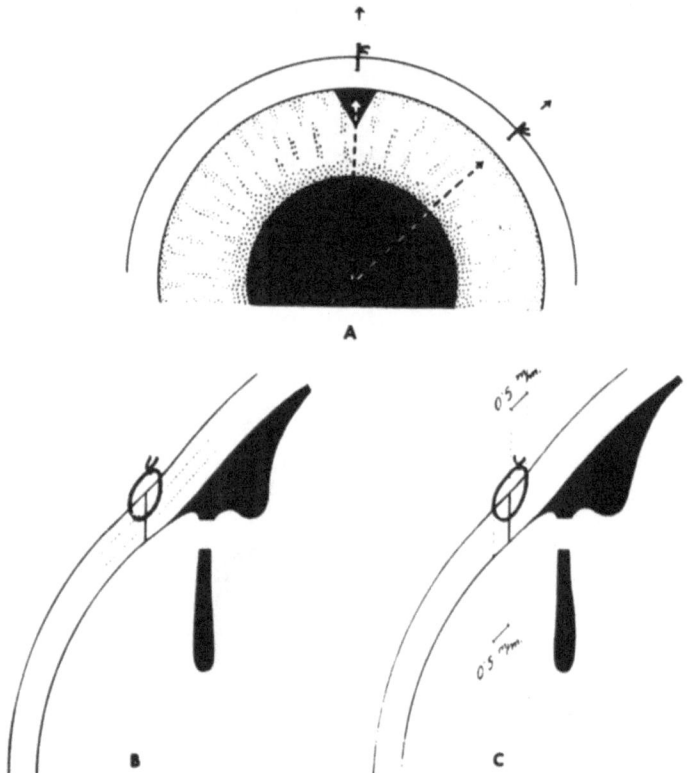

Fig. 14. The sutures are placed radially. b. They are passed through the middle third of the corneoscleral thickness. c. A bite of 0.5 mm. is taken at each side of the incision.

The needles and the sutures should be of the smalles calibre compatible with sufficient strength in order to cause as little trauma and inflammatory reaction as possible.

A suture that is not exactly radial will cause lateral displacement of the wound edges (Fig. 15). This displacement produces folds in the cornea, which are seen best when the corneal surface is dry

A too superficial suture will cause the incision to gape posteriorly (Fig. 16). Aqueous enters between the lamellae of the corneal stroma, and wound healing is delayed. The defect may lead to filtration, and because of its small bite, the suture may even cut through the tissue.

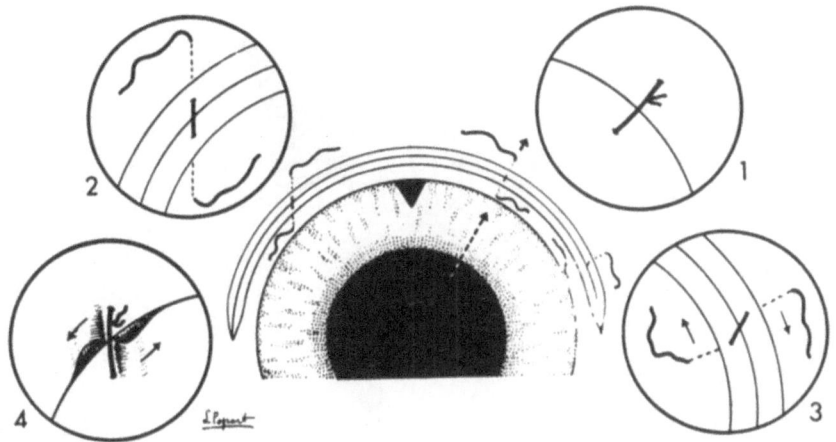

Fig. 15. 1. Radial suture. 2. and 3. Nonradial sutures. 4. Distortion of the wound edges by nonradial suture.

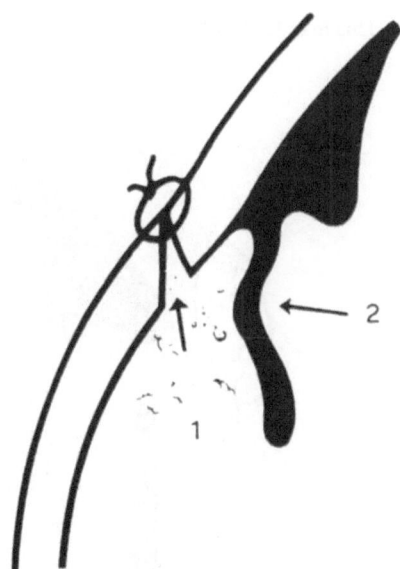

Fig. 16. Superficial suture causing posterior gaping of the wound. This may lead to filtration. (1) and iris incarceration in an area away from the iridectomy (2).

A too deep suture may penetrate the anterior chamber as it is placed, or later as result of necrosis of the deep layers (Fig. 17). The necrosis is promoted by the strangulation of the tissues on becoming edematous (Fig. 18). Excessive vascularization may further weaken the cicatrix.

A suture placed at unequal depths, superficial in one edge and deep in

115

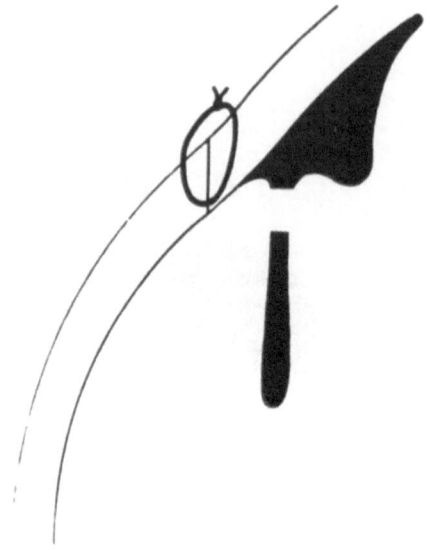

Fig. 1 7. Too deep suture. This may lead to fistulization.

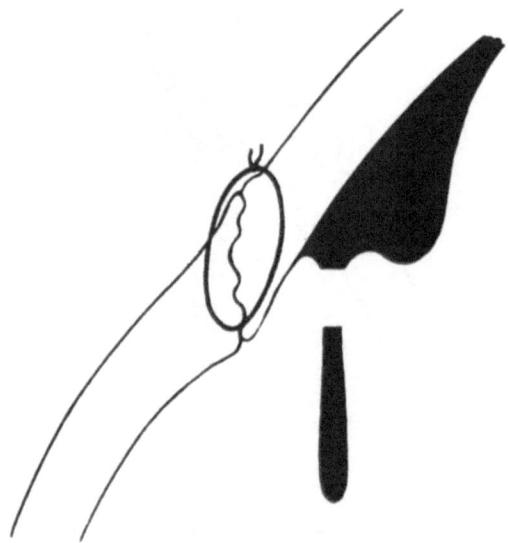

Fig. 18. Too deep suture. The tissues are strangulated on becoming edematous.

the other, causes poor apposition (Fig. 19), and the above complications may occur in combination.

A suture placed too close to the wound edges may cut through the tissue (Fig. 20). A bite that is too long tends to cause the tissue to wrinkel when

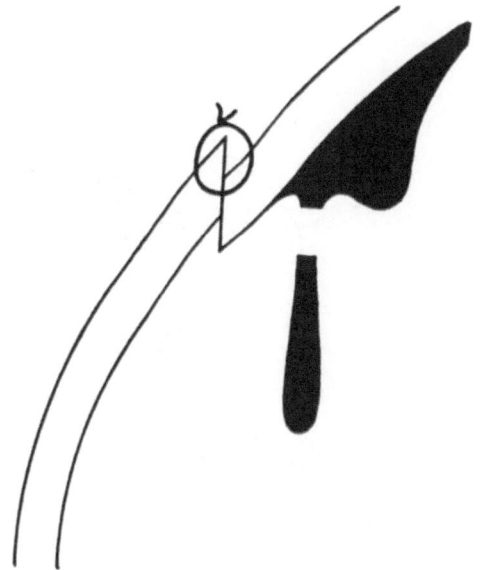

Fig. 19. Suture at unequal depths causing poor apposition.

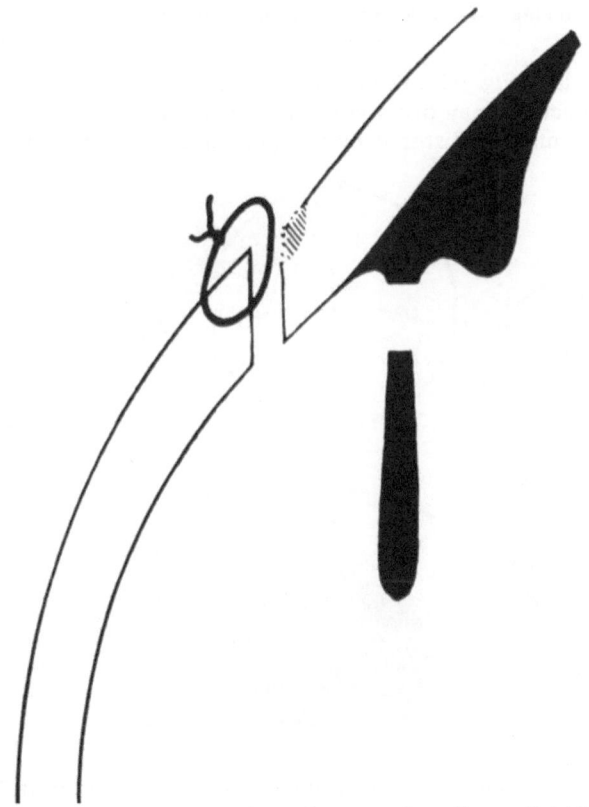

Fig. 20. Suture cutting through the tissues because of small superficial bite.

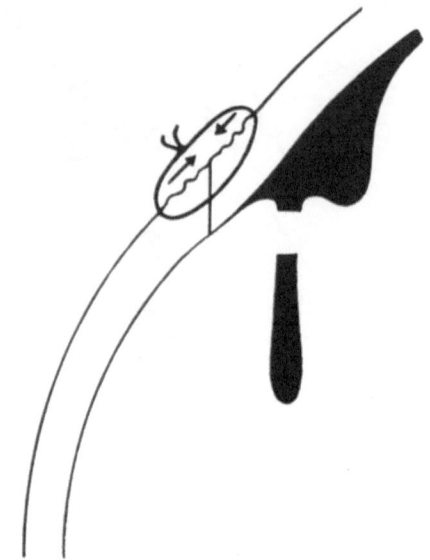

Fig. 21. Suture taking too long a bite and wrinkling the tissue.

the suture is tied (Fig. 21); the poor apposition may lead to excessive astigmatism, and necrosis may occur as a result of strangulation.

The wound may be distored by unequal tension of the sutures (Fig. 22).

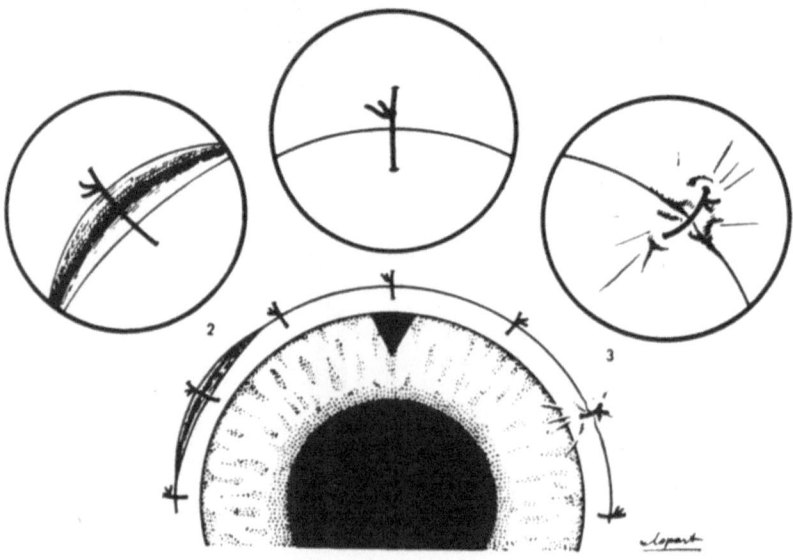

Fig. 22. Wound distorsion by unequal tension of the sutures: 1. Correct, 2. Too loose, and 3. Too tight.

Tight sutures compress the tissues excessively and may lead to necrosis and posterior gaping. Loose sutures do not produce sufficient apposition of the wound edges, which may immediately become evident when the anterior chamber is being re-formed with artificial aqueous humor.

Although a small number of sutures may produce good coaptation, increased intraocular pressure may cause the wound closure to fail. An excessive number of sutures, however, produces considerable trauma and unnecessarily prolongs the operation.

In routine intracapsular cataract extraction we use postplaced subconjunctival sutures with a limbus-based flap (Fig. 23). Only one suture is placed before the extraction and another six are placed afterwards.

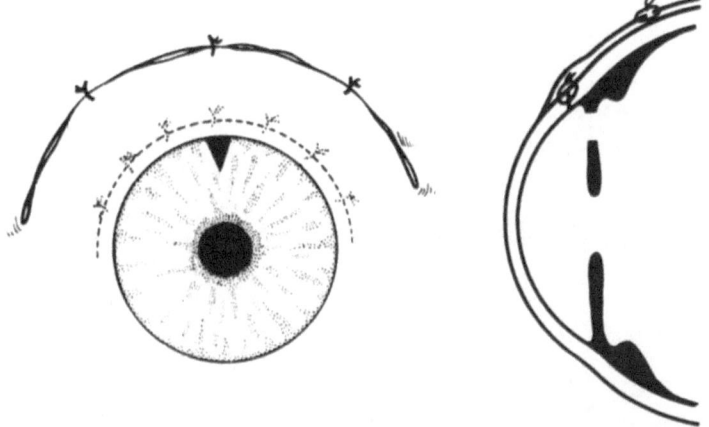

Fig. 23. Subconjunctival corneoscleral sutures. The limbus-based flap is sutured separately.

The limbus-based flap is turned over on the cornea. The corneal wound lip is grasped with the colibri forceps. An 83/4 Grieshaber needle with virgin silk is held with the mosquito needle holder. The needle is made to enter the cornea near the tips of the forceps, 0.5 mm. anterior to the incision but behind the insertion of the conjunctival flap at the limbus. If applied too far from the forceps, the needle will take an oblique course. The point of the needle must penetrate the corneal surface almost perpendicularly. The point is then directed radially to the middle third of the cut surface of the corneal lip (Fig. 24). As the needle emerges from the corneal lip, the colibri forceps in transferred to the scleral lip and the needle is passed into the latter. The point of the needle is directed to emerge from the sclera 0.5 mm. posterior to the incision. Thus each corneoscleral suture is placed in one stage. As the needle is passed across the incision the radial and vertical alignment must be perfect. For this alignment, the corneal lip is held with the needle in the needle holder and the scleral lip with the colibri forcpes (Fig. 25). When enough of the needle has emerged form the sclera to be grasped with the needle holder (Fig. 26), it is pulled through. The silk has a

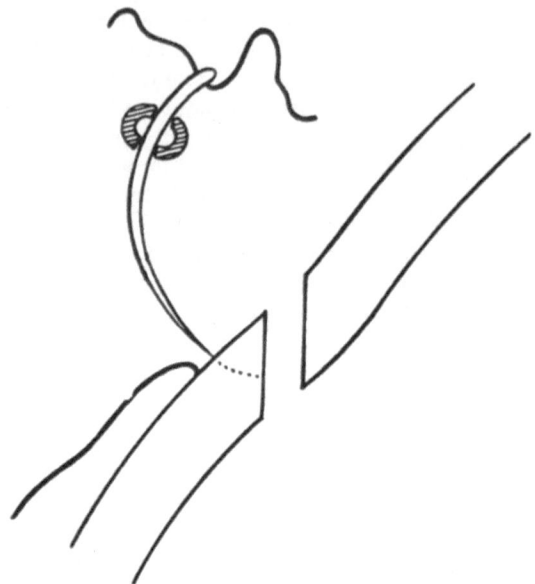

Fig. 24. Perpendicular puncture with the 83/4 Grieshaber needle.

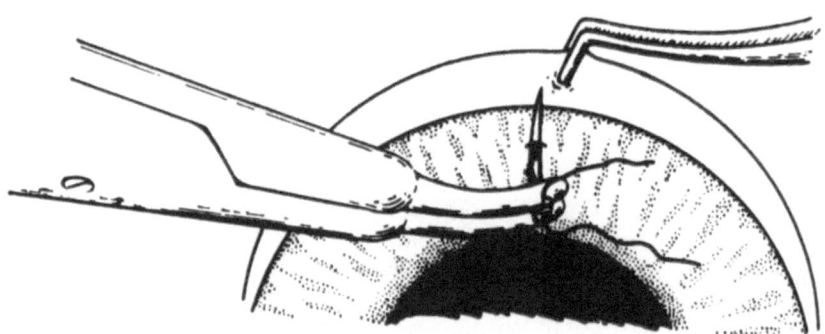

Fig. 25. The needle is passed through the aligned wound lips.

tendency to catch and invaginate subconjunctival tissue on being pulled through. The limbus-based flap is held away with the colibri forceps to prevent this.

A correctly placed suture does not produce folds in the cornea (radial apposition), and it maintains both wound edges at the same level (vertical apposition). To prevent overriding, the slanting wound edges of the von Graefe knife incision require particular care in placing the sutures at equal depths. These details are better appreciated when the wound edges are dried with a marten hair brush.

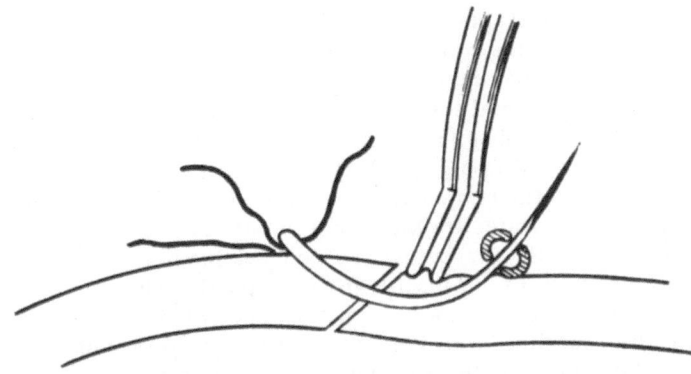

Fig. 26. The emerging needle is grasped with the needle holder far enough behind the point not ot injure the cutting edge. The jaws of the needle holder are shown in cross section.

The first part of the knot should always be a double hitch to prevent it from becoming loose (Fig. 27). The suture ends are pulled in opposite radial directions to obtain good apposition of the wound edges without overriding and without producing folds in the cornea. The second part of the knot should be a single hitch creating a square knot. This part is tied without much tension especially if virgin silk is used, to prevent the first part of the knot from tightening.

The knot is placed on the scleral side of the incision. The conjunctival flap is thicker and provides a better permanent covering here than at the limbus. This also prevents the suture ends from getting between the wound

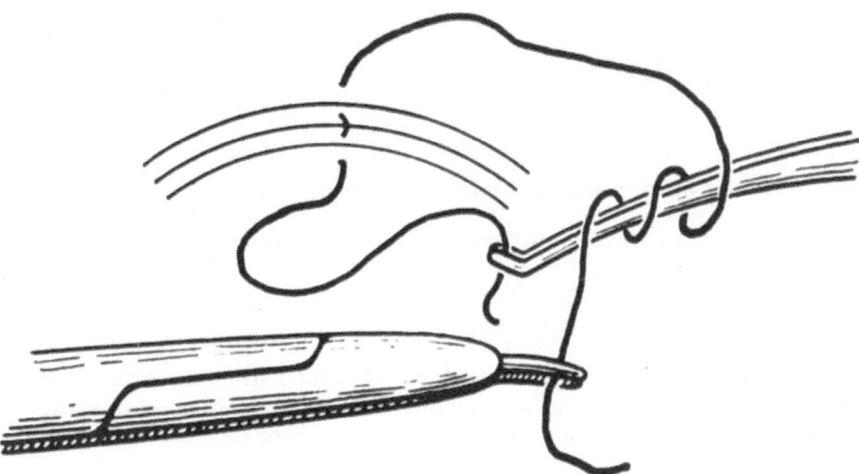

Fig. 27. Instrument tie with the colibri forceps and the mosquito needle holder.

edges. The ends must be left relatively long. about 2 mm., or they will bristle and perforate the conjunctiva postoperatively. When the ands are cut very short, the knot may become untied.

After the corneoscleral sutures have been placed, the anterior chamber is re-formed with artificial aqueous humor or with air, which should be retained readily. If the wound appears well closed and free of iris tissue and other extraneous matter, the conjunctiva is closed with 3 to 5 virgin silk sutures. The corneoscleral sutures are thus buried under the conjunctiva. (Fig. 23).

After closure of the first suture at 12 o'clock the injection of air into the anterior chamber is of diagnostic and therapeutic value in regard to the vitreous. When the pupil cannot be constricted or when it remains distorted, there may be a mushroom of vitreous protruding into the anterior chamber (Fig. 28). Air will push the vitreous back enabling the pupil to contract (Fig. 29). Once miosis has been obtained the air is replaced by artificial

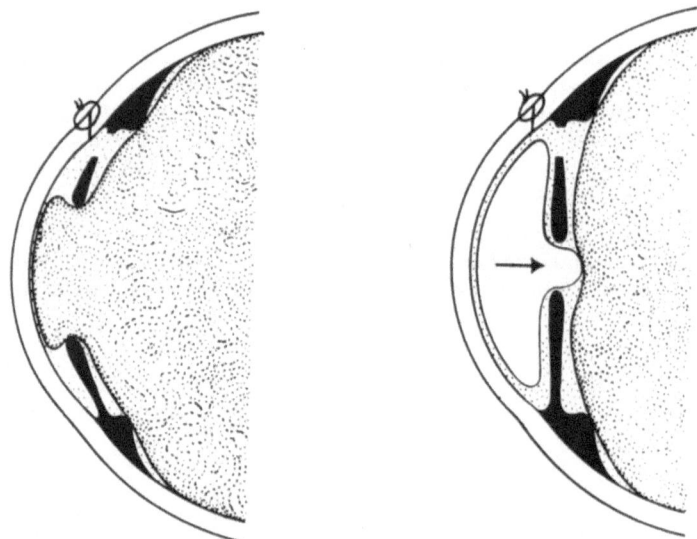

Fig. 28. Mushroom of vitreous interfering with constriction of the pupil.

Fig. 29. Air injected into the anterior chamber pushes the vitreous back and allows the pupil to contract.

aqueous humor. It is of great importance that the solutions which are used for irrigation of the anterior chamber should be isotonic and without impurities which could cause important alterations of the corneal endothelium and the iris.

In special cases the use of a Flieringa ring and osmotherapy are very useful. Our technique has changed very little during the last 20 years.

122

Docum. Ophthal. Proc. Series, Vol. 21

DIRECTIONS FOR THE USE OF ALPHA-CHYMOTRYPSIN IN ENZYMATIC ZONULOLYSIS.

J. TEMPRANO

(Barcelona, Spain)

Alpha-chymotrypsin is a proteolytic enzyme that attacks the very close linkages of aromatic amino-acids (phenylalanine, thyroxine, tryptophan, norleucine and norvaline).

Injected in the posterior chamber of the eye, its fibrinolytic and proteolytic action affects selectively the zonule and causes its lysis.

It is obtained from bovine pancreas through activation of chymotrypsinogen by means of trypsin, and is purified until crystallisation after dialysation and lyophilyzation.

When using it as an agent for chemical zonulolysis to facilitate lens

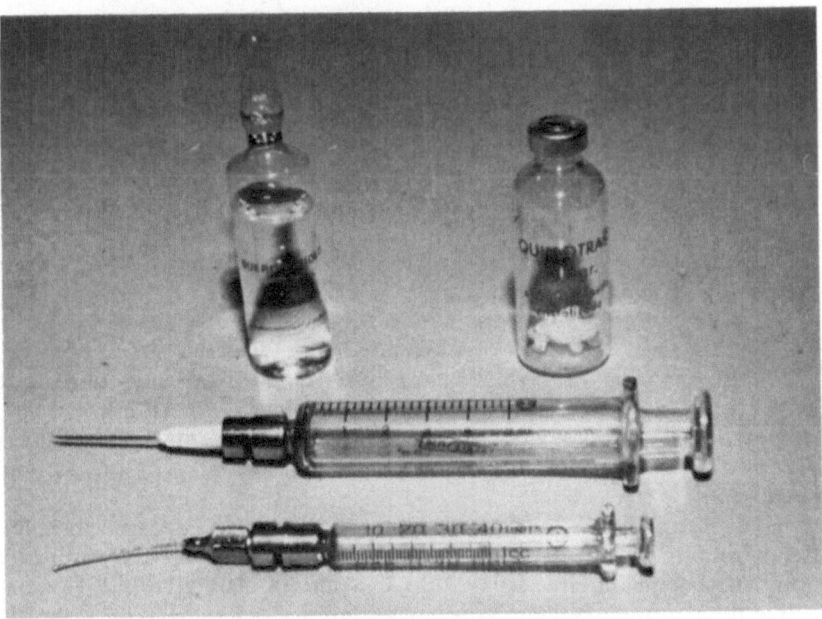

Fig. 1. Lyophilyzed alpha-chymotrypsin and balanced salt solution, with the syringe for preparation of the solution and the syringe for use with the olive-shaped cannula.

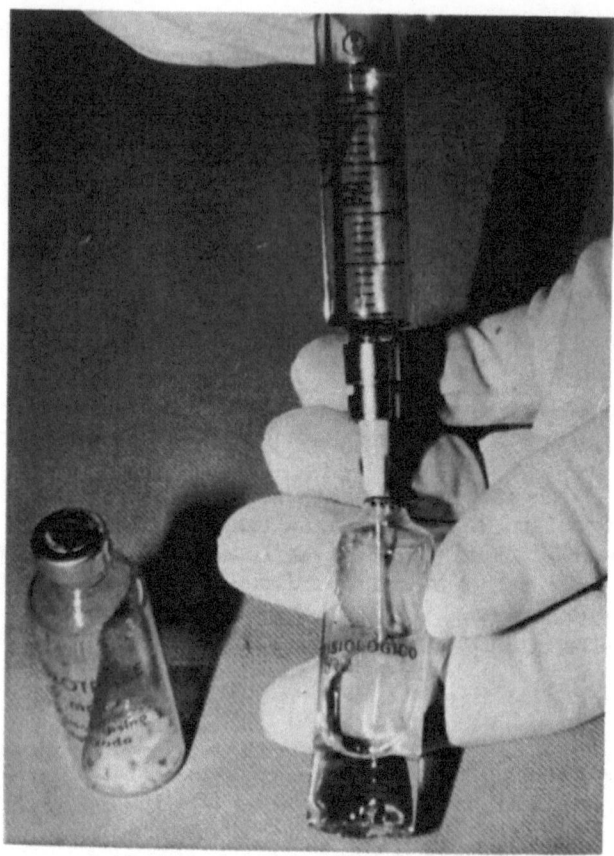

Fig. 2. Aspiration of 5 ccm balanced salt solution with the syringe.

extraction, we must keep in mind some fundamental factors which we are going to outline hereafter.

The commercial product is supplied as a crystalline powder and a diluent in form of a vial with balanced salt solution. Due to its thermolability, it must be protected against heat and also against humidity until the moment of preparing the solution, in order to preserve its effectiveness.

When preparing the solution, we must use syringes and cannulae that have been sterilized by means of dry heat and have not been in contact with alcohol or detergents which — besides affecting the corneal endothelium — would inactivate the ferment; throw-away syringes may be the preferable choice.

The solution must be fresh and should be prepared in each instance at the beginning of the surgical session, because the dissolved product will otherwise become ineffective (within 3 to 6 hours after dilution).

On the contrary, calcium salts enhance its activity by increasing the stability of the ferment, thus increasing likewise the time of action within the eye and causing delayed wound healing, wherefore we must always use balanced

124

salt solution or artifical aqueous humour to prepare the solution.

As temperature, too, acts upon alpha-chymotrypsin enhancing its zonulolytic activity while reducing its stability, we must avoid the use of material (syringes, etc.) at temperatures above 37° Celsius when preparing the solution.

The actual preparation is done using a syringe with a perforating needle, aspirating 5 ccm of balanced salt solution or artifical queous humour and introducing it into the vial that contains 5 mgm of the lyophilyzed product.

With the same syringe, we then aspirate again 4 ccm of balanced salt solution and 1 ccm of the alpha-chymotrypsin solution, thus obtaining a concentration of 1/5000 which is best for zonulolysis without causing corneal alterations, delayed wound healing or dispersion of iris pigment.

One of the most important details to be kept in mind for prevention of complications is the purity of the product; only alphachymotrypsin of great

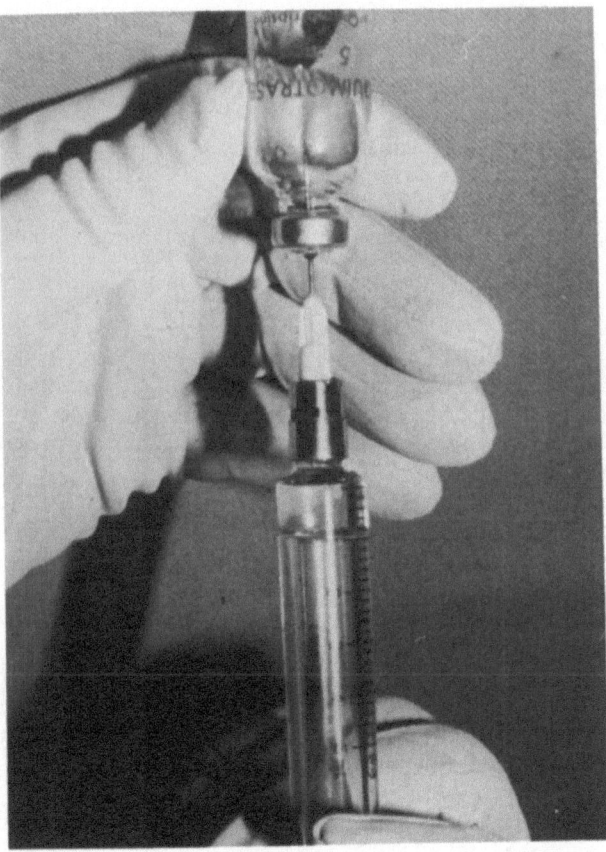

Fig. 3. Injection of the balanced salt solution into the vial with lyophilyzed alpha-chymotrypsin.

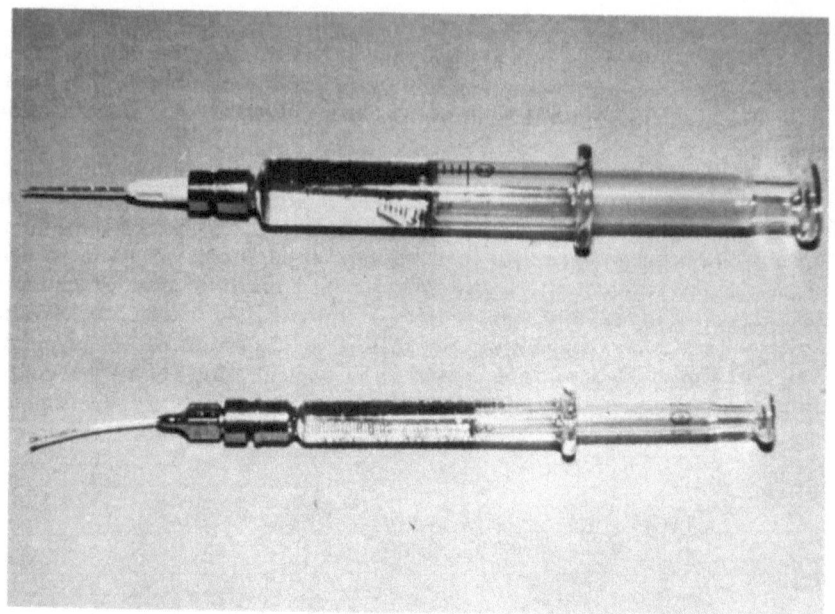

Fig. 4. Both syringes with the solution ready for use.

purity should be used. Nowadays, trustworthy commercial preparations are available in all countries.

SURGICAL TECHNIQUE

In addition to adequate preparation of the solution, at the moment of using it there are further details that require attention in order to obtain the maximum benefit of the advantages of zonulolysis and to prevent possible complications.

1. Corneoscleral conjunctival incision in two planes, which has the advantage that the more posteriorly placed incision thus obtained favours wound healing (avoiding delays in re-formation of the anterior chamber), a feature which is moreover enhanced by the conjunctival flap.

2. The scleral incision implies the need to cauterize the bleeding spots — which are visualized by irrigation with artificial aqueous humour — to avoid formation of blood clots in the anterior chamber which by incorporation of the alpha-chymotrypsin would increase the duration of its activity.

3. A peripheral iridectomy is then performed at the 12 o'clock meridian, to facilitate the passage of aqueous humour from the posterior to the anterior chamber and to prevent pupil block.

4. A corneoscleral suture is placed — but not tied — at the 12 o'clock meridian and its ends are hooked aside.

5. The 1/5000 solution of alpha-chymotrypsin is then applied:

   a. A precision syringe is used, making sure that the plunger is gliding

126

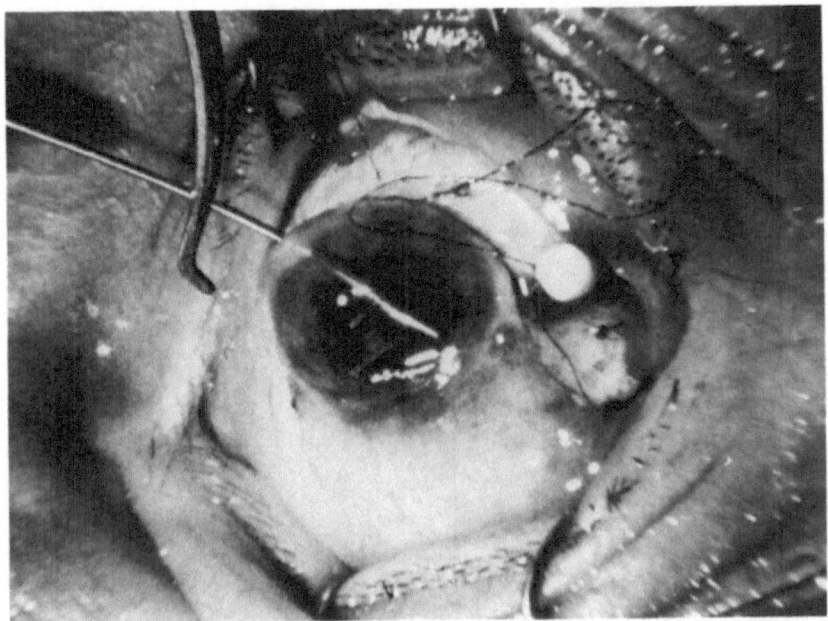

Fig. 5. The preplaced suture is visible, while the hold on the olive-shaped cannula with the forceps improves fixation.

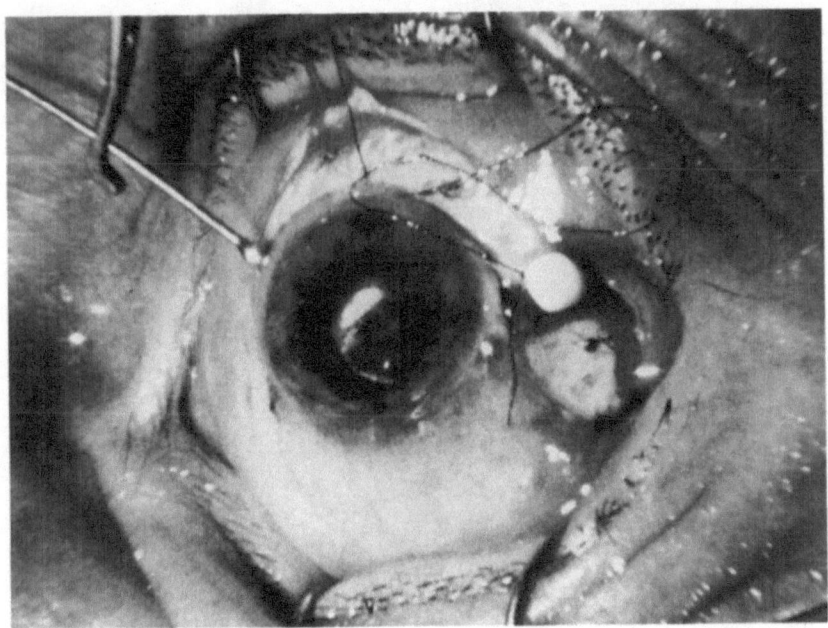

Fig. 6. Irrigation of the lower quadrants through the pupil.

127

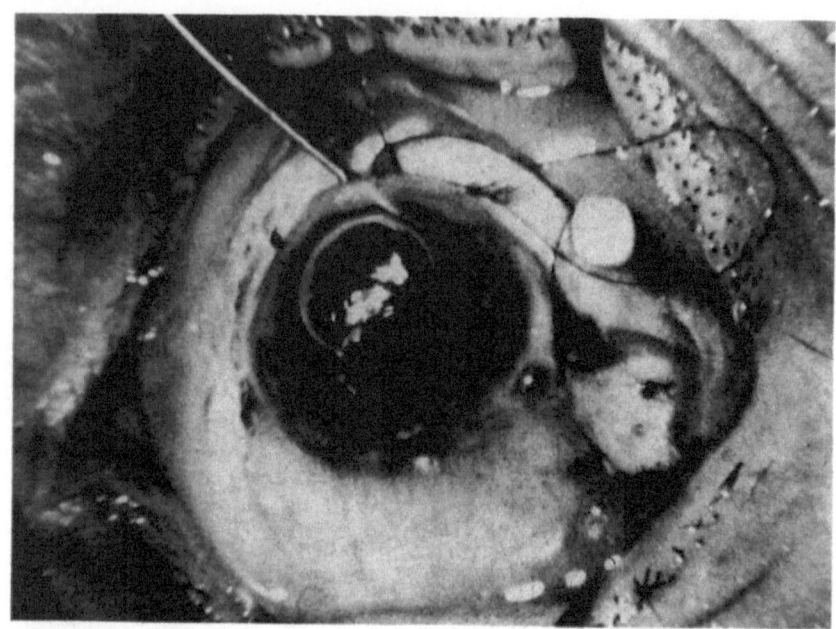

Fig. 7. Irrigation of the upper quadrants through the peripheral iridectomy.

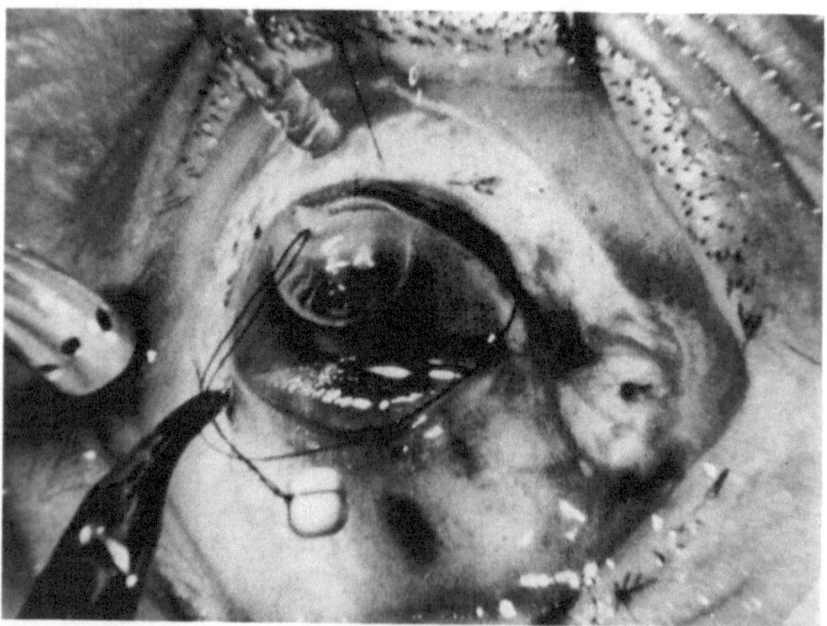

Fig. 8. Gentle but abundant perfusion of the anterior chamber with artificial aqueous humour to wash away the residues of the ferment.

128

very smoothly to avoid any abruptness and traumatism during the injection. This syringe is fixed to a cannula with an olive-shaped ending — thus avoiding traumatism of the pigment layer of the iris — and outflow orifice underneath so that the alpha-chymotrypsin solution can be applied directly to the zonule.

b. When introducing the cannula into the anterior chamber, we hold it with a forceps for a better control of movements to avoid damage of endothelium, iris or crystalline lens.

c. The cannula is introduced between the iris and the lens, and directed into the posterior chamber, with a slight downward pressure on the lens to protect the anterior crystalloid when irrigating the zonule.

d. 0,5 ccm of the alpha-chymotrypsin solution are injected through the pupil to act on the lower half of the zonule, and through the peripheral iridectomy to act on the upper half, taking care not to tear it with this manoeuvre, and verifying thus its permeability at the same time.

6. To wash away any possible excess of alpha-chymotrypsin from the area of the corneoscleral incision, we close the anterior chamber with a forceps and perfuse the lips of the wound with balanced salt solution or artificial aqueous humour.

7. In adult cataract patients, we permit the alpha-chymotrypsin solution to act during two minutes; in young patients — and also whenever we suspect or have verified that the zonule is very resistent — irrigation with the same solution can be repeated for another two minutes. The anterior chamber is then gently washed out with artificial aqueous humour, to expel any remaining ferment.

8. The cataract is removed by the usual method of the surgeon's choice (erysophake, cryostylet, forceps or expression) and the preplaced suture is tied.

9. Using a cannula, we irrigate the anterior chamber with 1/10.000 acetylcholine to contract the pupil and to expel the very last residues of alpha-chymotrypsin that might still be present.

10. We then inject air for diagnostic purposes, to make sure that there is no vitreous, and coapt the corneo-scleral wound with 7 additional sutures. Finally, the air bubble is replaced by artificial aqueous humour and with the anterior chamber of normal depth, we then suture the conjunctival flap.

With this technique and adequate care in the preparation of the alpha-chymotrypsin solution, the incidence of complications which we have met is not higher than in those cases in which the ferment was not used, while its use greatly facilitates cataract extraction.

SUMMARY

1. Only completely pure alpha-chymotrypsin must be used.
2. Make a 1:5000 dilution, using a fresh sterile (throw-away) syringe.
3. The solution should be used no more than 2 hours after it has been prepared, to prevent it inactivating.
4. Introduce the solution into the anterior chamber, between the iris and the crystalline lens, using a cannula fitted onto a syringe.

5. Place 0,5 ccm in the lower half of the zonule, and through the peripheral iridectomy, and leave to activate for two minutes.

6. Finally, thoroughly wash the anterior chamber with artificial physiological solution, before extracting the crystalline lens, and again with the same solution or acetylcholine in 1:10.000, after extraction and once you have tied the 12 hour starting point of the suturing.

Authors's address:
Instituto Barraquer
Laforja 88
Barcelona 6
Spain

Docum. Ophthal. Proc. Series, Vol. 21

PHACOEMULSIFICATION TECHNIQUE – SPECIAL CONSIDERATIONS

CHARLES D. KELMAN

(New York, U.S.A.)

Other papers have adequately covered the basic principles of emulsification. This paper will deal with the technique as related to avoidance of complications during surgery.

ANESTHESIA

The first cases of emulsification performed should be done under general anesthesia. These cases may take the surgeon slightly longer to do and hopefully the surgeon will be assisted by someone with experience with the technique. Under these circumstances, general anesthesia is advisable. Once the surgeon has totally mastered the technique, local anesthesia is, in my opinion, preferable.

Position of surgeon

The surgeon can not sit directly at the head of the operating table. It is important that his right hand (if he is right-handed) be in a comfortable position. This can only be achieved if the surgeon sits somewhat to the left side of the patient, with the corner of the operating table between his knees. This places his right hand approximately in the 11 o'clock position for the incision. If the eye to be operated on is the right eye, this places the incision away from the highest point of the brow and is ideal. On the left eye, the surgeon must sit even more to the left of the patient so that the phacoemulsifier doesn't have to pass over the highest part of the brow. If the patient has a deep-set eye, the incision should be placed more laterally. Trying to place the emulsifier in the deep set eye in the 12 o'clock position is an almost certain way to burn the cornea at the sight of the incision.

WILLINGNESS TO CONVERT

Most of the serious complications such as loss of the lens in the vitreous, vitreous loss, etc. are due to the surgeon's unwillingness to convert the procedure to a planned extracapsular extraction. The beginning surgeon should expect to convert about 50% of his early cases to a planned extracapsular case. The results of a planned extracapsular extraction are excellent and the surgeon should not fear enlarging the incision.

TWO-HAND SUPPORT

Especially in the surgeon's early experience with phacoemulsification, two hands should be used on any instrument which is placed inside the eye. With the emulsifier handpiece, for example, the right hand holds the emulsifier like a pencil, while the index finger of the left hand is placed close to the needle to stabilize the tip. The left hand index finger acts almost like a fulcrum but not quite; the true fulcrum is the incision. With experience, it is possible to use two instruments inside the eye, for example, the emulsifier and a spatula as described by Dr. Little and Dr. Kratz.

CONJUNCTIVAL FLAP

If the conjunctival flap is too large, it may fall down over the cornea during emulsification and prevent visualization in the anterior chamber. Too small a flap can tear. It should be (Fig. 1) approximately 4 mm at its base at the limbus with the sides of the triangle also 4 mm (Fig. 2). Tenon's capsule is incised with the scissor before dissection is made down to the limbus (Fig. 3). It is important to cut the flap down to the limbus on both sides. If this is not done, fluid escaping from the anterior chamber will dissect under the conjunctiva and cause a large chemosis. While this is not serious, it can affect visualization into the anterior chamber, and certainly leads to a more irritated eye.

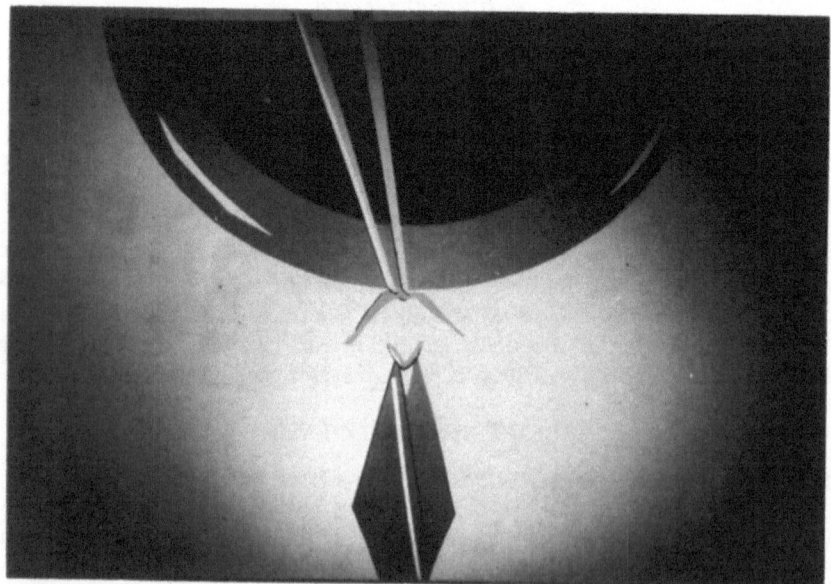

Fig. 1. Incision through conjunctiva

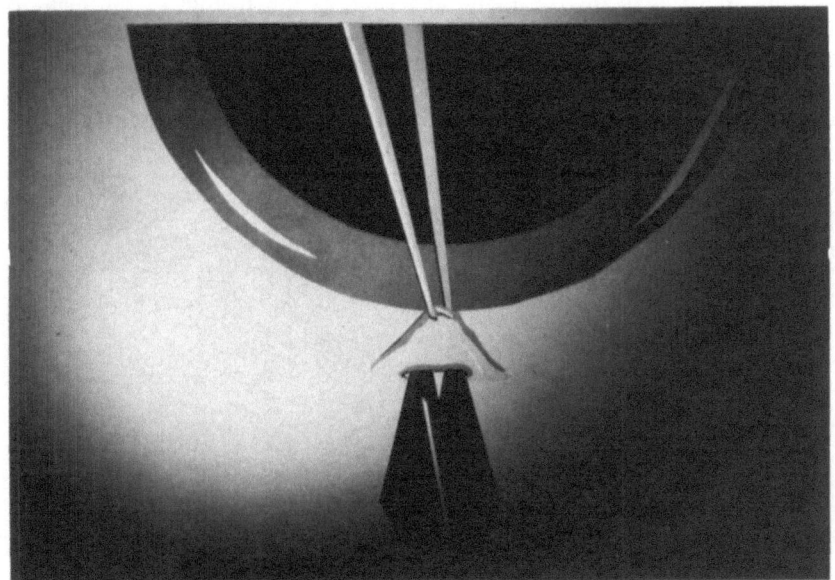

Fig. 2. Incision through Tenon's and spreading

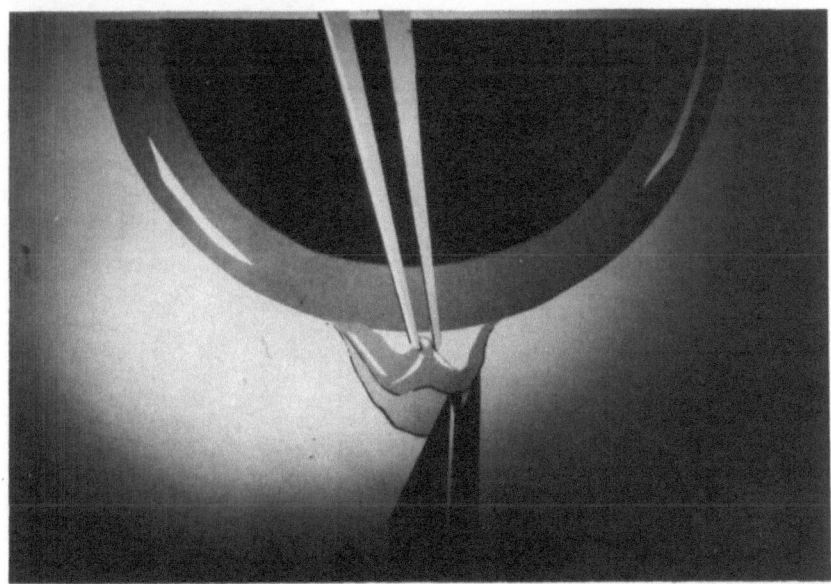

Fig. 3. Dissection of Tenon's and conjunctiva to limbus

CORNEAL-SCLERAL INCISION

It is important that the corneal scleral incision be one plane, shelved and almost parallel to the iris (Fig. 4). A sharp razor is pressed against the limbus with the sharp edge on the tissue and then as the handle of the blade is rotated to the left, the point of the blade enters the eye (Fig. 5). The incision is then enlarged with short sawing strokes to approximately 3 mm. If the incision is made too far posteriorly, the iris will prolapse through the incision during emulsification. Also, the iris will be caught by instruments

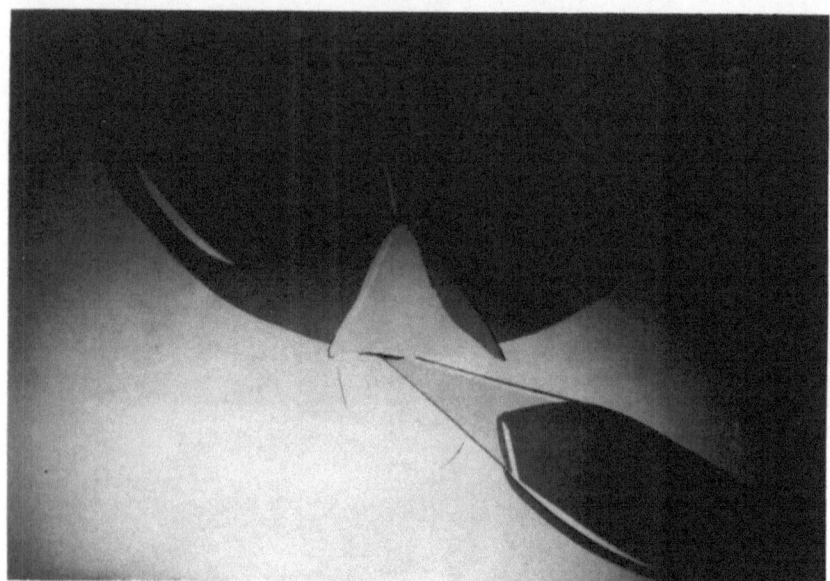

Fig. 4. Razor edge applied to limbus

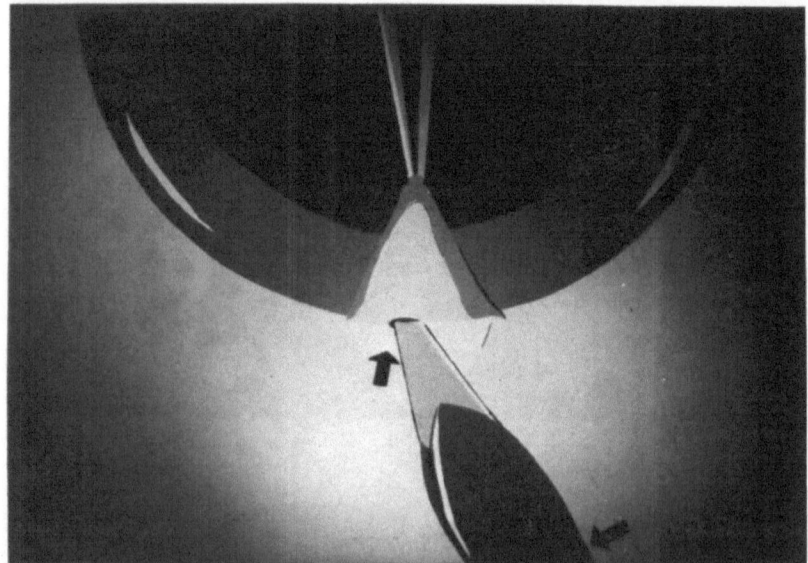

Fig. 5. Handle turned to penetrate

134

going into the eye and could be dialized. If the incision is too corneal, a disinsertion of Descemet's is possible. The incision should be made at the junction of the posterior third and the anterior two-thirds of the limbus.

ANTERIOR CAPSULOTOMY

The main principle in opening the anterior capsule is to get it open; widely open. It doesn't matter if the triangulation technique is used or the 'can-opener' technique is used as long as it is widely opened its periphery. Without this, the lens cannot be brought into the anterior chamber except with difficulty. The method I recommend for anterior capsulotomy is as follows: The cystotome is gently placed on the capsule 4 mm from the optical center of the lens (Fig. 6). The anterior capsule is gently engaged with the point of the irrigating cystotome so as not to perforate the capsule but merely to tend it (Fig. 7). The cystotome continues to be withdrawn toward the incision during which time the capsule opens in the form of a triangle (Fig. 8). This triangle is continued down toward the incision. Additional peripheral slits are made in the capsule (Fig. 9) to widely open it to allow for a maximum exposure of the anterior surface of the lens.

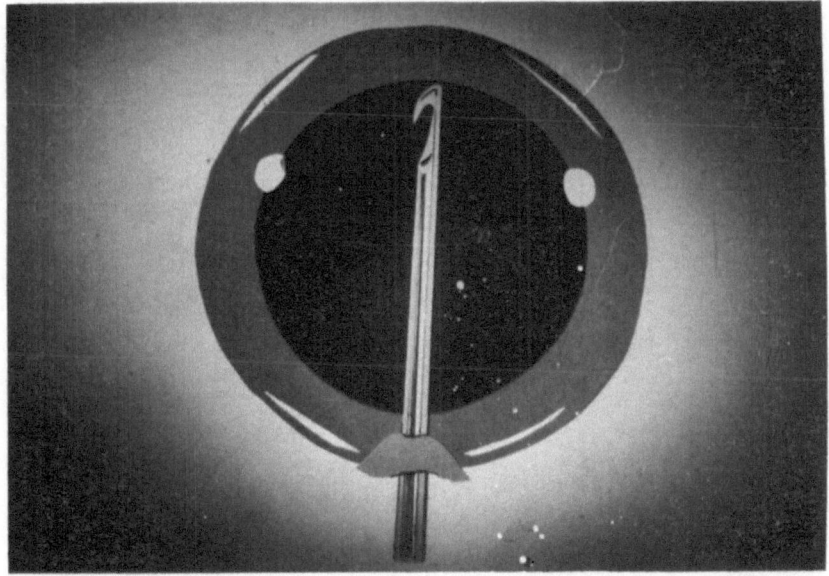

Fig. 6. Cystotome gently touches capsule

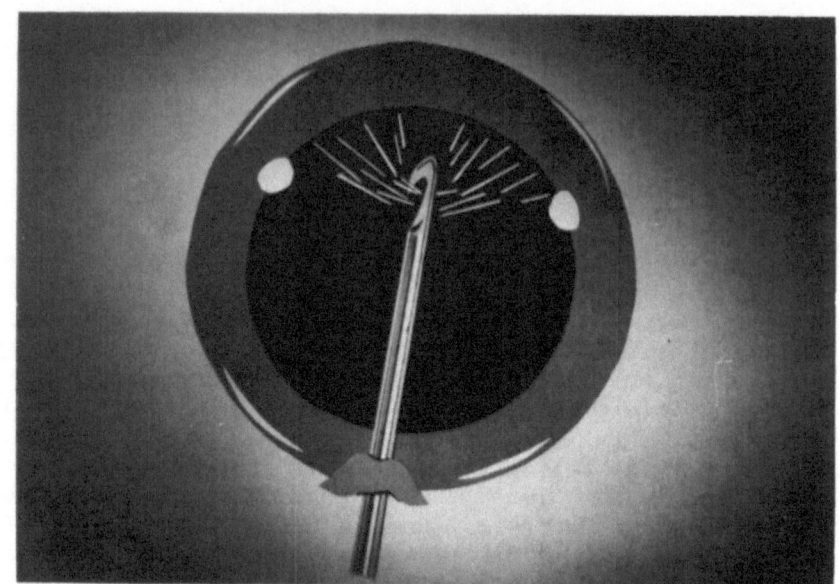

Fig. 7. Cystotome engages capsule with traction lines

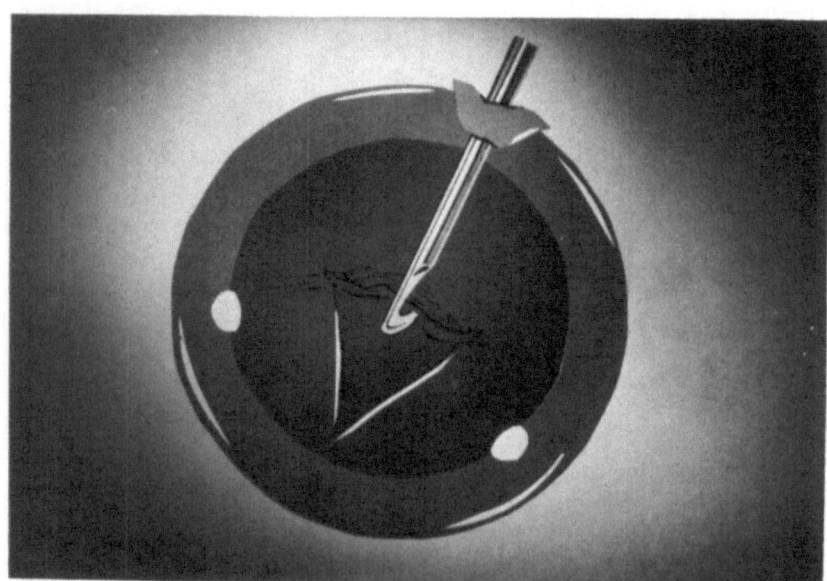

Fig. 8. Triangulation of capsule

136

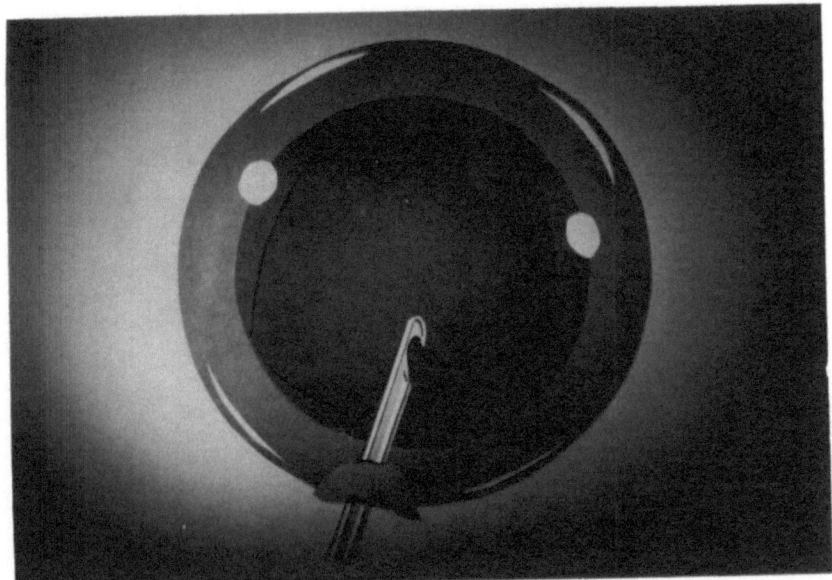

Fig. 9. Additional peripheral slits in capsule

PROLAPSE OF THE NUCLEUS

Bringing the lens into the anterior chamber is considered difficult by many beginning surgeons but actually it is easy if two factors are kept in mind. The pupil must be widely dilated and the anterior capsule must be widely opened. With these fundamentals provided for, prolapse of the lens is simple. The cystotome is placed on the nucleus and the lens withdrawn toward the incision (Fig. 10). The lens should be continued to be withdrawn toward the incision until the exposed pole is at the 3–9 o'clock position. The lens is then released with the cystotome, the cystotome is placed close to the incision (Fig. 11) and the lens is then pushed away from the incision bringing it over the iris below and out of the capsule above. Figure 12 shows the beginning of this maneuver called the 'see-saw' maneuver in cross-section. It shows how the lens is rocked out of the capsule below and then pushed away and out of the capsule above in Figure 13. A softer lens will not respond well to the vertical see-saw technique because the sharp point will just slice through the soft tissue. In this case a lateral see-saw technique (Fig. 14) is used. The principles are identical to the vertical see-saw except that the lens is moved laterally to the right and then once out of the capsule on the left side of the lens, the lens is moved to the left (Fig. 15).

The mistake that most surgeons make in prolapsing the lens is one of timidity. The pole of the lens must be brought to the midline. If this is not accomplished, the lens may well slip back into the capsular bag during which time the pupil is constricting. As the pupil further constricts, it becomes more and more difficult to bring the lens into the chamber. Another frequent mistake is that of not using the incision as a fulcrum. If

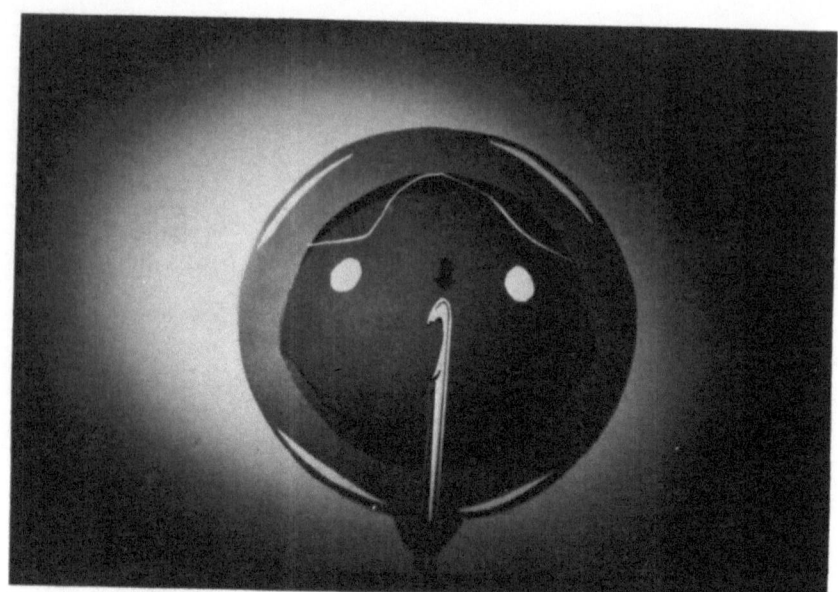

Fig. 10. Lens displaced toward incision

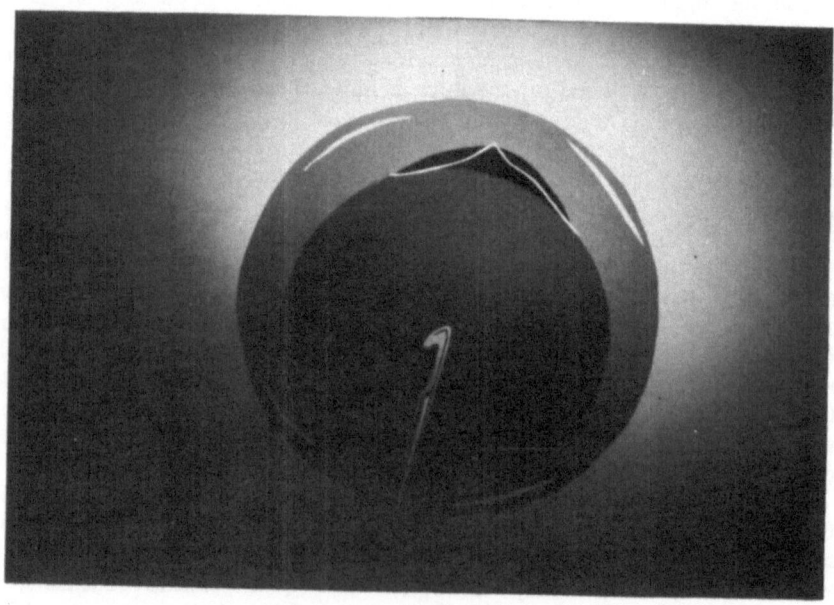

Fig. 11. Lens out of capsule inferiorly, now displaced away from incision

138

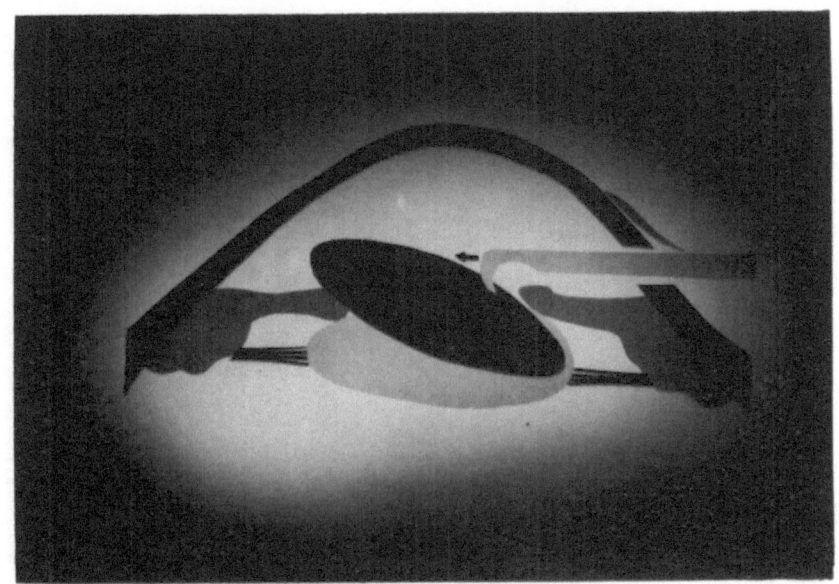

Fig. 12. Cross-section of see-saw maneuver

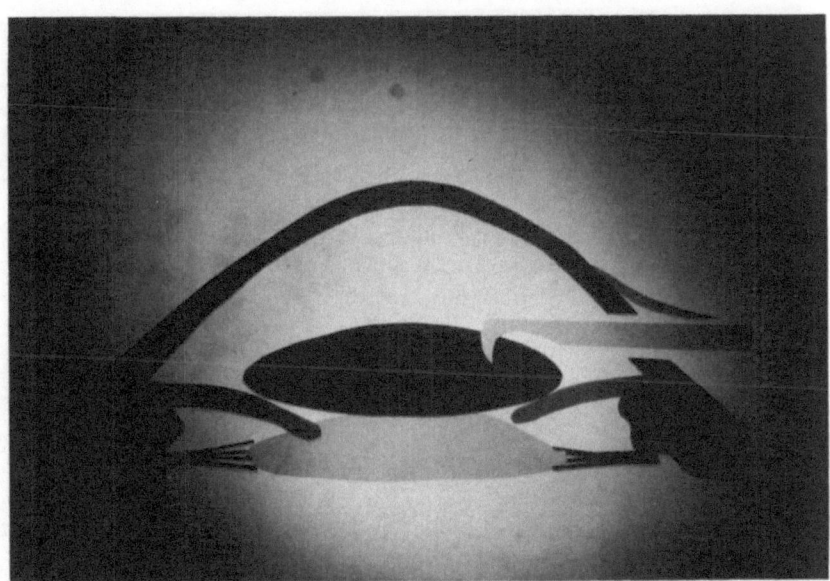

Fig. 13. Lens in anterior chamber

139

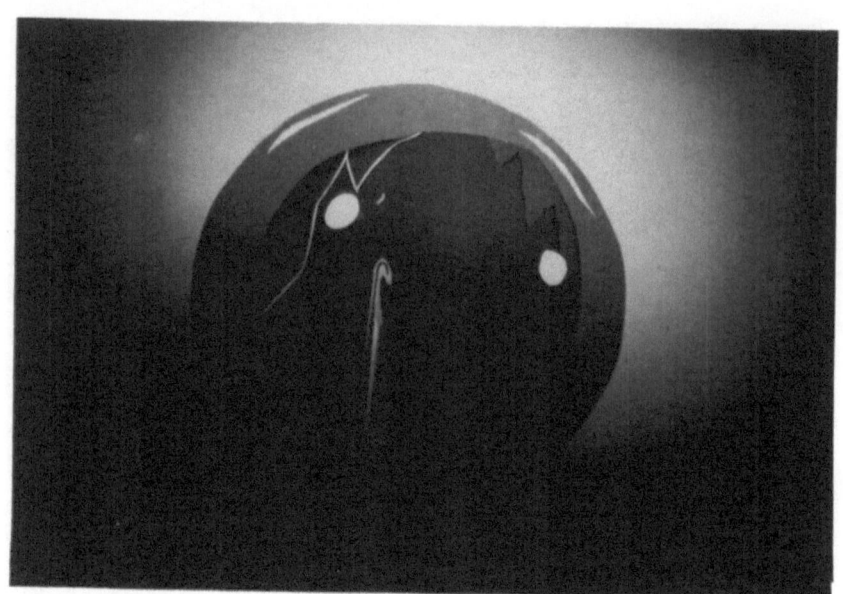

Fig. 14. Lateral see-saw first maneuver

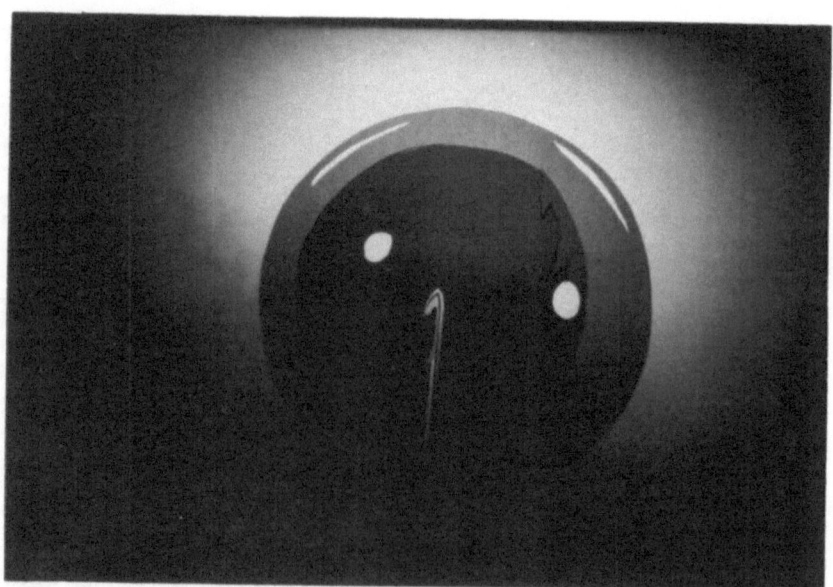

Fig. 15. Lateral see-saw second maneuver

140

the surgeon is moving the eye by pressing the cystotome against the incision while he is trying to manipulate the lens, all the force of the cystotome is transmitted to the incision and not the lens. In this case, the eye moves rather than the nucleus.

EMULSIFICATION OF THE LENS

With the lens in the anterior chamber, the emulsification of the lens is quite simple. The surgeon must learn not to press the lens against the endothelium but merely to touch the lens with the emulsifier tip allowing the lens to come into the tip. Care must be taken also not to press the lens against the posterior capsule and of course, not to touch the posterior capsule or the cornea with the vibrating tip. There are two basic approaches to emulsification of the lens. A) Carousel Technique: Here the lens is attacked from the periphery first leaving the nucleus until the end (Fig. 16). The edge of the lens is engaged and the lens slowly rotates into the emulsifier. Care must be taken with this maneuver not to let the lens rapidly spin as this spinning could remove endothelial cells. B) Croissant Technique: Here the nucleus is attacked first (Fig. 17), sculptured away and hollowed-out and then the peripheral cortical material is easily removed.

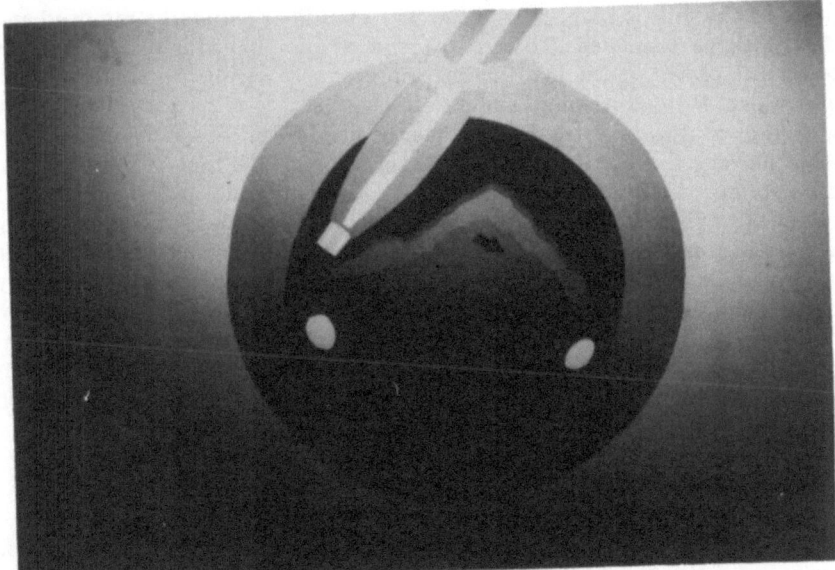

Fig. 16. Carousel technique of emulsification

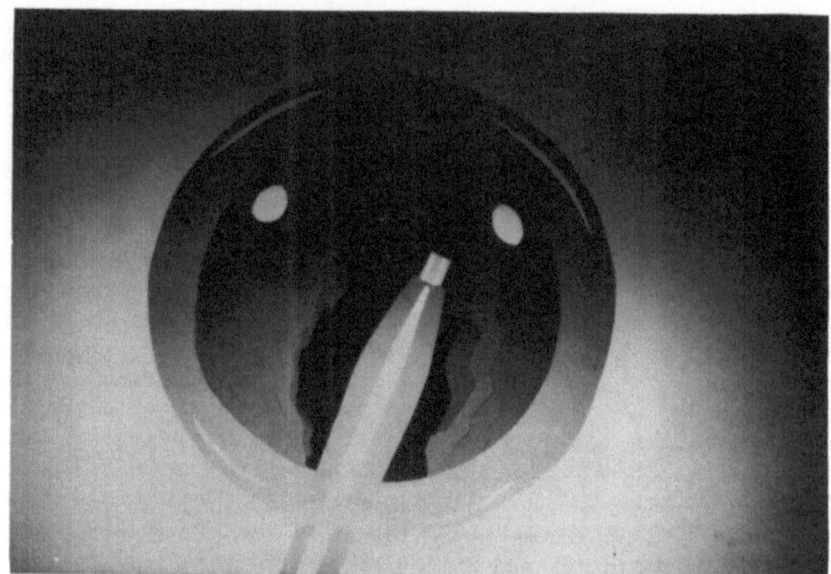

Fig. 17. Croissant technique of emulsification

All through the emulsification the surgeon should be aware of heat build-up. This can be readily seen by first an innocuous clouding in the anterior chamber. This cloudiness represents emulsified lens particles which have been freed but not aspirated. Since they were not aspirated, it means that a piece of the lens is plugging the tip. The emulsifier should be removed and the blockage remedied. Toward the end of the emulsification, one must lower the power of the instrument to prevent shattering of small lens parti-cles against the endothelium and also to avoid engaging the posterior capsule with the emulsifier. Vitreous loss must be handled in the following manner: A) If nucleus is present in the anterior chamber at the time of vitreous loss, the eye must be opened up to 180 degrees and the nucleus spooned out of the eye. At this time, a shallow anterior vitrectomy is performed, removing any cortical material as well. If only a small piece of nucleus is left when the vitreous face is ruptured, careful emulsification of the remaining pieces may be attempted without opening the eye. B) After the nucleus has been removed be sure all of the cortex has been removed: once the nucleus has been removed it is no longer necessary to open the eye if there is vitreous loss. A simple vitrectomy including any remaining cortical material will suffice to clear the eye and to give a good visual result.

ASPIRATION OF REMAINING CORTICAL MATERIAL

Using the irrigation/aspiration handpiece, the rest of the cortical material is easily removed. Care must be taken not to turn the lumen of the tip down to the posterior capsule since this might engage it (Fig. 18). If this does

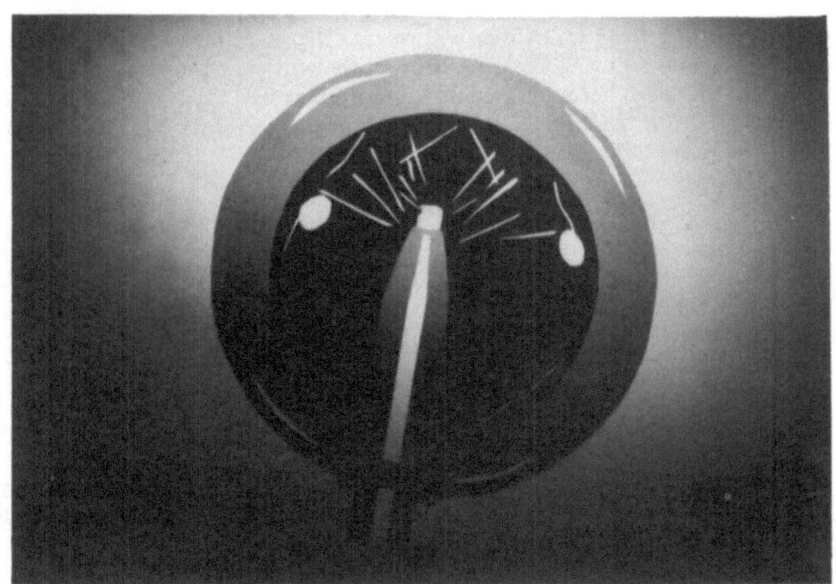

Fig. 18.   Posterior capsule engaged in irrigation/aspiration tip

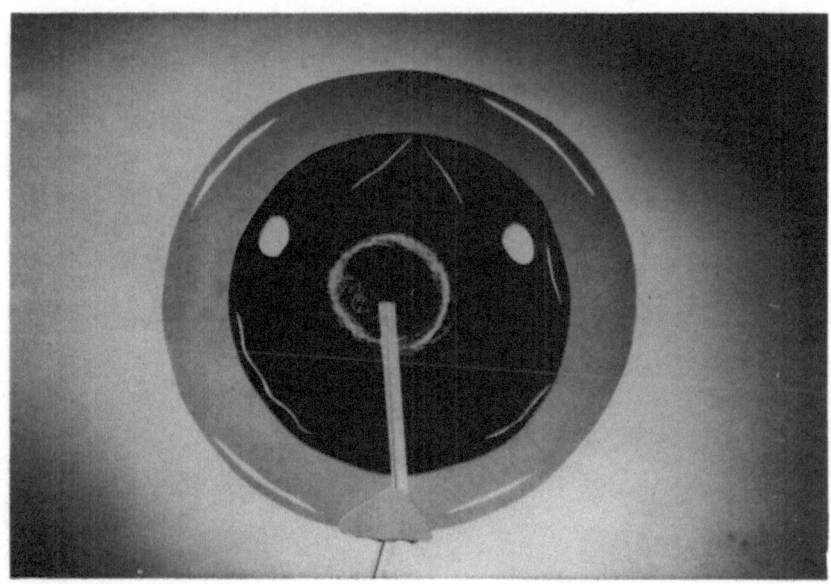

Fig. 19.   Halo around air injection needle

occur, releasing the foot switch will release the posterior capsule. The most common mistake during the aspiration of the cortical material is attempting to grasp the peripheral fragments of cortex rather than placing the irrigation/aspiration handpiece under the iris in the very fornix of the capsule to get the root of the material.

POSTERIOR CAPSULE

When a instrument is placed on the posterior capsule, a halo appears around the instrument (Fig. 19). This permits the surgeon to know when he is touching the posterior capsule so that he can clean off any remaining cells. These cells should be removed if possible, even if the posterior capsule is going to be opened since it will reduce fibrosis of the peripheral fragments of posterior capsule. After the incision is closed, a Ziegler knife is passed adjacent to the suture (Fig. 20) and the capsule is gently depressed with the knife. As the knife is swept to the side, the posterior capsule opens usually leaving the vitreous face intact (Fig. 21).

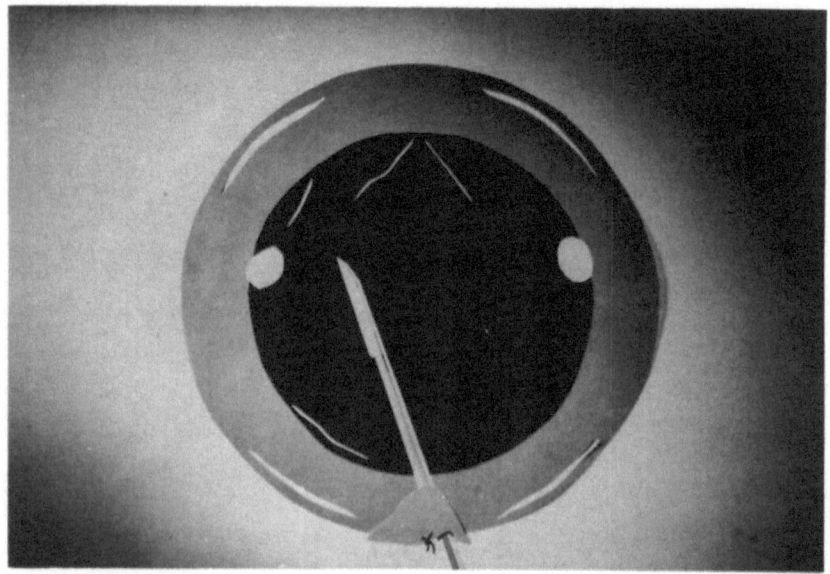

Fig. 20. Ziegler knife inserted

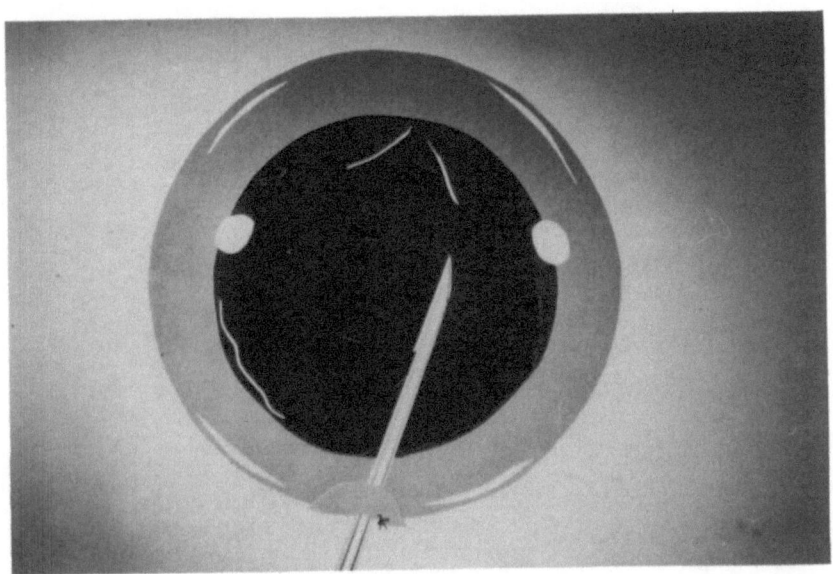

Fig. 21.   Posterior capsule opened

Author's Address:
150 East 58th Street
New York, N.Y. 10022
U.S.A.

PHACOEMULSIFICATION – INDICATIONS, CONTRA-INDICATIONS AND RESULTS

CHARLES D. KELMAN

(New York, U.S.A.)

INDICATIONS FOR PHACOEMULSIFICATION

According to Cleasby, the advantages of Phacoemulsification are as follows:
1) **Visual Advantages,** (a) Earlier rehabilitation. A small incision severs fewer corneal nerves than a large incision. Corneal anesthesia following phacoemulsification is therefore extremely limited, and a contact lens can safely be worn almost immediately post-operatively. In some cases, it is possible to place a hard contact lens on the eye immediately following the emulsification. If the patient has worn contact lenses prior to surgery, he'll have no difficulty accomodating the hard lens. Soft lenses can also be used immediately post-operatively, however, they require the use of post-operative medication without preservatives. In most cases, contact lenses are prescribed 2-3 weeks following the surgery. The refractive error stabilizes sooner because of the small incision, the cornea returns to its normal curvature usually in a matter of hours or days. (b) Less astigmatism. Where pre-operative k-readings have been taken in a large series of patients, the average induced astigmatism following phacoemulsification was 0.37 diopters. This is considerably less than the astigmatism generally reported using a larger incision.
2) **Physical Advantages** – (a) Earlier return to normal activities. Following the procedure no restrictions are imposed on the patient. Within hours of the operation, the patient is allowed all of his normal activities including working at his job, traveling, etc. without a shield or a patch being required. (b) Less physical deterioration from inactivity. The well-known fatigue following hospitalization is absent with this procedure since the patient is performed under local anesthesia, the patient can walk back to his room and immediately be ambulatory. (c) Less discomfort. There is usually little irritation from the one suture covered by a small conjunctival flap. (d) Less redness and swelling. Because of a lack of trauma to the conjunctiva and cornea, the eyes are relatively quiet without lid edema.
3) **Safety** – (a) Less danger from post-operative trauma. Because of the shelved incision and because of its size, even a severe blow to the eye will not generally cause loss of the anterior chamber. (b) Less danger from and earlier performance of postoperative diagnostic procedures, e.g. gonioscopy, scleral indentation, and ophthalmodynamometry. (c) Less danger from and earlier performance of post-operative surgery, e.g., retinal reattachment, photocoagulation, and posterior vitrectomy. (d) Earlier and better post-ope-

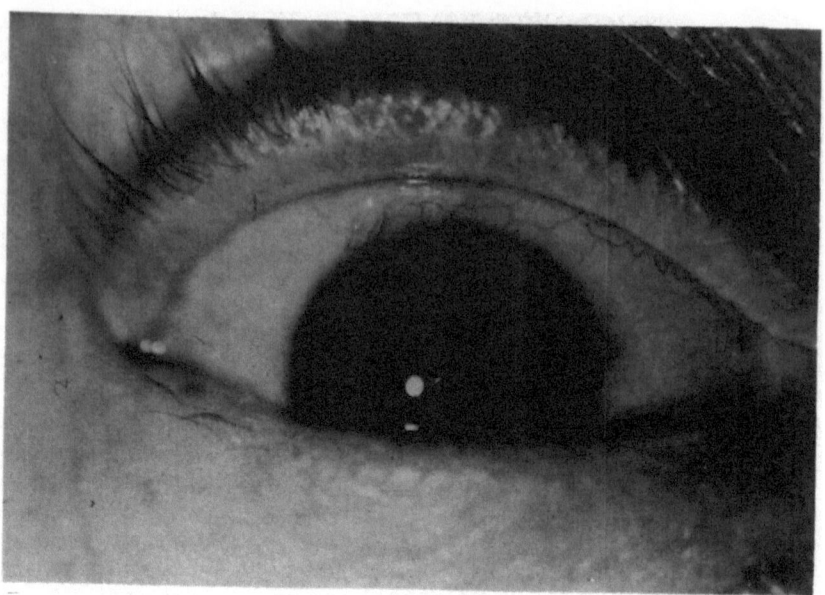

Fig. 1.

rative fundus view than obtained with standard intracapsular surgery since the intraocular pressure returns to normal sooner. (e) Much safer in the presence of diseases associated with poor healing, e.g., trachoma, rheumatoid arthritis, malnutrition and diabetes. (f) Reduced operative complications. (g) Vitreous disruption or 'loss' is easier to correct and to obtain a wound free of strands. (h) Bleeding – lesser incidence and magnitude of bleeding from the wound and elsewhere, including expulsive choroidal hemmorhage. (i) Definitely lesser incidence of flat anterior chamber, iris prolapse, wound separation, vitreous touch, updrawn pupil and hyphema. (j) Probably lesser incidence of cystoid macular edema, pupillary block, hypotony, infection, and retinal detachment.

4) **Versatility** – (a) Easier and safer lens removal in posterior vitrectomy, and penetrating keratoplasty. (b) Easier and more effective correction of postoperative astigmatism by suture manipulation. (c) With intraocular lenses – phacoemulsification may prove to be the technique of choice in many cases.

5) **Financial Advantages** – (a) Immediate return to work is possible if circumstances and the condition of the other eye permit. (b) In general, less hospitalization. (c) Fewer changes in correction. (d) Fewer post-operative visits with resultant decrease in the amount of time away from work and travel expense. (e) Reduction of expense for organizations and agencies providing disability benefits.

CONTRA-INDICATIONS TO PHACOEMULSIFICATION

1) **Brunescent cataracts.** Although theoretically, any cataract no matter how brunescent can be emulsified, the amount of time it would take (5–10

minutes) makes it much more expedient to do a planned extra-capsular extraction through a 100—110 degree incision. The harder the lens the more potential damage is possible to the corneal endothelium. Some might prefer to do a brunescent with emulsification in the posterior chamber. 2) **Dislocated of subluxated cataract** in the patient over 40 years. In the child or young adult, the lens is soft enough to perform an emulsification intracapsularly, that is to say within the capsular sack. This allows the lens to be aspirated without mixing lens material with vitreous. In older patients, the lens is too firm-it would be further subluxated and possibly dislocated due to the motion of the tip against the hard nucleus. The procedure of choice in a subluxated or dislocated due to the motion of the tip against the hard nucleus. The procedure of choice in a subluxated or dislocated lens in a patient over the age of 40 is usually an intracapsular cataract extraction. 3) **Shallow anterior** chamber. A shallow chamber is usually associated with difficulty in prolapsing the nucleus in the anterior chamber. Even if the nucleus can be brought into the chamber, there is little room to maneuver the emulsifier tip. 4) **Miotic pupil**. Except in the hands of a very experienced surgeon, a miotic pupil is a contra-indication. It is impossible to bring the lens into the anterior chamber and a posterior chamber emulsification cannot be done since the surgeon cannot visualize most of the lens. The surgeon having sufficient experience can do a sphicterotomy, then bring the lens into the anterior chamber, emulsify it, and finally re-suture the iris with 10—0 nylon. 5) **Endothelial disease**. This is a relative contra-indication. An experienced surgeon can emulsify a fairly soft lens and have no difficulty even in the face of endothelial disease. A harder lens will certainly cause endothelial damage if the emulsification is performed in the anterior chamber. Some surgeons prefer to do emulsification in the posterior chamber in the face of endothelial disease, provided the pupil is widely dilated. 6) **Non transparent cornea**. When the surgeon cannot see into the anterior chamber through the cornea, emulsification is contra-indicated. 7) **Age of patient vs. experience of surgeon**. The older patient, the less his cornea will tolerate the experience of the surgeon. An experienced surgeon will generally be more careful of the endothelium where a beginner is apt to brush the lens against this delicate layer. Naturally, the harder the lens, and the older the patient, the more experience is required on the part of the surgeon.

SPECIAL INDICATIONS FOR PHACOEMULSIFICATION

1) **High induced astigmatism** in first eye with intracapsular extraction. 2) **Retinal detachment** in the first eye with intracapsular extraction. 3) Retinal detachment in cataractous eye. 4) CME in first eye with intracapsular extraction. 5) Congenital cataracts. 6) Young adult cataract. 7) Traumatic cataracts with ruptured capsules. 8) Super-active individuals to prevent endophthalmodonesis. 9) Medical conditions — (a) Bleeding, (b) Poor healing such as diabetes, rheumatoid arthritis. (c) Psychoses.

WHY PHACOEMULSIFICATION IS
'DIFFICULT' TO PERFORM

In fact, phacoemulsification is quite easy to perform. Learning **how** to do it is what's difficult. Once the technique is mastered, it can be performed with ease and with great speed. It is difficult to learn for the following reasons: 1) Margin for error and variation is small whereas with the standard intracapsular extraction the surgeon is permitted great latitude regarding all steps of the procedure, but with phacoemulsification, there is practically no latitude. With intracapsular surgery the incision can be shelved or vertical, it can be slightly too large, or slightly too small, it can be slightly too far corneal or slightly too scleral, the cyro-probe can be placed almost anywhere on the lens, etc, etc. With phacoemulsification, each step of the procedure is much more critical. If the incision is one millimeter too large, there will be excessive leakage of irrigating fluid and the chamber may collapse. If the incision is one millimeter too small, there will not be sufficient irrigation going into the chamber due to constriction of the silicone sleeve. In every step of the emulsification, this narrow margin of error and variation is apparent. If the capsulotomy is one millimeter too narrow, the surgeon will have great difficulty in prolapsing the lens. If the phacoemulsifier is placed one millimeter too close to the iris, the iris may be aspirated to the tip through the small localized area of atrophy. Every step of the way demands the most minute concentration on the details of the operation. Once these details are learned and are part of the surgeon's routine, and only then does the operation become facile. 2) Prior surgical experience of little value. Except for the iridectomy, none of the maneuvers in phacoemulsification are familiar to the surgeon. The delicate placement of the

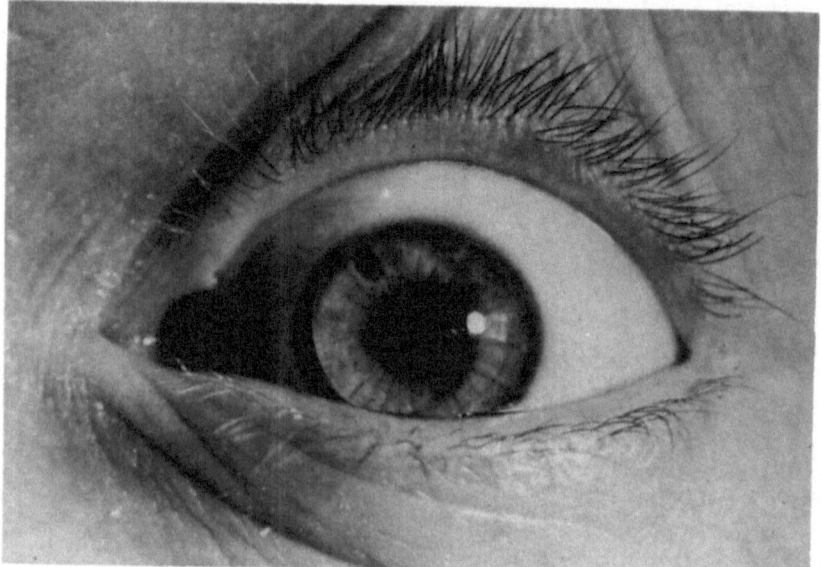

Fig. 2.

150

cystotome on the anterior capsule so as to tent rather then to tear is new to him. The technique of prolapsing the lens in the chamber using the incision as the focum is new to him. The gentle motion of the emulsifier against the nucleus without pressing that nucleus against the endothelium is new to him. All through the operation, new skills are required which do not spring from any prior training the surgeon has had. 3) Surgeon's awareness of equipment is imperative. In the operating room, the surgeon must be the captain of the ship. He must know the equipment better than the technician so that he can sense malfunction or an improper connection before anyone else. This requires an intimate knowledge of the principles or irrigation/ aspiration and emulsification and a complete familiarity with the equipment. Any less than this places the surgeon at the mercy of the technician or nurse who is assisting him. 4) Prior expertise with the microscope is essential. Trying to learn phacoemulsification while at the same time becoming familiar with the operating microscope is like learning to drive a car and write your name at the same time. The surgeon should be adept with the operating microscope before undertaking phacoemulsification. 5) Controversy places the surgeon under added pressure. Because there is and will be for some time a certain amount of controversy about phacoemulsification the surgeon, especially the beginning surgeon may be faced with resistance from his peers. Being well-trained and extremely knowledgable about the technique alleviates this condition considerably. 6) Additional time required in the operating room in first cases. In the beginning it will take longer to do phacoemulsification than an intracapsular extraction. With experience, this is reversed. Most surgeons who are highly skilled with emulsification can do two, three, or sometimes four cases in one hour. 7) Ego problem. It is important for the surgeon to realize that in his first cases, he may have to convert some of them to a larger incision planned extracapsular extraction. If the pupil constricts quickly, and the surgeon cannot bring the lens into the anterior chamber, if the patient becomes restless, etc, the surgeon must be willing to forego an emulsification and to enlarge the incision. Some surgeons take this as a sign of incompetence with the technique, while in fact, it is exactly the opposite. The experienced surgeon realizes that a planned extracapsular extraction is an excellent procedure and when conditions are not perfect for a phacoemulsification will readily convert saving himself and possibly the patient a great deal of discomfort.

RESULTS OF PHACOEMULSIFICATION

1) **Visual Results.** In the cataract survey of the Cataract Phacoemulsification Committee by Richard C. Troutman, M.D., et al, published in the transactions of the American Academy of Ophthalmology and Otolaryngology, January-February, 1975, it was concluded that extracapsular cataract surgery done by phacoemulsification is, at one year follow-up level, in all probability, as effective in restoring vision after cataract as our currently practiced intracapsular techniques, but certainly no more so ... Those of you who wish to may cautiously adopt extracapsular technique, realizing that there are instances where it is particularly to be recommended. 2) **Com-**

plications of phacoemulsification. This paper will deal with the most important complications of cataract surgery, i.e., retinal detachment and macular edema. The other complications such as iris prolapse, wound dehiscence, infection, etc. are really so minimal with this procedure, that they will not be dealt with here.

For the purpose of this presentation 1000 consecutive cases of phacoemulsification were examined. These patients had a minimum follow-up of 1.5 years with a maximum follow-up of 3 years. Of the 1000 charts examined, 819 were included in this study. 181 charts belonged to patients referred from out of town where there was no adequate follow-up. None of these 181 patients when examined in the office following emulsification had any post-operative problems at that time. Only local patients which we could follow or referred patients with adequate follow-up from the referring physician noted on our charts are included. The average age of these patients was 59 years. This average age is low because other cataract surveys, since an unusual high number of congenital and young adult cataracts were included in this study. In most other cataract surveys, only senile cataracts were included. Since congenital juvenile and young adult patients usually have more complications post-operatively than the garden-variety senile cataract, it would tend to weigh the results of this study unfavorably regarding phacoemulsification. If these young patients were eliminated from this study, the statistical analysis would have proven even more favorable to emulsification. a) Retinal detachments. There were 13 detachments in the group. One patient was a Marfan's, who had had a detachment on the first eye following an attempted intracapsular extraction.

The second eye of this patient was operated on because the intraocular pressure was high, the vision was extremely poor and I anticipated a good result with a careful emulsification and aspiration. A detachment ensued in this eye, leaving me with a feeling of dispair regarding the removal of lenses in Marfan's patients by any technique. One detachment, although not proven by ultrasonigraphy was probably pre-existing to the extraction. Both of these patients were included in this series of complications. The average age of the 13 detachment patients was 53 years, 6 years younger than the average age of all of the charts examined. The incidence of retinal detachment despite these two cases being included and in spite of the young age group of the patients was only 1.58%. In a recent paper by Montague Ruben, M.D., et al in the British Journal of Ophthalmology 1976, 944 consecutive intracapsular cataract patients were evaluated. The average age in his group was considerably older, 65, since he had eliminated any patients in the younger age group, ie the higher risk patients. The total incidence of aphakic detachment in Dr. Ruben's series was 5.7% on intracapsular cataract extractions. Two-thirds of the detachments in his series occured in the first year and most of the other detachments occured in the subsequent year. Clearly a much higher incidence of retinal detachment following intracapsular surgery than with phacoemulsification. Of the 13 detachments, 9 patients had posterior capsulotomies, and 4 had intact posterior capsules. At first glance, this might seem to indicate that there is twice as much chance of a patient with a posterior capsulotomy to have a detachment. This is not so. More than twice as many of the patients in this series had posterior capsulotomies than those who did not. One would therefore suspect to have more detachments in the posterior capsulotomy group. This would indicate that although the incidence of retinal detachment is significantly reduced with Phacoemulsification, it makes no difference whether the central capsule has been opened or not. This is entirely consistant with my feeling that the advantage of the extracapsular surgery lies in the support of the base of the vitreous by the peripheral capsule. Ruben, moreover, quotes Shapland in a study conducted in 1934 of the incidence of retinal detachment following extracapsular extraction (In 1934!) the incidence was only 2.2%. It is also interesting to note that of the retinal detachments, 38% were cases of -5 diopters or more refractive error. This is also consistant with Ruben's finding of an incidence of retinal detachment being considerably higher in the high myopes.

CENTRAL MACULAR EDEMA
FOLLOWING PHACOEMULSIFICATION

This study was not entirely finished at the time of the preparation of this paper. A maximum of 18 patients from the group of 819 studied had permanent CME. It is possible that some of these patients had acutally macular degeneration instead of CME since all the patients did not have a confirmation of the diagnosis by fluorescein. In spite of this, for the purposes of this discussion, we will include 18 patients or 1.8% permanent CME. What is of interest and importance is that 12 patients had posterior capsulotomies and 6 had intact posterior capsules. Again one might assume that an intact capsule but again we must be reminded that more than twice as many of the patients studied had capsulotomies and we would therefore expect twice as many patients to have CME. It seems conclusive from this study that CME, whatever the cause, is no more or no less prevalent whether or not the posterior capsule has been opened following surgery.

In summary, the incidence of retinal detachment following phacoemulsification is considerably lower than reported from intracapsular extraction. Both the incidence of retinal detachment and CME is uneffected by the condition of the central posterior capsule.

Author's address:
150 East 58th Street
New York, N.Y. 10022
U.S.A.

Docum. Ophthal. Proc. Series, Vol. 21

SMALL INCISION INTRA–OCULAR LENS

CHARLES D. KELMAN

(New York, U.S.A.)

This paper deals with the need and the rational behind a small incision intraocular lens. There are two basic reasons for persuing such a lens. 1- With a small incision, the lens can be inserted safely while the chamber is maintained by irrigation. With this system there is practically no chance of endothelial touch to the intraocular lens. 2- The benefits of a small incision for cataract surgery have been presented elsewhere. They include rapid rehabilitation, few wound complications, practically no astigmatism, rapid wearing of a contact lens, etc.

In reviewing the possibilities of placement of such a lens, let us consider first the posterior chamber. There were several disadvantages to working in the posterior chamber. 1- The insertion of the lens in the capsular bag through a small incision was somewhat difficult. 2- A fairly large inferior capsular bag had to be maintained. 3- Centration of such a lens was a serious problem. Unless the lens was sutured to the iris, centration could not be maintained. Even when sutured to the iris, the suture had to be placed exactly in order to guarantee centration. Placing the suture through such a small incision was extremely difficult. 4- Because the lens was in close proximity to the posterior surface of the iris, there were frequent deposits of pigment on the surface of the lens reducing the patient's vision. 5- Posterior synechia of the iris to the pseudo-phakis were common. 6- A late capsulotomy was practically impossible to perform. The capsule would often times adhere to the lens, and when the capsule would cloud at a later date, even through the pars plana, a capsulotomy was performed only with great difficulty. All of these cases therefore had to have capsulotomies performed at the time of surgery. These capsulotomies were extremely difficult to perform also because they were behind a pseudo-phakis, and it was often times difficult to be certain that an adequate opening was made. 7- Removal of the pseudo-phakis was also difficult. The lens would become bound to the iris and to the capsule. In the one case where the posterior chamber lens had to be removed, only the optic was removed, the haptics were left in place. (Fig. 1–3).

IRIDO-CAPSULAR LENSES

These lenses because of the thickness of the lens, were impossible to insert

155

through a very small incision. A large enough incision is required for these lenses so that the cornea can be bent backwards out of the way of the entering pseudo-phakis. The incision required is so large that the chamber cannot be adequately maintained with irrigation.

IRIS PLANE LENSES

These lenses were considered but rejected because of the high incidence of central macula edema.

The anterior chamber seemed particularly well-suited to a small incision lens. Lenses implanted by Choyce almost two decades ago were still in place, with little or no irritation. In investigating his results, it was apparent that some patients did very well and others had more complications. I was convinced that this was not a matter of a chance and that there were certain reasons for discrepancy in the results.

GEOMETRIC SHAPE

The ideal placement for the Choyce lens is at the scleral spur. With four feet in the anterior chamber, unless the measurement of the lens was exquisitely perfect, and the scleral spur were in a perfect geometric plane, only three feet would be well seated. The fourth foot, outside of the plane (A plane is defined by the junction of three points) would be improperly placed. Furthermore, this fourth foot would move, rocking from one position to the other as various pressures from blinking, rubbing, etc. were placed on the eye. Only if the lens were too large and therefore wedged into the scleral spur would the lens be immobile. In this case, however, there would be a tendency toward erosion and significant tenderness on touch. With one of the feet moving, the tendency toward corneal endothelial touch, iritis and hyphema would be increased. When one tries to make the Choyce lens narrower so that it can go through a small incision, all of the above drawbacks are accentuated. As the lens was made narrower, the tendency for canting or displacement around the central vertical axis became increased. Simply taking the Choyce lens and making it narrower to fit through a small incision was therefore not possible. The narrower the Choyce lens, the less stability and more rocking of the feet one will encounter (Fig. 4).

In looking for the most stable geometric design it is obvious that a triangle is the most suitable. A four-legged chair (Fig. 5) will rock if the floor is even slightly unstable. A three-legged chair or stool, howeverm will find a plane common to all three feet and will remain stable regardless of the irregularities of the floor. Why not then make the Choyce lens triangular? This was tried and the stability was insufficient. The explanation is that a wide tripod is much more stable than a narrow tripod (Fig. 6). Clearly then the ideal shape for an anterior chamber lens would be wide triangle (Fig. 7).

Insertion of wide triangle through a small incision seems at first glance impossible. The unique shape of the Kelman Anterior Chamber lens however, makes wide triangular fixation in combination with a small incision feasible. (Fig. 8).

156

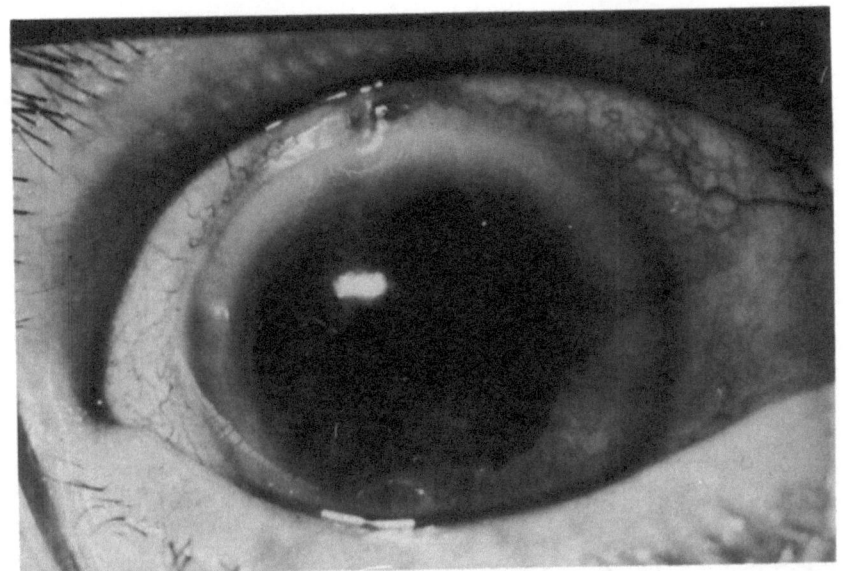

Fig. 1. Post-op eye, posterior chamber lens

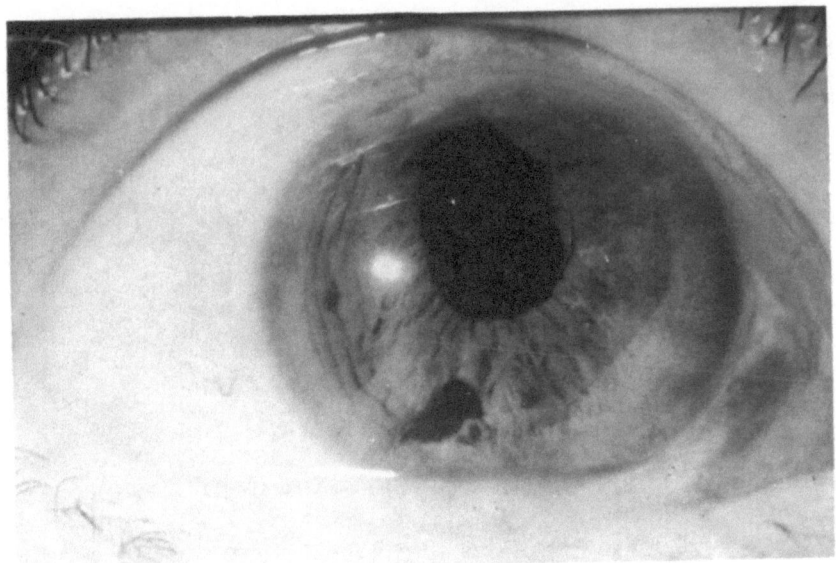

Fig. 2. Post-op eye, posterior chamber lens

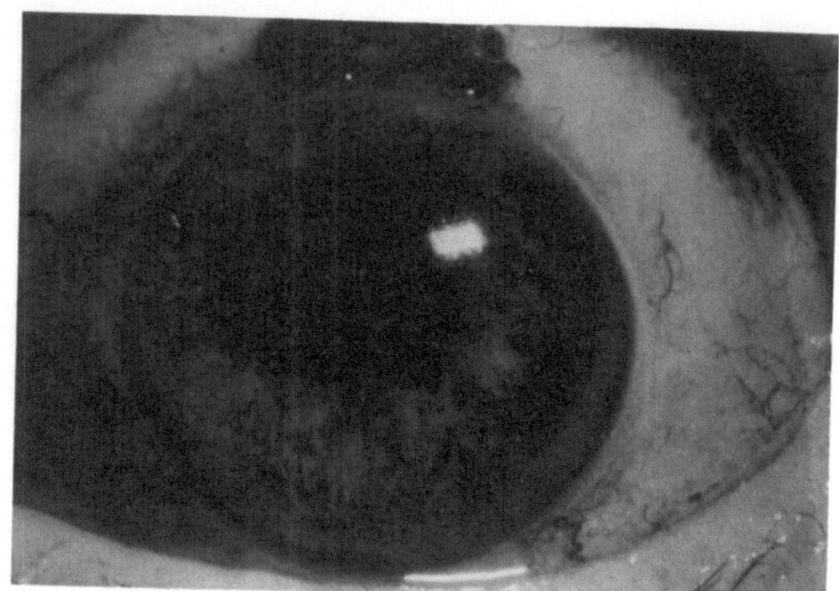

Fig. 3.   Post-op eye, posterior chamber lens

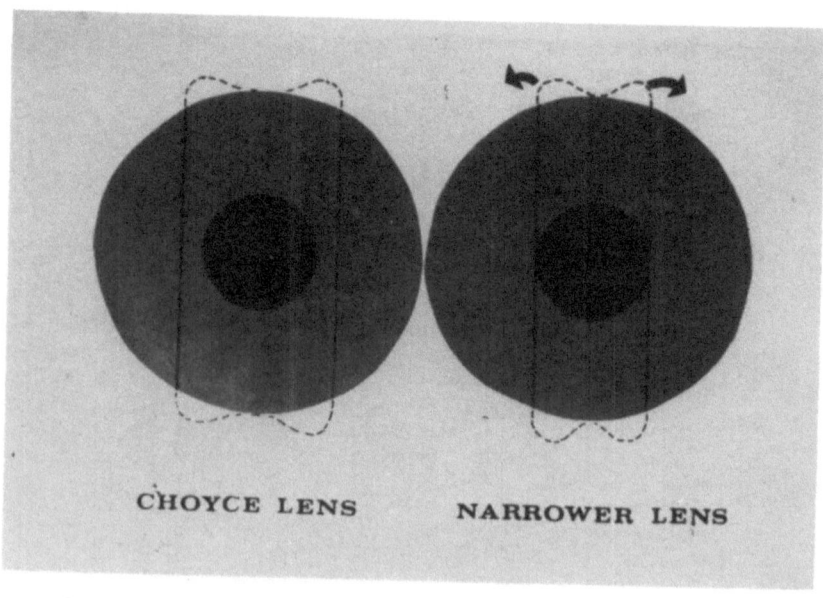

CHOYCE LENS   NARROWER LENS

Fig. 4.   Choyce lens problems accentuated by making lens narrower

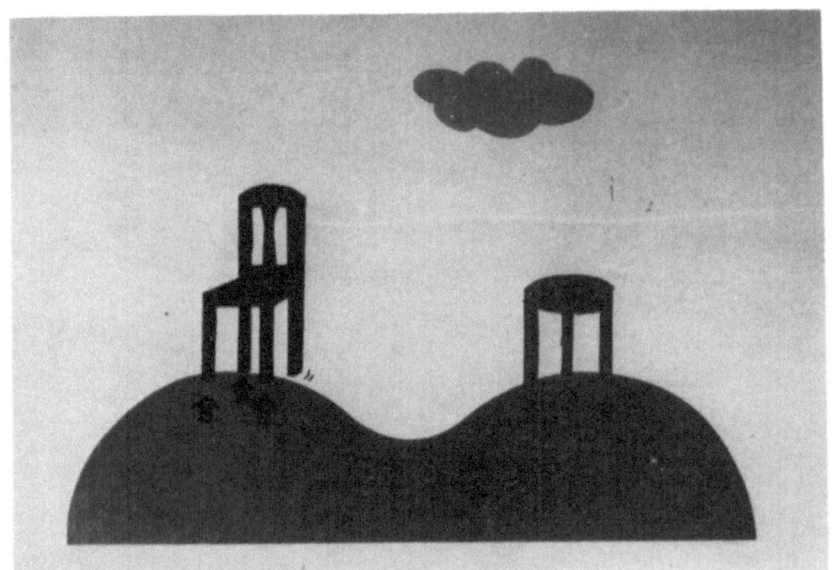

Fig. 5. Comparison of three-legged to four-legged stool

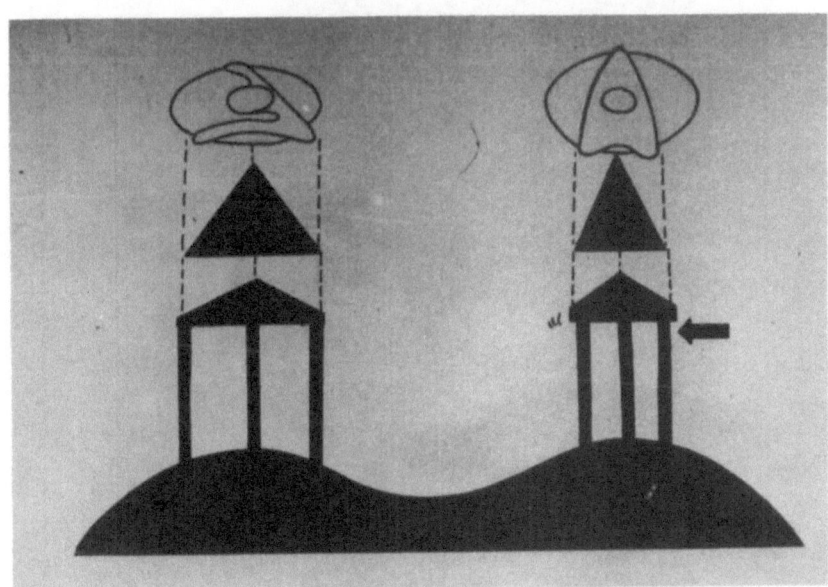

Fig. 6. Comparison of wide three-legged stool to narrow three-legged stool

159

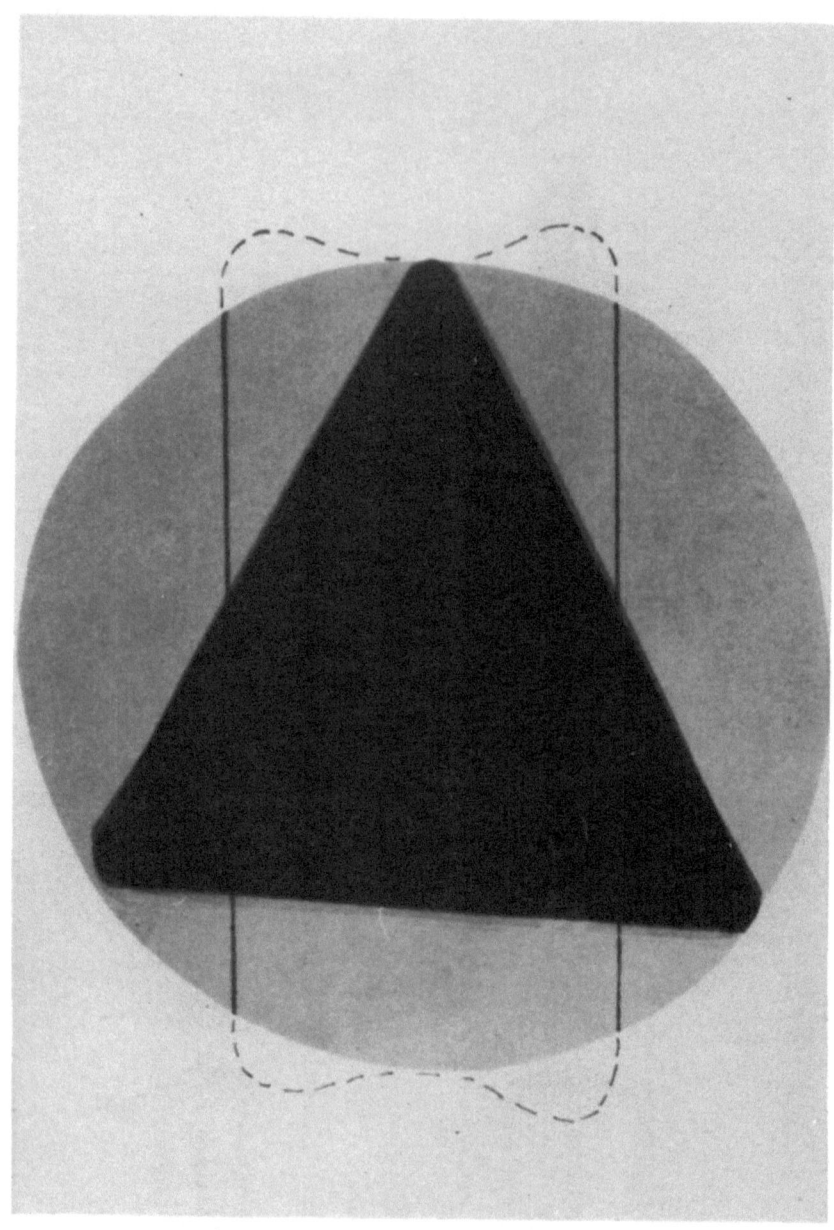

Fig. 7. Ideal shape of anterior chamber lens

Determination of what size Choyce lens to use was previously made by measuring white to white and adding one millimeter. It occured to me that this might lead to inaccurate lens size inside the eye if the relationship of the scleral spur diameter was not always one millimeter larger than the white to white diameter.

Measuring the white to white on cadever eyes, then disecting away the cornea and measuring the actual scleral spur to scleral spur dimension, a significant discrepancy was found in 20% of the eyes examined. In the operating room, measuring white to white and then measuring the internal diameter with the Kelman Dip Stick showed the same discrepancy (Fig. 9 & 10). The anterior chamber dip stick measures the distance from the scleral spur to the center of the pupil. This distance doubled accurately reflects the size lens required. This instrument has irrigation to maintain the chamber during the measurement. It is placed against the scleral spur until the eye just barely moves. This is the end point of insertion. Obtaining a reading at the center of the pupil is quite easy. The dip stick is measured in millimeter and half a millimeter markings. Looking at figure 11, we note that there are several cases of discrepancies of more than one millimeter. Putting in the wrong size anterior chamber lens could certainly lead to movement of the lens with iritis, hyphema and some of the late complications described with the Choyce lens.

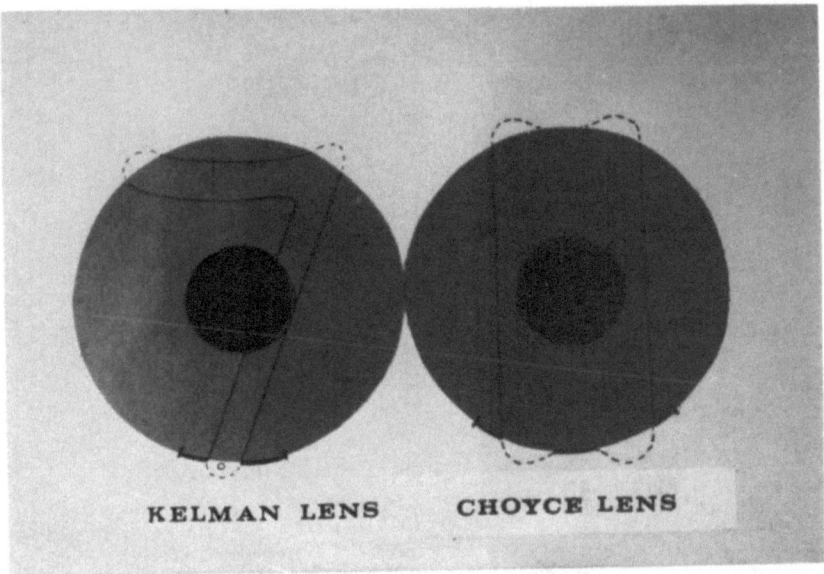

KELMAN LENS   CHOYCE LENS

Fig. 8. Comparison of Kelman lens to Choyce lens

161

INFLEXIBILITY OF IMPLANT

The Choyce lens is a rigid piece of plastic put into the anterior chamber. During blinking, rubbing of the eye, pressure from the pillow during sleep, etc., the shape of the anterior chamber can change slightly. With a rigid piece of plastic in the anterior chamber, it seems more than likely that undue pressures can be exerted on ocular tissue. It seems obvious that a lens must be flexible in addition to the above mentioned qualities in order for it to be tolerated in a very high percentage of cases. The shape of the lens which I designed, not only allows for insertion through a small incision, with wide triangular fixation, but is flexible. When the eye is deformed by external pressure the lens easily bends and then returns to its original shape.

TECHNIQUE OF INSERTION

In order to prevent the cornea from touching the lens, a separate inflow system was devised to keep the anterior chamber full of fluid at all times. Even if the lens should touch the endothelium, this is a **wet touch** as opposed to a **dry touch** which we have when air is in the chamber. It is obvious that less damage will be done to the cornea when there is fluid serving as a lubricant in the anterior chamber. The insertion is as follows: After a phacoemulsification, the incision is enlarged to 4 mm and the chamber maintainer is introduced through a separate small incision. If the lens is being used after intracapsular extraction, the incision is sutured closed, leaving only a 4 mm area for insertion of the lens (Fig. 12). The lens is held with a forceps as the fluid is introduced in the anterior chamber and the lower foot is inserted (Fig. 13). The insertion continues as the 8 o'clock

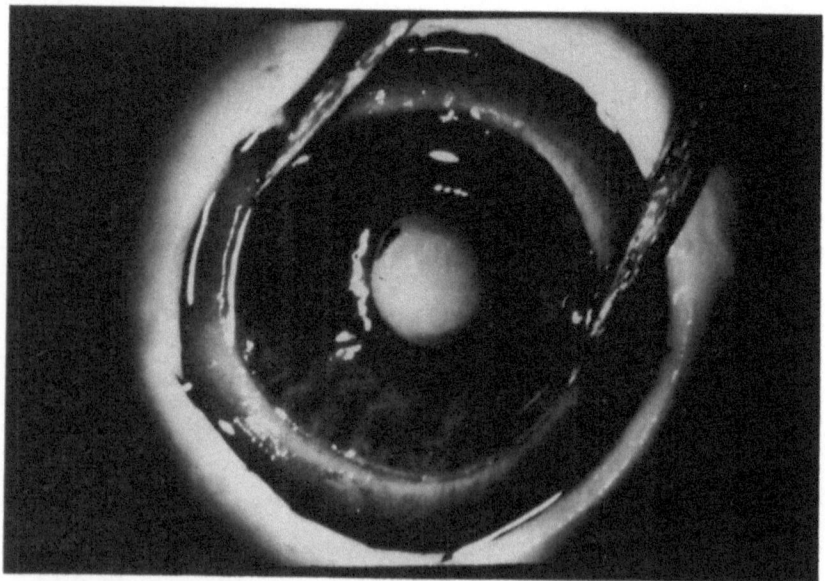

Fig. 9.   Measurement of scleral spur to scleral spur with calipers

Age/sex	Caliper white to white	Estimated internal diameter	Measured diameter (dip stick)	difference
57 ♀	12.0	13.0	12.5	−0.5 mm
69 ♂	11.5	12.5	13.0	+0.5 mm
10 ♂	12.0	13.0	12.0	−1.00 mm
58 ♀	12.0	13.0	13.0	0
64 ♀	11.2	12.2	12.5	+0.3 mm
60 ♂	12.5	13.5	13.0	−0.5 mm
66 ♀	11.5	12.5	12.5	0
72 ♀	11.5	12.5	12.5	0
48 ♀	11.5	12.5	12.0	−0.5 mm
81 ♀	10.5	11.5	13.0	+1.5 mm
73 ♀	11.5	12.5	12.5	0
70 ♀	11.5	12.5	14.0	+1.5 mm
51 ♀	12.0	13.0	13.0	0
60 ♂	11.5	12.5	13.0	+0.5 mm

Fig. 11. Discrepancy between white to white and actual internal measurement

foot is inserted (Fig. 14). When the optic is at the incision, the lens is re-positioned slightly to the right and the insertion continues (Fig. 15, 16) & 17). The upper foot of the lens is inserted by inserting a small forceps in the hole of the lens provided for this, retracting the sclera with a cystotome or other hook, and gently pressing the lens posteriorly. It is important not to push the lens toward the inferior angle (Fig. 16, 18). A cystotome can be used to gently retract the iris away from the feet to make certain that there is no iris incarceration (Fig. 19).

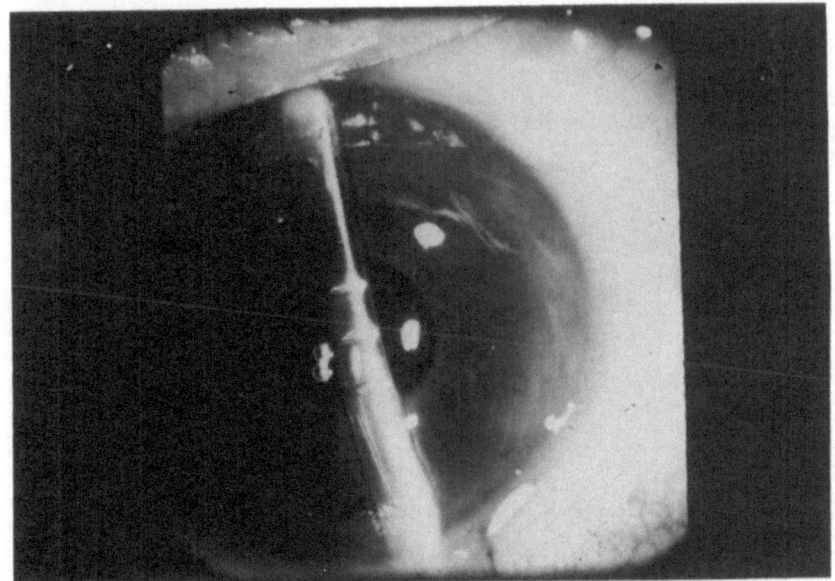

Fig.10 Dipstick in place.

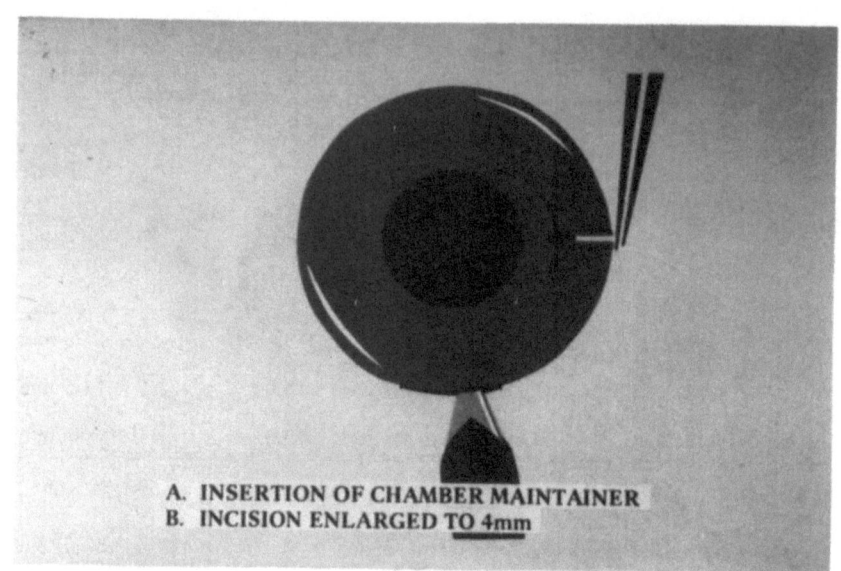

Fig. 12. 4 mm incision.

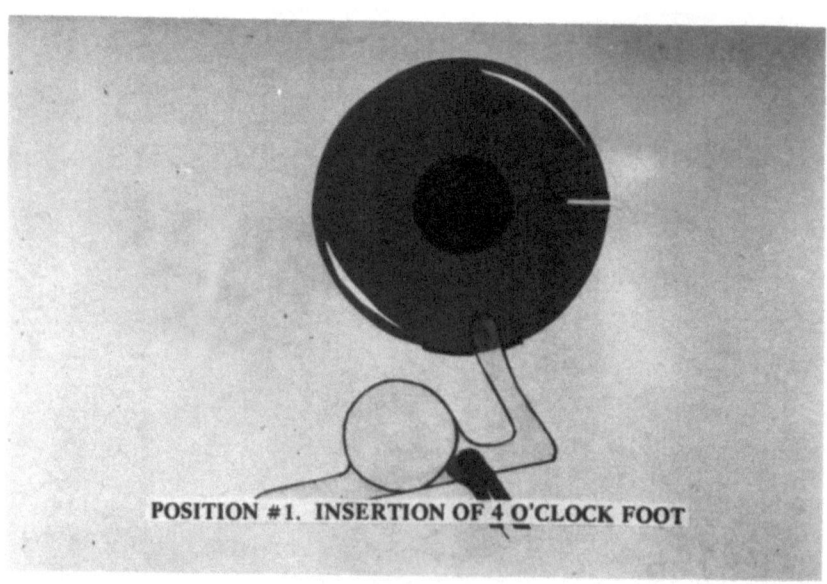

Fig. 13. Insertion of 4 o'clock foot.

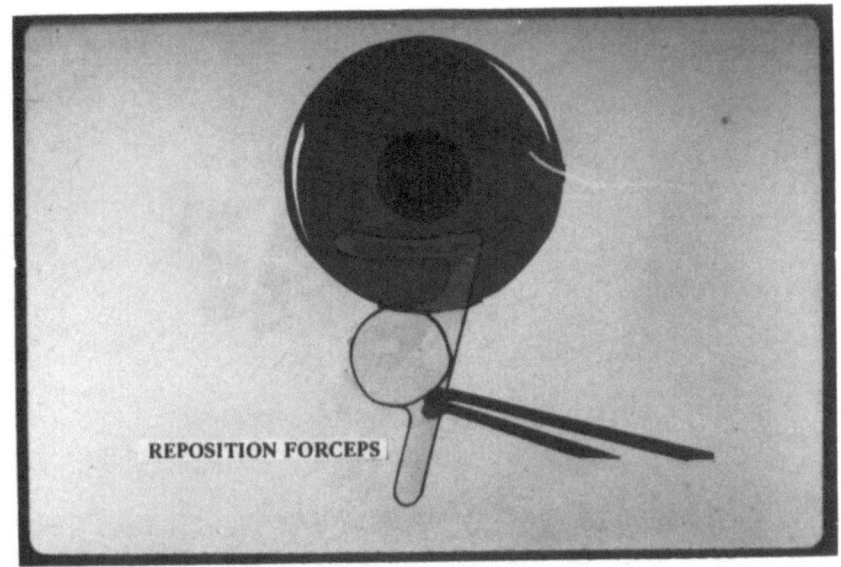

Fig. 14. Insertion of 8 o'clock foot.

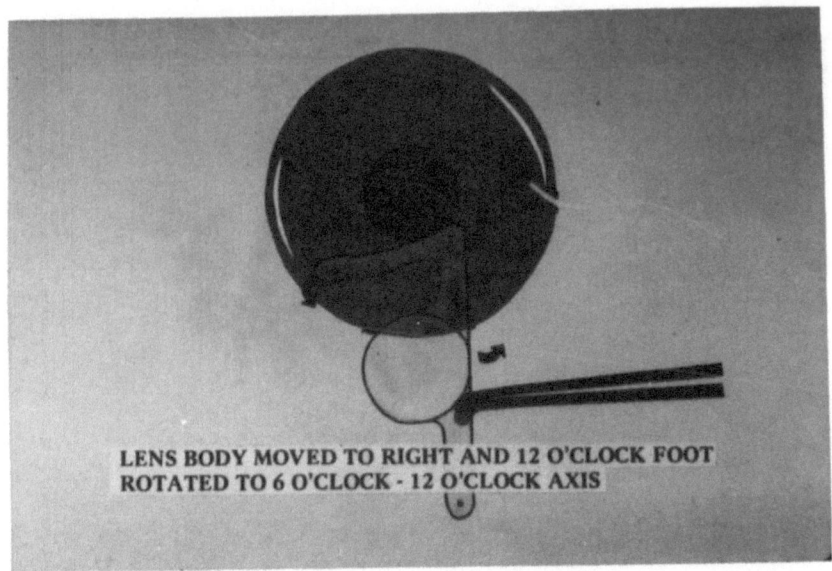

Fig. 15. Insertion of lens continues.

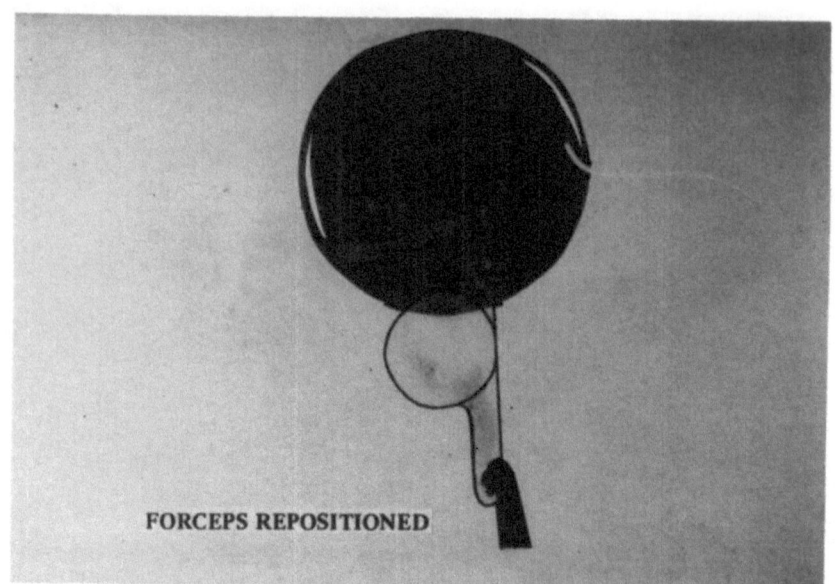

Fig. 16. Insertion of lens continues.

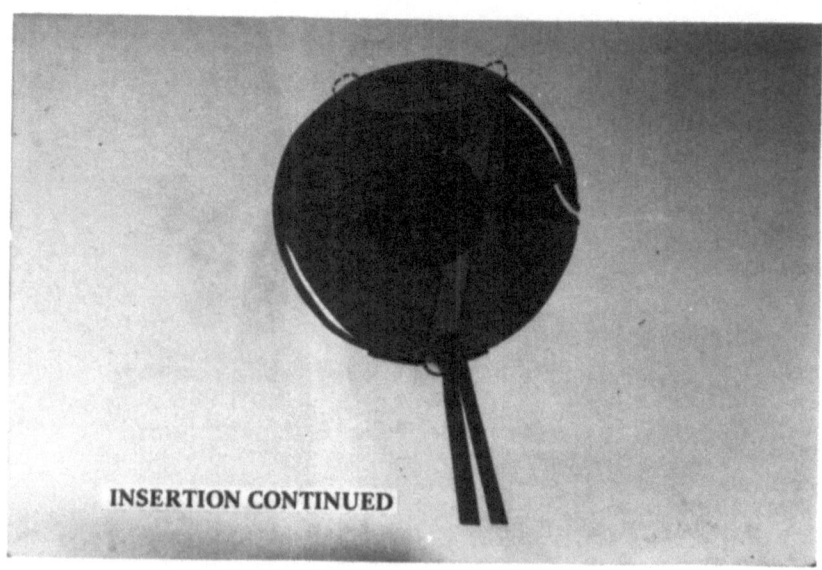

Fig. 17. Insertion of lens continues.

166

RESULTS

Several hundred cases of this lens were performed by myself and other investigators. With the accurate size determination of the lens, there were no late complications, (with a year follow-up) such as late hyphema, uveitis, or glaucoma. Because of the small incision and atraumatic insertion the eyes are white and quiet almost immediately, with usually excellent vision on the first day post-operatively. The incidence of cystoid macula edema fell within the normal range for cataract surgery. The same was true with the incidence of retinal detachment (Fig. 20 & 21).

Only a few patients complained of slight tenderness on touch, but this definitely be ascribed to the intraocular lens. In no case did this tenderness on touch persist for more than 2–3 weeks post-operatively, and could certainly be related merely to an incision with suturing.

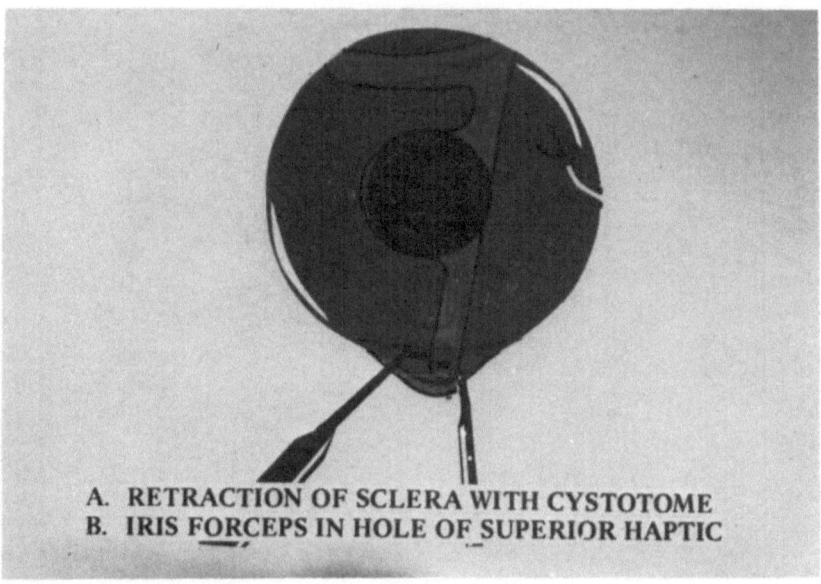

A. RETRACTION OF SCLERA WITH CYSTOTOME
B. IRIS FORCEPS IN HOLE OF SUPERIOR HAPTIC

Fig. 18. Insertion of lens continues.

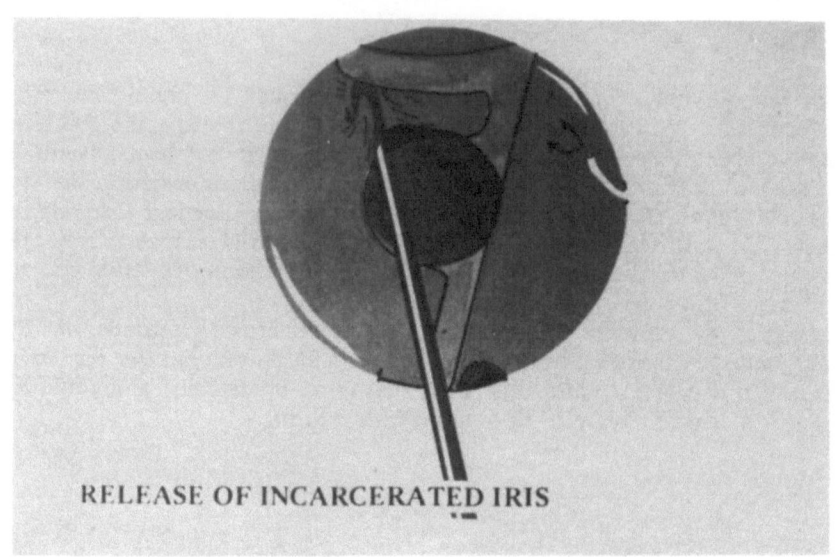

Fig. 19.   Release of incarcerated iris.

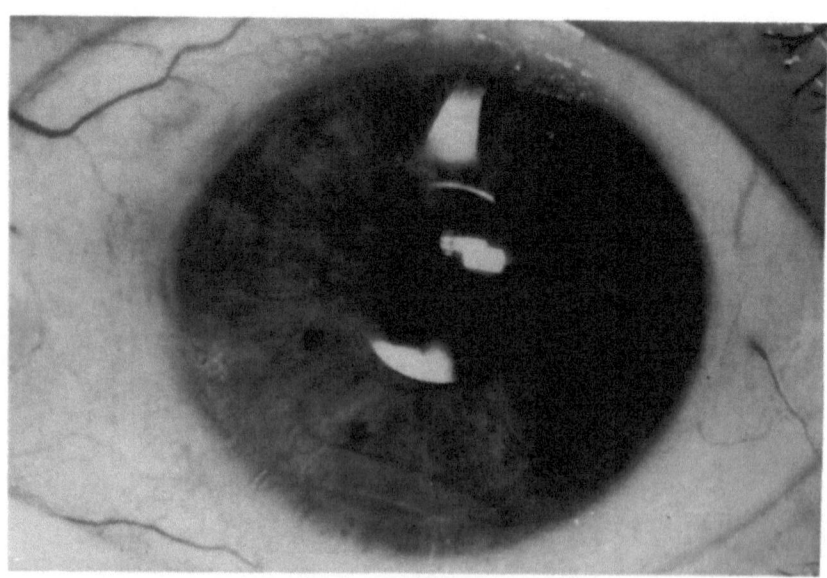

Fig. 20.   Post-op eye, Kelman Anterior-Chamber lens.

168

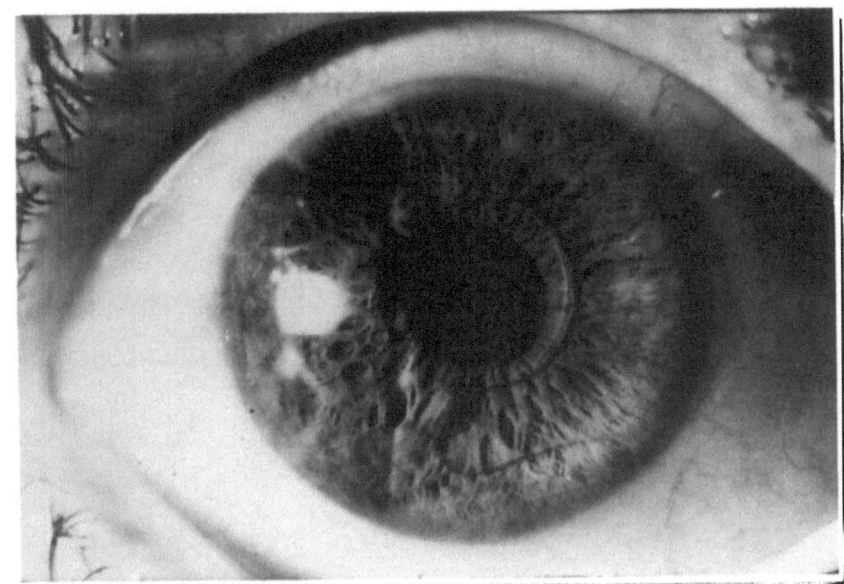

Fig. 21. Post-op eye, Kelman Anterior-Chamber lens.

Author's address:
150 East 58th Street
New York, N.Y. 10022
U.S.A.

Docum. Ophthal. Proc. Series, Vol. 21

EXTRACTION BY ULTRASONIC PHACO EMULSIFICATION

R.P. KRATZ

(Los Angeles, California, U.S.A.)

It has been said that phaco-emulsification is dying out but the opposite is true. In 1971 there were only 5 machines whereas in 1977 there were 644. Beginning and advanced courses are offerred at several institutions on a regular basis. In 1971 only 47 surgeons were trained and by 1977, 2634 surgeons in the U.S. and 183 abroad. The equipment is used in 34 clinics in Europe. In 1971 only 230 procedures had been performed but by 1977 over 120,000 procedures had been done. The new model 8000 delivered 35% more power than the first model and 15% more power than the 7007 model.

The small incision size which is only 3 mm minimizes wound disruption, iris prolapse, bleba, flat anterior chamber, peripheral synochiale and corneal astigmatism. The small incision permits shorter hospitalisation, greater postoperative comfort, rapid physical rehabilitation and lower total disability expense. Usually contact lenses are fitted in 3 or 4 weeks and fewer total postoperative visits are required. Kelman phaco-emulsification has special advantages in the young patient with strong zonular and collapsible sclera. It has particular advantages in patients with a bull neck. Filtering bleba are not collapsed if pheco-emulsification is used to remove the cataract. Phaco-emulsification with an intact posterior capsule is helpful when the fellow eye has suffered vitreous loss, retinal detachment or visual impairment from cystoid macular edema. Phaco-emulsification may be combined with vitrectomy at the time of primary surgery.

Operative and postoperative advantages include decreased vitreous loss, no expulsive haemorrhage and little likelihood of an epithelial ingrowth. Persons with poor ability to heal such as blood dyscrasia, collagen disease, steroid induced tissue abnormality or posterior capsule vitreous face adhesions are helped by the small incision.

The intact capsule acts as a physiological barrier and even with a central posterior capsulotomy there is excellent support of the vitreous base and virtual elimination of endophthalmodenisis.

The capsule provides support for intraocular lenses. It protects against cornea-vitreal touch and retains the vitreous when keratoplasty or glaucome procedures are used. A 4 or 5 mm posterior capsulotomy is large enough to view the peripheral retina and yet give 87% or 80% support to the vitreous base.

If the capsule is left intact 19% will cloud the first year, 20% the second year and 13% the third year. The capsulotomy may be done under sterile conditions in the office with only topical anaesthesia. In 1400 cases followed for over 2 years the retinal detachment rate was 0.5% with an intact capsule, 1.5% when the capsule was opened and 7.0% when vitreous was lost. Clinically significant cystoid macular edema was present 0.5% with an intact capsule and 4.5% when the capsule was opened. Endothelial cell loss was 8% when the phaco-emulsification was done in the anterior chamber and less when done in the posterior chamber. Other complications were rare.

Author's address:
15225 Vanowen Street
Van Nuys, Calif. 91405
U.S.A.

CATARACT EXTRACTION BY ULTRASONIC FRAGMENTATION (USF)

LOUIS J. GIRARD

(Houston, Texas, U.S.A.)

INTRODUCTION

Ultrasonic fragmentation (USF) is a technique for fragmenting the lens into small particles that can be aspirated through a 23 or 20 guage needle. The surgical technique is an outgrowth of a closed, bimanual system of aspiration/irrigation which was introduced by the author in 1966. The addition, in 1972, of ultrasonic fragmentation to the technique increased the age range of cataracts that could be aspirated. It was also found that other ocular tissues such as iris, vitreous and ciliary body could be removed in the same manner.

MECHANISM OF FRAGMENTATION

The Ultrasonic Fragmentor console contains a high frequency oscillator which activates a piezoelectrical crystal system in the handpiece. The crystals vibrate and these vibrations are transmitted by resonance to the tip of the metal needle. The needle vibrates longitudinally 0.09 to 0.11 mm at approximately 40,000 vibrations per second or 40 kHz. When the vibrating needle is brought in contact with various materials and with certain intraocular tissues fragmentation occurs by 1) mechanical pulverization, 2) cavitation and 3) microstreaming.

High frequency vibrations with only a small amplitude of displacement can produce great stress within a solid vibrating body. The acceleration obtained can be as great as 72,000 times that of gravity.

Cavitation is a specific phenomena by which sonic shock waves are generated with high frequency power. When a solid vibration is placed in a liquid medium and when certain threshold values are reached vaporization of the medium occurs. The shock waves produced can enhance fragmentation.

Microstreaming refers to currents in the medium set up by the vibrating solid which brings the particles back to the tip for further fragmentation.

In ultrasonic fragmentation for intraocular surgery the stream of irrigating solution is constantly aspirated by the aspirating/fragmenting needle. When the fragmenting needle is brought in contact with certain intraocular tissues, the tissues are fragmented into small particles and aspirated. The size of the irrigating and aspirating cannulas is either 23 or 20 guage needles.

173

INDICATIONS FOR THE USE OF ULTRASONIC FRAGMENTATION

There is a wide variety of indications for the use of ultrasonic fragmentation that includes: 1) cataract extraction (congenital, traumatic or senile, subluxated, dislocated, secondary or retroimplant membranes) either by the anterior chamber or pars plana approach; 2) complications of intraocular surgery such as vitreous loss, aphakic bullous keratopathy, hyphema, pupillary block glaucoma, updrawn pupil, iridocapsular membranes and cystoid macular edema from vitreous incarceration; 3) vitrectomy for any type of vitreous opacification such as uveitis, hemorrhage, etc; 4) treatment of fresh or late trauma such as cataract, hyphema, obstruction of the visual axis by iridocapsular membranes or vitreous opacification and intraocular foreign bodies; 6) combined lensectomy and vitrectomy for such conditions as diabetic retinopathy, RLF, and PHPV.

TECHNIQUE

A. *Pars Plana Approach*

1. Lensectomy

Pars plana lensectomy with ultrasonic fragmentation is performed in the following manner: the conjunctiva is incised and the sclera exposed in the superior temporal and superior nasal quadrants. Sclerotomy incisions are made with a Girard knife at the 10 and 2 o'clock positions 4 mm from the limbus. The knife is passed through the sclera, through the equator of the lens and into the nucleus. The irrigating and aspirating/fragmenting cannulas are inserted through these openings into the lens. An attempt is made to keep the anterior and posterior lens capsules intact as long as possible while, methodically, the nucleus, the anterior cortex and the posterior cortex are first removed. Next, the anterior capsule is removed by a combination of fragmentation and aspiration. It may be necessary to use the two needle chopping-block technique because the anterior lens capsule can be very durable. In this technique the capsule is caught between the two needles when the fragmentation is activated. It produces a sharp shearing action which will fragment the anterior lens capsule so that it may be aspirated. The posterior capsule is easily fragmented and aspirated and an anterior vitrectomy is part of this procedure. Lens remnants beneath the iris can be brought into view by scleral depression where they can be fragmented and aspirated.

Should lens fragments drop into the vitreous they can be retrieved by aspiration against the aspirating cannula, brought into the middle of the eye where they can be fragmented and aspirated. A flat contact lens is essential in viewing the posterior pole of the eye (Girard flat contact lens).

The needles are withdrawn and, if vitreous herniates through the wound, this is fragmented and aspirated. The scleral wounds are closed with a single suture of the surgeon's choice. The conjunctiva can be closed with a single or running suture of the surgeon's choice.

2. Subluxated lenses

Subluxated lenses are best removed by pars plana lensectomy. Usually the lens has some zonular attachments which stabilize the lens while it is being fragmented and aspirated. Scleral depression should be utilized to visualize the portion of the lens beneath the iris.

3. Dislocated lenses

Lenses dislocated into the vitreous or into the anterior chamber are best removed by the pars plana approach. If the lens is lying against the retina it is necessary to use a flat contact lens for visualization. Once the lens capsule is ruptured the lens cortex and nucleus are methodically fragmented and aspirated with particular care that no fragmentation takes place while the lens material is in contact with the retina. The technique is to aspirate the material, bring it to the middle of the eye where it is aspirated and fragmented. The process is repeated until all of the lens is entirely removed.

4. Secondary and retroimplant membranes

Secondary membranes and membranes behind intraocular implants are best removed through the pars plana approach. If the membrane consists mainly of posterior capsule and Elschnig pearls, it is easily fragmented and aspirated. If the membrane is composed of both anterior and posterior lens capsules usually a tough, fibrous membrane results. It can be very resistant to fragmentation and it is necessary to employ the two needle chopping-block technique to fragment the membrane before aspiration.

In retro-implant membranes it is important to explore the membrane first without aspiration or fragmentation, to be sure of its position and durability. Then the membrane is aspirated, brought away from the implant before being fragmented and aspirated. Care should be taken not to bring the fragmenting needle against the implant during fragmentation or etching of the implant will take place.

5. Combined lensectomy and vitrectomy

In patients who have cataract and vitreous opacification a combined lensectomy and vitrectomy may be performed through the pars plana. The technique is particularly valuable in cases of diabetic retinopathy, penetrating wounds and intraocular foreign bodies, both magnetic and non-magnetic.

6. Combined lensectomy and glaucoma filter

After pars plana lensectomy or after pars plana vitrectomy, a filter can be created by leaving one of the incisions open and carefully closing Tenon's capsule and conjunctiva over the opening. Essential to the technique is the free flow of aqueous through the incision without being blocked by formed vitreous. If formed vitreous prolapses into the wound it will stop the filter.

175

Therefore, during the procedure vitrectomy must be continued until no **formed vitreous prolapses into the wound.** During this time irrigation is continued and when there is a free flow of BSS from the wound, the surgeon knows that the formed vitreous has been removed.

B. *Anterior Chamber Approach. Extracapsular Extraction.*

Extracapsular cataract extraction can be performed with ultrasonic fragmentation in the following manner. Two beveled incisions are made 1 mm inside the limbus of the cornea at the 10 and 2 o'clock positions. The irrigating cannula is inserted through one incision and the anterior chamber is kept formed. The aspirating/fragmenting needle is inserted through the second incision. Using a combination of fragmentation, irrigation and aspiration, the anterior lens capsule is first removed, attempting to remove as much as possible. The anterior cortex is then removed. Next the nucleus is fragmented and aspirated. The posterior cortex can usually be removed by aspiration alone without using fragmentation. This allows preservation of the intact posterior capsule. Particular care must be taken in removing the cortex at the equator of the lens which is aspirated without fragmentation. Scleral depression can aid in obtaining lens material underneath the iris.

If a posterior subcapsular opacity is present it can usually be scraped off with the aspirating needle which has a smooth surface.

It is important to do all fragmentation in the pupillary area as far as possible from the corneal endothelium and the posterior capsule.

Should the posterior capsule inadvertently be ruptured, the Ultrasonic Fragmentor will perform a vitrectomy. All vitreous and lens material should be carefully removed, in other words, a total lensectomy and anterior vitrectomy. Nuclear material dropped into the vitreous should be retrieved by aspiration, brought to the center of the eye and fragmented. For retrieval of lens fragments from the retina it is necessary to use a flat contact lens to visualize the posterior segment of the globe.

SUMMARY

Ultrasonic fragmentation with USF is a technique for fragmenting the lens into small particles that can be aspirated through a 23 or 20 guage needle. The needles can be inserted through small incisions in the sclera in the region of the pars plana (pars plana approach) or in corneal limbus (anterior chamber approach). Extracapsular extraction leaving the posterior capsule, subtotal lensectomy leaving the anterior lens capsule intact or total lensectomy can be performed by either approach. The technique is applicable to all types of cataracts: congenital, traumatic, senile, subluxated, dislocated or any type of secondary membrane. Ultrasonic fragmentation can also be used for iridectomy, cyclectomy or vitrectomy. For this reason it can be used for the treatment of a variety of conditions such as the complications of intraocular surgery (vitreous loss, aphakic bullous keratopathy, pupillary block glaucoma, etc.) for vitrectomy (vitreous hemorrhage, diabetic vitritis, etc.) and for trauma (cataract, vitreous hemorrhage, removal of intraocular foreign bodies, etc.).

Author's address:
59 Tiel Way
Houston, Texas 77019
USA

PHACOEMULSIFICATION

A. EDWARD MAUMENEE

(Baltimore, Maryland, U.S.A.)

As a preface to my discussion of phacoemulsification I would like to make a few remarks about the changing attitude of physicians and the lay public in the United States in regards to self promotion and advertising. In the late 1800's following the Flexner Report there was a marked improvement in the medical schools in our country. Concurrently strict regulations were established to prevent physicians from advertising. During the past 30 years there has been a gradual erosion of this ethical principle. This has occurred for multiple reasons, some of which are as follows. First, the involvement of litigation in our daily lives has become a much more frequent occurrence. Thus, the failure of a patient to respond favorably to medical therapy frequently has been called malpractice. Also, attempts of medical organizations to regulate the ethics of their members has been construed as defamation of character or restraint of trade. During this same period governmental or third-party payment for medical care has increased and for this reason it has been thought by many that the public should be more fully informed of medical progress. For this reason there has been a proliferation of news articles in all media about medical accomplishments. Finally, the Federal Trade Commission has ruled that organized medicine is acting as a monopoly in preventing physicians from advertising. It is the Commission's opinion that if advertising is allowed, competition among physicians will increase and the cost of medical care will be reduced.

It is within this atmosphere that phacoemulsification was first introduced. Instead of finding its place in ophthalmology through the scientific medical journals, claims for the advantage of this procedure were widely publicized in newspapers, weekly magazines, radio, and television. These articles cited the names of physicians who were performing this procedure and stated that it was a revolutionary improvement in cataract surgery. The lay public frequently obtained the impression that the cataracts were removed with a "laser beam" without surgery. This often resulted in an instantaneous development of a large cataract surgical practice for the physician who obtained an instrument that cost approximately $30,000.

This hitherto unaccepted method of introducing a surgical technique into the practice of medicine immediately polarized ophthalmologists about the procedure. The most frequent question that I had from my colleagues was, "Should I purchase a phaco-emulsification machine in order to protect my practice?".

I introduce my presentation with this non-scientific discussion to make you aware of the circumstances which have made this procedure so controversial.

SCIENTIFIC EVALUATION OF PHACOEMULSIFICATION

Recently several excellent reports have been presented on the complications and visual results of this operative procedure. Emery (1978) has reviewed his findings on 200 consecutive carefully selected patients. Wilkinson (1978) has reviewed the incidence of retinal detachment in 1,500 eyes on which phacoemulsification cataract extraction was performed by one of the most skillful surgeons now using this instrument in our country. Unfortunately, these two physicians, who were to present their material at this meeting, were not able to attend and I will therefore attempt to summarize some of their findings.

In Emery's series of patients, 155 of the eyes had posterior subcapsular cataracts and 45 nuclear. The average was 57 with a range from 30 to 92. One hundred twenty three were males and 77 females. The right eye was involved in 97 instances and the left eye 103. The duration of follow-up is indicated in Table 1. Only 44 (22%) of the patients were followed for less than one year.

Table 1. Duration of follow-up

	Number of patients
Less than 6mo	29
6mo – 1yr	15
1 to 2yr	80
2 to 3yr	53
3 to 4yr	18
4 to 5yr	5

Complications at the time of surgery were few. Descemet's membrane was stripped in one patient. Three patients had cosmetically noticeable trauma to the iris. Vitreous was lost in seven eyes (3.5% of the cases). There were no choroidal hemorrhages or loss of the nucleus into the vitreous. In six cases (3%) the incision had to be enlarged from 3 mm to approximately 18 mm.

Immediate postoperative complications involved central corneal edema which lasted for more than one week in three cases; wound leak with the formation of a filtering bleb in two cases; a flat anterior chamber in one patient; transient glaucoma in two patients; and transient hypotony in one.

Only one patient suffered persistent low-grade iridocyclitis. There were no cases of hyphema, endophthalmitis, or sympathetic ophthalmia.

There were four patients who suffered reduced visual acuity from cystoid maculopathy, but the final visual acuity was reduced to 20/40 in only one instance.

Retinal detachment occurred in two patients, one three years postoperatively and a second patient eight months after operation.

The posterior capsule of the lens was left intact in 185 cases (82.5%). Thirty two of these cases (19.4%) developed capsular opacification with reduced visual acuity to less than 20/40. The longer the follow-up the higher the incidence of capsular opacification (Table 2). Thirty two percent of the patients with intact posterior capsules developed significant opacification after three to five years follow-up. Clouding of the capsule occurred more frequently in the younger age groups. Secondary discission of the posterior capsule was carried out in 27 cases with a resultant rupture of the vitreous face in two patients, and a retinal detachment in one case. This patient had been cited previously.

Table 2. Rate of capsule opacification

Less than 1yr	3%
1 – 2yr	20%
2 – 3yr	28%
3 – 5yr	32%

The visual acuity at the time of last follow-up was 20/40 or better in 94% of the cases. The causes of visual acuity less than 20/40 at the latest follow-up are noted in Table 3.

Table 3. Causes of visual acuity less than 20/40

Opacified capsule	5
Senile macular degeneration	4
Retinal detachment	1
Macular edema	1
Corneal edema	1

COMMENT

These results are indeed excellent. Emery is one of my former residents and is one of the most careful, meticulous surgeons that I have ever observed. He informs me that his patients not infrequently have 20/20 vision with proper refraction within the first week after cataract extraction. This is unquestionably a more rapid recovery than usually occurs after routine intracapsular cataract extraction. The final visual acuity in the patients, however, is essentially the same as that reported by experienced surgeons using the intracapsular technique. Likewise, the long-term follow-up of major complications is essentially the same as reported by both techniques. (Stark, Hirst, Snip & Maunemee 1977; Maunemee & Meredith 1974).

RETINAL DETACHMENTS FOLLOWING PHACOEMULSIFICATION

In a second study Wilkinson (1978) reviewed a consecutive series of 1,500 eyes in which phacoemulsification had been performed by one of the most experienced ophthalmic surgeons in the use of phacoemulsification. The lenght of follow-up in these case is given in Table 4. It will be noted that 58% of the patients had been followed for a year of less. The overall incidence of retinal detachments was 3.6%. Vitreous loss occurred at the time of surgery in 63 of the 1,500 eyes, an incidence of 4.2%, and in this group of 63 eyes, the incidence of detachment was 14%. The time of retinal detachment following phacoemulsification is listed in Table 5. It is important to note that only 46% of the detachments occurred within one year following operation. Thus, it would seem logical that with a longer duration of follow-up than is listed in Table 4, the percentage of retinal detachments will increase. It is worth noting that this series of patients was not selected for phacoemulsification as was the previous series, but was rather an unselected group of individuals who needed cataract surgery.

Table 4. Length of follow-up obtained in 1,500 consecutive cases of phacoemulsification

Follow-up Time	Number of Patients	Percentage
lmo & less	685	46
lmo – 1 yr	185	12
1 – 2 yrs	128	8
2 – 3 yrs	162	11
3 yrs +	340	23
	1,500	100%

Table 5. Time of retinal detachments following phacoemulsification in the consecutive series of 1,500 eyes.

Time	Percentage of Patients
0 – 6wks	7%
6wk – 3mo	13%
3 – 6mo	7%
6 – 12mo	19%
lyr – 2yr	26%
2yr – 3yr	16%
3yr +	6%
Unknown	6%
	100%

Posterior capsulotomies or capsulectomies were performed in 94.7% of the eyes. One-third of the cases in which the posterior capsule was left intact required discission within three years.

In a second series of patients reported by the same authors the results of reattachment operations in eyes in which lens removal had occurred by phacofragmentation were reported. The types of retinal breaks which produced the detachments were essentially the same as those found in other eyes with aphakia, 71% having tears in the superior temporal quadrant. Most

180

of the tears were located along the posterior insertion of the vitreous base, but in 46% of the eyes at least one tear was located at the equator or posteriorly.

Surgery was performed on 74 of the 76 eyes with detachment. Several aspects of phacoemulsification frequently made surgery more difficult by reducing the view of the fundus. The most important of these were residual lens capsule, retained peripheral lens cortex, and a relative miosis due to posterior synechiae. The primary surgical procedures in these 74 eyes are listed in Table 6. The reattachment rates following retinal detachment surgery are listed in Table 7. The visual results following successful surgery are listed in Table 8.

Table 6. Primary surgical procedures (74 eyes) for retinal detachment

Transconjunctival cryothermy	11
Segmental buckle (90 degrees +)	6
360 degree buckle (Exoplant)	54
Vitrectomy + buckle	3
	74

Table 7. Reattachment rates following retinal detachment surgery (74 primary and 3 secondary operations)

Overall Success Rate 91%	
Transconjunctival cryo	100%
Segmental buckle	100%
360 degree buckle	91%
Vitrectomy + buckle	0%

Table 8. Visual results following successful surgery

Visual	All cases	Cases with macular involvement
20/50+	40 (60%)	20 (49%)
20/59 – 20/200	18 (27%)	12 (29%)
20/400 & less	9 (13%)	9 (22%)
	67 (100%)	41 (100%)

In still another series, Wilkinson has performed vitrectomy for complications of phacoemulsification in 25 patients (Table 9). The cataract surgery performed on these eyes with phacoemulsification had been done by several ophthalmic surgeons, rather than by the single surgeon who had performed the series of 1,500 cases.

COMMENT

It would appear from the two large consecutive series mentioned in this presentation that when phacoemulsification is performed by an experienced, skilled ophthalmic surgeon that the major complication is retinal

Table 9. Vitrectomy for complications of phacoemulsification

Corneal edema with vitreous touch		10
Pupillary membranes (usually capsule)		8
Vitreous opacification		2
Retained lens material		4
Media cloudy	1	
Phacolytic glaucoma	1	
Severe uveitis	2	
Irvine-Gass syndrome		1
		25

detachment. The incidence of retinal detachment is comparable to that which occurs after routine intracapsular cataract surgery. Other complications such as those listed in Table 9 will occur during the first hundred or so phacoemulsifications with skilled surgeons, and will probably be more frequent with the ophthalmologist who operates only occasionally, as would occur with intracapsular surgery.

A FOLLOW-UP OF OPHTHALMOLOGISTS TRAINED IN PHACOEMULSIFICATION

Emery has verbally reported another very interesting survey. He sent questionnaires to 250 ophthalmologists who had received training in phacoemulsification. Two hundred twenty one of these replied. Of these trainees, 61% were doing phacoemulsification, 20% planned to use this technique, 9% would not try, and 10% had given it up. The total number of operations done by this group ranged from one to 400 cases, with an average of 43. The percentage of cataract cases done by phacoemulsification in the group ranged from 0.5% to 95%, with an average of 19%. The annual number of cataracts performed by the respondents were as follows. Those performing phacoemulsification ranged from 10 to 500, with a mean of 121. Those who would not try the procedure ranged from 50 to 350 cases, with a mean of 120; and those who had tried the procedure and given it up ranged from 12 to 400, with a mean of 96 extractions per year.

The complication rate with phacoemulsification as compared with intracapsular cataract extraction reported by this group of ophthalmologists is listed in Table 10.

Table 10. Complications with phacoemulsification compared with intracapsular cataract extraction

	Still Doing	Gave Up
More with phacoemul.	37%	79%
Same	46%	16%
Less	17%	5%

COMMENT

It would appear from the results reported in the series of cases listed in this presentation that they are essentially the same with the use of phacoemulsification in skilled hands as with the intracapsular cataract extraction. The exaggerated claims made in the lay press in the United States of the revolutionary advance in cataract surgery are not proven to be true. The patients are rehabilitated slightly earlier, and their best visual acuity following surgery occurs sooner; however, with modern wound closure and adequate suturing, outpatient cataract surgery is being performed in the United States by some physicians and most patients remain in the hospital only two to four days following cataract surgery. Emery does not give his patients contact lenses following phacoemulsification until a month or longer after surgery, and this is the same time that I give contact lenses following routine intracapsular cataract operation.

The phacoemulsifer as designed by Kelman unquestionably is a better instrument for aspiration of soft lenses in young patients than is a simple syringe. However, the cost of the instrument ranges from $20,000 to $30,000. In the United States the aspiration needle following phacoemulsification needs to be returned to the manufacturer after each operation, and this is an added expense of $150. Likewise, the time required by the operating room staff to clean and prepare the instrument adds several hundred dollars to the cost of cataract extraction in our country.

I would therefore conclude that this is an operation and a technique that might be preferred by individual surgeons. In skilled hands the results are certainly comparable to those of intracapsular cataract surgery. The added cost involved in the use of the machine is unquestionably a factor that should be taken into consideration.

Over the years many fads, minor modifications, and real improvements have been made in cataract surgery. Only time and adequately documented clinical studies published in scientific ophthalmic journals will determine whether this technique is merely a fad or is a true advance that will remain in the armamentarium of the ophthalmic surgeon.

REFERENCES

Emery, J.M., Wilhemus, K.A., & Rosenberg, S. Complications of Phacoelmulsification. Symposium: Complications of Modern Surgical Procedures. *Ophthalmology* 85:141-150, Feb. 1978.

Wilkinson, C.P., Anderson, L.S. & Little, J.H. Retinal Detachment Following Phacoemulsification. *Ophthalmology* 85:151–156, Feb. 1978

Stark, W.J., Hirst, L.W., Snip, R. & Maumenee, A.E. A Two-year Trial of Intraocular Lenses at the Wilmer Institute. *Amer. J. Ophthal.* 84:769–774, Dec. 1977

Maumenee, A.E. & Meredith, T.A. A Survey of 500 Cases of Cataract Extraction. *Current Concepts in Cataract Surgery.* Selected proceedings of the Third Biennial Cataract Surgical Congress; Emery, J.M. & Paton, D. (eds.) Chapter 67, pp. 423-426, C.V. Mosby Co., St. Louis, 1974.

Author's address:
The Wilmer Institute
Johns Hopkins Hospital
601 N. Broadway
Baltimore, Md 21205
U.S.A.

183

Docum. Ophthal. Proc. Series, Vol. 21

PARS PLANA LENSECTOMY WITH ULTRASONIC FRAGMENTATION (USF)

LOUIS J. GIRARD

(Houston, Texas, U.S.A.)

INTRODUCTION

Intracapsular cataract extraction has been the standard operation for extraction of the lens throughout the world for the past 75 years. The operation has become highly sophisticated with newer technical developments such as the use of the operating microscope, finer instruments and sutures. In spite of the degree of sophistication there are still many complications which occur with intracapsular cataract extraction. In his book on the subject, Jaffee (1976) devotes 307 pages to the complications of intracapsular cataract extraction. As the age of the population increases, the number of postoperative years after intracapsular cataract increases and more complications develop.

There have been a number of attempts to replace the intracapsular cataract extraction with a different type of operation. The extracapsular extraction was revived (Shoch et al. 1978) and the technique of extracapsular cataract extraction was modified by Kelman but the results of a survey (Troutman 1975) showed that the extracapsular cataract extraction does not produce any better results than intracapsular cataract extraction. In addition, ECCE requires discission of a secondary membrane in 35-50% of cases after 2 years.

Lensectomy through the pars plana is a completely new approach to the removal of cataracts. It eliminates the corneal sections, improper closure of which accounts for so many complications of intra and extracapsular cataract extraction. It uses a closed system which eliminates the "moment of truth" when the surgeon must deliver the lens without loss of vitreous. It eliminates the large incisions which cause the postoperative astigmatism and prolonged convalescence.

Lensectomy through the pars plana was an outgrowth of vitrectomy through the pars plana. (Girard & Hawkins 1974). When both cataract extraction and vitrectomy were indicated, it was found simpler to do both procedures through the pars plana. The appearance of eyes operated on with this technique was so good that it was decided to use this for routine cataracts.

Ultrasonic fragmentation (USF) was used primarily for extracapsular extraction through the anterior chamber approach. This in turn was an outgrowth of a technique of aspiration and irrigation introduced by the author in 1966. Even though smaller incisions were used, extracapsular

185

extraction by USF required corneal incisions with all of the possible complications of corneal incisions such as anterior synechia, vitreous incarceration, wound dehiscence, epithelial downgrowth or stromal downgrowth, etc.

Vitrectomy by ultrasonic fragmentation through the pars plana was first introduced by 1972 and has been highly successful. It was a natural development to use the Ultrasonic Fragmentor for removal of cataracts through the pars plana as well.

The results of lensectomy through the pars plana appear to be very encouraging. Many of the complications of intracapsular cataract extraction are eliminated by this approach. The technique will be described and the advantages and disadvantages will be discussed.

TECHNIQUE

A. *Patient preparation*

The patient is prepared in the usual way for intraocular surgery. The pupil is maximally dilated. Anesthesia can be either local or general; however, because of the closed system technique it is unnecessary to have "perfect" anesthesia and analgesia because the pressure can be controlled by the surgeon. It is unnecessary to use digital pressure, aqueous inhibitors or osmotic agents preoperatively.

B. *Incisions*

An assistant rotates the eye downward; no superior rectus suture is necessary. Conjunctiva and Tenon's capsule are incised at the 10 and 2 o'clock

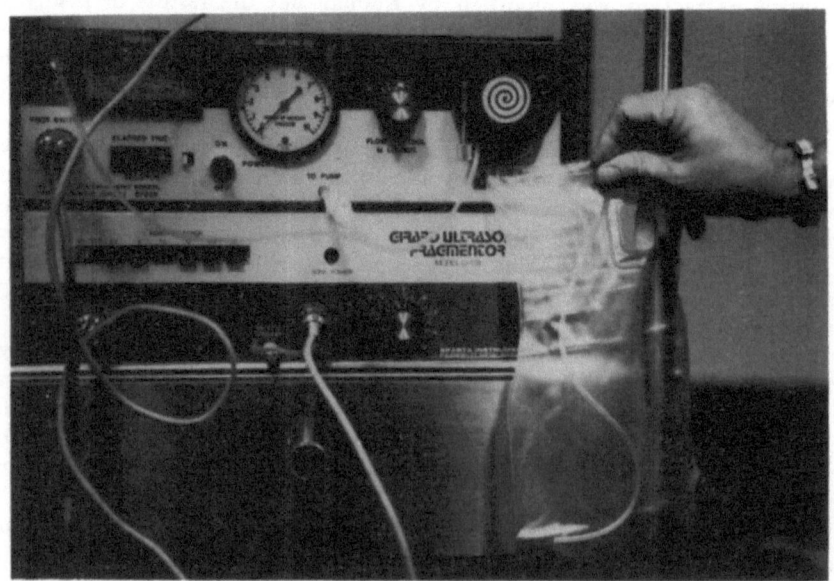

Fig. 1. The Ultrasonic Fragmentor and aspirator. (Courtesy of C.V. Mosby Co.)

186

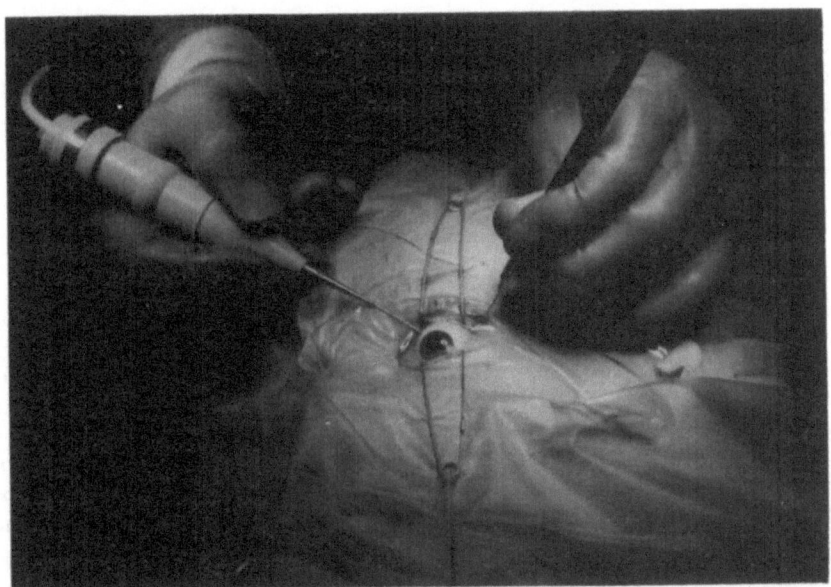

Fig. 2. Pars plana lensectomy by ultrasonic fragmentation. The surgeon holds the irrigator in his left hand and the fragmentor/aspirator in his right hand. (Courtesy of C.V. Mosby Co.)

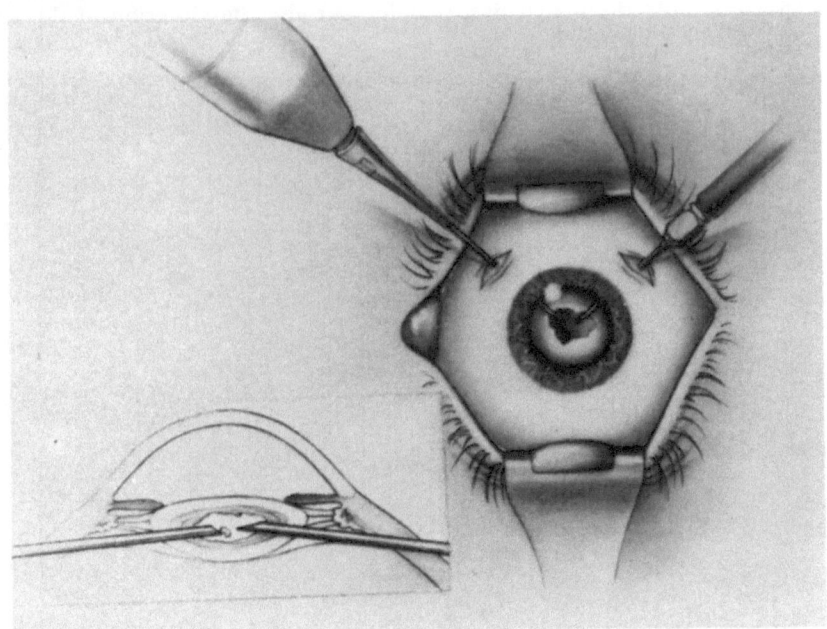

Fig. 3. Through incisions in conjunctiva and sclera. The irrigator is inserted into the lens at 2 o'clock and the fragmentor/aspirator at 10 o'clock. By a combination of fragmentation, irrigation and aspiration, the lens is removed. (Courtesy of C.V. Mosby Co.)

187

positions and the sclera exposed. Usually there is little or no bleeding. A caliper is used to mark 4 mm from the limbus and a small cautery mark is made. A sclerotomy incision is made at 10 and 2 o'clock with a small knife such as a Girard knife. The incision at the 10 o'clock position (if the surgeon is right-handed) might have to be enlarged slightly to accommodate the rather blunt tip of the fragmenting/aspirating needle.

C. *Subtotal lensectomy*

A 20 guage irrigating needle of the Ultrasonic Fragmentor is inserted through the 2 o'clock position into the lens and the fragmenting/aspirating cannula is inserted through the 10 o'clock incision into the lens. Fragmentation is begun and the two needles are brought into close proximity in the nucleus. **Nuclectomy** is first achieved by creating a cavity in the necleus and then gradually enlarging it. When all of the nucleus has been removed a **cortectomy** is performed attempting to keep both the anterior and posterior lens capsules intact. Cortex in the equatorial region beneath the iris can be brought into the view of the surgeon by the help of scleral depression by an assistant. When all or a majority of the cortex has been removed the posterior capsule and anterior vitreous are removed.

The anterior lens capsule should be left intact if possible. The posterior surface of this lens capsule should be scraped using the fragmenting/aspirating cannula. The anterior lens capsule is very durable and usually withstands not only the mechanical scraping but also the vibration of the activated fragmenting needle.

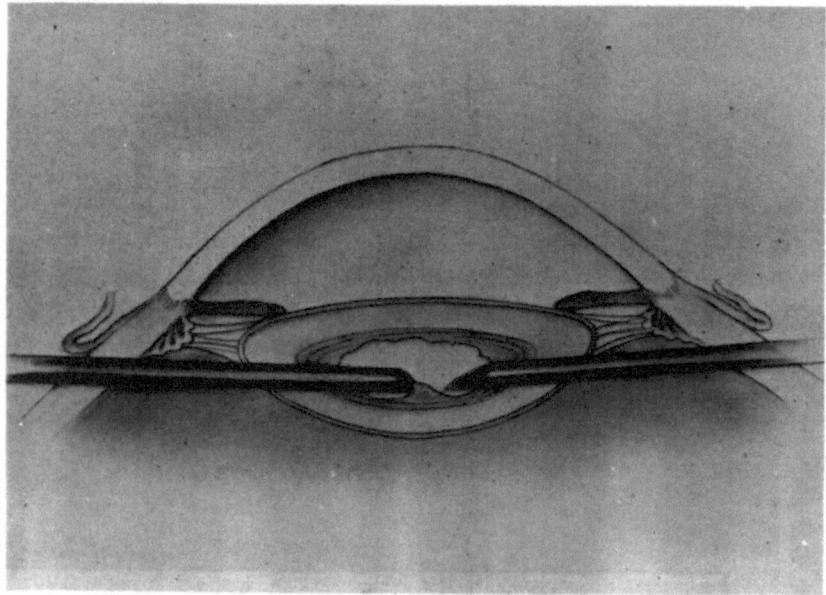

Fig. 4. Nuclectomy (Courtesy of C.V. Mosby Co.)

188

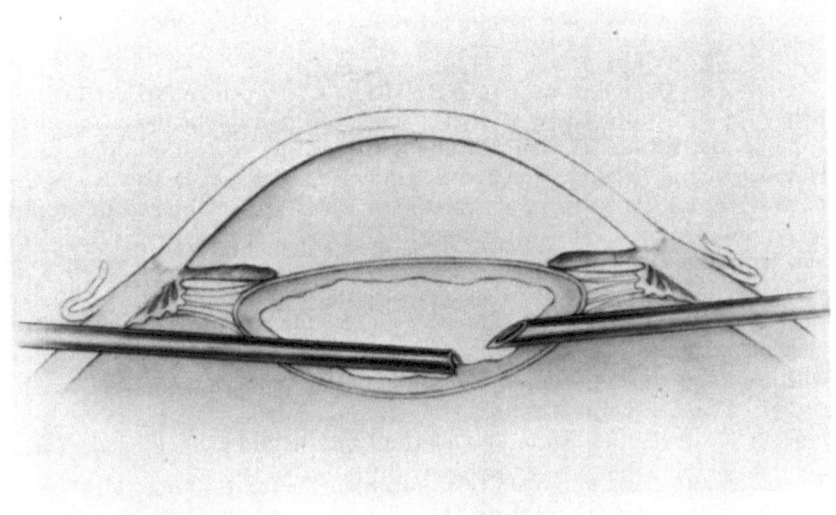

Fig. 5. Cortectomy. (Courtesy of C.V. Mosby Co.)

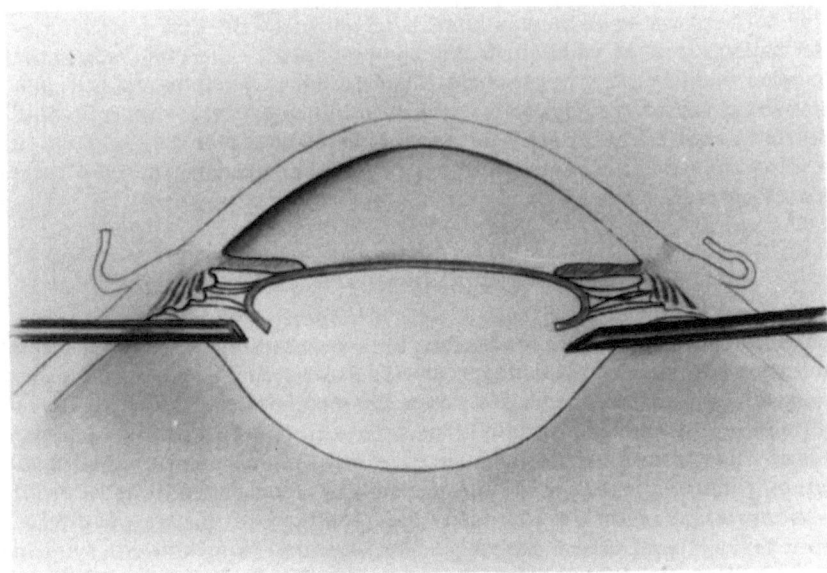

Fig. 6. After removal of the nucleus, cortex, posterior capsule and anterior vitreous, the procedure is completed by closure of the incisions. The anterior capsule is left intact. (Courtesy of C.V. Mosby Co.)

189

If any lens fragments drop into the vitreous they can be retrieved with the help of a flat contact lens whitch extends the view of the operating microscope to the retina. The microscope is focused down to the retina and the lens fragments located. The fragmenting/aspirating needle is then inserted posteriorly with aspiration activated, the lens fragment picked up from the retina and brought to the central portion of the globe where it is fragmented and aspirated.

The fragmenting/aspirating needle is withdrawn first and then the irrigating needle. The wound should be checked for the presence of prolapsed vitreous. If there is any prolapsed vitreous this should be carefully removed with the fragmenting/aspirating needle.

D. *Examination of the fundus*

This is an excellent opportunity to examine the fundus under ideal circumstances. The indirect ophthalmoscope and scleral depression can be performed and the retina carefully checked. Any pathology should be given appropriate treatment, i.e., cryotherapy for retinal holes, etc.

E. *Closure*

Scleral incisions are closed with deep sutures of the surgeon's choice. The author prefers a 9-0 nylon interrupted suture. The conjunctiva can be approximated or can be sutured.

F. *Postoperative care*

The patients can be ambulated immediately. Usually the first postoperative day there will be no corneal changes and perhaps a 1+ flare and cells in the anterior chamber. Prophylactic local antibiotics, a cycloplegic and a mild steroid are sufficient. Usually the patient can be corrected to 20/20 the first postoperative day. Because there are no corneal incisions the final correction of spectacles can be given within a few days or the patient can be fitted with a contact lens.

DISCUSSION

Lensectomy through the pars plana with ultrasonic fragmentation has many advantages over intra or extracapsular cataract extraction. The pars plana approach eliminates vitreous loss, impending and actual, rupture of the lens capsule, epithelial and stromal downgrowth, scleral collapse, expulsive hemorrhage, wound gaping or dehiscence, iris prolapse, loss of the anterior chamber, detachment of Descemet's membrane, corneal endothelial proliferation, prolapse of the vitreous into the anterior chamber, keratopathy from vitreous incarceration or adherence, keratopathy from anterior synechia, postoperative astigmatism and prolonged convalescence. Vitrectomy prevents such complications as pupillary block glaucoma, aphakic glaucoma, prolapse of the vitreous into the anterior chamber, keratopathy from vitreous incarceration and adherence.

There are certain complications of intracapsular cataract extraction which are shared by pars plana lensectomy such as retinal detachment, cystoid macular edema, uveitis and infection.

Cystoid macular edema has not been a problem in our experience and has been successfully controlled by keeping the pressure normal or slightly elevated by the use of local steroids. Retinal detachment has approximately the same incidence as intracapsular cataract extraction but it is hoped with the careful scrutiny of the fundus at the end of the procedure, this complication can be greatly reduced or eliminated.

Uveitis can occur because pars plana lensectomy is an extracapsular extraction. Two cases of phacoanaphylactic uveitis have occurred in patients who have had both eyes operated on one week apart. No cases of infection have occurred.

SUMMARY

Lensectomy through the pars plana with ultrasonic fragmentation (USF) is a new operation for the removal of cataracts. It is applicable to any type of cataract; congenital, traumatic, senile, subluxated, dislocated, secondary or any type of membrane such as a retroimplant membrane. The operation requires the skilled use of the operating microscope, coaxial illumination and the skilled use of the Ultrasonic Fragmentor. Many of the complications of intracapsular or extracapsular cataract extraction are eliminated with the use of this procedure; however, it will have to stand the test of time and experience by many surgeons before it has the possibility of replacing intracapsular cataract extraction as the treatment of choice.

REFERENCES

Girard, L.J.: Aspiration-irrigation of congenital and traumatic cataracts. *Arch. Ophthalmol.* 77:387, March 1967.

Girard, L.J., Ultrasonic Fragmentation (USF) for Intraocular Surgery. St. Louis. The C.V. Mosby Co, (In Press).

Girard, L.J., Hawkins, R.S: Cataract extraction by ultrasonic aspiration. Vitrectomy by ultrasonic fragmentation. *Trans Am. Acad. Ophthalmol. Otolaryngol* 78:OP-50, 1974.

Jaffee, N.: Cataract Surgery and Its Complications (2nd ed), St. Louis, The C.V. Mosby Co, 1976.

Shoch, D. et al.: Symposium: modern aspects of cataract operations, *Ophthalmology* 85: 39, 1978.

Troutman, R.: Cataract survey of the cataract phacoemulsification committee, *Trans Am. Acad. Ophthalmol. Otolaryngol.* 79:OP-178, 1975.

Author's address:
59 Tiel Way
Houston, Texas 77019
USA

Docum. Ophthal. Proc. Series, Vol. 21

INDICATIONS AND TECHNIQUES OF BILATERAL
CATARACT EXTRACTION

F. PINTUCCI

(Rome, Italy)

In this article on bilateral cataract operation I will only discuss pre-senile and senile cataract.

1. Loss of binocular vision
2. Difficulty in using glasses or contact or intracameral lenses.

The greatest trouble in a patient operated for cataract in one eye is the loss of binocular vision. Contact lenses and intracameral lenses do not resolve the problem in all cases because, apart from tolerance of the first and risks of the second, these lenses are not always able to remove anisometropia or to completely correct the refractive defect.

Patients operated in one eye only often prefer to use the unoperated eye, even with less vision, rather than resort to glasses or a contact lens. Thus it is obvious that it is best to perform the two operations within a short period of time and, if possible at the same time.

1. Recovery of binocular vision
2. Reduction of psycho-physical stress
3. Shorter time of hospitalization

The bilateral cataract operation in which both eyes are operated at the same time, does not only give the advantage of immediate recovery of bilateral vision but also less psycho-physical stress for the patient and a shorter time of hospitalization.

1. Risk of surgical infection
2. Need of general anaesthesia
3. Necessity of binocular occlusion
4. Lack of observation of post-operative recovery in the first eye

The reasons which up to now have induced most surgeons to forego bilateral operation may be summarised as follows: fear of surgical infection, the need to resort to general anaesthesia, the necessity of binocular occlusion, the lack of observation of post-operative recovery in the first eye.

These reasons, which have led many surgeons to give up the advantages of bilateral operation, are, in the light of present day medical knowledge, no longer valid, since careful ocular and general study of the patient together with proper antibiotic treatment practically guarantee freedom from infection. Moreover, general anaesthetic techniques have been brought to such perfection, that they can be used in the majority cases. The binocular occlusion, with the application of safe techniques, can be removed after 48 hours and if necessary, even sooner. Finally, any suggestions which may be obtained from observation of post-operative recovery in the first eye are not in themselves important enough to lead the surgeon to forego the advantage of the bilateral operation.

Bilateral cataract extraction is an important operation and specific conditions must exist if it is to be performed:

Surgery indications   1. short- and long-focus vision in both eyes
                       2. evolution of the cataract
                       3. profession
                       4. age

If the cataract has a fast evolution, it is useless to postpone the operation; if, instead, evolution is very slow, the operation may be postponed. Often it is better to wait until the cataracts have reached a certain evolution and operate on both eyes together rather than operate only one eye, the latter method leaving the patient with a sense of uncertainty due to the loss of binocular vision.

Cataracts in both eyes which do not prevent the patient from continuing his usual activity and profession should not be removed, but in other cases, even with superior visual acuity, the loss of binocular vision due to increase of the cataract in one eye may, in view of the patient's profession, make necessary a bilateral operation.

The age of the patient is quite important; if, on one hand, it is difficult to estimate the possibilities of survival in a very old patient, on the other hand, his advanced age will not allow the adaption necessary for overcoming the spatial troubles caused by loss of binocular vision. However, if the cataracts show a tendency to increase, it is better to operate at the age of 80 with a good general health condition than to wait several years and operate when these conditions will certainly be worse, or at least uncertain.

Pre-operative objective   1. Anterior segment
clinical examination   2. Fundus oculi and functional tests
                          3. Ocular refraction (severe myopia)
                          4. Ocular pressure (tonometric curve, tonography)
                          5. Ocular adnexa

The clinical examination, though routine, must be performed with the greatest care. Particular attention should be given to the fundus oculi in view of connection between cataract extraction and retinal detachment. If possible an examination in maximum mydriasis should be performed, with particular regard to peripheral and central degenerative lesions. The presence of the first may make a cataract operation unadvisable and may suggest the necessity for a prophylactic operation on the retina; the second may give, although in terms in which cannot be strictly estimated, various data for the prognosis. If macular lesions exist, it is even more advisable to perform a bilateral operation because if only the better eye is operated, the other may never be operated, while if both are operated, even if the visual acuity in one eye is very low, the patient may recover a good vision-field and binocular balance with more satisfactory final results.

Of course, the slighest doubts as to the presence of more or less latent infections involving the adnexa is an absolute contraindication to the operation.

MEDICAL AND PSYCHOLOGICAL EXAMINATIONS

The general surgical indications depend on assessment of the results of the various examinations requested by the internist and the anaesthesist. Special attention must be given to focal infections in order to prevent the outbreak of highly dangerous infections. Not to be overlooked are the patient's psycological balance and the necessity for establishing an atmosphere of trust and confidence which can help the patient to overcome a shock which is certainly greater than is commonly supposed. Obviously the patient must fully accept the operation, and it may be wise for the surgeon to consider the possibility of stopping after the operation of the first eye if there are any complications. Actually this is almost never necessary, but this possibility seems to reassure the patient rather than alarm him.

CHARACTERISTICS OF OPERATIVE ROOM AND VARIOUS TECHNIQUES

In the operating room special attention must be given to the sterilization of instruments, operation field and any substances used. A quite important part in the outbreak of infections is played by surgical trauma and by the introduction into the anterior chamber of instruments and solutions which should be reduced to the absolute minimum. At the end of the operation on the first eye, the surgeon should change his gown mask and gloves, should use new instruments and new solutions.

CHARACTERISTICS OF THE SURGEON AND HIS TECHNIQUE

If advising a bilateral operation, the surgeon must have reached an excellent

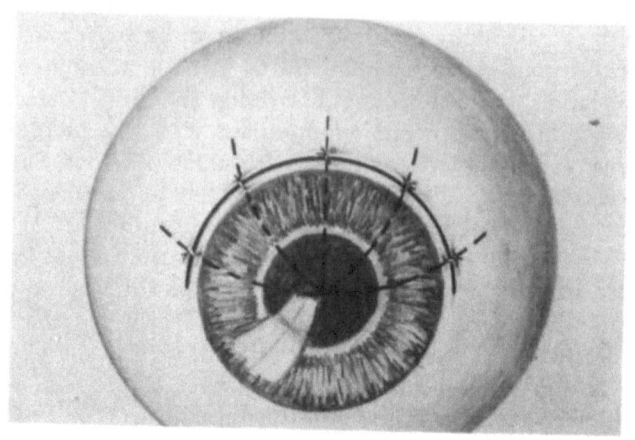

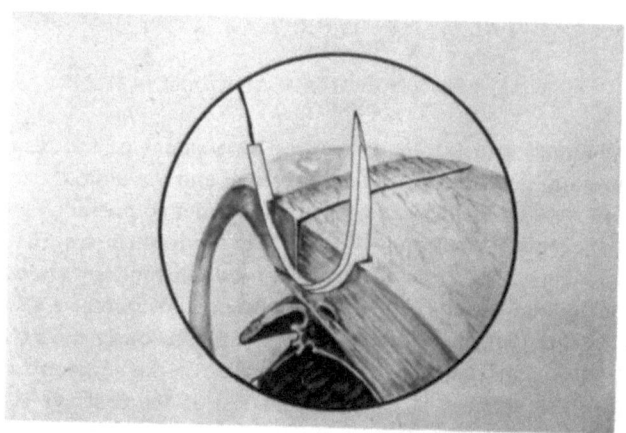

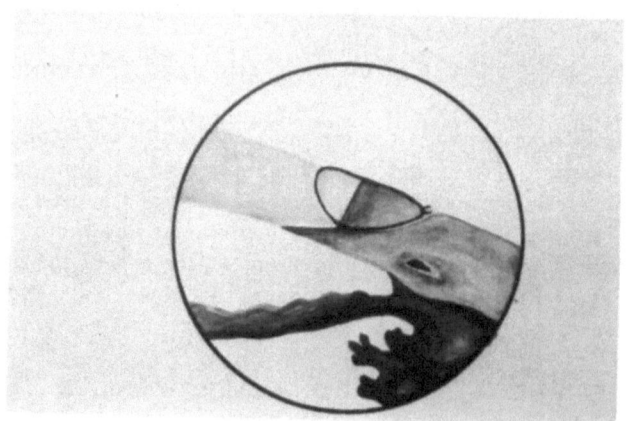

Figs. 1–2. See text.

technical level, must have wide experience and must have obtained good results over a long period of time. Certainly self-criticism and decision on this matter are never easy; the decision to undertake a bilateral operation must be made spontaneously, and it would be a mistake to perform such an operation without profound conviction.

Obviously, operative technique is very important; in this regard, a few personal technical details should be mentioned here. Special importance must be given to opening and closing the anterior chamber, because most complications depend on this. The opening of the anterior chamber should be as circular as possible and should be placed parallel to the limbus and the sutures along the meridians (Fig. 1). I prefer the limbus, since the stiches will be covered by the conjunctiva.

The incision made in the external 2/3 is vertical to facilitate the application of the sutures, and in the internal 1/3 it is bevelled to increase the contact surface and to create a uniform posterior limit for the depth of the sutures. Two sutures placed before opening the anterior chamber have con-

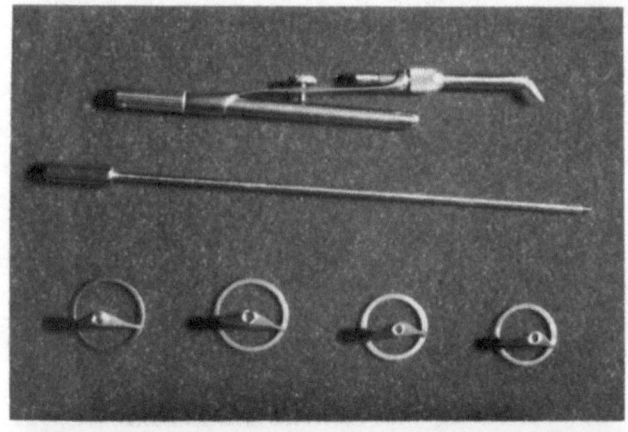

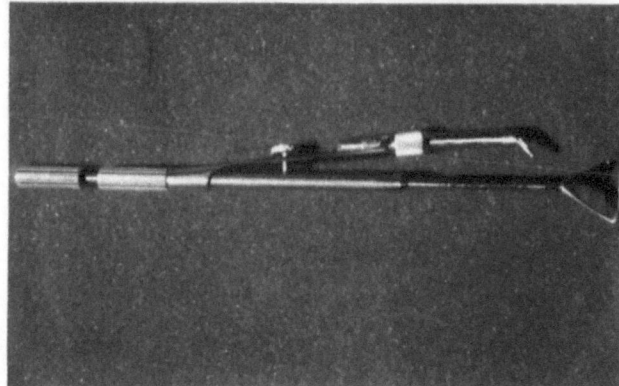

Fig. 3. See text.

siderable importance because at the end of the operation they confront corresponding stiches with reduction of astigmatism, while during the operation they allow the surgeon to close the anterior chamber at any moment (Fig. 2–2^1). To give nylon a certain manoeuvrability, caudate sutures may be used. These are made of 15 cm. of 7/0 Kalt silk mounted on a corneal needle and by a nylon tail at the lower end. In the middle third of the silk, a loop which works like the Gomez-Marquez stop is prepared with the aid of a watchmakers forceps. At the end of the operation, traction applied to the Kalt thread is enough to untie the loop and to make the nylon slide within the passage.

To perform a semicircular incision allowing sutures to be preplaced, the compass keratotome is used (Fig. 3) a diamond scalpel + scissors are used for opening the anterior chamber.

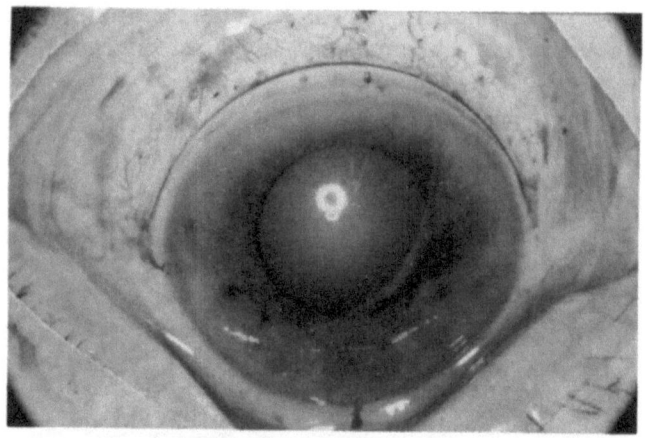

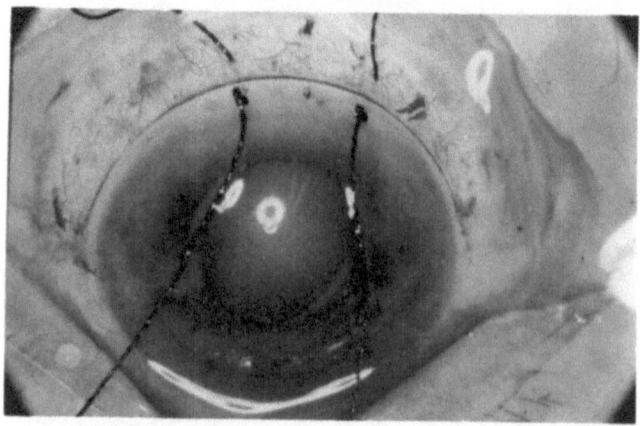

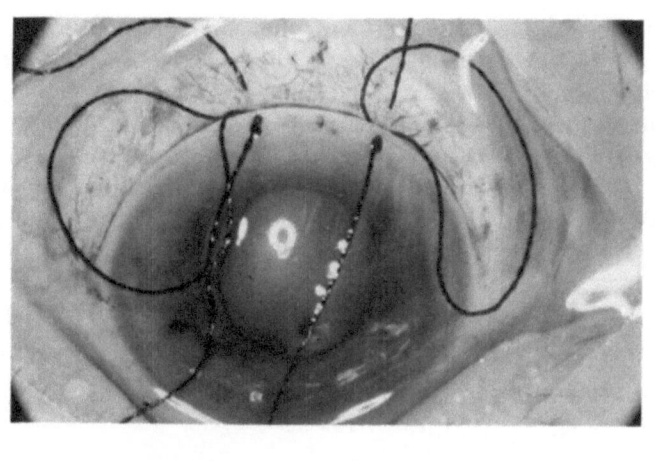

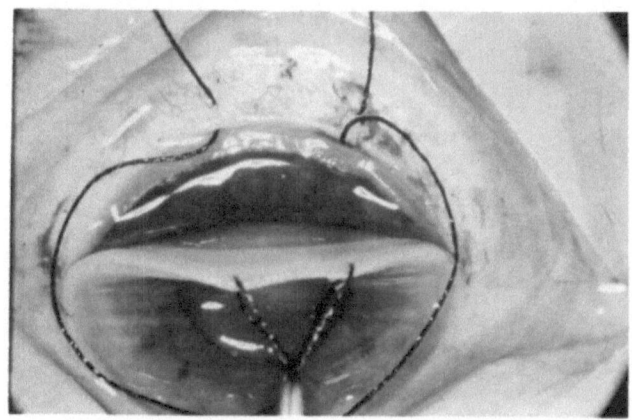

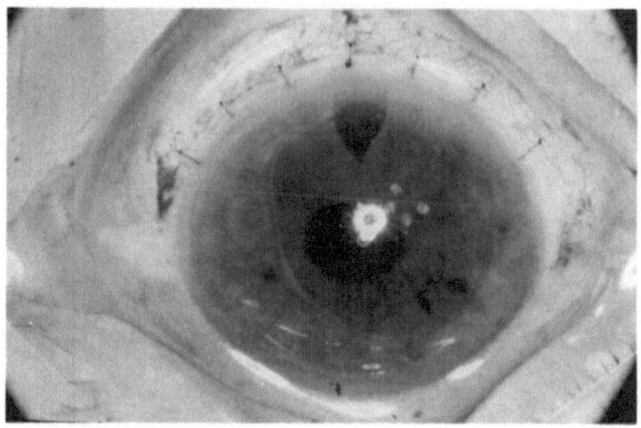

Fig. 4. Operation techniques.

Since October 1965, 170 bilateral extraction operations have been performed using this technique on patients whose ages ranged from 51 to 85 years, with an average age of 70 years and 6 months. Complications were the same as those met in uni-lateral operations. Personally, the author has never regretted having performed a bilateral operation. If, in some rare cases, a complication has arisen involving one eye, the other eye immediately could be used. In the author's experience, his patients have never shown complications depending directly or indirectly on the bilateral operation.

Author's address:
F. Pintucci
Primario Ospedale Oftalmico
Via Bertoloni, 37
Rome
Italy

EXPERIMENTAL IMPLANTATION OF CRYSTALLINE LENS

SHUZO IWATA

(Nagoya, Japan)

Ever since the demonstration that lens opacification can be induced as experimental cataract in various animals, many important aspects have been delineated concerning the cataract formation. In order to clarify the cause of the trigger reaction as one of the initial processes in lens turbidity, it is important to investigate and understand the nature of the surroundings of the crystalline lens as well as its inner-environment (Iwata, Ikemoto & Takehana 1976).

The present paper deals with an attempt at implanting the young mouse lens into the aphakic eye of an adult mouse. This experimental lens implantation implies the long term system of in vivo culturing, and may confirm the property and behavior of the lens itself at organ level which is incorporated in the eye.

For that reason, the present experiments were attempted to determine the growth situation of implanted lens in its environment (Yamamoto & Iwata 1974), and to investigate whether the hereditary mouse cataract is due to a gene-induced alteration of the lens itself or due to changes of the outer-environment of lens (Yamamoto & Iwata 1972, 1973).

MATERIALS AND METHODS

In the first implantation experiments of the crystalline lens, the mice of the ICR strain were used. The donor lenses to be implanted were always 6 to 8 days old animals, and the adult mice, approximately two months old, were used as the recipients. The recipient mouse was anesthetized with intravenous 0.5% sodium pentobarbital (1.0 ml/100 g body weight), and a topical anesthesia (0.4% benoxinate hydrochloride solution) was induces in the right eye. The left eye was always untouched to use as a control. After the pupil was opened with a mydriatic (0.5% tropicamide and 0.5% phenylephrine-HCl) the cornea was incised along the upper limbus for one-third of the corneal circumference. Alpha-chymotrypsin solution (2,000 units per ml) was injected into the posterior chamber through the corneal wound, and about 3 minutes later, the crystalline lens of the recipient eye was removed using forceps, and the anterior chamber was irrigated gently with the balanced salt solution. The donor lens, which had been taken in a similar manner from the eye of the young mouse without the anesthesia treatment, was

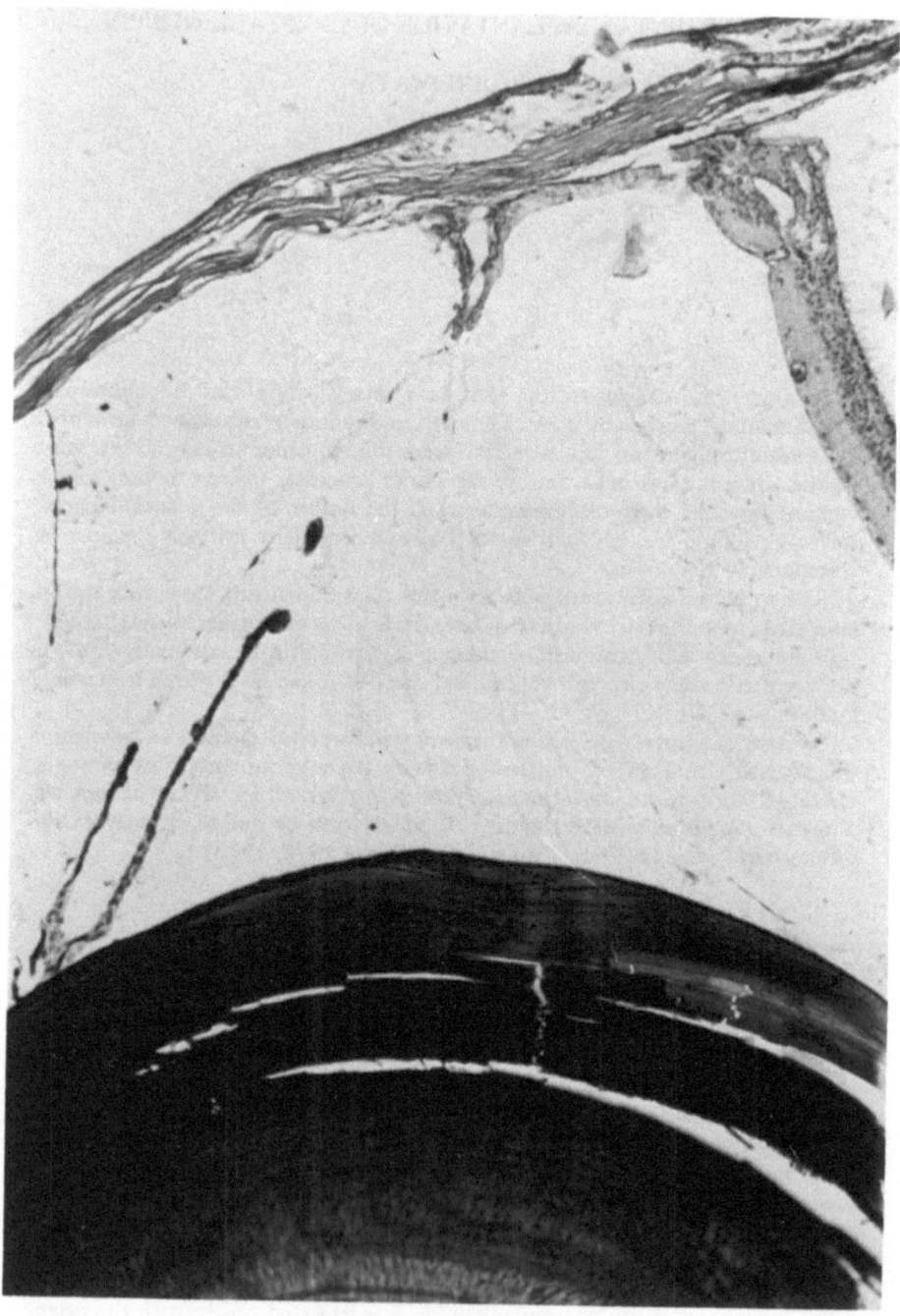

Fig. 1. The regenerating zonular fibers between the surface of implanted lens and the ciliary part of the recipient eye, x 60.

immediately implanted, using a blunt-tipped spatula, into the space from which the recipients lens had just been removed.

It was important, in placing the donor lens into the aphakic eye, to assure the antero-posterior direction, in both normal and reverse orientations. After lens implantation, the corneal wound had two stitches with 10-0 suture, 6 mm/0.15 mm needle, and chloramphenicol ointment was applied topically.

RESULTS AND DISCUSSION

Growth behavior of implanted lens in orientation

In the first orientation experiment, the young lens of normal mouse was implanted in normal orientation and position into the aphakic eye of the normal adult mouse to examine the behavior upon the growth of the implanted lens.

Five days after implantation, the connection between the implanted lens and the ciliary part of the recipient was well recognized with the regeneration of zonular fibers from the recipient in the histological observation (Fig. 1 and 2a), and the implanted lens grew normally in the increase in the diameter of lens is shown in Fig. 3, and its transparency was kept for more than 150 days after implantation.

When the young donor lens was implanted in reverse orientation into the normal aphakic eye to study the polarity of lens in the ocular environment, the epithelial cells of the implanted lens elongated to the center of lens on the side of retina, and the new epithelium was formed on the corneal side of the lens (Fig. 2b). The lenses implanted reversely into the recipient eyes did not grow and appeared opaque.

The first experimental result, in the normal orientation, indicates the feasibility of crystalline lens implantation in mouse. The normal young lens of the mouse can grow normally and maintain its transparency when implanted into the healthy eye, and regenerating zonular fibers are observed between the surface of implanted lens and ciliary body. The partial opacities and the failure of lens growth found in some cases were thought to be due to a slight physical damage to the donor lens at the time of the implantation.

In the second experiment, it was observed that when the young lens was implanted in the reverse orientation, the differentiation of the original epithelial cells to fiber cells led to elongation in the portion facing the neural retina of the recipient eye. This result suggests that the differentiation of the epithelial cells to lens fiber cells has polarity in the ocular environment, or is dependent on the chemotaxis of the some substances in the neural retina of the aphakic eye.

Ocular environment in hereditary mouse cataract

Success in the above lens implantation studies allowed further ocular environmental investigations on the implanted lens to be made.

Recently, a study was made on preliminary evidence suggesting that an apparent deficiency of Na-K ATPase may be included in the initial factors

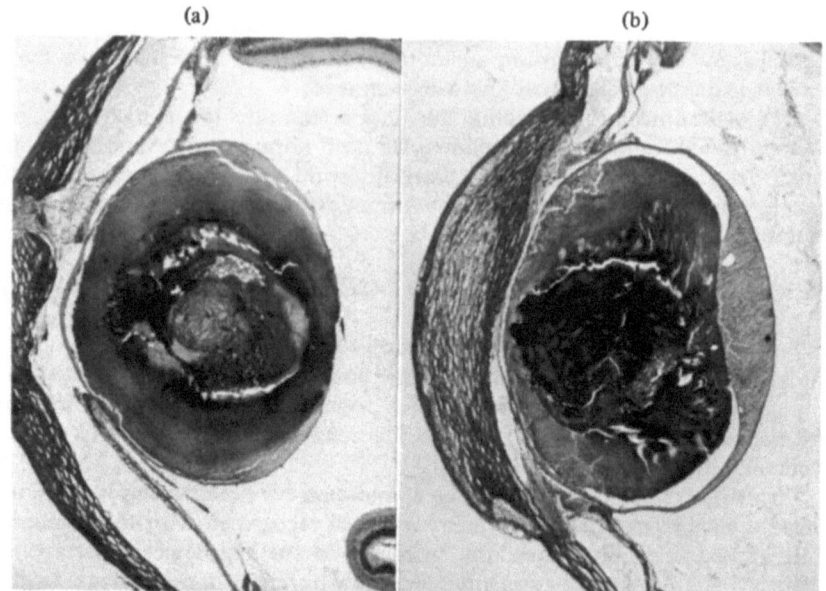

Fig. 2. The lenses implanted into the normal eyes in the two orientations. (a): A young implanted lens in the normal orientation, x 25. (b): A young implanted lens in the reverse orientation, x 25, Note the elongated original epithelial cells on the side of retina.

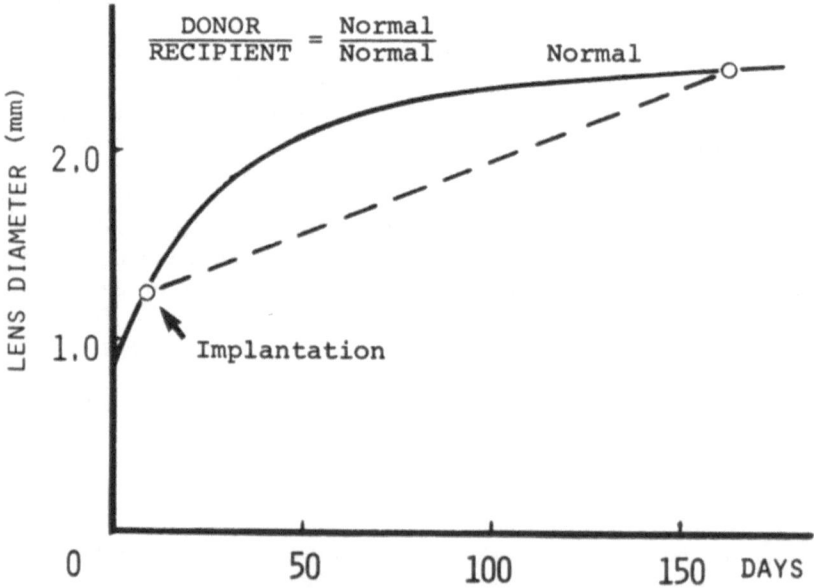

Fig. 3. Growth curves (lens diamters) of the normal lens and the normal implanted lens in adult mice.

of hereditary cataract of cac strain mice (Iwata & Kinoshita 1971). An important result of a defect of this cation-pump is an interaction between the sign of enzyme deficiency and the environment surrounding the crystalline lens. One possibility for an explanation of this interaction may be confirmed with the lens implantation experiment.

This hereditary cataract (cac strain) was found as a mutation in mice in Japan by Nakano et al. (1960). The normal and the hereditary cataractous mice open their eyes on the 14 postnatal days. At the eye open-time, the lenses of defective mice are still clear. The lenses become opacified at the age of about 24 days after birth, and the opacity appears as a 'pin-head' opacity in the lens nucleus. This lens opacity then slowly enlarges until the entire lens is involved and the mature cataract is formed. The fact that the lenses keep transparency for a certain length of time, and then become opaque over a certain period, makes them suitable and convenient experimental models for elucidative study of the ocular environment.

Lenses were inplanted in four different ways in the mice of ICR and cac strain. These were as follows (Fig. 4):

I. The young normal lens was implanted into the adult normal eye for the experiment of lens implantation as already described in above.

II. The young normal lens was implanted into the aphakic eye of hereditray cataract mouse for the check of intraocular environment.

III. The young cataractforming lens while transparent was implanted into the eyeball of the mature cataract for the reaffirmation of congenital cataract.

IV. The young cataractous lens while transparent was implanted into the adult normal eye for the confirmation of genetic defect.

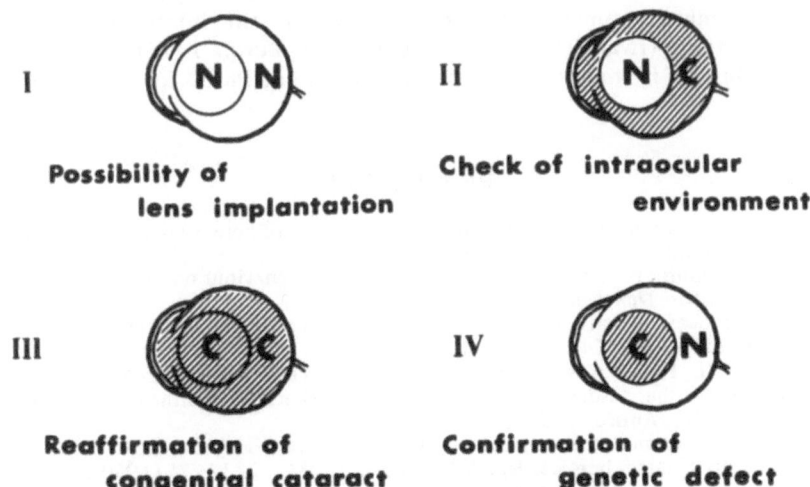

Fig. 4. Lens implantation of four different ways in the mice of ICR and cac strain. N: the normal young implanted lens or normal recipient eye, C: The young donor lens of hereditary cataract or the adult recipient eye of hereditary cataract.

Table I. Results of the lens implantation in the four different ways.

Type of Implantation DONER RECIPIENT	State of Implanted Lens	Diameter of Lens Normal : 2.14 mm Cataract : 1.79 mm
1 Normal / Normal	Transparent	2.17 mm
2 Normal / Cataract	Transparent	1.93 mm
3 Cataract / Cataract	Opacification	1.75 mm
4 Cataract / Normal	Opacification	1.76 mm

In these four different procedures, the postoperative follow-up was made for 100 to 150 days. The overall results are given in Table 1.

In the second experiment (Fig. 4,II), the normal growth and transparency of young normal lens would indicate that the intraocular environment of the mice of the cataractous trait did not play a decisive role in the process of the hereditary cataract.

On the other hand, the third and fourth experimental results would point to the gene-induced mechanism of the cataract development residing within the lens tissue itself. This suggests that the opacifying factor or factors are not present in the outer-environment surrounding the lens, but that the trigger reaction exists in the inner-environment of lens. It is now assumed that a membrane function factor is involved in the inhibition of Na-K ATPase activity (Iwata 1974; Kinoshita, Fukui & Merola 1976).

The author is indebted to Dr. Y. Yamamoto, Ph.D. for his technical assistance.

REFERENCES

Iwata, S. & Kinoshita, J.H.: Mechanism of development of hereditary cataract in mice, *Invest. Ophthal.,* 10, *504-512* (1971).
Iwata, S., Ikemoto, F. & Takehana, M.: Environmental behaviour on the lens opacification, *Acta Soc. Ophthalm. Jap,,*
Iwata, S.: Process of lens opacification and membrane function, A review, *Ophthal. Res.,* 6, *138-154* (1974).
Kinoshita, J.H., Fukui, H.N. & Merola, L.O.: Na-K ATPase inhibitor in Nakano mouse cataract, In the Association for Research in Vision and Ophthalmology, Spring Meeting, USA, April 26, 1976.
Nakano, K., Yamamoto, S., Kutsukake, G., Ogawa, H., Nakajima, A. & Takano, E.: Hereditary cataract in mice, *Jap. J. Clin. Ophthal.,* 14, *1772-1775* (1960).
Yamamoto, Y. & Iwata, S.: Implantation of the crystalline lens in mous, A preliminary report, *Jap. J. Ophthal.,* 16, *300-303* (1972).
Yamamoto, Y. & Iwata, S.: Implantation of crystalline lens in mouse – As one of the approaches for cataract study –, *Acta Soc. Ophthalm.,* 77, *888-896* (1973).

Yamamoto, Y. & Iwata, S.: Some problems concerning lens implantation, *Acta Soc. Ophthalm. Jap.*, 78, *957-961* (1974).

Author's address:
Laboratory of Biophysical Chemistry
Faculty of Pharmaceutical Sciences
Meijo University
Nagoya 468, Japan

Docum. Ophthal. Proc. Series, Vol. 21

CONGENITAL CATARACT-SURGICAL PROBLEMS

G. SCUDERI - S. M. RECUPERO

(Rome, Italy)

INTRODUCTION

General criteria for the choice of the most appropriate time for surgical operation of congenital cataract are based on the following clinical factors: the type of cataract (partial or total, unilateral or bilateral) and its possible assocation with other ocular alternations (strabismus, etc.). From an examination of table I, it can be deduced that small stationary opacities of the lens, which, especially when peripheric, cause only slight visual disturbance, are not particularly significant. On the contrary, the large central opacities and, even more, the total ones, necessitate early operation, never in any case to be postponed beyong the fifth year of age. In bilateral forms, it is very important to operate on the second eye only a few months after the first in order to provide binocular vision as soon as possible and to avoid establishment of an irreversible amblyopia.

Concerning judgement as to operability, great caution and reserve must be used when inflammation or ocular or associated general malformations exist. Therefore it is indispensable, in the pre-operative period, that the patient be routinely subjected to careful medical examination and above all to a complete ocular check-up with:

pharmacodynamic tests for pupillary mobility; tonometry; gonioscopy; ecography; electroretinography; ophthalmoscopy (when possible). etc.

Table I. Indications for the best time for the operation

Total cataract	
monolateral	— early operation (7-9 months old)
bilateral	— early operation; the second eye 2-3 months after clinical healing of the first eye.
Partial cataract	
monolateral	— with vision inferior to 2-3/10 operation within 5 years of age.
bilateral	— with vision inferior to 2-3/10 operation within 4 years of age; the second eye 2-3 months after clinical healing of the first eye.
Cataract and strabismus	— operate first on the cataract.

With a practically complete clinical picture of the eye for operation, the surgeon will have available all of the necessary data for a wise choice of the type of technique to be used and can thus program the various phases of the operation. Success is largely dependent on the application of some general rules which are valid no matter what the type of cataract or the kind of technique employed. Good rules for the surgeon to follow are to operate: in deep general anesthesia; in maximum mydriasis; in bulbar hypotonia; under microscopic control.

Maximum pupil dilation and optimal tonometric values (8-10mm Hg.), remaining constant for the whole duration of the operation, are essential factors for correct and total removal of the cataract and for reducing to a minimum the occurence of the most common pre-operative complications (vitreous loss, etc.). The methods for obtaining such conditions are outlined in Table II.

The systematic use of the binocular operation microscope, with the magnification and illumination (coaxial or through a slit) which are most appropriate to the need, offers the irreplaceable advantage of perfect visualization of the field of operation and perception of some essential details otherwise impossible to detect (for example, the persistence of minute residual lenticular fragments, of vitreal fibres, of thickening of the posterior capsule of the lens, etc.).

It would seem essential to repeat again some basic principles, which, variously expressed (Cordes, J. François and others) summarise the characteristics and final aims of the 'ideal' operation for congenital cataract. These are:

— The utility of operating in one single sitting;
— strict respect for the integrity of the corneal endothelium, of the iris, and when possible, of the posterior capsule and of the hyaloid.
— practically total removal of the cataractous masses.

Table II

	Mydriasis
Several hours before operation	— 1%atropin sulphate collyrium (repeated instillations)
Half an hour before operation	a) 1%atropin sulphate collyrium b) 10% phenylefrin collyrium c) adrenal in + atropin (infraconjunctivally in the more obstinate cases)
	Bulbar Hypotonia
90 minutes before operation	Intravenous injection of 20% mannitol
Few minutes before operation	a) non-depolarizing drugs (used for anesthesia) and, if necessary: b) ocular massage for 10-15 min. c) 1.5 cc. of 2%carbocain by retrobulbar injection.

It is well known that congenital cataract is notably polymorphic for the extreme variability of its location and for the degree of extension of its opacity. The numerous and sometimes discordant clinical classifications mentioned in the literature refer the most part to these parameters. In reality, the semeiological datum of greatest interest to the surgeon is the consistency of the crystalline lens. In general, in fact, we speak of surgical therapy of soft congenital cataracts and of membranous on cretaceous congenital cataracts, i.e., those grouped by François under the generic terms of 'regressive'.

This subdivision is fully justified on a practical level by the substantial difference in problems and thus in surgical solutions existing between the two great categories.

Rubella cataract must be treated in a separate discussion, owing to the large incidence of complications probably linked to its etiopathogenesis.

SURGERY OF SOFT CONGENITAL CATARACTS

Discussion of this subject is characterized by contrasting opinions, decisions and directions, as a definitive surgical solution is not yet found.

Nevertheless simultaneous irrigation and aspiration, though with various different methods and instruments, is the principle inspiring almost all modern surgery of soft congenital cataract. In practise, it can be achieved by:

— two needles employed separately for the two functions (Cirard, Phillips Wang, Etienne-Donné, Barraquer, Dardenne, etc.).
— a single double-barreled cannula (Wolfe & Wolfe, Fuchs; Fink; Ferguson, Atchoo, etc.).

In 1968 the authors devised a method based on the use of an instrument entirely designed and created, in its original version, by the Eye Clinic of the University of Bari; its technical characteristics and mode of use are outlined in fig. 1 and 2. The double-barreled cannula is illustrated in fig. 3.

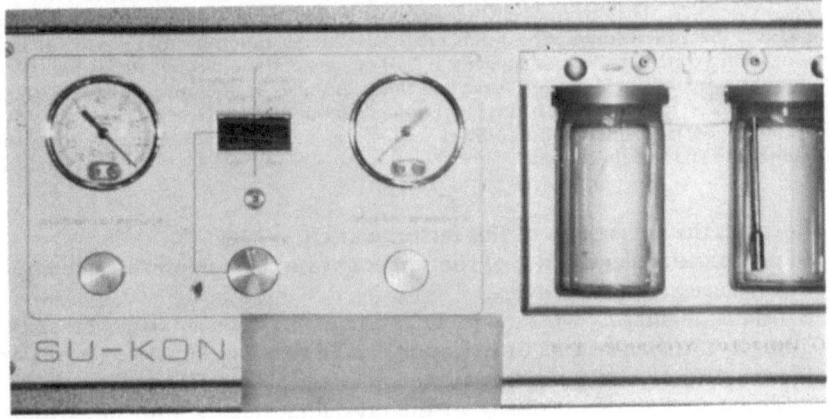

Fig. 1.

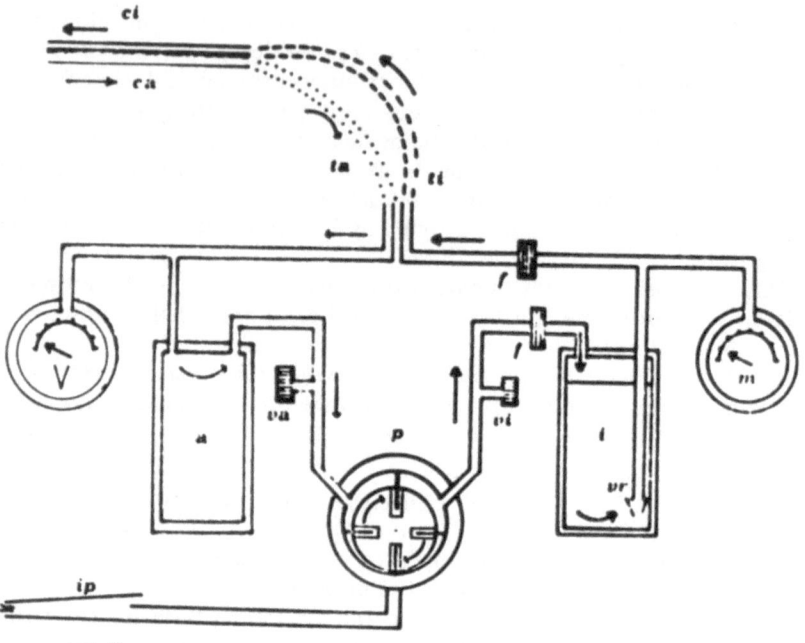

p	:	rotative pump			
va	:	adjustable aspiration valve			
vi	:	adjustable irrigation valve			
a	:	aspiration container (hermetic sealing)			
i	:	infusion container (containing artificial aqueous humour)			
v	:	vacuum-gauge			
m	:	manometer	ca	:	aspiration cannula
f	:	filters	ci	:	infusion cannula
ta	:	aspiration tube	vr	:	retention valve
ti	:	infusion tube	ip	:	pedal switch

Fig. 2. The pedal switch ip starts the rotative pump p, operated by an electric motor; this produces a system of compression and aspiration controlled respectively by the valves Vi and Va. The hermetically closed glass container A is empty and serves for aspiration; the other container I holds artificial aqueous humour and is used for irrigation. Both containers, whose capacity is 150 cc., are extractable and sterilizable. The vacuum-gauge v indicates suction force and the manometer m the pressure of the liquid for irrigation. f indicates the filters, bateriologically active, replaceable, necessary for the sterility of the aqueous humour. ta and ti are the silicon tubes connecting the instrument to the needle-cannula.

In short, the advantages of this instrument are:
— the absolute independence of the surgeon, who can perform alone almost of the necessary manoeuvres.
— constant, regular hydrostatic preservation of the anterior chamber, as the intensity of suction and of irrigation can be varied separately. These two forces, in fact, must be in 'variable equilibrium', since, due to the different size and consistency of the crystalline masses, they must sometimes be used with different intensities in some stages of the operation.

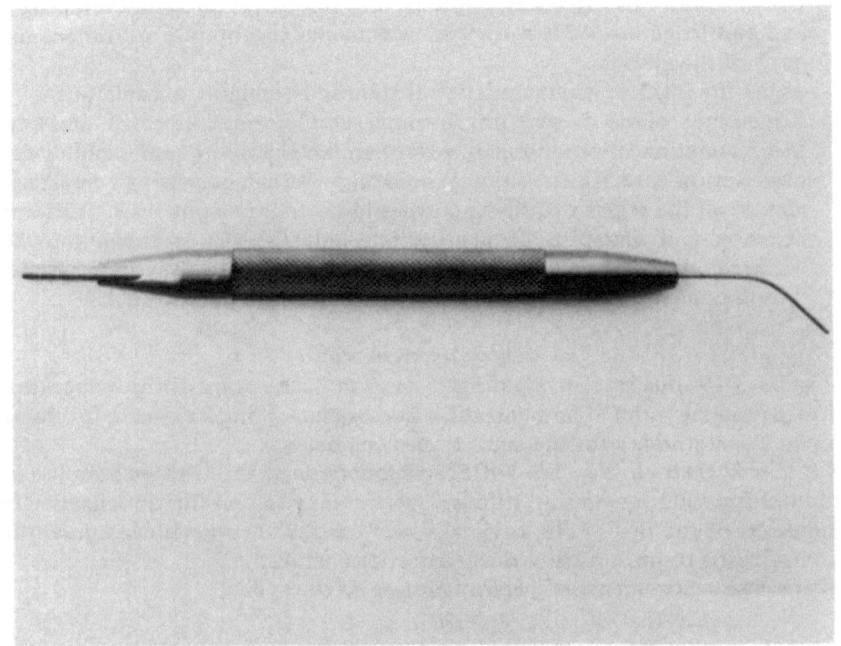

Fig. 3. the needle-cannula has a rough-finished handle and a point with two openings of different diameters: the larger for aspiration and the smaller for irrigation. The opening for aspiration has different sizes and locations in the various models (Fig. 4).

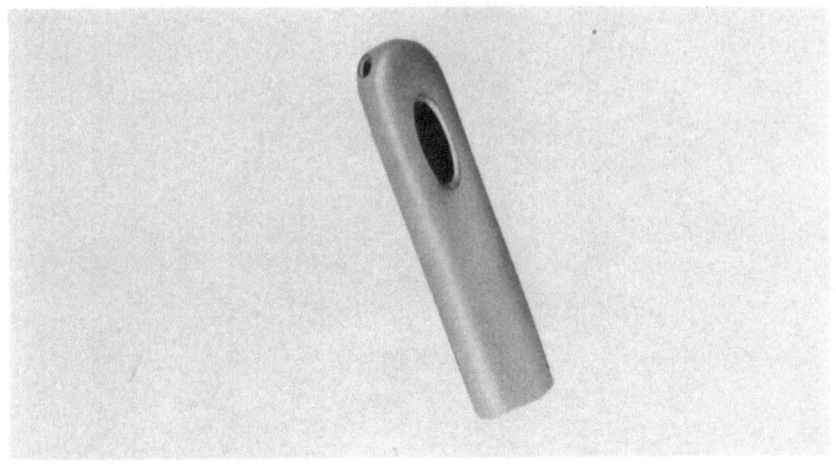

Fig. 4.

- the possibility of using only aspiration or only irrigation and even aspiration and irrigation with two separate cannulas appropriately connected to each of the systems.
- as for the intrinsic characteristics of the needle-cannula, its small dimensions allow it perform through keratotomies of small diameter; the inclination of the point in respect to the handle permits rapid, easy penetration through the surgical opening, with the possibility of reaching almost all the regions of the anterior and posterior chamber; the different location and diameter of the suction hole (fig. 4), according to the different models available, permits aspiration even in the case of hard, voluminous residue or of peripheral masses located under the iris.

Operative technique

Figures 5-19 illustrate in rapid succession the basic stages of the operation. The following brief comments the more salient points explain in greater detail the methods and final aims of the manoeuvres:

Pre-placed U-stitch (Fig. 5-6-7-8): the application of the U-shaped loop has a double function: to obtain, through traction exerted on the threads, perfect adhesion of the lips of the surgical wound around the needle-cannula, thus contributing to preservation of the anterior chamber.

To perform movements of passive piloting of the eyeball.

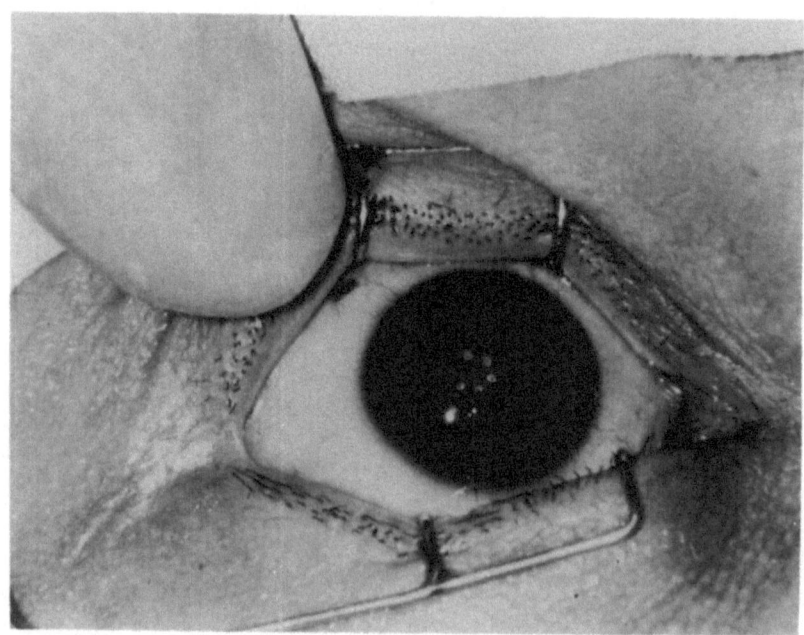

Fig. 5.

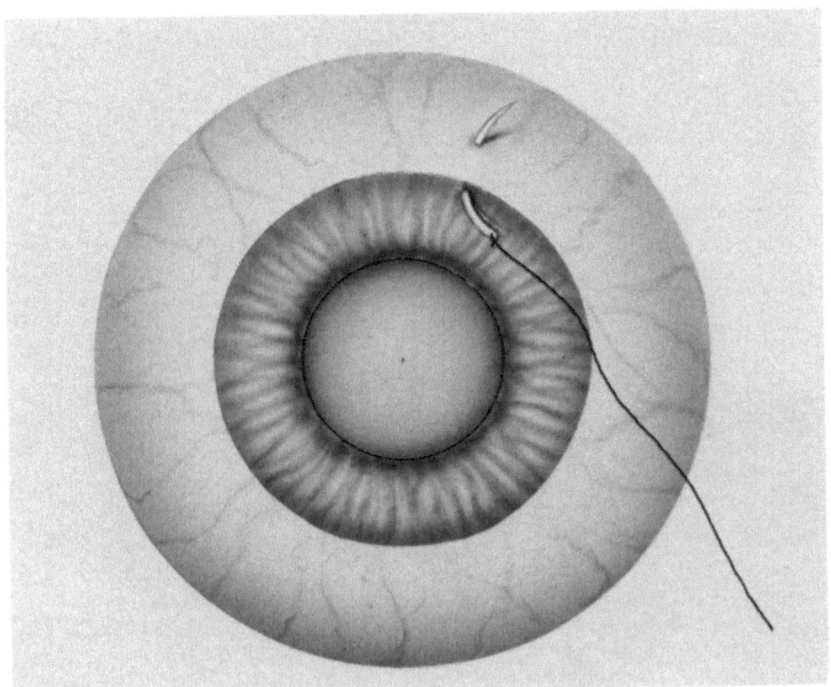

Fig. 6.

Contralateral paracentesis (Fig. 9): contralateral keratomy, valve–like may serve in the following stages of the operation for introducing air or water into the chamber, for the introduction of a spatula and, after further enlargement of the incision, of the cannula of the instrument for extirpation of infra-iridean residue otherwise reached with difficulty.

Keratotomy (Fig. 10): the cut must be made in the space within the looped stitch, either with a lancelet or a two-way cutting knife, it must be corneal (at half a mm. from the limbus); it must not be wider than 3-4 mm.

Anterior capsulotomy (Fig. 11-12-13-14): this must be ample. For this purpose, after opening of the anterior chamber, the surgeon can reach with the point of the same cutting instrument in proximity to the edge of the pupillar foramen opposite the corneal incision and then slowly pulls back the blade, giving it a slight back-and-forth movement in such a way as to open the capsule with a large gash, which may be made in the form of an inclined M (during these manoeuvres the surgeon must take great care, and the microscope is a valuable aid in this, not to harm the camerular structures, especially the corneal endothelium and the iris). Having done this, it is a good rule to introduce an irrigating spatula to perform gentle friction on the masses, and then to wait a few minutes until the more transparent crystalline fibers have absorbed the liquid and become visible.

215

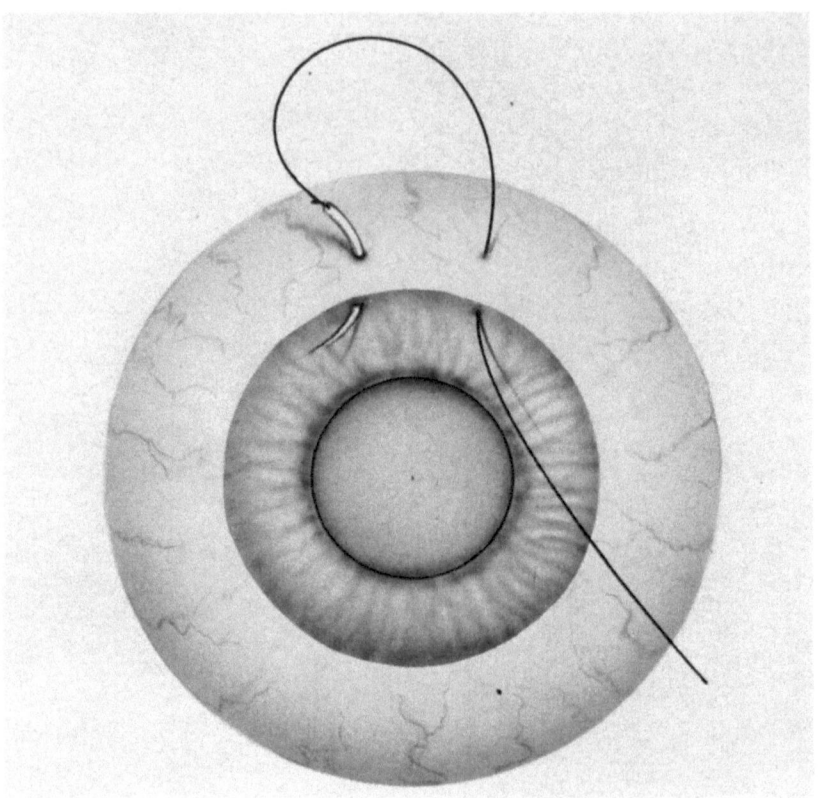

Fig. 7.

Suction and irrigation (Fig. 15-16-17-18): initially it is necessary to set the instrument on the lowest rating and to regulate the two forces separately, according to necessity. Moreover, it is preferable that the action not be made continuously but rather at more or less brief intervals, turning the electric current on and off with the pedal-operated switch and constantly checking the level of the iridean diaphragm so as not to exceed in intensity. Such important precautions serve to avoid serious accidents such as the involvement or the prolapse of the iris in the wound and the rupture of the posterior capsule; consequently the hydrostatic preservation of the anterior chamber is assured. At the end, if the suction has been complete, the pupil will appear free. At this point, abundant irrigation should be made, taking great care that no masses or fibres remain at the level of the irido-corneal angle; then miosis is induced by the instillation of a 1% solution of acetyl-cholin.

216

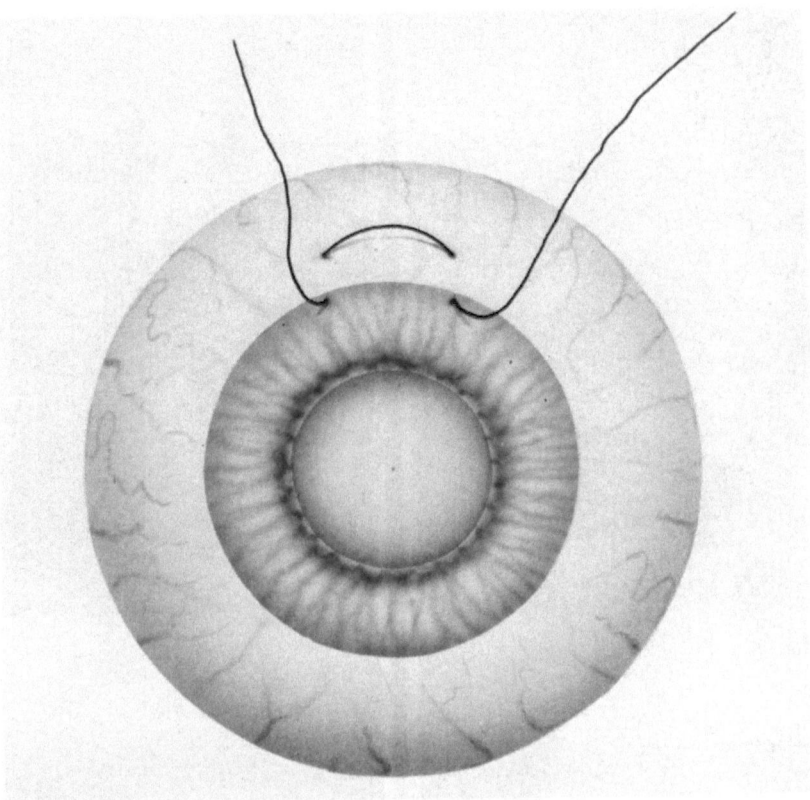

Fig. 8.

Sutures (Fig. 19): the surgical wound is hermetically closed with 2-3 stitches in virgin silk. The anterior chamber must then be reformed with artificial aqueous humour or better with an air bubble, taking care to leave it a meniscus of liquid of at least 1-1.5 mm. for the purpose of keeping the periphery of the iris away from the keratotomies, of re-enforcing the miosis and of assuring the correct depth of the anterior chamber.

Iridian involvement and vitreous prolapse represent the infrequent and almost always remediable operative complications of this technique. In the first case it is sufficient to replace this iris with a fine spatula, using very gentle movements so as to avoid tearing and hemorrhage and the later appearance of achromic patches of atrophy of this tissue. In the case of vitreous loss it is necessary, as previously discussed, to proceed to reduction of the prolapse in its various phases (anterior vitrectomy, cleansing of the wound, peripherial or sectorial iridectomy if necessary). Finally, it must be pointed out that the posterior capsule, if transparent, is left intact in situ; if instead it is opaque the techniques explained in the following paragraph should be used.

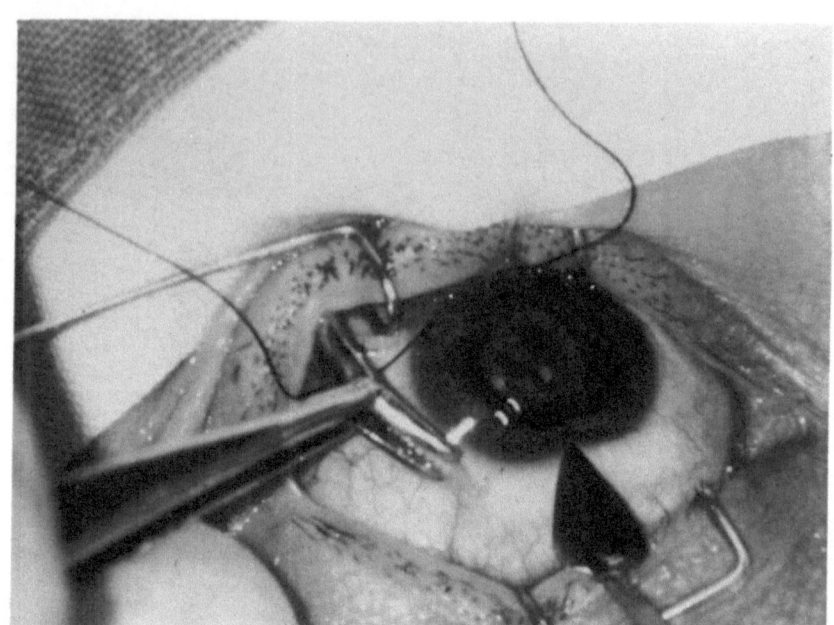

Fig. 9.

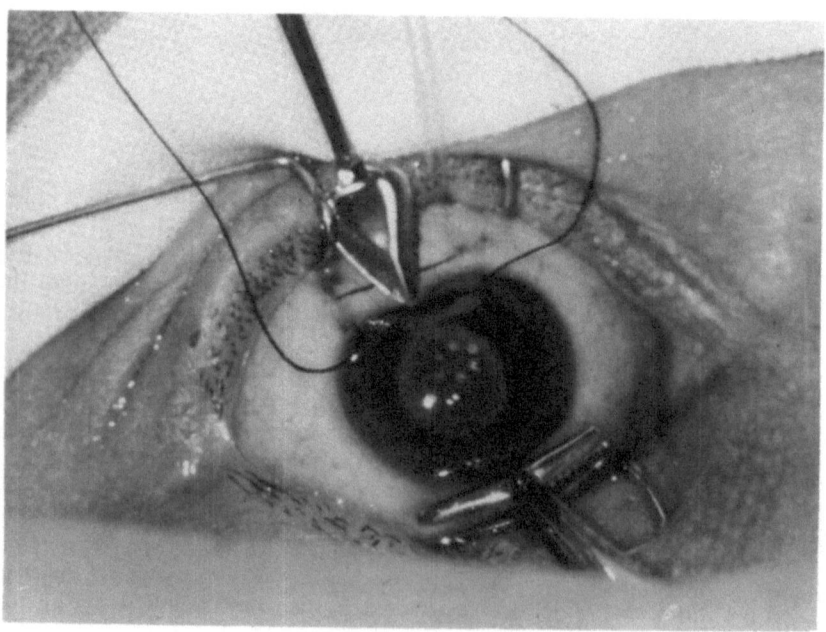

Fig. 10.

218

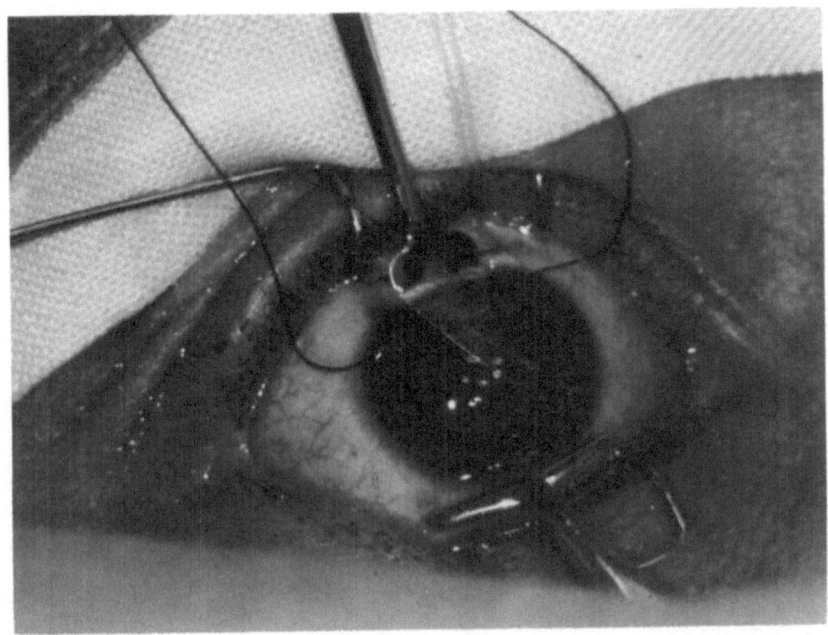

Fig. 11.

SURGERY OF CONGENITAL MEMBRANOUS CATARACTS AND OF SECONDARY CATARACTS

Though simultaneous irrigation and aspiration with the 'globe fermé' is the preferred technique, and certainly the least traumatizing with the lowest risks, for soft congenital cataracts, it is obvious that its utilization is very limited as regards the extraction of 'hard' (membranous or cretaceous) cataracts. Only very thin membranes, in fact, can be removed by aspiration and even these often block the cannula. Thick, hard, crystalline membranes, often closely adherent to the iris or to the vitreous by vast, tenacious synechiaes make the employement of this instrument practically useless, and even sometimes harmful.

The treatment of membranous cataract and that of secondary cataract are here discussed together, not only because the latter is the most common late complication of congenital cataract, but also and more important because, although their pathogenesis is totally different, they are both susceptible to practically analogous surgical solutions. Substantial differences exist, however, as regards the best time for the operation. While the indications given in the general scheme are valid for the creataceous, for the secondary cataract it is useful, and even indispensable, to let a certain lapse of time elapse, usually not less than 3-4 months after the first operation. Various reasons justify this: not to subject the patient, almost always a young child, to further operation stress under anaesthesia while

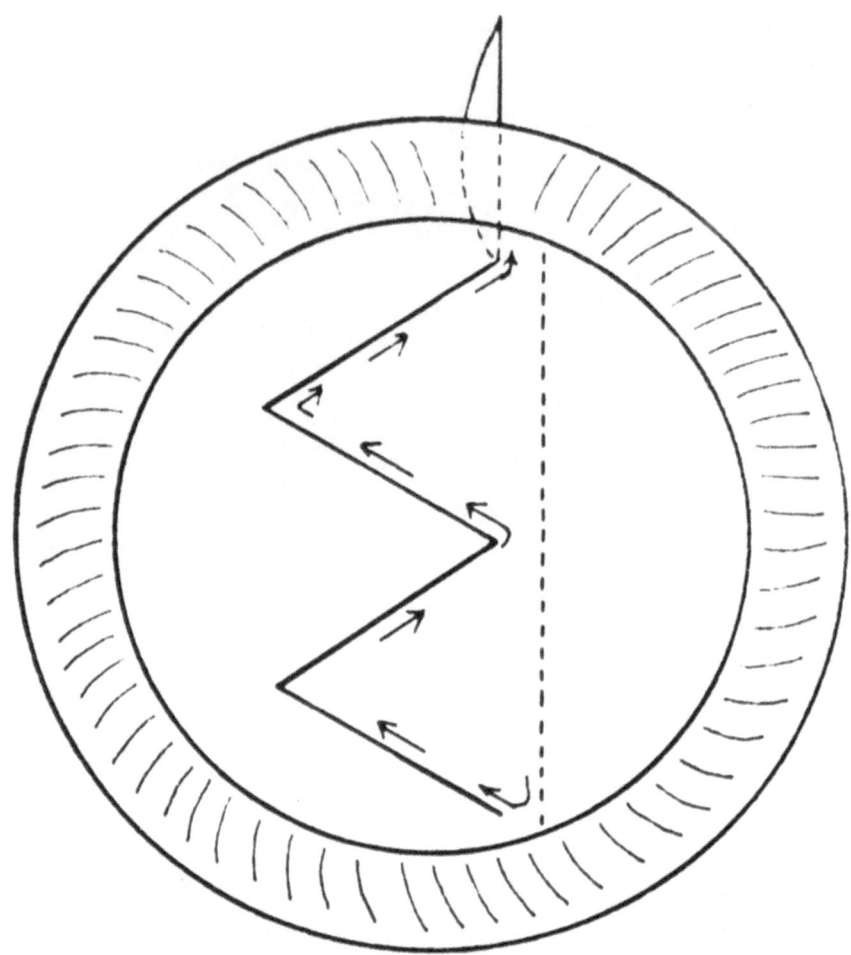

Fig. 12. method of performing anterior capsulotomy.

still in the period of convalescence; to avoid the serious and dangerous reactive processes which may easily take place in an organ disturbed by previous operative manoeuvres while the phenomena of cicatrization and recovery are not yet completely consolidated in the various ocular districts; to have the absolute certainty that spontaneous re-absorption of masses with acceptable improvement of visual acuity, as sometimes takes place, is no longer a possibility.

It is, moreover, indispensable to emphasise the absolute necessity that, in similar circumstances, the operation be performed only after careful objective examination conducted in maximum mydriasis and preferably with the biomicroscope, in order to have an exact evaluation of the

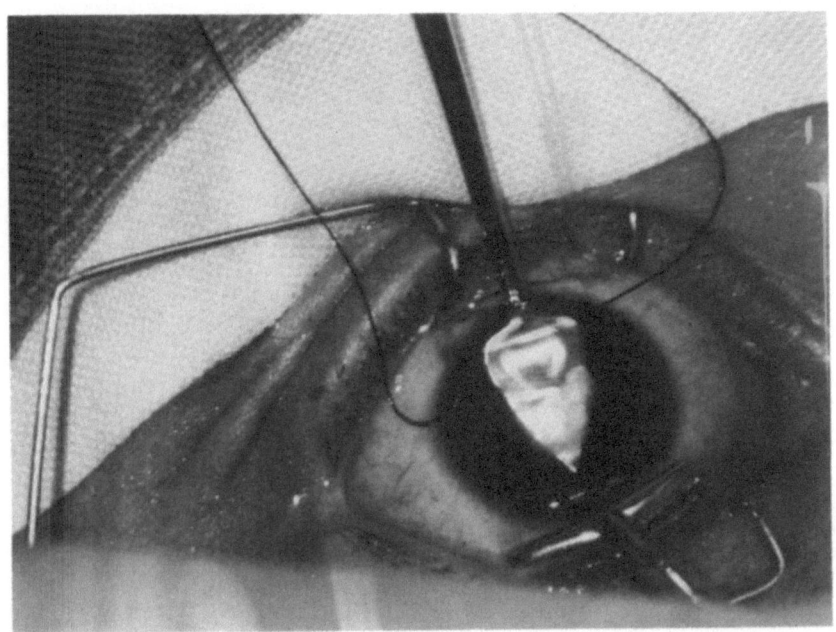

Fig. 13.

anatomical conditions of the eyeball (presence of synechiaes, etc.) and above all of the consistency and thickness of the cataract. These, in fact, are the two elements conditioning the choise of the type of operation. In the case of tenuous membranes or in the so-called pure secondary capsular cataract (Paufique and coll.) it is advisable to perform a simple discission with one or two needles, or at the most, sectioning of the membrane with a fine, well-sharpened Graefe.

When instead the cataract is thick and consistent (membranous) or in the the case of a secondary capsulolenticular cataract, i.e., one made up of abundant crystalline residues massed in a partially re-formed capsular sac, extraction is without doubt preferable. This surgical technique, when well performed, has the indubitable advantage of freeing the pupil almost completely; however, it always implies a more or less extensive opening of the anterior chamber and sometimes a loss, though limited, of vitreous. After the preparation of a small conjuctival flap, an incision of about 5-6 mm. is made in the surgical limbus with a lancet. Previous study of the case permits choice of the sector (usually the superior or the temperal) where it is most advantageous to open in order to get the best grasp of the cataract. When synechiaes are present, they must be gently freed with a spatula, (two-way cutting spatula is best) so as to avoid later harmful traction which could cause severe iridean hemorrhages. The surgeon then proceeds to extraction with the forceps. For this purpose, Von Mandach's forceps is an

221

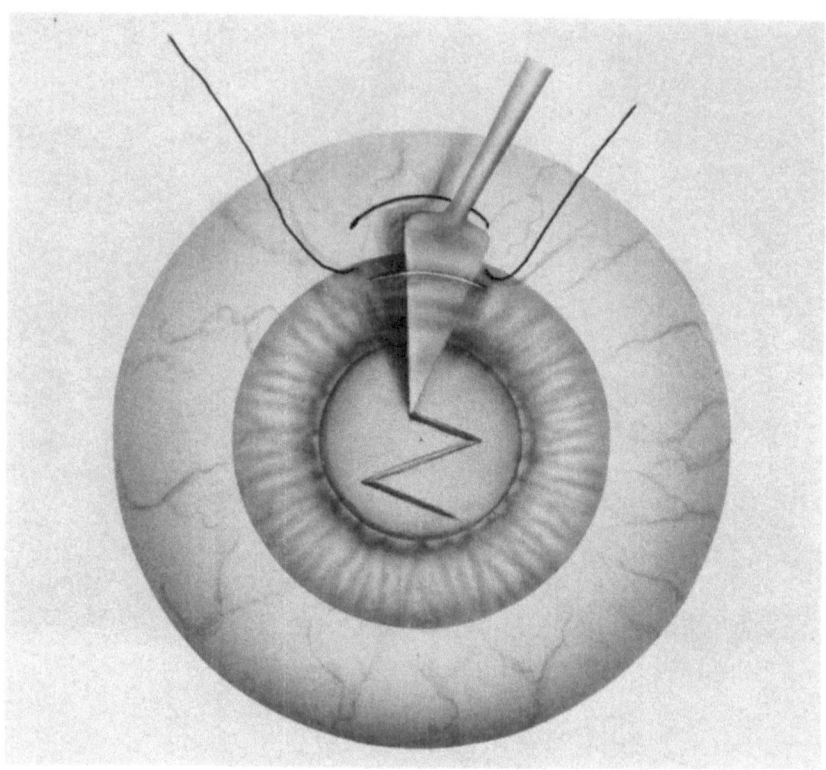

Fig. 14.

extremely valuable instrument, different models of which are utilized: the standard type for cataracts with a knobbly or irregular surface, the model with toothed or grooved ands for the others with a more or less tightly-stretched surface. The forceps is introduced shut into the anterior chamber. Upon reaching the pupillar margin opposite to the incision, it is opened slightly and the cataract is grasped; then it is pulled back gently with slight lateral left-and-right movements to detach any tenuous adhesions.. Usually the entire cataract can be extracted in this manner. Sometimes however it is necessary that the assistant, with an iris scissors forceps or a Vannas, cuts off on the level of the wound the vitreal strand which almost always adheres to it. Analogous manoeuvres must be repeated if the extraction has been incomplete and residue remains. However, it is a good rule not to persist when confronted with strong resistance to traction because, as Paufique affirms, this would be extremely harmful to the future of the eye. In such cases, when numerous and massive adhesions exist, the surgeon must know when to stop, giving up the hope of an 'in toto' extraction and falling back on the possibility of removal of a greater or less part of the membranous cataract. This can be achieved by cutting in situ and by using the 'emporte-piece' Vacher type forceps, of which the authors have designed a new

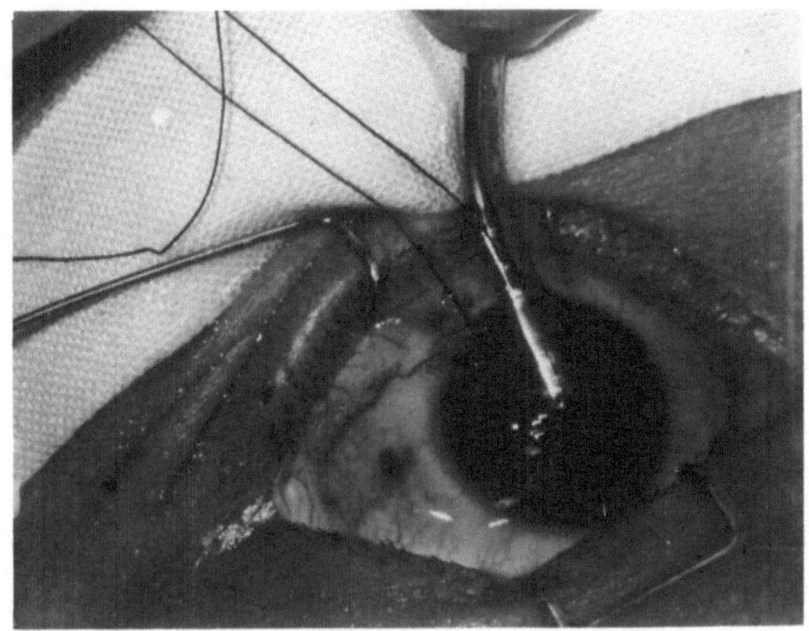

Fig. 15.

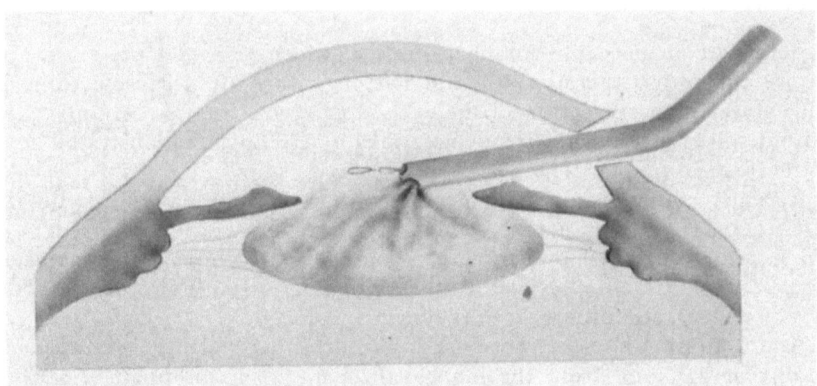

Fig. 16.

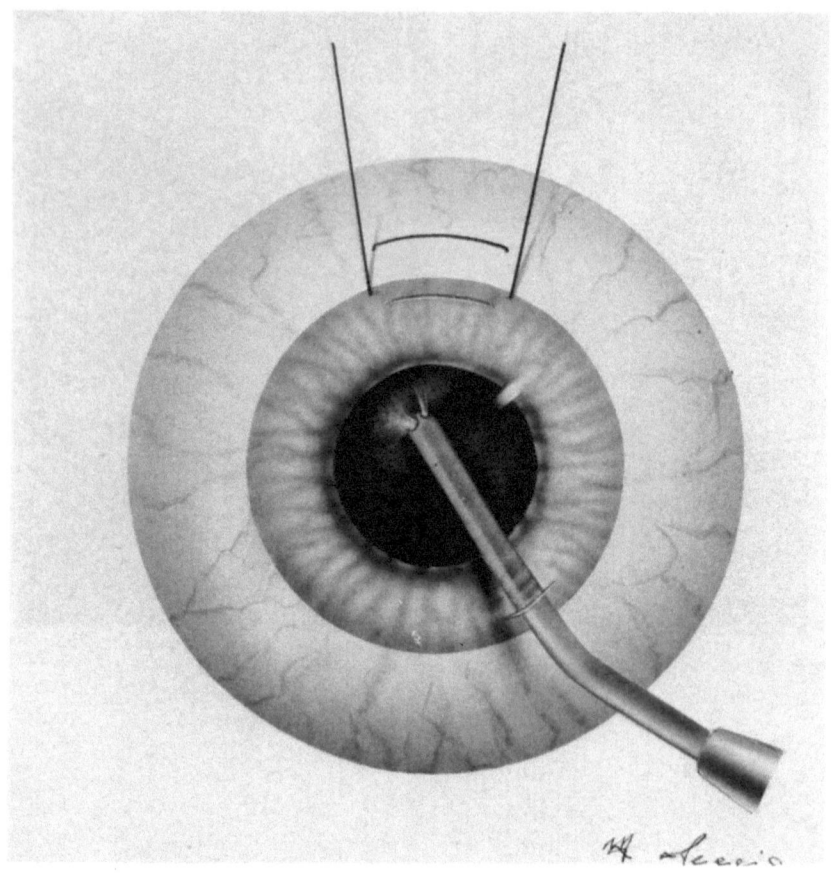

Fig. 17.

model, more manageable for microsurgery, which gives a more exact and precise cut and is therefore less traumatising. More often capsulectomy in three stages with extraction of the excised tract practised, according to the old but still efficacious technique described by Elschnig and illustrated in all of the treatises on ocular surgery, should be considered.

Recently, these forms of hard cataract have been treated also with the vitreotome. This technique has already been used in therapy of membranous and secondary cataract by various surgeons, some of whom prefer access by the pars plana (Michels en coll.), others the anterior path (Douvas, Goddé-Jolly, Ruellan), still others, both (Peyman and coll.).

As regards the authors' personal experience, they perform a small kera-totomy at 2-3 mm. from the limbus, through which the point of a Kloti vitreotome or better of a Drews phacotome is introduced. In this way one can easily cut and break up even thick, resistent membranes; remove them

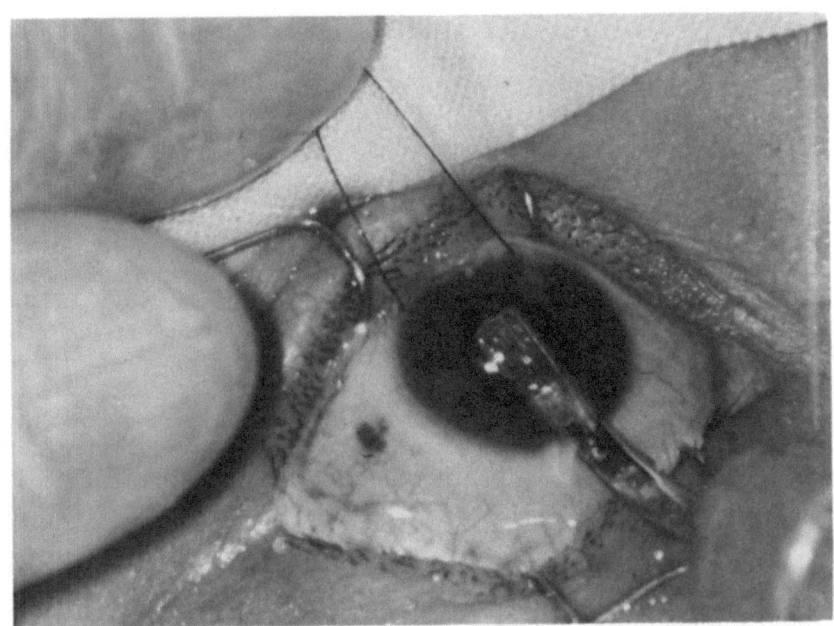

Fig. 18.

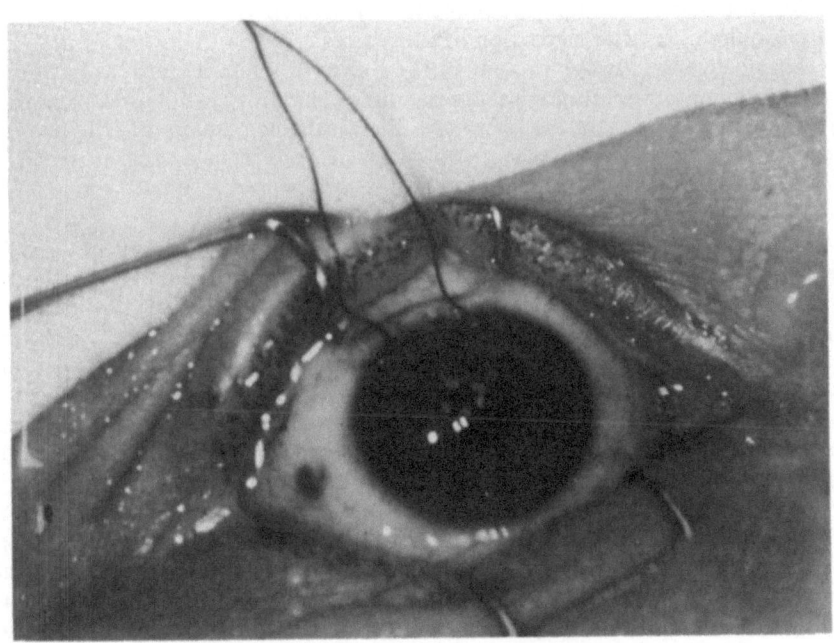

Fig. 19.

by suction; preserve an anterior chamber of constant depth, thanks to the contemporaneous introduction of artificial acqueous humour.

Although present experience is still quite limited, this surgical approach seems most useful, especially for eliminating large cataractous masses, hard and cretaceous, mixed with vitreous, which, as the surgeon well knows, are slippery and hard to remove with the forceps.

SURGERY OF RUBELLA CATARACT

Surgery of rubella cataract is complicated and difficult, as shown by the high percentage of failures reported in the world literature, attributable to very serious per and post-operative complications; of these, phthisis of the eyeball is perhaps the most sadly famous (Cotlier 10%, Boniuk V. and M. 5%, Wolff 8%, Scheie 24%). This can be ascribed to three factors: the anatomophathological characteristics of the lenticular lesion; the frequent severe ocular alterations associated (microphthalmia, shallow anterior chamber, restricted pupillar dilation, glaucoma, etc. . . . .); the presence of the virus in the crystalline lens even up to the third year of age (Hertzburg).

Two observations of a general nature can be derived: the necessity that abscission of the lens masses be really precise and total and that it be performed in one single stage. It is evident that both of these conditions are fully satisfied by the authors' technique.

The persistence of cataractours residue parasited by the virus is largely responsable for post-operative inflammations; therefore it is extremely useful to perform a lengthy, abundant irrigation of the whole region of the anterior chamber after aspiration of the masses.

Torpid uveitis, always present in these eyes in a latent state (as has been proved on anatomopathological bases) and the immunity cellular reaction to a new liberation of viral antigen are the probable causes of the severe reactions following on a second operation. Interference is therefore justifiable only in the case, unfortunately not rare, where a fibrous membrane of secondary cataract forms.

Unlike the therapy of soft cataract, in which it is only rarely practiced, sectorial iridectomy is always a useful measure here, both from the technical point of view of the restricted or in sufficient dilation of the pupillar aperture, and as prophylaxis in preventing glaucoma due to pupil blockage, a dangerous and recurrent complication. It must, moreover, constitute the rule in the case of microphthalmia. Contrary to the opinion of Scheie, who advises this therapy several weeks before the cataract operation, the authors believe it better, for the above-mentioned reasons, to perform it during the operation, of course before beginning aspiration of the cataract.

As for judgement of operability, it is strictly correlated to the patient's general conditions and to satisfactor ERG and ecography tests. The choice of the best time for the operation is dependant, not only on those general parameters expressed above, but also on factors of a virological and immunological order. In fact, the observation of a high concentration of specific antibodies does not present, as is now recognized, a sure indication of operability, since in these circumstances the viral agent can still be detected,

Table III Institute of Ophthalmology of Bari University
Congenital cataracts: Results obtained on 87 cases operated from 1968 to 1971

AGE	ANTERIOR-POLAR -NUCLEAR -ZONULAR CATARACTS		CAPSULO-LENTICULAR -TOTAL CATARACTS		POSTERIOR CAPSULAR -POSTERIOR POLAR CATARACTS		MEMBRANOUS CATARACT		RUBEOLAR CASES		favourable	unfavourable
	operated eyes	results	operated eyes	results	operated eyes	results	operated eyes	results	operated eyes	results		
from 7 months to 5 years	4	2*** 2**	22	5*** 9** 5* 3°	3	2** 1*			4	1*** 1* 2-	28	5
from 6 years to 15 years	15	6*** 5** 2° 2-	9	4*** 2** 2° 1-	8	3*** 2** 2* 1°	2	1*** 1-			29	5
from 16 years to 29 years	6	2*** 2** 1* 1°	4	1*** 3**	5	1*** 2** 1* 1-	5	2*** 1** 1* 1°			17	3
	25		35		16		7		4		74	13
											85,05%	14,9%

*** very good result ** good result * poor result - negative result
° cases with associated ocular malformations.

227

Table IV Institute of Ophthalmology of Bari University
Congenital cataracts: Results obtained on 210 cases operated from to 1972 – to 1977

AGE	-ANTERIOR POLAR -NUCLEAR -ZONULAR CATARACTS		-CAPSULO LENTICULAR -TOTAL CATARACTS		-POSTERIOR CAPSULAR -POSTERIOR POLAR CATARACTS		-MEMBRANOUS CATARACT		-RUBEOLAR CATARACT		CASES	
	operated eyes	results	operated eyes	results	operated eyes	results	operated eyes	results	operated eyes	results	favourable	unfavourable
from 7 months to 5 years	30	15*** 14** 1-	45	15*** 18** 8* 4°	12	6** 4* 2-			11	2*** 2** 2* 3- 2°	86	12
from 6 years to 15 years	30	10*** 10** 3*° 5* 2-	21	8*** 7** 5* 1°	15	4*** 5** 3* 3-	9	1*** 4** 4-			65	10
from 16 years to 29 years	9	3*** 4** 1* 1-*	10	3*** 5** 2*	9	1*** 4** 2* 2-	9	2*** 1** 3* 2-° 1-			31	6
	69		76		36		18		11		183	27
											87,14%	12,85%

*** very good results ** good results * poor result -negative result
° Cases with associated ocular malformations

Table V Institute of Ophthalmology of Bari University

Congenital cataracts. Complications (On 297 cases)

	-ANTERIOR POLAR -NUCLEAR -ZONULAR CATARACTS	-CAPSULO-LENTICULAR -TOTAL CATARACTS	-POSTERIOR CAPSULAR -POSTERIOR POLAR CATARACTS	MEMBRANOUS CATARACT	RUBEOLAR CATARACT	TOTAL Complications
	94	111	52	25	15	
Serious hyphema	1	1	–	–	–	2
Synechiae:						
anterior	3	3	1	3	1	11
posterior	2	4	4	4	5	19
Iridocyclitis	–	–	–	–	3	3
Loss of vitreous	2	2	4	3	–	11
Hemorrhage into the vitreous	–	1	–	1	–	2
TOTAL	8	11	9	11	9	48 (16.16%)

due to an immunological phenomenon which is still not wholly understood. Important, instead, is the clinically-based finding (Scheie) of a conspicuous reduction in the number of complications, especially reactive phenomena, with the increasing age of the patient. It can therefore be maintained that the operation should be postponed until after the second year of age.

RESULTS

Results obtained in the period from 1968 to 1977 are subdivided in Tables III and IV. In particular, Table III includes operations performed from 1968 to 1971, a period in which the authors at first used a modified Fuchs two-way syringe (in 66 eyes) and later an experimental model of their own instrument (in 21 eyes).

Since 1972 the authors have been routinely using, with rare exeptions, their instrument in its present version. (Table IV).

It is important, moreover, to point out that only results checked periodically for a period of time varying from 6 months to 1 year have been considered valid.

The immediate and late complications founds in the 297 eyes operated are listed in Table V.

A critical analysis of these figures gives rise to some brief considerations:
— the real practical validity of the author's method of aspiration and irrigation, which for simplicity of method and striking reduction of risks, can be considered an efficacious and very advantageous technique for the treatment of soft congenital cataract;
— the satisfying results obtained, following the method and technique described, with membranous cataracts, also in consideration of their frequent association with other ocular malformations;
— the higher percentage rate of complications in rubella cataract, a fact confirmed by comparative analysis with other authors, and moreover independent, for the above-mentioned causes, of correct performance of surgical technique.

REFERENCES

Atchoo P.D. - Double-barred anterior chamber irrigating needle *Arch. Ophthal.* (Chicago), 79,580,1968.

Barraquer J.I. - Cataract surgery in children *Japan J. Ophthal.*, 18,213,1974.

Boniuk V. & Boniuk M. The incidence of phtisis bulbi as a complication of cataract surgery in the congenital Rubella syndrome - Rubella and other intraocular vitrea diseases in Infancy. Little Brown & company, Boston.*Int. Ophthal. Clin.* 12,771972.

Chansel J.M. & Polack F.M. Phacoemulsification utilisant l'appareil de Girard. Etude expérimentale des effects sur l'endothélium cornéen du lapin. *Arch. d'Ophtal.*, 36,595,1976.

Cordes F.C. Evaluation of the surgery of congenital cataracts - A Acad. od Med. Section of Ophthal. 16 Avril 1951.

Cotlier E. Surgical results in Rubella and non Rubella congenital cataracts. *Amer. J. Ophthal.* 66,539,1968.

Dardenne M.V. Techniques of surgery for congenital cataracts - Atti 10° congresso Panellenico di Ottalmologia, Creta 1977

Binder P.S., Sternberg H., Wickham M.G. & Worthen D.M. Corneal endothelial damage associated with phacoemulsification *Am. Jour. Ophthal.* 82,*48*,1976.

Douvas N.G. The cataract roto-extractor. *Trans. Am. Acad. Ophthal. Oro-Rhino-Laryngol, 77,792*,1973.

Etienne R. Le traitement chirurgical des cataractes congénitales - *Arch. Opthal. (Paris)* 32,779,1972.

Etienne R. & Donné M.R. Microchirurgie des cataractes congénitales ou traumatiques. Opération en un temps par irrigation-aspiration ('push-pull') *Arch. Ophtal. (Paris).* 32,189,1972.

Ferguson E.C. A modified instrument for aspiration and irrigation of congenital or soft cataracts. *Am. J. Ophthal.,* 57,*596*,1964.

Fink A.I. & Weinstein G.W. A modification of the Fuchs syringe *Am. J. Ophthal.,* 58,129,1964.

François J. Les cataractes congénitales. Masson et c^ie, édit. Paris, 1959.

Fuchs J. Die Zweiwegespritze, ein neuartiges Instrument zur Absaugung weicher Stare. *Klin. Mbl. Augenheilk.* 121,592,1952.

Girard L.S. Aspiration-irrigation of congenital and traumatic cataracts *Arch. Ophthal.,* 77,387,1967.

Girard L.J. & Hawkins R.S. Aspiration-irrigation of senile cataracts with ultrasonic fragmentation. *Trans. Am. Ac. of Ophthal. and Otolaryng.* 78,*OP50*,1974.

Goddé Jolly D. & Ruellan M.Y.M. Note pratique sur l'utilisation du vitréotome de Kloti dans le traitement des membranules épaisses et des cataractes secondaires après cataractes congénitales. *Bull. Soc. d'Ophtal.* de France, 76,*141*,1976.

Hertzburg R. Comunicazione personale, Citato da Scheie - 1969.

Kelman C.D. Phaco-emulsification and aspiration: A new technique of cataract removal: A preliminary report. *Amer. J. Ophthal.,* 64,23,1957.

Krasnov M.M. Laser-phacopuncture in the treatment of soft cataracts - *Brit. J. Ophthal.* 59,96,1975.

Leonardi E. Chirurgia dell'apparato oculare - Ed. Arte della Stampa, Roma, 1947,I,267.

Legrand J., Hervouet F. & Baron A. Knejev - L'alpha-chymotrypsine dans l'opération de la cataracte. *Bull. Soc. Ophtal. Fran.* 59,*695*,1958.

Michels R.G. - Machemer R. & Mueller-Jensen K. Vitreous surgery: history and current concepts. *Ophthalmic Surgery, 5,13*,1974.

Paufique L., Guillaumet L. & The Saint Martin R. Traitement chirurgical des affections oculaires. Vol. I ed. Doin Parigi 1971.

Peyman G.A., Huamonte F. & Goldberg M.F. Management of cataract in patients undergoing vitrectomy. *A.J.O. P.A.A.* 80,(1),30,1975.

Phillips C.I. & Wang M.K. Cataract aspiration-irrigation (through separate needles with push-pull syringe). *Brit. J. Ophthal.* 55, 361, 1971.

Polack F.M. & Sugar A. The phacoemulsification procedure. II. Corneal endothelial changes. *Invest. Ophthal.* 15,6,458,1976.

Scheie H.G. Aspiration of congenital or soft cataracts: a new technique *Amer. J. Ophthal.* 50,*1048*,1960,

Scheie H.G. Cataract surgery in children. *Acta Cong. Ophthal., Mexico,* 1,345,1970.

Scuderi G. & Sborgia G. Problemi chirurgici nel trattamento della cataratta congenita. Atti VI° congresso S.O.M., Bari, Marzo 1972.

Scuderi G. Terapia chirurgicalà a cataractei congenitale *Oftalmologia,* 17,*15*,1973.

Scuderi G., Sborgia G. & Recupero S.M. Comportamento nelle complicanze della chirurgia della cataratta congenita e traumatica - Relazione al VII° congresso S.O.M., Cagliari, Maggio-Giugno 1973.

Scuderi G. & Sborgia G. La cura chirurgica della cataratta congenita Relazione al congresso del Collegium Biologicum Europeo, Roma, Dic. 1973.

Scuderi G., Ranieri G. & Sborgia G. Problèmes soulevés par la chirurgie de la cataracte congénitale. Présentation de nouvelles techniques. *Bull. Soc. Belge Ophtal.,* 157,*573*,1974.

Scuderi G. & Recupero S.M. La cataratta congenita Prospettive in pediatria 18,179, 1975.

Scuderi G., Sborgia G. & Recupero S.M. Une expérience faite sur 210 cas de patients opérés par une technique chirurgicale originale di extraction linéaire par lavage et aspiration *Bull. et Memo. Soc. Fr. Ophtal. pag. 174, 1975.*

Scuderi G. & Recupero S.M. Results and considerations on 250 cases of congenital cataract operated with original techniques - Atti 10° congresso Panellenico di ottalmologia, Creta 1977.

Vail D. The zonule of Zinn and its clinical significance - *Trans. Oph. Coc. U.K., 79,485,1959.*

Wolfe O.R. & Wolfe R.M. Removal of soft cataract by suction. New double barreled aspirating needle. *Arch. Ophthal. (Chicago). 26,127,*1941.

Authors' address:
Università Clinica Oculistà
Rome
Italia.

Docum. Ophthal. Proc. Series, Vol. 21

CATARACT IN THE YOUNG

WERTHER DUQUE ESTRADA

(Rio de Janairo, Brazil)

The surgical techniques used in surgery of congenital and of juvenile cataract have undergone a beneficent evolution. From optical iridectomy to phacoemulsification, a series of new methods have been providing ever better surgical results, making the operation safer, and reducing the complications.

Practically all the most modern methods are based on simultaneous aspiration-irrigation, and for this purpose various surgical instruments and various techniques have been devised. I would cite, merely as examples, the double-way syringe of Fuchs, the infusion-suction device pf J.D. Gass, the instrument of J. Berrocal, the apparatus of Scuderiranieri among others equally efficient. As to more sophisticated devices and techniques, mention should be made as examples of the apparatus of Girard and the phaco emulsifier 'Cavitron' of Kelman.

If on the one hand the technology has improved, thus leading to better surgical results, the visual results, on the other hand — although also improved by reduction of the complications during and after the operation — have not enjoyed a success proportional to the development of technology. This is owing to the fact that functional success depends on other ocular changes also, especially sensorial. Papers by Paton and by Maumenee, as well as observations by Parks, concerning children operated on for congenital cataract before completing the first year of life, bear witness to the extremely poor visual results, even when these babies were fitted with contact lenses after the surgery. Deprivation amblyopia was not avoided, at least to the extent one might naturally expect.

Fortunately, the visual results obtained following surgery of juvenile cataracts are very good. A visual acuity of 20/40 to 20/20 is generally achieved, and this is also the experience in my service.

Various techniques have been used over the years in the service I direct: optical iridectomy (which still has its place), discission, linear extraction and various aspiration techniques, among them that of Scheie and of Scuderi. One of my assistants, A. Fatorelli, made a long study of this subject and wrote a thesis, 'Cataract in Child and Youth', where he emphasizes surgical investigations making use, in particular, of the aspiration-irrigation technique.

Today the aspiration-irrigation technique continues to be the most used by my assistants. Meanwhile, one group of my collaborators, led by P. Moacyr Aguiar, devotes itself especially to phacoemulsification (Cavitron), and

233

the present tendency is to apply this technique to all cases of congenital and of juvenile cataract. Indeed, there is a strong tendency in this group to use the same process also in senile cataracts, which I consider indicated when it is not a question of hard cataracts. A number of senile cataracts have already been operated on with excellent visual results, and few complications.

The beginning of phacoemulsification in Brazil took place in 1975, when Robert Sinskey carried out, in my service, a series of operations with the Cavitron, all with excellent results to date. These operations included juvenile and adult cataracts. No complications were observed in the follow-up, and the recovery of visual acuity was very good.

SOME POINTS TO EMPHASIZE

It is of extreme importance, in any of the techniques used, to remove from the eye all the cortical material. Sometimes the surgeon has the impression that the posterior capsule is clean; however, careful observation with the surgical microscope — which should systematically be used — may reveal a scanty part of the cortex. This should be removed by scraping, which is greatly facilitated by use of instruments that are a part of the Cavitron.

However, even when the greatest care is used there sometimes persist, on the surface of the posterior capsule, epithelial pearls. These pearls may later give rise to a fibrous growth, and cause partial opacification and reduction of visual acuity. There is a tendency with those who make use of the Cavitron to execute a small incision in the posterior capsule at termination of the surgery, thus avoiding the necessity of doing it later.

In all cases operated on I always try to leave a small quantity of saline as well as a small quantity of air in the anterior chamber, so as to keep it always present in the postoperative period.

Although the habitual aspiration-irrigation techniques are efficient, there is no doubt that one advantage of the Cavitron is to permit permanent and automatic maintenance of the anterior chamber during the surgical act. The surgeon does not have to worry about protecting the chamber.

If, in a juvenile cataract — generally a soft cataract — a hard nucleus is encountered during the operation, it can be emulsified with relative ease. A greater difficulty is the presence of subcapsular plaques that neither aspiration nor phacoemulsification can fragment. However, they can be dissected under the microscope and removed in toto without damage to the eye.

Author's address:
Department of Ophthalmology
University of Rio de Janeiro
Brazil

234

TRAUMATIC CATARACT

O. –E. LUND

(München, F.R.G.)

Traumatic cataract represents a very frequent complication of penetrating injuries of the eye and is less frequently found with contusions. Ruptures of the lens capsule from minimal to large extensions occur, sometimes combined with a dislocation (Luxatio lentis).
We separate different groups:
1. Simple traumatic cataract
2. Complicated traumatic cataract
a. with lesion of the iris
b. with vitreous loss
c. with vitreous haemorrhage
d. with lens luxation
The therapeutic procedure has to be orientated according to:
1. The degree of the traumatic cataract
2. The age of the patient
3. Additional complications
    The time for surgery of a traumatic cataract is influenced by the following factors:
With a minimal lens opacity without visible rupture of the capsule we wait until visual acuity decreases by increasing swelling of the lens.
    With a dense opacity of the lens and dislocation of the lens fragments into the anterior chamber we operate after 3 to 7 days after the penetrating injury to avoid the phase of posttraumatic infection.
    With heavy penetrating injuries with a complicated traumatic cataract and vitreous loss or vitreous prolaps into the anterior chamber the lens or its resdues will be removed with the primary surgical procedure.
    With a phacogenetic or phacolytic secondary glaucoma the cataract has to be removed as soon as the tension rises.
    With a combination of traumatic cataract with vitreous haemorrhages we tend to operate after 2 to 3 weeks.
    For an individual case no rigid scheme can be applied according to the varying sequels of the trauma. So this time table must be understood as a basic rule only.

SURGICAL TECHNIQUE:

The surgical procedure differs with the simple and complicated cases and

235

with the age of the patient. With juvenile and adolescent patients up to the 40th year we perform a lens aspiration. Should the case be complicated by vitreous prolapse an open sky-vitrectomy will be combined with a lensecto-my (phacectomy). Lens aspiration can be executed with a single or a double-channel-system. The aspiration of an uncomplicated traumatic cataract with juveniles is technically rather simple and the optical results are normal-ly good. 3 to 4 weeks after the operation corrections with a contact lens should be executed to restore binocular function. If possible an iridectomy should be executed. A secondary cataract will frequently occur and can be easily treated with a discission.

The surgical situation is more difficult with traumatic cataract of patients older than 40 years. The procedure here depends on the swelling of the trau-matized lens. With a broad aperture of the capsule and liquified lens masses we try an aspiration. The expression of a denser nucleus often has to be ad-ded.

In cases of small capsular ruptures a primary intracapsular lens extraction with zonulolysis should be tried.

Severe and complicated lens injuries should be oprated with a simultane-ous revision of the anterior vitreous body. If possible this revision should be done at the primary intervention, i.e. removing of the lens tissue and anterior vitrectomy should be combined with the corneal suture.

Iris and anterior chamber angle must be repositioned and cleaned from vitreous body.

All different situations represent the combination of vitreous haemorrhage with cataract and an intact anterior chamber. If the lens opacities are not too dense and some details are still visible behind the lens a pars-plana-vi-trectomy should be executed, combined with a lensectomy. This should be done with the vitrotom. To avoid secondary damage by haemosiderosis this procedure should be performed 3 to 4 weeks after the trauma. The progno-sis remains uncertain with heavy and complicated injuries. Ultrasonography should be executed in all cases to exclude a retinal detachment.

Intralental foreign bodies should be operated with the onset of cataract formation.

Postoperative treatment

Mydriatics and local antibiotics are necessary; sometimes a combination with corticosteroids is advisable.

Iris-Clip-Lens after operation of a traumatic cataract? Finally the implan-tation of an Iris-Clip-Lens or an iridocapsular Clip-Lens after traumatic cata-ract should be discussed. Possible infection, complications from the vitreous body and lesions of the iris in our opinion are arguments against the use of intraocular lenses.

The presentation will be completed by film scenes.

Author's address:
Direktor der Augenklinik
der Universität München
Mathildenstr. 8
D-8000 München 2
F.R.G.

PREFERRED SURGICAL METHODS IN POST-INFLAMMATORY CATARACT IN YOUNG PEOPLE AND ADULTS

G. SCASSELLATI SFORZOLINI

(Bologna, Italy)

Complicated post-operative cataracts are progressive lenticular opacities developing in consequence of inflammatory ocular diseases.

Most often these are cataracts dependent on local inflammatory processes of different etiology, distinguished as cataracts due to juvenile or adult uveitis, which require different surgical methods, and cataracts following anterior and posterior uveitis, having particular biomicroscopic characteristics and different problems of prognosis and operative techniques.

In other cases, we may find a senile or pre-senile cataract in an eye which has been altered by anterior or posterior uveitis, and more rarely a cataract due to Fuch's cyclitic heterochromia, or exceptionally, one due to sympathetic ophthalmitis. A less common eventually is an isolated posterior subcapsular cataract following cortisone treatment which may be local (for an anterior or posterior silent uveitis) or general (for a posterior uveitis); cataract extraction in this case does not present particular difficulties, except for the age of the patients, often young.

From a surgical point of view, the pre-existence of an intraocular inflammatory process poses two orders of problems:
— firstly, the presence of sequelae of the inflammation concerning the anterior or posterior segment and the ocular tension.
— secondly, the possibility that the inflammation is still active, or may flare up again in consequence of the surgical intervention.
The oculist must therefore:
— study the entire eye very fully from the anatomofunctional point of view.
— eliminate the origin of the uveitis.
— pre-treat the inflammation so as to operate on a non-inflamed eye.
— reduce to a minimum pre- and post-operative complications (first among them the recurrence of uveitis).
— choose the right moment for the operation.

Once the operation is decided, the objective in adults and, if possible, in young people, is intracapsular extraction; in the very young, it is extracapsular extraction. Both methods must be practiced with techniques which reduce to a minimum post-operative inflammation so as to avoid new syne-

237

chiae, secondary and tertiary cataracts and secondary glaucoma. In the post-operative period, it is essential that observation be more careful than in routine cases, for quicker recognition and treatment of complications, which are usually more frequent.

PRE-OPERATIVE SEMEIOLOGY

This serves to establish the evolutive stage of the uveitis and the cataract; the degree to which the vitreous and the retina are compromised; the functional visual prognosis; the most appropriate operating technique. It makes use of the following instrumental examinations: biomicroscopy of the eye for operation, of the cornea, of the anterior chamber, of the iris, of the pupil, of the crystalline lens, and, in the contralateral eye, of signs of inflammation and of atrophy; gonioscopy; Kalt test; diaphanoscopy or transillumination of the iris; tonometry and tonography; and A-scan of the vitreous and of the retina. Other instrumental examinations include study of the hemato-ophthalmic barrier by fluorometry, fluorophotometry, and iris fluoroniography; and radiographic research for intrabulbar foreign bodies.

Functional examinations include testing of visual acuity (for distance and near, with stenopaeic hole or slit: for the D.D. between visual diminution of lenticular or vitreal origin); testing of pupillar reflectivity; testing of perception and projection of light; and chromatic tests and electro-oculography, electro-retinography, evoked visual potentials.

In vitro examination includes paracentesis of the anterior chamber with cytological examination and albumin concentration count.

PREPARATORY TREATMENT

Medical preparatory treatment includes corticosteroid, A.C.T.H., anti-hemorrhagic, immunodepressive and climatic therapies.

Surgical preparation includes preparatory iridectomy, indicated as being anti-inflammatory diagnostic and prophylactic of seclusio and occlusio. Its advantages are that it is prophylactic of pre-operative hemorrhage; it permits evaluation of iridociliary surgical tolerance: and it provides transitory hypotonia. The minimum interval between operations is 2 to 3 months.

Operating technique may be sectorial (preferred) or peripheric. Other surgical preparatory treatments are iridocorneal laserdevascularization, perforating keratoplasty, or enuclation of the blind contralateral eye (if it shows cyclitic signs).

CHOICE OF THE BEST TIME FOR THE OPERATION

The choice of the best time for the operation depends on several factors, among them the condition of the anterior segment; the operation can be performed even in the presence of a slight uveitis (in these cases, preparatory iridectomy is particularly indicated). It is not always possible to suppress the inflammation completely. Aqueous flare does not always disappear.

The condition of the lens is important too. Post-mature cataracts must be extracted without waiting too long, in order to prevent uveitis and phacolytic glaucoma.

Another important factor is the condition of the tension. The operation may be performed even with slight hypotonia. In the presence of hypertonia, or sectorial iridectomy a combined operation is advisable, while cataract extraction alone is sufficient with phacolytic glaucoma. The interval of time necessary for operation after uveitis ranges from 3 months to 1 year.

PRE-OPERATIVE EVALUATION OF THE PATIENT

The following elements should be carefully studied;
— cardio-circulatory function
— respiratory function
— hepato-renal function
— neuro-psychic condition

PREMEDICATION AND GENERAL ANESTHESIA

The objective is a reversible reduction of the capacity of the uveal vascular bed to keep ocular tension as low as possible; this is achieved by:
— variations on osmotic pressure (mannitol, urea, glycerol)
— local venous hypotension (postural drainage)
— prevention of hypertensive venous incidents (coughing, vomiting, endobronchial hyperpressure)
— prevention of hypertensive arterial 'poussées' (pre-operative sedation; correct induction, maintenance of uniform narcotic mental effect).
— reduction of peripheral resistance (ganglioplegics, anesthetics)
— positive pressure respiratory ventilation (reduction of venous return, reduction of cardiac range, cranio-facial ischemia from hyperoxygenation).

LOCO-REGIONAL ANESTHESIA

Executed following the classical technique, together with orbicular akynesia, is limited to those cases were general anesthesia is contra-indicated.

STANDARD OPERATIVE TECHNIQUE

Standard operative technique includes:
— hypertonization of the eyeball
— external canthotomy

239

— fixation suture in the tendon of the superior rectus muscle
— Flieringa's ring
— conjunctival flap
— sclero-corneal ab externo incision (on the corneal side)
— pre-placed sutures
— sectorial iridectomy (12 o'clock): the technique is classic; advantages are that it facilitates extraction. prevents seclusio and occlusio, has an anti-inflammatory effect, permits better post-operative ophthalmoscopic exploration and facilitates extraction of the lens material (in capsular rupture and in extracapsular extraction).

An alternative technique is complete radial iridotomy (12 o'clock). This may be simple, following peripherial iridectomy and it may be temporary, since it is followed by an iris suture.It has optical and anatomical advantages. It is prophylactic of anterior synechiae and of contact of the anterior chamber with the vitreous.
— synechiotomy:
this includes synechiotomy of anterior s., of posterior s. and of s. at the camerular angle (peripheral iridectomy on both sides is preferable).
— sphincterotomy:
sphincterotomy may be single (6 o'clock) or multiple (5—7 o'clock). Its advantages are that it prevents updrawing of the pupil, facilitates extraction by sliding (if the pupil does not dilate, or the lens is intumescent), facilitates extraction by rotation (by giving better access to the lower equator of the lens), prevents pupillary block, and allows better post-operative ophthalmoscopic exploration. Its disadvantages include the introduction of an instrument into the anterior chamber, hyphaema, pupil deformation, bad utilization of pupillomotor drugs.
— hemostasis:
this must be careful and continuous.
— enzymatis zonulolysis:
this is necessary only in the young, as the zonule is usually very fragile. The effect takes rather a long time as the zonule is usually covered with exudate.
— capsulectomy:
capsulaectomy may be an isolated procedure, or it may be associated with iridectomy, with the extraction of the lens after synechiotomy, or even with anterior vitrectomy.
— extraction of the lens:
the classis intracapsular method may be chosen for adults (over 50 years of age) and also younger people (35—50). It is the obligatory method in the precense of phacolytic hypertensive uveitis and preferred in hipotony.

Methods used are traction, either simple or combined with compression, and expression (intumescent cataract). Manoeuvres used for the three methods are tumbling, which may be simple, or with compression, direct or inverse; and sliding. Often necessary is resection of the hyaloideo-capsular

ligament or of inflammatory hyaloideo-capsular adhesions (inverse tumbling). Instruments used are the cryode, the erysiphake or the forceps.
– extracapsular extraction is indicated for the very young (10–35 years of age), and the young (35–50). It is the obligatory method in the presence of irido-lenticular cyclitic membrane, especially if this is vascularized. Techniques used include discission of the anterior capsule, washing and aspiration of the lens material, phacoemulsification and phacophagia with vitreotome (if the nucleus is not hard). Injection of air or balanced salt solution into the anterior chamber is also practiced. Corneo-scleral or corneal and, if necessary, conjunctival sutures, subconjunctival injections of bactericidal antibiotics, soluble corticosteroids and mydriatics are administered after extracapsular extraction.

Indication of some particular cases;

1. Cataract associated with severe alterations of the corneal stroma – This requires perforating keratoplasty which may be previous, simultaneous or successive.

2. Cataract associated with endothelial dystrophya – the technique used here requires an ample scleral incision and particular respect for the endothelium.

3. Inflammatory cataract in juvenile reumathoid arthritis (the evolution can be accelerated by treatment with high-dosage cortisones); simple discission of anterior capsulae with suction-irrigation under anti-inflammatory and steroid protection; prognosis is unlucky, especially if band shaped cheratopathy and ipotony coexist.

4. Fuch's heterochromic cyclitis – the prognosis is generally good. The technique followed is standard; it is necessary to respect the atrophic iris and to avoid abnormal vessels. The course of recovery is favourable (it must be remembered that this is a degenerative reaction, late-appearing secondary glaucoma, and withish vitreal opacity.

5. Cataract associated with organization of vitreous – here vitrectomy is practiced; it may be anterior (pre-operative) or via the pars plana, pre-operative associated with phacophagia of a soft cataract (post-operative in not acknowledged organisation of the vitreous).

6. Cataract associated with detachment of retina – prognosis is generally unlucky; non-surgery is advisable.

7. Cataract originated by uveo-papillitis – prognosis depends upon the anatomo-functional conditions of macula, papilla and pupil, as well as of intraocular tension; extraction (possibly intracapsular) should be done with surely quiet eye, not simultaneously in both eyes and with steroid and/or immunodepressor protection.

8. Cataract associated with secondary glaucoma – this can be treated by a combined operation or a successive operation. Indicated in glaucoma due to pupillary block are: chiefly sectorial iridectomy (which may simple or associated with encleisis of one pillar), in less severe forms peripheral iridectomy,

and in selected cases iris laser-transfixation. Chandler hyaloids discission is indicated in the forms secondary to tertiary cataract. Indicated in glaucoma due to blockage of the chamber angle, or to trabecular dysfunction are: trabeculectomy, fistulizing scheie, cyclodialysis or cyclodiastasis, retrociliarydiatermy or cido-cryo-treatment.

9. Cataract originating from sympathetic ophthalmitis — prognosis is fair. The interval required before operating is at least 3 years of ocular silence. The technique demends great caution, preparatory iridectomy, steroid protection and the use of immunodepressors.

10. In selected cases, the secondary implant of intraocular lenses is possible after the extracapsular procedure.

POST-OPERATIVE MEDICAL TREATMENT

This includes the use of large range bactericidal or specific antibiotics, steroid or non-steroid antiphlogistics (in case of association with A.C.T.H.), mydriatics, anti-hemorrhagics, fibrinolysis inhibitors and immunodepressors.

POST-OPERATIVE RECOVERY

In the post-operative recovery, outcomes of previously undiscovered lessions may be observed. These may be connected with uveitis or independent of it. They may also involve the vitreous, the retina or the papilla

POST-OPERATIVE COMPLICATIONS PECULAR TO UVEITIC CATARACTS

These may include: persistance or recurring hyphemas, synechiae, immediate or late-appearing iridocyclitis, endophthalmitis, phacoanaphylactic uveitis, 'growing up' pupil, bullous keratopathy, hypertonia, persistant hypotonia, secondary or tertiary cataract, atrophy of the eyeball and, in exceptional cases, sympathetic ophthalmitis.

CONCLUSIONS

Prognosis is better in elderly and adult patients in relation to vitreo-retinial alterations which are usually less severe; better still in senile cataract in eyes already affected by uveitis. In young patients the prognosis is not so good owing to the severity of the uveitis, and also in relation to stronger individual reaction, which frequently determines macrocystic macular modifications. Prognosis is even worse in Still's disease.

Recent surgical techniques, in particular vitrectomy via pars plana, seem to bring real progress to the treatment and prognosis of cases with severe vitreous alterations but adherent retina, and cases with marked hypotonia. Even the purely cosmetic indication, controversial and usually badly accepted, may perhaps meet with greater favour.

Before closing, I think it is necessary to emphasize that experience, skillfulness and technical preferences of each surgeon are extremely important in this particular branch of pathology, where different problems are always encountered, so that programs, methods and behaviours must fit every case.

It follows that the operation will frequently be atypical, apparently in contradiction with standard technique; only apparantly however, as procedure is always based on that patrimony of knowledge which the author has tried to condense in this brief discussion. This knowledge, when well applied, permits the expert ophthalmologist to obtain functional results which are often good, and almost always quite acceptable to the patient, and, at the same time, to free the patient from those recurrent inflammatory attacks which frequently afflicted him before.

Author's address:
Ospedale Policlinico S. Orsola
Via Massarenti, 9
40138 Bologna
Italy

Docum. Ophthal. Proc. Series, Vol. 21

CATARACT WITH RETINAL DETACHMENT

R. WITMER

(Zurich, Switzerland)

The presence of both cataract and retinal detachment in the same eye is always a serious problem and careful evaluation is necessary. At the first instance most of us will have the tendency to operate on the cataract first and then deal with the retinal detachment at a later date. There are certainly many instances where this sequence of procedures is the only possible way. But there are cases where it may be wrong.

The second problem, which has to be discussed is the patient, who already has had a retinal detachment (phakic or aphakic) on one eye and now has a cataract in his second eye. What should be done first, extraction of the lens or prophylactic treatment of the retina?

CATARACT AND RETINAL DETACHMENT

The diagnosis of the presence of both diseases in the same eye should be easy. Vision is poorer than one would expect from the opacity of the lens. If the cataract is mature, then light projection is usually defective. A history of a recent drop of vision and of a detachment of the vitreous is very suspicious. Echography is of utmost importance, and electroretinography also is very helpful.

In the presence of a mature dense cataract, extraction of the lens should only be performed if the eye still has light perception. The ERG may be negative, but echography should at least reveal a flat and not a funnel shaped detachment. The history of the loss of function should not be older than one year. In some cases it may not be possible to have an acurate history, mainly in children or patients with trisomy.

For the purpose of this study we have analyzed a group of 36 patients. We felt in all these cases, that proper retinal surgery could not be performed without removing the cataract. The extraction of the lens was performed with the use of alpha chymotrypsin in 22 patients and without the enzyme in 14 patients. Retinal surgery was usually performed 4-6 weeks later and consisted always in an encircling procedure, 15 eyes required repeated surgery.

The results were as follows: 20 retinas were fully, 6 partially attached. The remaining 10 eyes were failures. The success rate of 64% is much lower

245

than in a comperative group of primary aphakic retinal detachments (77-81%).

The conclusion therefore is, that retinal surgery should be performed prior to cataract surgery if at all possible. An eye with a retinal detachment made aphakic will have a very poor prognosis; the success rate will be lower than in a simple aphakic retinal detachment.

The situation of the retinal detachment apparently becomes much worse after removal of the lens. We know, that the incidence of retinal detachment in the aphakic eye is very high. It runs around 1-2% in all clinical statistics. It is likely that the traumatism of cataract surgery and the inevitable prolapse and alteration of the vitreous due to the leaking of hyaluronic acid are reponsible for this fact. If a retinal detachment is already present, then the extraction of the lens may lead to a further deterioration of the vitreous, vitreous retraction may occur and a morning glory type of detachment develops within a very short time of a few weeks. The detachment becomes inoperable.

Since vitrectomy has become a very fashionable procedure, the next logical step will be to combine the extraction of the lens with vitrectomy and retinal surgery. If, however, vitrectomy is postponed 4-6 weeks after cataract surgery, it seems to be of no value. We cannot remove the shrinking layer of pathologically altered vitreous laying closest to the retina, which is responsible for the symptome of the funnel shaped detachment. Vitrectomy should therefore be immediately combined with the extraction of the lens and retinal surgery. In other words, the operation of the cataract should be followed at once by vitrectomy through the pars plana and an encircling procedure with possibly an episcleral plombage and cryocoagulation. After the removal of the vitreous it has to be decided, whether to fill up the eye with saline, air or some other gas. In our experience air seems to be satisfactory, since it does not produce secondary glaucoma. But despite such heroic surgery, which is certainly only indicated in rather desperate cases, the final results are statistically discouraging and so far not better than with the above mentioned standard procedures.

THE PROBLEM OF THE CATARACT IN THE SECOND EYE

There are some authors (Hudson 1977; Regnault 1977), who are very much in favor of a prophylactic circumferential cryocoagulation of the second eye of every patient with a history of aphakic retinal detachment in the first eye. This treatment should be done either prior to the extraction of the lens or immediately afterwards.

We have studied a series of 32 cataract patients with a history of a retinal detachment of the first eye. In half of these patients the retinal detachment occurred after cataract surgery. Only two patients were treated prophylactically on the second eye prior to cataract surgery.

All the cataracts of this series were extracted with enzymatic zonulolysis to reduce the surgical trauma. Despite the use of the Flieringa ring in most cases, anterior vitrectomy had to be performed in 4 cases.

Of the 32 eyes 10 never developed any tears or detachment over an observation period from one to ten years. 6 patients had tears without detachment. These were all treated either by light or cryocoagulation. These 16 eyes have good vision.

14 patients (40%) developed a retinal detachment despite all precautions and thorough biomicroscopic examination after cataract surgery. Most of these detachments had very small retinal tears, which could have been overlooked. 10 of these detachments were treated with succes and ended up with good vision; in 4 caes, however, we failed to reattach the retina. 2 eyes suffered a severe vitreous hemorrhage after the extraction of the lens.

From the total of 32 patients therefore 6 (19%) lost their second eye, 26 patients (81%) kept good vision, 16 of them after successful retinal surgery.

From our small series we can deduce that the risk of a retinal detachment in the second eye after removal of a cataract is very high indeed. The poor functional results of detachment surgery in aphakic eyes and the high incidence of bliaterality serve to emphasize the need for careful prophylaxis to the second eyes, especially when the risks are further increased by the presence of myopia or vitreous loss.

From the study of Hudson & Kanski 1977 we can take it that 28% of second eyes developed retinal detachment with new retinal breaks occuring in normal retina despite selective local prophylaxis. The 40% incidence of our series is even higher. Something should be done to bring this number down.

Hudson now treats these second eyes with circumferential cryopexy, which has given good results in his hands. But his number of cases and observation time are still too short for statistical evaluation. Regnault & Brégeat conclude that every eye with definite equatorial degeneration has to be treated prophylactically either before or immediately after the extraction of the lens. In eyes without apparent peripheral degeneration one should at least watch very carefully and perform perhaps a circumferential cryocoagulation, according to the study of Hudson and Kanski.

REFERENCES

Hudson, J.R. & Kanski, J.J.: Prevention of aphakic retinal detachment by circumferential cryotherapy. *Modern. Probl. in Ophth.* 18, *530* (1977).

Regnault, F. & Brégeat, P.: Traitement préventif du décollement de la rétine dans les yeux aphaques. Mod. *Probl. in Ophth.* 18, *538* (1977).

Witmer, R.: Cataract operation and retinal detachment. *Modern Probl. in Ophth.* 18, *477* (1977).

Author's address:

Rämistrasse 100
8091 Zurich
Switzerland

Docum. Ophthal. Proc. Series Vol. 21

CATARACT EXTRACTION AFTER FILTERING OPERATION

M. BONNET
(Lyon, France)

SPECIAL PROBLEMS

The extraction of the cataract from an eye with a filtering antiglaucomatous wound is fraught with a number of special problems. These are linked to two different factors, which are as follows: a. the anatomical and functional disorders following on the glaucoma and the anti-glaucomatus operation; b. the risk of a secondary obstruction of the antiglaucomatous bleb.

Lesions following on the glaucoma and the antiglaucomatous operation

1. Modifications of the anterior segment
The modifications of the anterior segment lead to special operating problems. The most important modifications as regards operating consequences are as follows:
   The filtering wound itself. Here is needed a special type of incision.
   The shallowness of the anterior chamber in the eyes operated for glaucoma of the closed angle type. This has repercussions on the technique of the incision.
   The lesions of the iris: a bad pupillary dilation due to rigidity of the iris, posterior synechiea or post-inflammatory membrane in front of the lens; updrawn pupil after iridencleisis; goniosynechiae; atrophy of the iris. Lesions of the iris increase the risk of a rupture of the capsule, and they are also responsible for inflammatory reactions after the operation.
   Modifications of the lens. The lens rarely gives rise to problems of itself. Yet it is advisable to take into account its size which often is relatively important in the small hypermetropic eyes operated for closed angle glaucoma. In addition, in some cases a subluxation with bulging of the superior pole towards the fistula is to be observed.
2. Alterations of the posterior segment..
The alterations of the posterior segment have no consequences on the operating technique. But optic atrophy following on glaucoma works against the functional results after surgery.

249

The risk of secondary obstruction of the antiglaucomatous belb

The secondary obstruction of the antiglaucomatous bleb is the most serious risk at the operation can lead to. In effect, the reappearance of ocular hypertension in an eye by now aphakic poses therapeutic problems which are difficult.

1. Causes for the obstruction of the bleb.

The principal causes for secondary obstruction of the bleb are three in number:

— Imperfect coaptation of the incision. This imperfection plays a major role. It must be understood that by imperfect coaptation is not only meant the major abnormalities of coaptation which are responsible for the flattening of the anterior chamber, synechiae and inflammatory reaction, but also the simple delay of coaptation and healing of the deepest layers.

— Inflammatory reactions after surgery. Such reactions are due to the alterations of the iris. They will take on catastrophic dimension in the case of extra-capsular extraction, loss of vitreous humour, or of a serious delay in cicatrization of the wound.

— The secondary rupture of the hyaloid membrane after surgery. The secondary rupture of the hyaloid after surgery may be followed by an embedding of the vitreous humour into the fistule. Among all the causes of obstruction of the fistula, only this one cannot as of yet benefit from a satisfying prophylaxis. But it might be well to observe that this cause is rare on the one hand, and that, on the other hand, late ruptures of the hyaloid do not, generally, lead to the obstruction of the fistule, even when the vitreous humour invades the whole anterior chamber.

2. Means to avoid obstruction of the fistule.

The means to avoid obstruction of the fistule above all are related to the technique of incision. This technique is very important. Nevertheless it does not resume the prophylaxis. Inferior incision has been advised. In fact, this method considerably increases the difficulties involved in the operation due to the unusual and uncomfortable position which the surgeon must adopt, and due also to the trouble caused by the pupil when it is drawn up. Inferior incision should not be advocated because it increases the risk of rupture of the capsule, loss of vitreous humour and imperfect coaptation of the incision. Superior incision, very posterior, which passes through the filtering bleb gives rise to so many risks that it should not be advocated but in cases of an unpatent fistule. The best incision remains the upper corneal incision 2 mm. distant from the fistula.

ADVISED OPERATING TECHNIQUE AND CARE AFTER SURGERY

Operating Technique

The advised operating technique is obviously done under the microscope, and, except contraindication, under general anesthesia. This technique consists of the following steps:

1. Suture of a Flieringa's ring
This step has the purpose of avoiding a collapse of the eyeball due to high hypotony which sometimes occures after the extraction of the lens.
2. Upper corneal incision
The incision is made with an 11 mm. corneal trephine which goes through the upper superficial third of the cornea. It passes 2 mm. distant from the fistula at 12 o'clock. The anterior chamber is then opened 'ab externo' with a knife few mm. away from the site of the iridectomy. The incision is then completed with Troutmann-Barraquer scissors. The blade of the scissors is held at an oblique angle in order to obtain an incision with two slopes. The incision made is large; it goes beyond the horizontal meridian up to 4 o'clock and 8 o'clock.

The advantages of this type of incision are the following ones: The incision is perfectly round; this incision increases the thickness of the edges of the wound and makes easier the localization of the predescemetique layers at the level of which the perlon sutures have to be placed. The incision should be long enough in order to avoid rupture of the lens capsule during the extraction. In addition to this, the longest incision is the less is the astigmatism against the rule after surgery.

3. The Iris
The preliminary antiglaucomatous iridectomy, when it is peripheral, is not systematically completed because the persistence of the sphincter of the iris at 12 o'clock ensures a certain protection against the protrusion of the vitreous humour into the anterior chamber.

The iridectomy is completed only when the iris is rigid and the dilation of the pupil is not sufficient to allow an easy extraction of the lens. When the pupil is not large enough two sphincterotomies can be performed at 5 and 7 o'clock. When the iris is not too abnormal, a suture of the iris re-establishes the continuity of the sphincter at 12 o'clock, at the end of the operation.

The posterior synechiae, when present, are cut by means of a spatula which is passed behind the iris through the iridectomy. When a membrane covers the pupil, it is detached with a spatula, and then cut with blunt Vanas' scissors.

4. Extraction
The extraction, of itself, does not give rise to any particular problems. It should preferably be performed with the cryode, after irrigation with alpha-chymotrypsin.

5. Sutures
Three corneal sutures with 8/0 virgin silk will have been pre-placed before extraction. These remain in place. A running with perlon 10/0 monofilament completes the closure of the incision. This suture is passed at the predescemetic level so as to obtain perfect coaptation of the edges of the wound, along the whole of its thickness, without any separation whatsoever of the deep layers. The suture is knotted on both its ends. It is stretched and

tightened on a re-formed anterior chamber so as to avoid all excessive tension which can bring about serious astigmatism. It would seem that that running suture is preferable to separate sutures, as the former makes it possible to better control astigmatism after surgery.

Care after surgery

In the period following surgery, two points particularly deserve our attention. They are as follows: the control of the inflammatory reaction after surgery; the removal of the sutures.

1. Control of the inflammatory reaction after surgery
Control of the inflammatory reaction after surgery is ensured with topical mydriatic and corticoids on the very next day. Contrary to what is required after the extraction of senile cataracts, these extractions need mydriatics and corticoids given for six weeks after the operation, or at least until any Tyndall has vanished from the anterior chamber.

2. Removal of the sutures
The three virgin silk sutures have been left in place with the purpose of activating the healing of the wound. In effect, this healing is slower with the use of perlon. Virgin silk sutures are removed by the third of fourth week. The perlon suture must be left in place for a minimum of four months. If by the second month the astigmatism is too important to prescribe optic correction, the knot on each end of the running suture is cut out. In this case the astigmatism is rapidly reduced. A suture having both free ends buried can be left indefinitely; usually, however, it ends by going up outside the wound, and it is best to remove it by the fourth month at the latest.

Results

1. Study material
Sixteen eyes (ten patients) bearing an antiglaucomatous filtering wound were operated with the above described technique. The age of the patients ranges from 48 to 72. The antiglaucomatous operation was an iridencleisis in two cases, a Lagrange iridosclerectomy in 8 cases, a trabeculectomy in 4 cases. The technique was unknown in 2 cases. The interval between the antiglaucomatous operation and the extraction of the cataract varied from 18 years to 6 months (an average of 5 years and a half). The follow up after cataract extraction varies from 5 months to 2 years.

2. Results
In this series no complication during surgery was observed. A post-operative adhesion between the iris and the wound was observed in one eye where the suture was removed too early, that is, at the second month. A peaked pupil due to a secondary rupture of the hyaloid membrane in the third month was observed in an other case.

252

All of the eyes operated retained a functional filtering wound, with a normal ocular pressure without treatment. The ocular pressure after surgery varied from 11 mm. Hg to 20 mm. Hg. In 8 cases the ocular pressure was the same as that before lens extraction. In 8 cases the pressure was somewhat higher, though remaining less than 21 mm. Hg. In the latter cases the tensional elevation after surgery varied from 3 mm. Hg to 10 mm. Hg (average of 7 mm. Hg).

The astigmatism after surgery before removal of the sutures was, on an average, 3 diopters (Min. = 0, Max. = 8.5 diopters). It was usually against the rule. In the fourth month, after cutting the knots on the two ends or after removal of the sutures, the average astigmatism was 0.8 diopters, the maximum astigmatism was 2.5 diopters. The astigmatism was zero in 50% of the cases.

Visual acuity after optical correction varied from 1/20 to 10/10. It was equal to or higher than 0.6 in only 68% of cases. Poor visual acuity is due to optic atrophy secondary to glaucoma. In addition, one eye showed a thrombosis of the central retinal vein one year after cataract extraction.

CONCLUSION

In 1968, F. Hervouet wrote that 'We know that upon removing the lens from a previously fistulized eye, the cystoid wound almost immediately disappears after the operation, with the consequences which we are all acquainted with'. In 1978, the following may be said: 'Upon removing the lens from a fistulized eye, the cystoid wound, in almost all cases, remains after the operation, maintaining a normal ocular tension'.

This radical change in the prognosis is due to the improvement allowed by microsurgery. Nonetheless, the visual results of cataract extraction in an eye previously fistulized are not so good as those of the extraction of the senile cataract, as the former depend on the state of the optic disc prior to the antiglaucomatous operation.

Authors's address:
Clinique Ophthalmologique Universitaire
B. de Lyon – Hopital de la Croix Rousse
Lyon
France

Docum. Ophthal. Proc. Series, Vol. 21

THE SURGICAL TREATMENT OF SUB—LUXATED LENSES

H. SAUTTER & U. DEMELER

(Hamburg, F.R.G.)

This lecture is going to concern the surgical treatment of subluxated lenses, and we suggest dividing the report — which covers 160 cases operated between 1971 and 1977 — into two parts.

In the first part, we shall deal with the surgical treatment of subluxated lenses in childhood and adolescence. The second will cover surgery of subluxated lenses in adults.

First, then for **lens dislocation in children.**

As we know, in childhood lens and vitreous are so closely attached to each other around Berger's space along the ligamentum hyaloideo-capsulare Wieger that attempted lens extraction would inevitably cause vitreous loss. This is the reason why until now surgery of subluxated lenses in children was regarded with reservation. The recent development of a suction-technique has so reduced the considerable risks involved, that surgery of these cases has now acquired new importance.

Let us, therefore, **report on 71 eyes in 39 patients.**

Their ages ranged from 3 to 21 years. The distribution of the sexes was roughly equal.

The causes of lens subluxation were:

in 16 patients - 31 eyes - marfan - or marchsanti - syndrome,

in 3 patients - 3 operated eyes - a homocystinuria,

in 3 patients - 3 eyes - a trauma, and

in 17 patients - 34 eyes - no obvious reason for lens subluxation nor any other anomaly.

SURGICAL TECHNIQUE:

An operating microscope with a coaxial light beam is of extreme importance for the surgical technique of lens suction. The canula (fig. 1) is attached to a handle and connected to our microsurgical unit via an intermediate tube analogous to the erysiphake.

A manometer measures the suction energy according to a water-columm as with the erysiphake. Usually, suction strenght of only 2 to 3 m water-column is necessary here, compared to the much stronger of approximately 9 m used with the erysiphake.

255

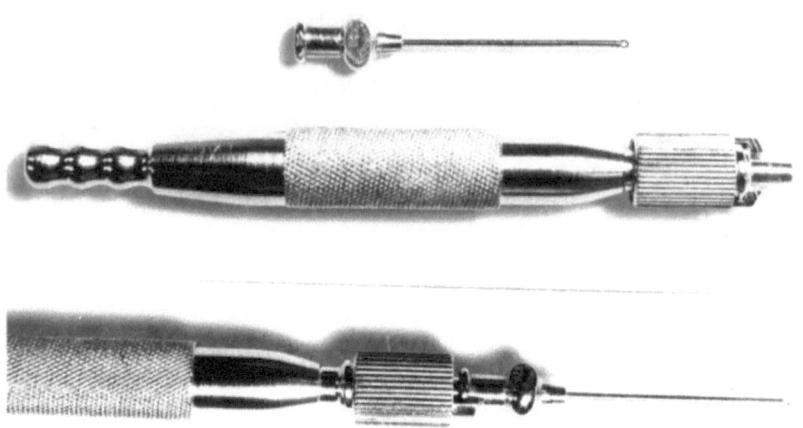

Fig. 1.

Suction can be controlled and interrrupted by a pedal attached to the chair of the operating unit.

This construction is superior to an ordinary manually worked canula, because
1. the suction can be varied in intensy and interrupted instantaneously by foot-control
and
2. in this way only one hand is needed for suction,
the other remaining free to hold or rotate
the globe.

We use a blunt needle because a pointed one can easily traumatize the posterior lens capsule especially during manipulation behind the iris.

Maximal mydriasis is of utmost importance to prevent pupillary constriction during surgical procedure. Parasympathicolytic agents are especially useful in the marfan- and marchesani-syndromes, where the dilatator muscle is almost aplastic.

We prefer a subconjunctival approach because:
1. it enables us to reach the upper part of the lens;
2. the postoperative astigmatism is ususallly lower
than after corneal incision; and
3. the wound can be double-closed by a corneo-scleral
and conjunctival suture.

Also, the sclera is incised step by step limbally with a hockey knife, the innermost lamella remaining intact. A scheie- or sato-knife which is sharp on both edges is introduced and the lens capsule opened at a circumscribed point. The shaft of the knife closes the scleral opening so that loss of aqueous is prevented at this stage. As this is not possible during suction, the anterior chamber is constantly refilled with Ringer-solution by the assistent via a small lateral limbal incision prepared at the beginning of the operation. In this way, usually the entire lens masses can be removed and the lens capsule completely emptied. We do not attempt to extract the latter in order not to cause vitreous damage.

The operation is terminated by one 8x0 -virgin-silk-suture with water-tight closure of the corneo-scleral incision and by some conjunctival sutures with the same material. Normally an iridectomy is not necessary.

Postoperative result were: An improvement in visual acuity was obtained in 55 eyes; in 13 eyes vision remained unchanged - mostly due to amblyopia- and in 3 eyes there was a deterioration due to the optical characteristics of the lens capsule; vision, however, improved after a capsule discision.

An analysis of the improved visual acuity shows:
In 20 eyes vision increased from less than 0,1 to between 0,2 and 0,5; in 9 eyes from less than 0,1 to more than 0,5, in 21 eyes from between 0,2 and 0,4 to over 0,5; and in 5 eyes from 0,5 to over 0,8.

Indications for surgery can be regarded under the following aspects:
1. **Optical** ones, for instance in spherophakia and in cases of aberration and prismatic effects leading an indistinct retinal image, especially equatorial lens deformities, like the so-called lens coloboma and, of course, when there are lens opacities. Generally, we regard surgery as necessary when these optical properties of the lens reduce the visual acuity to less than 0,5.
2. A special **therapeutic** indication is given, for instance, in cases of pupillary-block or angle-closure-glaucoma due to dislocation or tilting of the lens; or in order to allow an exact examination of the retinal periphery to treat precursory signs of retinal detachment with xenon-light, cryo- or laser-coagulation. This is especially important in several congenital syndromes.
   Now, for lens dislocation in adults.
Our report covers 89 operated eyes in 75 patients between the ages of 22 and 82 years.
In 68 eyes the lens was subluxated, and in 21 eyes completely luxated; in 5 of them into the anterior chamber and in 16 posteriorly into the vitreous. **Causes** for lens displacement were: A contusion injury in 35 eyes - 36 eyes (One case with both eyes involved)-; a marfan- or marchesani-syndrome in 26 patients - 34 operated eyes-; other intraocular diseases in 14 patients - 19 eyes.

Indications for surgery were: First of all **optical** ones, for instance, to improve visual acuity, but also to allow exact funduscopy of the peripheral retina.
   Second range the **prophylactic** or **therapeutic** indications, for instance: secondary angle-closure-glaucoma or pupillaryblock due to dislocation of the lens anteriorly, or the presence of vitreous in the anterior chamber - usually in traumatic subluxation - causing a secondary open-angle-glaucoma; further-

more a phakolytic glaucoma with complete lens - luxation into the vitreous. Finally, a definite progression of subluxation may be a prophylactic indication too.

Regarding the **surgical technique**, the most important points are: Once again use of the operating microscope with coaxial-illumination; then a flieringa- ring onto the sclera and a corneal incision providing continous visibility during the operating.

We use a hockey- or a diamond-knife or an electric rotating knife.

Other points to be regarded are: vitrectomy if necessary; (the anterior chamber must be free of vitreous at the end of the operation!). In cases of luxation into the anterior chamber suction of nearly 5 ml vitreous via pars plana before corneal incision; injection of alphachymotrypsin in that area where the subluxated lens is still attached.

Extraction is performed with a cryo-probe. If the lens is completely luxated deep within the globe, we prefer sometimes to lift it up with a loop and then fix and extract it with the cryo-probe. The lens must be separated from adhering vitreous or, in younger patients, sometimes from the ligamentum hyaloideo-capsulare Wieger.

After lens extraction we make sure, by air injection, that the anterior chamber is free of vitreous. The operation terminates with a running 10x0 corneal suture. The **postoperative results** were: in 36 eyes with traumatic subluxation or luxation visual acuity improved in 28 eyes, remained unchanged in 7 eyes and deteriorated in 1 eye. In the 34 eyes with a congenital or syndrome-caused lens-luxation, visual acuity improved in 24, remained unchanged in 8, and worsened in 2 cases. In 13 eyes, where another ocular disease was present visual acuity improved in 15, remained unchanged in 4 and in no case worsened after operation.

To conclude, I venture to say that with the aid of the surgical technique available today, especially the use of the operating microscope with coaxial illumination, the treatment of subluxated or luxated lenses in children as well as in adults no longer presents severe problems.

Docum. Ophthal. Proc. Series, Vol. 21

CATARACT SURGERY AFTER PENETRATING KERATOPLASTY

DAVID PATON, M.D.

(Houston, Texas, U.S.A.)

There are three chief indications for cataract extraction performed after penetrating keratoplasty. The most common of these is the progression of a pre-existing, immature cataract. The other two causes are iatrogenic: damage to the lens capsule at the time of the keratoplasty (rare), and drug-induced cataract from the use of topical steroid.

Virtually any intraocular sugery is conducive to the progression of a pre-existing cataract. Topical steroids are an added incentive for senescent-type cataracts to advance. Cataracts originating from the use of topical steroid are dose-related. The larger the graft, the more steroid necessary for prevention or control of the allograft reaction. Thus, I tend to use grafts of 7.5-mm diameter; purely drug-induced cataracts should be unusual if not rare.

Although in the average case there is no significant difference in the long-range prognosis for an eye when the graft and cataract surgery are done as consecutive procedures rather than as a combined procedure, there are cases in which the surgeon's judgment should favor one or the other of these alternatives. For example, visual recovery time is less if the two operations are combined, particularly if an over-size graft (0.25—0.5 mm larger) is employed. Also, patients with shallow anterior chambers and moderately advanced cataracts (especially if there are a few peripheral anterior synechias) should have the combined procedure. In distinction, eyes with very early lens changes, borderline ocular tension control, irregular thickness of recipient tissue and moderate to marked vascularization are usually better served by performing penetrating keratoplasty first and waiting for the graft to become crystal clear before cataract extraction is accomplished. Several cases illustrating consecutive and combined surgery are shown in Figures 1 through 4. I should add, too, that there are cases when cataract surgery should precede the possibility of later keratoplasty — but for the most part the circumstances relate to stationary corneal opacity that is considered to be playing a minor role in vision loss.

There are three basic approaches to cataract surgery following keratoplasty: a large incision at the limbus for intracapsular cataract extraction; a small limbal incision for phacoemulsification (or its variants); and a pars plana approach, now popularly called lensectomy. It is the skill of the surgeon (meaning in large measure his surgical experience with these modalities) that should be the chief factor in determining the technique of cataract extraction elected. However, certain generalities can be made. In elderly

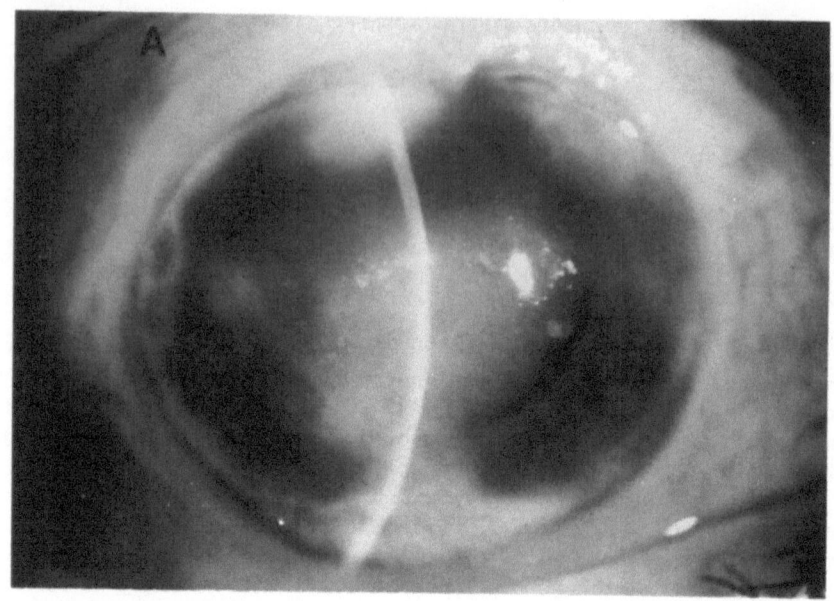

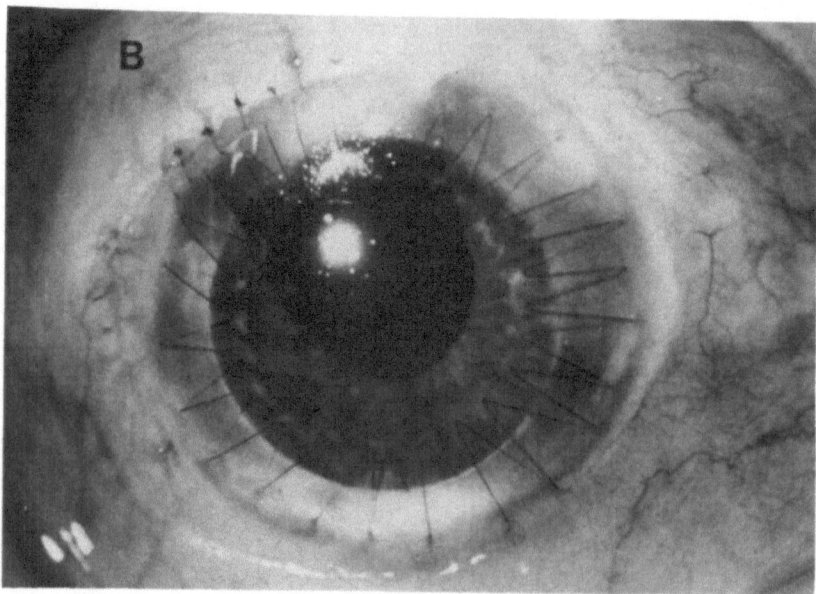

Fig. 1. A 70 year old patient whose only eye has post-inflammatory scarring as well as corneal thinning: A, sector iridectomy and filtering procedure was performed seven years ago; B, the same eye is shown one year following penetrating keratoplasty and two months subsequent to phacoemulsification. The filtering bleb has been undisturbed and the intraocular pressure is normal. The graft is clear. Consecutive surgery was considered the safer approach to the management of this patient's eye.

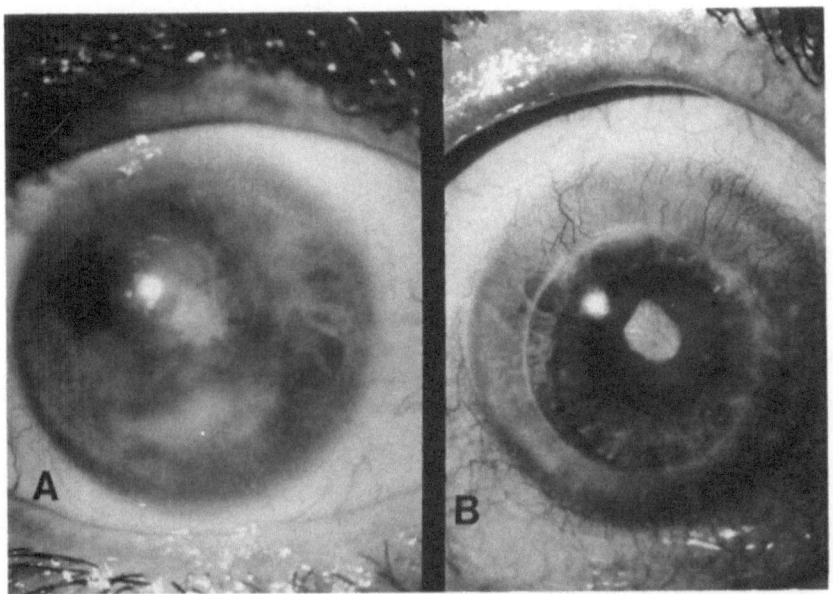

Fig. 2. A 54 year old patient with bilateral post-inflammatory corneal scarring has considerable vascularization and corneal thickness variability. A, there is an anterior polar cataract, but the extent of that cataract is difficult to assess preoperatively; B, penetrating keratoplasty was performed and the patient's acuity at eighteen months following surgery has improved to 20/50, despite the presence of the anterior lens opacity. With further progression of a nuclear cataract, cataract surgery may be indicated at a later date.

patients with nuclear cataracts (particularly if brunescent), the least traumatic way of removing the cataract is by intracapsular extraction through a large limbal incision. The surgery should not be done until the preceding keratoplasty has become 'crystal clear.' It is unusual for a graft to be crystal clear before six months into its postoperative course, and some grafts do not reach normalcy until a year following the keratoplasty. If nylon suture material has been used as a continuous 'buried' suture, the nylon should not be removed before the cataract procedure. Currently, I rarely remove the continuous nylon suture; experience has indicated no difficulty with subepithelial nylon or polypropylene suture despite the use of contact lens, often prescribed at six months following keratoplasty. In eyes with bullous keratopathy as the original indication for keratoplasty, removal of these sutures even as late as a year following keratoplasty can result in bulging of the graft and the need to resuture.

At the time of intracapsular extraction, folding back the cornea with its clear graft (and nylon suture in position) does not damage the graft any more than such folding damages the endothelium of the normal cornea. Maumenee has made that point and it is often unrecognized. However, to minimize direct trauma to the corneal endothelium it is my habit to use a

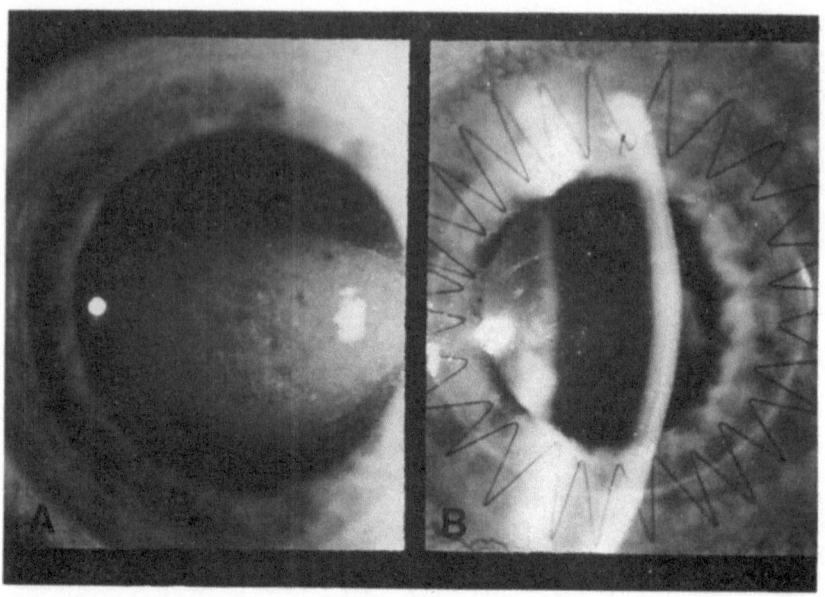

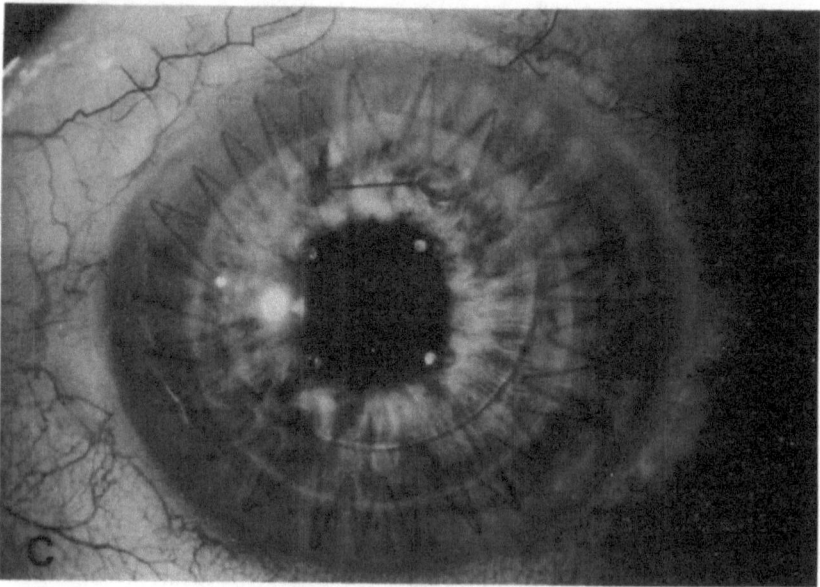

Fig. 3. A 78 year old patient with bilateral Fuchs endothelial dystrophy and early nuclear cataracts. Only the left eye is shown in these illustrations: A, preoperative appearance of bullous keratopathy; B, status following penetrating keratoplasty with early progression of the patient's senescent-type cataract. Keratometer measurements indicated minimal astigmatism. C, status of the eye following intracapsular cataract extraction and the placement of a medallion-type intraocular lens. The patient's acuity is 20/25 with +2.00+2.00 x 65°.

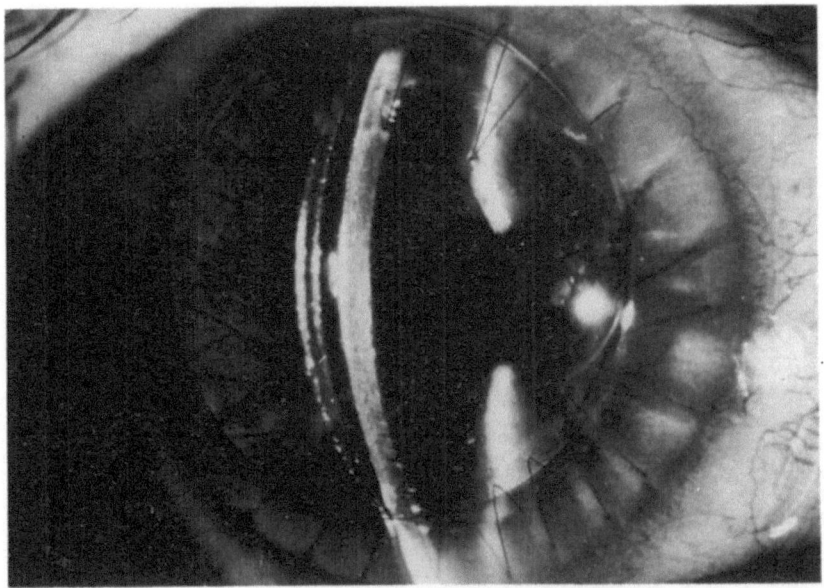

Fig. 4. A 78 year old female's right eye is shown 21 months following combined penetrating keratoplasty and intracapsular cataract extraction. The patient is wearing a hard contact lens. Due to the presence of bilateral bullous keratopathy from Fuchs dystrophy and also the advanced age of the patient, a combined procedure was performed. Somewhat irregular astigmatism however, requires the contact lens for 20/30 acuity.

posterior corneal section that is at least 160° in size when intracapsular extraction is performed on previously grafted eyes. That is approximately a 14-mm incision.

For cataracts in young adults and children, an extracapsular extraction procedure is preferable; I use the Kelman instrument for phaco-emulsification. Often it is possible to do the operation with simple aspiration and lavage without the use of ultrasound. Should there ever be a circumstance when cataract surgery is elected in the presence of a graft that is not completely crystal clear (such as localized microcystic edema near the graft periphery), I now believe that the least traumatizing surgery is phacoemulsification performed with the lens remaining in the posterior chamber, a technique championed by another good friend at this meeting, Dr. Richard Kratz.

Since I personally have no experience with pars plana lensectomy after keratoplasty, I can only mention this as one of the options. Dr. Louis Girard is a proponent of this technique and he is aware of my old-fashioned concern that with this method one necessarily damages the vitreous. I cannot put it from my mind that if one can perform cataract surgery without vitrectomy of any sort, it is safer for the eye in its future decades. Most surely there are times when pars plana lensectomy becomes the procedure

263

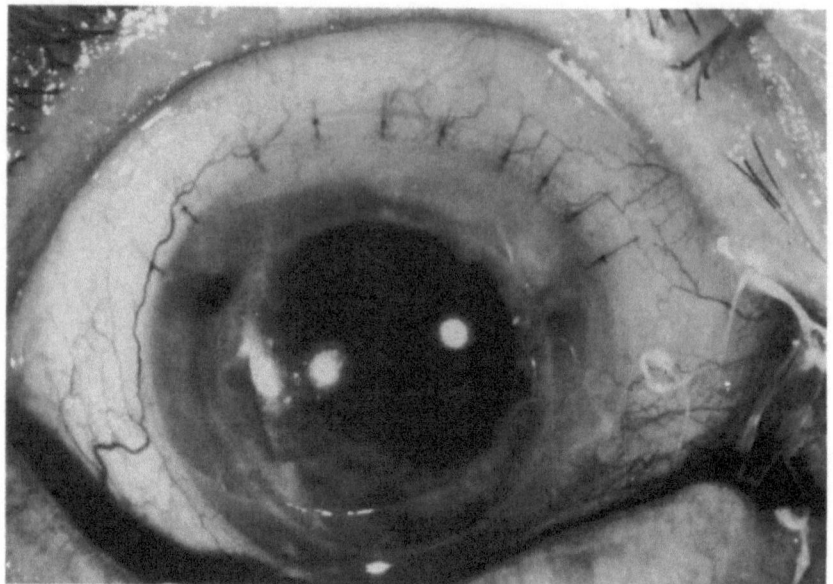

Fig. 5. A 77 year old woman had had previous penetrating keratoplasty followed by advancement of a cataract. The photograph shows the eye six months following intracapsular cataract extraction with placement of an anterior chamber lens. The graft had minimal astigmatism, justifying placement of the implant.

of choice – such as when lens removal is to be combined with an optical vitrectomy to remove hemorrhagic residues or other vitreous opacities of major visual significance.

The management options for coexistent corneal opacity and cataract have been discussed elsewhere (Paton & Jones 1976), and the indications and prognosis for keratoplasty based upon corneal morphology rather than disease entity have also been discussed (Paton 1976) – I refer to these papers for completeness of expression of personal opinions.

There is an added reason one might cite for consecutive rather than the combined procedure: the potential use of an intraocular lens. Rather than list the hypothetical circumstances in which one might employ such a device following keratoplasty, I will illustrate such circumstances by showing two cases (Figures 3 and 5). Both patients had had successful keratoplasty. Each patient, over 65 years of age, had advancement of cataract but normal intraocular pressure and evidently normal retina. In both cases, the keratometer indicated that there was no major astigmatism of the graft. Fortified by that knowledge, and because these patients were not good candidates for contact lenses, intraocular implants were placed at the time of intracapsular cataract extraction. In one case, an anterior chamber (Choyce–Tennant) lens was employed and in the other case a four-loop Binkhorst iris clip lens was selected. Monocular aphakia, central vitreous touch syndrome in the contralateral eye, and a few other indications such as those seem to justify the use of implants after keratoplasty if the graft is not highly astigmatic.

I have little to say about the so-called 'triple procedure' (penetrating keratoplasty-cataract extraction-intraocular lens placement) because I have had much less experience with it than have others, such as Kaufman (Pers. communication) who does not advocate it. Figure 6 illustrates a case of my own in which the eye has done exceedingly well but I also believe that I was exceedingly lucky that the recipient has little problem with the astigmatism of the graft. At times graft astigmatism can be irregular. Before keratoplasty, not only is it difficult to predict postoperative axial length of the eye (to estimate the power of the lens implant that should be selected), but the presence of high or irregular astigmatism remains an unpredictable factor in my hands – and, therefore, the value of an intraocular lens with a crystal clear but astigmatic graft is hardly beneficial if one also considers (as I do) that the implant has at least some statistical likelihood of late complications.

In the final part of this paper, I would like to describe my preferred technique for the combination of penetrating keratoplasty with intra- of extracapsular cataract surgery performed through the trephined cornea. Elements of this technique have been described elsewhere. (Paton and Jones, 1976). Routinely, I employ a 7.5-mm trephine on the recipient eye and a

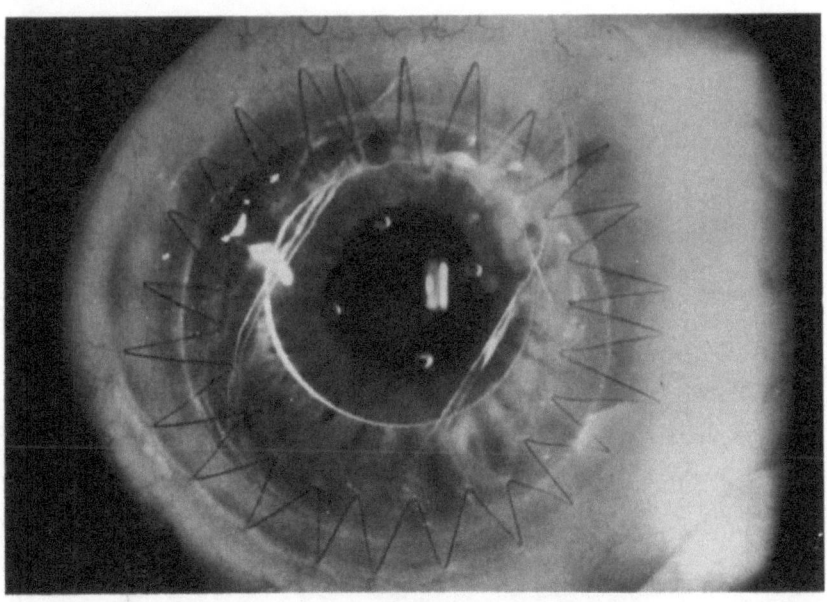

Fig. 6. The right eye of a 67 year old patient four months following 'the triple procedure': penetrating keratoplasty, cataract extraction, and placement of an intraocular lens. The acuity is 20/30 with +100+5.50 x 2 .

precut over-size graft (according to the recommendation of Troutman at the Second Corneal Congress in 1976). Donor tissue is stored in McCarey-Kaufman media containing tissue culture fluid, Dextran, penicillin and gentamicin. A history of penicillin sensitivity on the part of the recipient has not produced detectable effects (Liesegang & Paton 1978).

I use a 13-mm Flieringa ring, securing it at the limbus with eight interrupted 8–0 black silk sutures. There is no doubt in my mind that this gives optimal support for the peripheral cornea. Double rings and other varieties of scleral expanders are not necessary. The cornea is trephined with a disposable blade mounted on a simple tubing that permits centering of the trephine by observing the cornea through its hollow shaft (Figure 7). All steps of the procedure are done with the operating microscope. A small peripheral iridectomy is made and the lens is delivered by cryoextraction. Should the vitreous face be ruptured, an open-sky vitrectomy is performed with a motorized instrument (Ocutome). Vitreous is taken from the surface of the iris with cellulose sponges employing gentle technique. (Paton 1978) The posterior chamber is refilled with balanced salt solution and air is used in the anterior chamber as the pre-cut button is secured with interrupted 8–0 black silk sutures at the 12, 6, 3, and 9 o'clock positions. These sutures are removed as a continuous 10–0 nylon suture is run throughout the circumference of the graft and secured to itself at the 12 o'clock position. The suture is tightened to the point of gentle traction, the anterior chamber air replaced by balanced salt solution, and then the single knot is completed

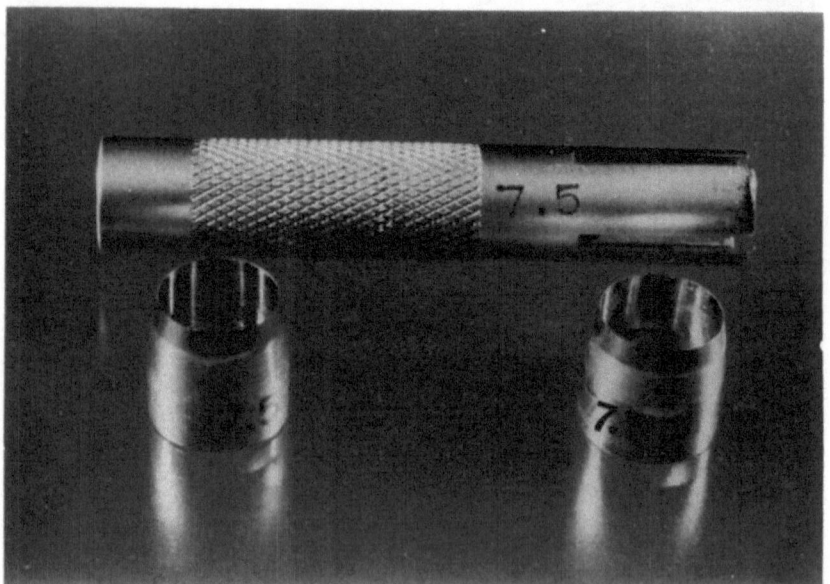

Fig. 7. Disposable trephine blades and the hollow-shaft handle to which they can be mounted, permitting optimal centering of the trephine by viewing cornea through the hollow tube. Storz Instrument Company, St. Louis, Missouri: #SP7–9270.

and advanced into the stroma of the graft. Extracapsular extraction (by open-sky-incision-and-lavage through the trephined cornea) constitutes no essential differences in the keratoplasty technique and is preferred in young patients.

As yet, I have not determined if there is less postoperative glaucoma in aphakic eyes when over-size grafts are employed; but routinely, acetazolamide is used in the early postoperative period, whether tension elevation is detected or not. Systemic steroids are employed only when vitrectomy has been necessary. Due to the skilled contact lens technologist in our department, Mr. Joseph Soper, most of these patients can be fitted with contact lenses six months following surgery, should that be preferred to spectacle correction.

REFERENCES

Kaufmann, H.E.: Personal communication.
Liesegang, T.J. & Paton, D.: The McCarey-Kaufman medium and penicillin allergy. *Ophthalmic Surg.* (In press)
Paton, D.: The prognosis of penetrating keratoplasty based upon corneal morphology. *Ophthalmic Surg.* 7:36−45, 1976.
Paton, D.: The management of vitreous by the anterior segment specialist. In Emery, J.M.: (ed.) Current Concepts in Cataract Surgery. Selected Proceedings of the Fifth Biennial Cataract Congress, February, 1977. St. Louis: The C.V. Mosby Company, 1978. (In press)
Paton, D. & Jones, D.B.: *Penetrating Keratoplasty.* Alcon Monograph Series, No. 1, October, 1976. Fort Worth, Texas: Alcon Laboratories, 1976.

Author's address:
Baylor College of Medicine
Department of Ophthalmology
Texas Medical Center
Houston, Texas 77030
U.S.A.

Docum. Ophthal. Proc. Series, Vol. 21

SIMULTANEOUS CATARACT EXTRACTION AND CORNEAL GRAFT

R.C. TROUTMAN

(New York, U.S.A.)

In the older patient, in particular when vision-compromising corneal pathology and cataract coexist, a simultaneous cataract extraction and keratoplasty often is the procedure of choice. In my experience, not only is more rapid rehabilitation possible, but also there is an increased opportunity for the graft to maintain clarity postoperatively. In our series of cases, approximately 88% of grafts remain clear during the period of follow-up. When an intraocular lens is added, there is 10% greater incidence of delayed opacification of the graft.

When the cataract is performed as a secondary procedure, even without lens implantation, graft clarity is found to be compromised in 22% of eyes, and with IOL in an additional 10%.

Sometimes the corneal pathology may not be sufficiently advanced to require keratoplasty and the cataract is performed first. In these cases, when a subsequent keratoplasty is performed, the results are about the same as when the operations are done simultaneously, the major compromise being the increased time required for rehabilitation.

A major problem following combined cataract and keratoplasty has been the time required for optimal optical rehabilitation. In many patients, spectacles can be used effectively within a few weeks postoperatively and are especially well tolerated when the patient is bilaterally aphakic. However, in the very old patient with Fuch's dystrophy, the spectacle distortion encountered with unilateral aphakia can curtail severely their already limited activity and function. Therefore, when surgery on only one eye can be done, the simultaneous introduction of an alloplastic lens substitute, the so-called 'triple procedure', is indicated. Precaution must be taken to prevent endothelial damage to the homograft by the implant or a marked increase of graft opacification will result. The triple procedure may not be required if the patient is axially myopic. Rather than submit the eye to the added risk of an intraocular lens, my disparate-diameter, graft-recipient opening technique can be employed. A donor button 1 mm larger in diameter than the diameter of the recipient opening, when healed in position, will induce 5 to 8 diopters of corneal myopia, obviating the necessity for high-power, aphakic postoperative spectacle correction. More commonly, however, especially in the patient with Fuch's dystrophy, the eye is hyperopic and an alloplastic lens substitute will be necessary, though one of correspondingly lower power is used with the disparate diameter technique.

Because of the added risk of lens implantation, the 'triple' operation never should be done if the patient does not have potentially useful vision in the fellow eye or is one-eyed. A combined penetrating keratoplasty and cataract extraction offers the least risk. Here, too, a graft larger in diameter than the recipient opening is used to reduce the amount of final hyperopic correction required.

In addition to the optical benefit from the disparate-diameter, graft-recipient technique, it has been shown that there is significantly less postoperative glaucoma, especially when the author's through-and-through technique is used to suture the graft. Olson has proposed the anatomic and mathematical reasons for this beneficial effect, simply stated, the retraction of the posterior lamella of the cornea toward the chamber angle meshwork that may occur when anteriorly placed, tightly tensioned suture loops are used, is prevented by through-and-through suture closure. Also, because of the firm, full-thickness apposition obtained by the through-and-through suture technique, excessive tightening of the wound is prevented and more physiologic healing takes place.

A second form of combined cataract graft surgery assuming increasing importance is lamellar refractive keratoplasty. The lamellar keratoplasty is done by one of two techniques, keratophakia, the interposition of an optically ground lamellar homograft lens between an excised lamellar corneal cap and the remaining posterior lamella of the cornea, or aphakic keratomileusis, where the stromal aspect of the resected lamellar corneal cap is ground to a plus power. Each of these techniques is designed to induce an increase in curvature of the anterior corneal surface. This increases the dioptric power of the cornea without decreasing the corneal diameter, thus effecting a correction of the aphakia.

This operation, conceived by José Barraquer, has been performed by us since October 1977, with uniformly good technical and vision results. This operation should not be used in a diseased cornea or following a successful penetrating graft. But for the cataract or aphakic patient with a normal cornea who cannot tolerate a contact lens or who wishes not to wear spectacles, the technique of Barraquer makes it possible to avoid the long-term risk of an alloplastic lens substitute. It can be performed on the fellow eye with relative safety or on the second eye of a patient corrected unilaterally with an intraocular lens. Some overrefraction may be necessary to correct small axial or astigmatic residuals. These patients usually require a period of months to attain maximum visual acuity. In the interim, our patients have been uniformly happy. Several patients have reported that, even though the acuity is slightly less, it seems more normal than that obtained with the fellow eye corrected by an intraocular lens or a contact lens. No serious complications have been encountered in the 16 cases that we have performed to date. Vision results have been uniformly good except in those patients with macular disease preoperatively. This latter group of patients, in fact, are among the happier ones since they retain peripheral field similar to that of the intraocular lens patient but without the associated glare.

Keratophakia or aphakic keratomileusis is currently being employed only on those patients where contact lenses or intraocular lens implants are contraindicated and spectacle correction is not acceptable.

SUMMARY

Combined cataract graft techniques, whether performed because of vision-compromising corneal pathology and cataract or to obviate the necessity for aphakic correction after cataract extraction, are made more safe and effective by microsurgery. Earlier visual rehabilitation is made possible by the selective use of alloplastic lens substitutes. However, more physiologic means, such as my disparate-diameter, graft-recipient technique or lamellar refractive keratoplasty, should be used preferentially when possible.

271

CHOICE AND CLINICAL EVALUATION OF SUTURAL MATERIAL

I. ESENTE, A. MOLINARA, G. LAGANA & G. AMBROSINI

(Florence, Italy)

INTRODUCTION

Since the majority of lens deliveries are done using ordinary techniques, **incision and wound closure** are still essential for good recovery of function.

As we have no yet accomplished immediate sealing of the entire wound, we still depend on material performance and tissue reaction.

Clearly no suture can be regarded as satisfactory unless the incision and closure are correct. Correct wound closure is based on the concept of obtaining an 'anatomical' reconstruction of the wound (Troutman) and of 'atraumatic surgery' (Paton). (see Fig. 1–2) Refinements of sutural material have widely contributed to improving results in cataract surgery.

A clinical selection of up-to-date sutural materials must be based on: a. patient's convenience, b. surgeon's requirements.

At present the patient's convenience, namely no discomfort and recovery of function, are fairly well catered for in a high percentage of cases. This percentage will increase in the future because it is often related to greater accuracy of procedure obtainable with a widespread use of microsurgery.

As for the surgeon's requirements, the term '**basic performances characteristics**' includes all of the most important properties of a sutural material such as (in short) the well known **operative evaluations** (visibility, strenght, pliability, pull-through, fraying properties, knot security, etc.) or the **postoperative ones** reaction, strength and wound healing time, recovery of function, etc.) (See Fig. 3).

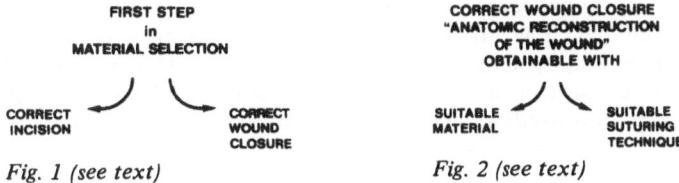

Fig. 1 (see text)   Fig. 2 (see text)

The basic performance characteristics can be classified as **excellent** (++), **good** (+) or **fair** (+−) in an attempt to give some schematic indications for selection.

273

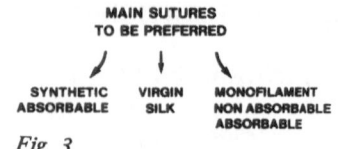

MAIN SUTURES
TO BE PREFERRED

SYNTHETIC ABSORBABLE   VIRGIN SILK   MONOFILAMENT NON ABSORBABLE ABSORBABLE

Fig. 3

ENUMERATION OF "BASIC PERFORMANCES" CHARACTERISTICS
OF MAIN SUTURAL MATERIALS

(°)

Operative	Silk 8 · 9/0	Synth. Absorbable 8/0	Synth. Monof. non Absorb. 10 · 11 · 12/0
1) Visibility	+ +	+ +	+
2) Strength (tensile)	+	+ +	+
3) Pliability	+	+	+ +
4) Pull-Through	+ −	+ −	+ +
5) Fraying	+	+.	+ +
6) Knot (security)	+ +	+	+
7) Tying (ease)	+	+	+ +
Postoperative			
8) Reaction (tissular)	+	+	+ +
9) Wound retention (strenght)	+	+	+ +
10) Wound healing time	+ +	+ +	+ −
11) Recovery of function	+	+	+ +
12) Suture disappearance	+	+ +	+ −
Excellent: + +	3	4	7
Good: +	8	7	3
Fair: + −	1	1	2

(°) In this evaluation we have omitted the synthetic monofilament absorbable (vicryl 9 or 10/0) and the needle performances.

Fig. 4

All sutures can be regarded as 'foreign bodies' in the wound, but nowadays this disadvantage has been minimized by reducing suture calibre.

The diameters can go from 13 to the more widely used 22-26 microns, which represent a real technical achievement and a consistent variety of choice.

The distinction between **nonpermanent or absorbable material** and **permanent or nonabsorbable material** can be maintained at present for clarity's sake but it is not completely pertinent from a clinical point of view which is mainly concerned with final functional results (see Fig. 4).

Anyhow, absorption is clinically advantageous and beneficial if it occurs at a 'uniform and predictable rate'[1] with minimal tissue reaction, ensuring

---

[1] The mechanism of degradation and absorption differs in natural and synthetic absorbable sutures. Absorption of collagen and surgical gut depends on cellular enzymatic activity (cellular collagenase and protease eventually degrade and remove protineaceous material). Absorption is more evident in vascular tissue and in the presence of infection or fever (more leukocytes and enzymes in loco).
The absorption in new synthetic material (dexon and vicryl) does not require special cellular activity: it is related to their hydrolysis (experimentally and clinically it occurs from 30 to 90 days) and depends only partially on tissue reaction.

good wound apposition and enabling permanent healing. Today these performance characteristics can be obtained with the absorbable synthetic derivates of polygycolic acid.

Other absorbable materials which, however, have an unpredictable or delayed rate' of absorption promoting possible antigenic and protinaceous tissue reactions, seem to be likewise unrecommendable. For this reason and in this category we must discard animal hair, cat-gut (first introduced in 1939) and collagen (1964).

These last two materials, even in their finest preparation (8/0 chromic or mild chromic) and clinically used extensively until 1970-72, now seem out of date, due also to their more delayed absorption, their obvious lack of uniformity and the manufacturing difficulties they involve.

So even surgeons not keen on microsurgery should give preference to the latest absorbable synthetics, dexon[2] (polyglycolic acid) or vicryl (polyglactin 100) in size 8/0.

These sutures, thanks to new refinements in needle, braids, colour, and reduced defects (fraying tendencies, fibrillation in tying, difficulty in pull-through and tissue incarceration) have become the best substitutes for cat-gut and collagen, and their clinical results must be considered important. Their most outstanding quality is their tensile strength and their absorption which is more predictable and generally quicker than with any other material (30-90 days).

A few problems still exist regarding their versatility, knotting problems (triple tying advisable), and their inelasticity.

Very recently the absorbable synthetic Vicryl has become available in the monofilament version (size 9 or 10/0). Originally prepared in monofilament form but due to its stiffness not clinically advisable, this newly refined product (not due to chemical variation) now appears to be indicated for all types of corneo-scleral closures. Its pliability is good and the time of disappearance is similar to that of the braid's product. It proves to be more effective when used in combination with another type of material (Vicryl 8/10, nylon or silk in one or more single sutures). The continuous suturing technique is preferable. The wound healing time and wound strenght contention seems to be sufficient but our clinical evaluation on this suture is not yet complete: therefore all preliminary and so far very favorable opinion must still be confirmed by more extensive experimentation.

Other materials, such as thin steel, the most inert material, can be considered to be completely **non-absorbable**. This is in fact seldom used and is only chosen by a few surgeons, an then only in conjunction with other material. Other material may be **partially absorbable** (by means of degradation, fragmentation or extrusion) at an unpredictable rate, from 30 to 180 days, but nevertheless clinically advantageous.

---

[2] Dexon is the registered trademark of Davies-Geck American Cyanamid Group. Vicryl is the registered trademark of Ethicon Comp.
Dexon is an homopolymere of polyglycolic acid and Vicryl is a copolymer of polyglycolic (90%) and lactic acid (10%).
The first should have easier hydrolysis.

This series includes virgin silk[3] whose general properties and performance characteristics must not be underestimated, especially by surgeons who do not require continuous suturing and do not neglect a controlled tissue reaction favoring the wound closure.

Silk is a partially 'protineaceous' substance, but is much better tolerated than cat-gut or collagen and has no antigenic reactions associated with it because it is not an animal derivate.

Clinically speaking, rare or exceptional partial wound separations, or erosion and micronecrosis may occur, but they are often to be blamed on poor quality material, irregular wound-apposition or excessive tightening.

Virgin silk (8 or 9-0) must be recommended only for scleral and covered flap procedure and it is contra-indicated in corneal wound repairs (neovascularisation and epithelialisation are possible). Interrupted sutures are obligatory as the material has no elasticity. 'Silk sutures can be tightened to a more precise and less changeable tension than is true of the more elastic nylon suture' (Paton).

Silk has an excellent 'hand' and ties securely with a single square knot.

In the experimental comparison between silk and absorbable synthetics (8/0), the latter have come out in a more favourable light as they do not promote significant tissue reaction: nevertheless, in our hands and experience, clinical and functional results have been very similar.

The sutural material most frequently used today, expecially when corneal wound closure or continuous and double suturing is required by the microsurgeon, is synthetic non-absorbable monofilament (nylon or perlon or prolene). Nylon was a fantastic discovery and it has contributed widely to the progress in ophthalmology and mocrosurgery.

Nylon suture is characterized mainly by its prominent elasticity (25% compared to the 2% elasticity of silk and collagen and absorbable synthetics.

Nylon made its first appearance in 1940 in the U.S.A. and in Germany as perlon (4). In ophthalmology it was first used in 1960 by Mackensen and Harms (sopramid or perlon) in a thread of approximately 40 microns in diameter.

It is the only material with a smooth exterior surface which does not catch

---

[3] Virgin silk is a virtually inelastic (2%) polypeptide (purified protein ± sericine), multifilamented (9/0 braided with 4 or 5 monofilaments, 8/0 braided with 8-9 monofilaments), giving mild tissue reaction (probably mainly due to sericine) more evident than with absorbable synthetics (Salthouse and Coll. 1977). Too deep suturing is neither necessary nor advisable (Paton) and can cause epithelialisation if it protrudes into the anterior chamber (Maumenee). Silk can produce a leukocytic tissue reaction or fibrosis. White 8/0 virgin silk is generally more satisfactory than the methilene blue which can cause slightly more annoyance. Twisted black and siliconized silk do not seem to present big disadvantages either, and they have the advantage of resisting enzymatic action.

[4] Nylon monofilament is a Polymid 66 and Perlon (registered trademark of Perlon Ass. Germany) monofilament a Polyamid 6. Nylon calibration goes up to 12/0 (more used 9-10/0) and exceptionally 13 microns. Supramid or Perlon are available in calibrations of 8-9-10/0.

CLINICAL CHOICE OF MATERIALS
BASED ON THEIR
"BASIC PERFORMANCES"

INTRACAPSULAR DELIVERIES	Vir. Silk	Synth. Abs.	Mon. non abs.
Corneal incision	– –	– +	+ +
Sclero-corneal incision	+ +	+ +	+ +
ALL TYPES OF DELIVERIES and incisions			
WITH INTRAOCULAR LENS IMPLANTATION	– –	– +	+ +

+ + Excellent   – + Usable   – – Unadvisable

Fig. 5

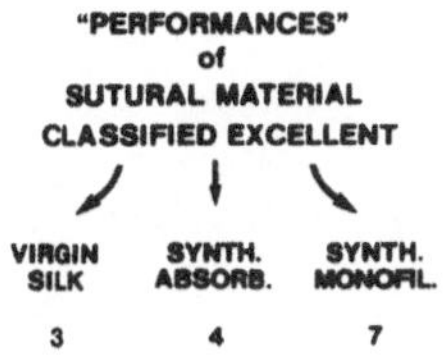

"PERFORMANCES"
of
SUTURAL MATERIAL
CLASSIFIED EXCELLENT

VIRGIN SILK	SYNTH. ABSORB.	SYNTH. MONOFIL.
3	4	7

Fig. 6

or abrade tissue, having a uniform diameter and tensile strenght. Its pliability and handling are unique. Nylon is capable of giving the wound its pre-operative configuration eliminating posterior gaps and ≪lambda≫ shaped profile (Troutman) and valuable for a 'through and trough' suturing technique.

Nylon can also be considered, in some way, a long-lasting and partially absorbable suture because it can undergo a very slow chemical degradation (depolymerization) over a period of one year or more. (5) In the other circumstance it remains encapsulated as a guest in the tissue without any apparent reaction.

The 9 or 10/0 (approximately 30 to 25 microns) preparations are most frequently used but 11 or 12/0 (that is a 14 microns diameter) are also available. The surgeon should become familiar with nylon and how to handle it properly. This requires the use of a microscope and microsurgical instrumentation. The monofilament polypropylene (prolene) (6) is more often indicated or preferred by some surgeons for corneal surgery and intra-ocular lens implantation.

Sophisticated requirements of the micro-surgeon can be met nowadays by another non absorbable monofilament of special calibration (13 m krous-nearly half the average monofilament and less than double the diameter of an erythrocyte) which requires particular handling.

This material seems to be a more important advance for microvascular surgery than for eye-wound closure, but at any rate it offers the subjective advantage to the patient of no suture sensation, no knotting problems and minimal inflammation of the wound.

Experimentally in animal sclera and muscle, the nylon is incapsulated within a thin band of fibrous tissue. This never happens in corneal tissue (T. Salthause and Coll. 1977) where this material produces a minimal inflammatory reaction covered by proliferating epithelial cells (R. Eve-R. Troutman 1976).

Prolene (the registered trademark of Ethicon Co.) is a polymerized propylene: it can be white or coloured (blue). Its knotting strenght is superior to other monofilaments and presents no capillarity, as some nylon does. It presents some differnt physical properties from nylon such as more elasticity.

277

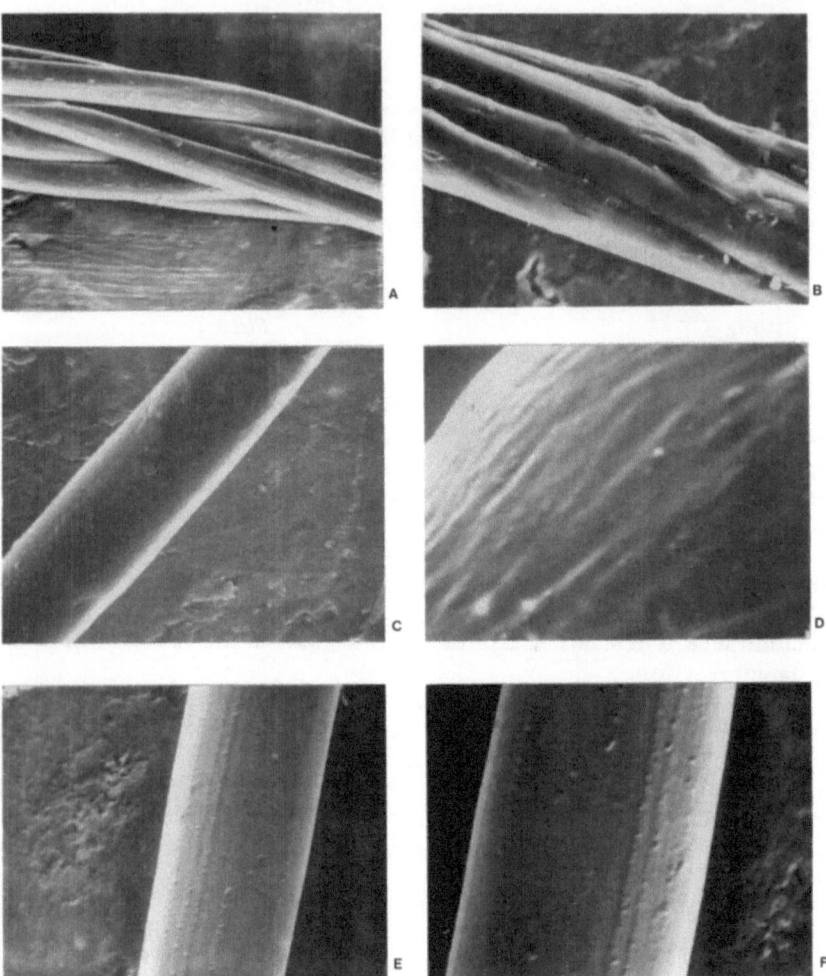

Fig. 7

Synthetic nonabsorbable monofilaments present some 'shortcomings', the main ones being a more delayed wound healing time and a more elaborate sutural technique, and preferably buried knots.

COMBINED SUTURAL MATERIALS

There are no speciale contraindications in the use of combined sutural material (silk, synthetics, monofilament, absorbable or non absorbable and in exceptional cases, steel).

Quite a number of surgeons are keen on this type of method, which should be considered from two points of view. We should first of all look at

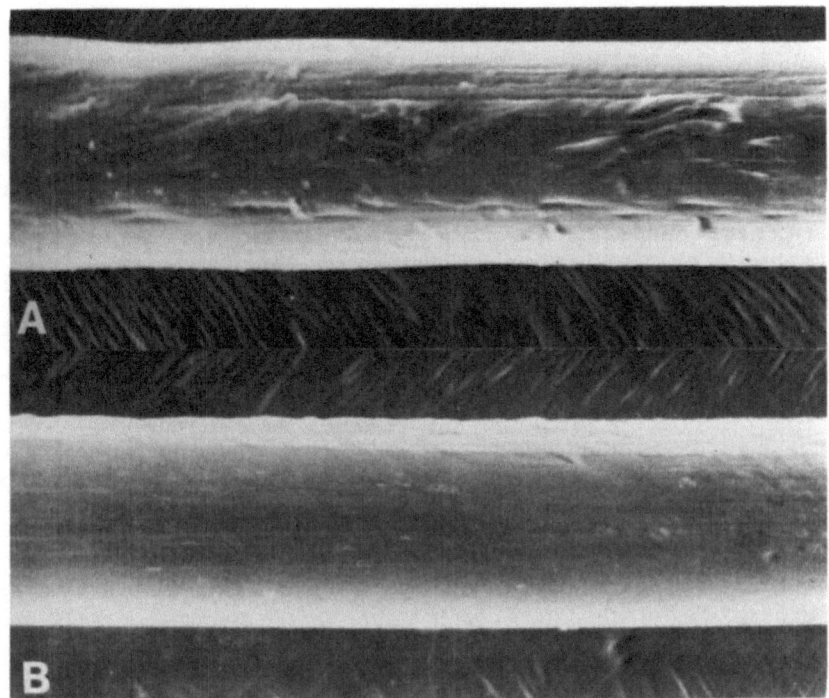

Fig. 8

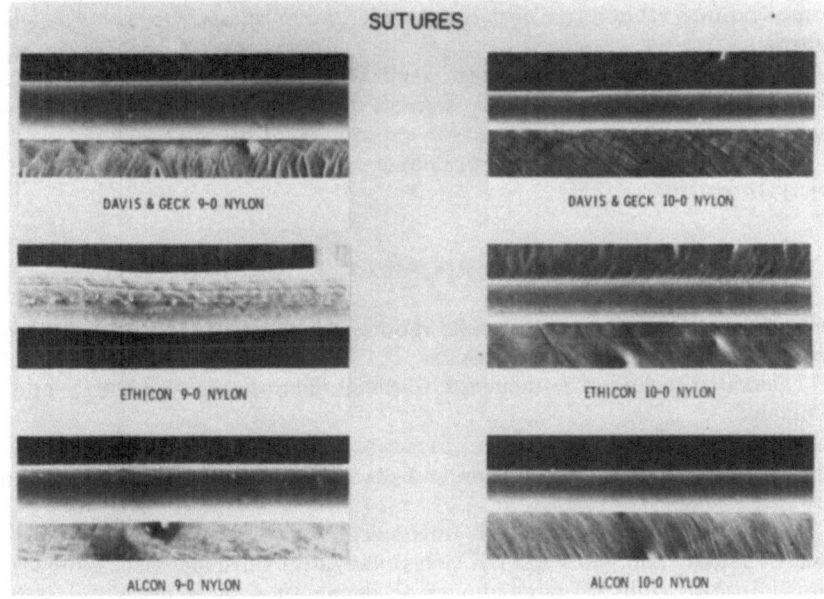

Fig. 9

it as an advantageous suturing technique, or as a useful integration of performance characteristics of two or more sutures. For instance, silk or absorbable synthetics are used as preplaced sutures and nylon or absorbable monofilament as additional postplaced sutures (which can close the profile of the wound deeper on the corneal side).

This first point of view, however, does not really concern us here, while the second seems mostly to do with the surgeon's personal preferences.

Use of combined materials can be advisable in cases where the surgeon is unfamiliar with the handling of monofilaments or double suturing. For instance, he could use some preliminary separated silk or absorbable sutures, and then acquire more skill, through practice, at using in the same procedure a different nylon suturing technique.

We have found that clinically speaking only a very few cases can be considered beneficial by the use of two or more materials in peculiar or unpredictable operative circumstances, and that it is generally more advisable not to say practical, to use a single material whose tissue reaction is easier to predict and therefore more under control.

Correlation between material used, macular cystoid degeneration, rupture of hyaloid or other inflammatory complication.

Paton's concept of 'atraumatic surgery' involves, among other factors, material, and so ideally this material should be virtually inert. With the use of a non-irritating suture, we can expect less post-operative inflammation and complications.

In our experience, we are unable to confirm a greater incidence of Irvine-Gass syndrome, or post-operative rupture of the hyaloid, or any other complications, related to a comparative use of monofilaments, or absorbable synthetics, or silk.

Nylon used in conjunction with a more refined microsurgical technique, should be considered the most suitable material, but nevertheless some incidence of hyaloid rupture has been reported with this material.

We do not yet have sufficient experience with absorbable monofilaments (vicryl 9 or 10/0).

ESSENTIAL NEEDLE PERFORMANCE CHARACTERISTICS

Ophthalmological sutural materials require needles with a combination of particular performance characteristics.

Thanks to technical refinements, excellent microsurgical needles are now available.

The main needle performance characteristics have already been perfected and these are: a. easy penetration and placement, b. minimal trauma without tissue drag.

A finer sutural material needs finer needle tailoring but the needle must be sufficiently rigid and must not change curvature during passage, while the wire should be thin but large enough to enable knot retraction (if needed).

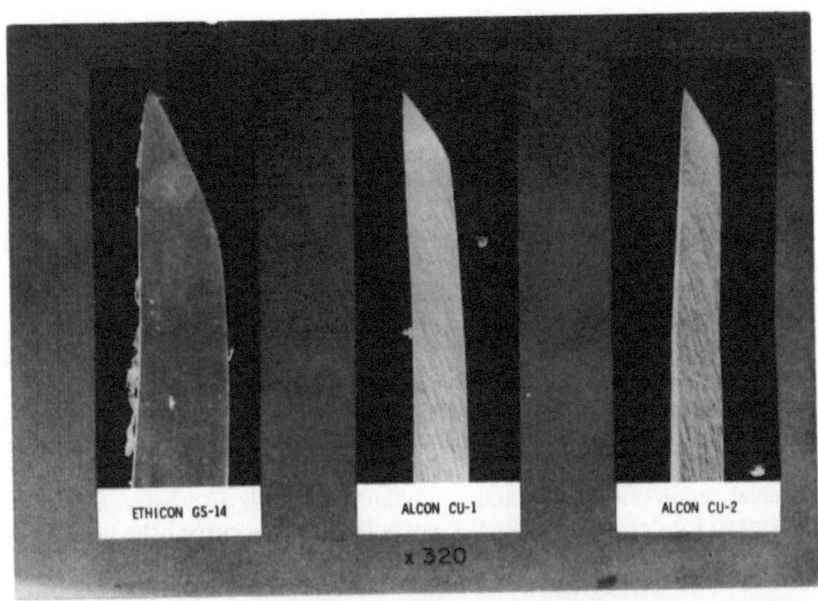

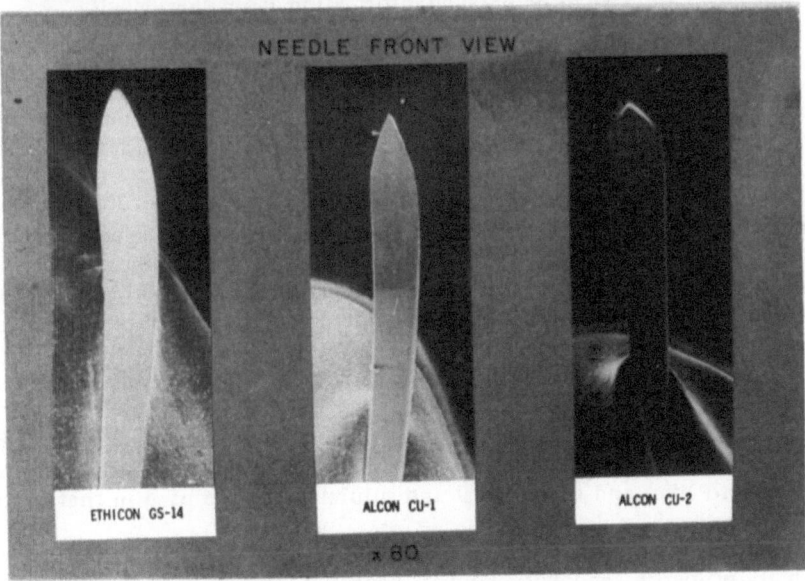

Fig. 10

Swaged needles are preferable, but eyed needles (still excellent in Barraquer's and Castroviejo's model) are useful mainly in emergencies when a swaged needle becomes damaged or separated from its thread.

The body of the shaft should have a wire diameter of about 0,1-0,2 mm, and be flattened or spatulated to give the holder a better grasp. The cutting point ad the cutting edge should take up nearly the first 1.4-1.8 mm of the needle. Micropoint needles with cutting spatulated edges (side cutting) are to be preferred (micropoint spatula needles). They should have a flattened back.

Less advisable are the **reverse cutting needles** (with an inverted triangular profile) which can cause deep placements or be too traumatic.
Preferable length: 5 to 7.5 mm.
Curvature or circle: 3/8 (135°-140°) or 1/2 (160°-175°)

The first is more eclectic and the second is preferable in deeper suturing. Circle 1/4 or 1/2 curved needles appear too flat.

In some cases (still insufficiently experimented) even flattened needles can be advantageous when used for intraparenchimal corneal continuous sutures (Charleux).

Special requirements can make bending the needle to a 'spear tip' useful (Troutman) for deeper placement (generally the more curved the needle, the more depth obtained).

It would be a good thing if the manufacturers could be produce uniform cutting edges and give more detailed information about their length.

CONCLUSIONS

Generally speaking, synthetic monofilament non absorbables appear to be the most eclectic materials available today and meet microsurgical requirements better than any other types.

Synthetic absorbable materials (diameter 8/0) represent a great step forward in cataract surgery and with their refinements may be considered a valid alternative but have a much more limited field of employment. The clinical experimentation of the monofilament synthetic absorbable (Vicryl 9 or 10/0) is presently insufficient and a precise evaluation of performances cannot yet be made.

Virgin silk is still a material which should not be discarded if used in definite circumstances and procedures.

In trying to select a sutural material, personal preferences must be taken into consideration, as well as the surgeon's capability and the equipment available to him, and the surgical and sutural technique used in that particular procedure.

Paton's suggestion to switch to a new suture only if you become familiar with its properties and with how to handle it, seem very wise too. Other factors to consider in selecting your material could be the progress of the surgical procedure (i.e. whether this is normal or whether it is complicated by unpredictable circumstances of lens delivery), the time at your disposal (it may become necessary to reduce or stop anesthaesia, and to shorten the operation due to the patient's condition or restlessness on his part). In such cases, the surgeon should try to be flexible and use an easier material to effect an early wound closure.

Selection of the material should also sometimes be based on the patient's age (there will be less tissue reaction in elderly people, while younger patients absorb the suture more easily and quickly), on his nutritional state, on clinical results obtained in previous lens delivery of the other eye, on the surgeon's experience, and on his foreknowledge of the performance characteristics of the material.

In conclusion, it must be said that the selection of the sutural material must be made taking into account all of the factors of a given clinical situation, which can differ during the procedure.

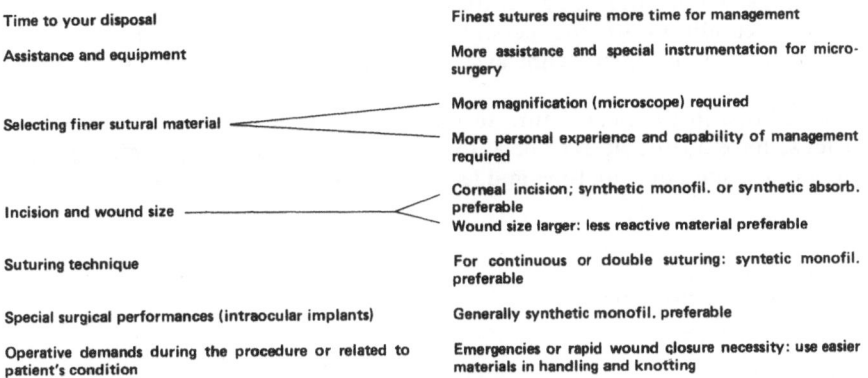

ADVICE ON SELECTING A SUTURAL MATERIAL

Time to your disposal	Finest sutures require more time for management
Assistance and equipment	More assistance and special instrumentation for micro-surgery
Selecting finer sutural material	More magnification (microscope) required
	More personal experience and capability of management required
Incision and wound size	Corneal incision; synthetic monofil. or synthetic absorb. preferable
	Wound size larger: less reactive material preferable
Suturing technique	For continuous or double suturing: syntetic monofil. preferable
Special surgical performances (intraocular implants)	Generally synthetic monofil. preferable
Operative demands during the procedure or related to patient's condition	Emergencies or rapid wound closure necessity: use easier materials in handling and knotting

Don't change sutural
material if you already
obtained an excellent
result in the first eye.

Fig. 11

SUMMARY

It can undoubtedly be affirmed today that cataract surgery has made greater progress in terms of functional results, among other things, by means of sutural refinements (better needling, minimum calibration, reduced tissue reaction). Clearly no suture can be considered satisfactory unless incision and closure are correct.

The most versatile material, especially for microsurgery, appears to be synthetic non-absorbable monofilament (nylon, perlon, or prolene), although it still presents certain shortcomings.

Absorbable synthetics (dexon and vicryl 8/0) offer a valid clinical alternative, mostly for surgeons not very keen on microsurgery. Vicryl, recently introduced as a new monofilament (9 or 10/0), should be a further advance, but the material has not yet been sufficiently experimented. However it is not expected to become an alternative of nylon.

Virgin silk (8 or 9/0), if properly used, can still be considered a valuable material although it has some disadvantages.

283

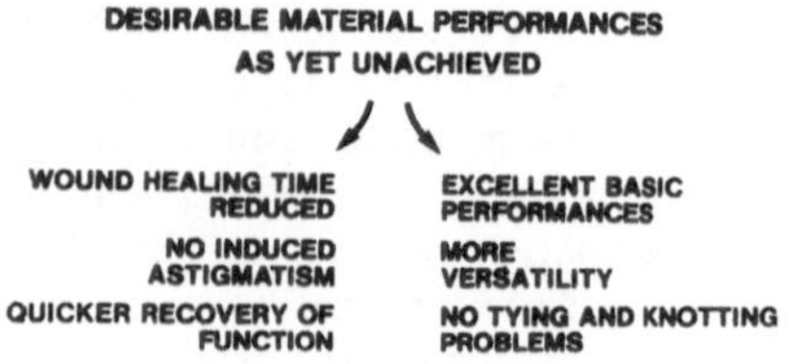

**DESIRABLE MATERIAL PERFORMANCES
AS YET UNACHIEVED**

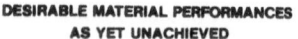

WOUND HEALING TIME REDUCED	EXCELLENT BASIC PERFORMANCES
NO INDUCED ASTIGMATISM	MORE VERSATILITY
QUICKER RECOVERY OF FUNCTION	NO TYING AND KNOTTING PROBLEMS

Fig. 12

In selecting sutural material, due weight must be given to specific personal preferences, the surgeon's capability, the equipment available to him and
the surgical procedure and suturing technique used, as well as the age and
general condition of the patient. The sutural choice should also be in
accordance with a given clinical situation which can differ during the procedure.

We hope in the near future to find a more 'ideal' sutural material which
should have a suitable rate of absorption, outstanding 'basic performances',
reduced wound healing time and less tying or knotting problems.

Author's address:
Societe Oftalmologica Italiana
Corso Italia, 2
Florence
Italy

Docum. Ophthal. Proc. Series, Vol. 21

AN EVALUATION OF 9-0 MONOFILAMENT POLYGLACTIN 910 SYNTHETIC ABSORBABLE SUTURE IN CATARACT SURGERY

J. ELLIOTT BLAYDESS,

(Bluefield, West Virginia, U.S.A.)

The synthetic absorbable suture has undergone continuous revision and refinement in the last half decade. Polyglactin 910, first developed as a monofilament, was redesigned as a braid and reduced in size so that it provided the cataract surgeon with a capably performing absorbable suture material. The braid eliminated the handling problems associated with early monofilament Polyglactin 910 and maintained the suture's high tensile strength, good knot security, batch-to-batch uniformity and provoked minimal reaction. However, the braided structure of Polyglactin 910 frequently incarcerated tissue and increased the incidence of premature tie (where a gap exists between the loop and throw).

In an effort to eliminate the pitfalls of braided Polyglactin 910 and at the same time maintain its positive qualities, a new monofilament form of Polyglactin 910 has been produced by Ethicon, Incorporated.

In a recently-concluded study, I compared 8-0 braided Polyglactin 910 to the same suture in 7-0 size in cataract surgery. The smaller 8-0 suture provided high tensile strength, production uniformity, knot security, minimal reaction, and the predictable absorption rate for which Polyglactin 910 is noted. It reduced the problems of tissue drag and fibrillation with 7-0 Polyglactin 910.

After my very favorable overall experience with 8-0 braided Polyglactin 910, I began a clinical evaluation of the 9-0 synthetic in monofilament form.

I anticipated that the smoother monofilament would pass through tissue easily, improving upon the braided suture's tendencies to incarcerate tissue and to tie prematurely.

Realizing the very exact tension needed to maintain wound coaption without suture cut-through, I was hopeful that experience gained in tying 8-0 braided Polyglactin 910 would be useful in avoiding tensioning errors when using the 9-0 monofilament.

It has been shown that the 8-0 braided Polyglactin 910 suture provided sufficient support to maintain wound coaption in the vital stages of healing. I anticipated that 9-0 monofilament Polyglactin 910 would also furnish adequate wound support.

Potential liabilities foreseeable with the 9-0 monofilament included inadequate knot security, difficulty in visualization, cut-through, handling problems associated with stiffness, brittle cut ends, premature tie, and premature absorption.

My evaluation of 9-0 monofilament Polyglactin 910 in cataract surgery began in November, 1976. It involved the clinical comparison of braided Polyglactin 910 in 8-0 size to monofilament Polyglactin 910 in 9-0 guage in 175 cataract surgical procedures.

MATERIALS AND METHODS

The criteria for evaluation of 9-0 monofilament Polyglactin 910 are shown in Table 1.

CRITERIA FOR EVALUATION OF 9-0 MONOFILAMENT POLYGLACTIN 910	
INTRAOPERATIVE OBSERVATIONS	POSTOPERATIVE OBSERVATIONS
Needle	Suture Disappearance
Visibility	Reaction
Strenth	Wound Healing
Pliability	Complications
Pull-Through	Recovery of Function
Fraying	
Knot	
Tying	

As far as possible, each patient was closely observed daily for the first three postoperative days, then again on the ninth day, and once a week thereafter for a total of six weeks. Many were observed more often.

At each postoperative visit, a microscopic examination was conducted. Drawings were made, illustrating the location of the remaining sutures and the position of the conjunctival flap. Serial photographs were taken of the operative eye at each visit for six weeks postoperative.

Constants maintained throughout the study included: 1) surgeon; 2) operating technique; 3) preoperative and postoperative medication: 4) suture manufacture; 5) approximately the same number of sutures; 6) type of knot; 7) all knots pulled to the scleral side.

Uncontrolled variables included: 1) age; 2) physical condition; 3) diet; 4) concomitant medication; 5) amount of reaction; 6) blink rate; 7) postoperative physical activity.

COMPARATIVE OPERATIVE OBSERVATIONS
8-0 BRAID VS. 9-0 MONOFILAMENT POLYGLACTIN 910

Needle: The GS-9 needle swaged to both 8-0 braid and 9-0 monofilament Polyglactin 910 possessed outstanding cutting quality and did not dull with repeated passage through tissue. Swaging was excellent.

Visibility: The violet color of 8-0 braided Polyglactin 910 made the suture readily detectible. Because of its smaller size, the 9-0 monofilament was less easily seen. The magnification of a loupe was satisfactory for handling both sutures.

Strength: The most outstanding characteristic of both Polyglactin 910 sutures was high tensile strength (Table II). Both sutures were stronger than the tissue into which they were implanted.

COMPARATIVE SIZES & TENSILE STRENGTHS*			
	DIAMETER (mils)	STRAIGHT PULL (lbs)	KNOT PULL (lbs)
8-0 braided Polyglactin 910	2.1	.34	.24
9-0 monofilament Polyglactin 910	1.5	.27	.17
9-0 Ethilon	1.3	.14	.11

*Ethicon, Inc.

Pliability: 8-0 braided Polyglactin 910 handled like silk. However, 9-0 monofilament Polyglactin 910 was significantly stiffer and more difficult to handle. I found that stretching the 9-0 suture to its elastic limit, short of elongation breaking point, improved its pliability somewhat. The smaller guage monofilament Polyglactin 910 suture was more pliable than its larger monofilament antecedents.

Pull-Through: In limbus-based flap procedures with 8-0 braided Polyglactin 910, an assistant had to retract the flap to prevent pronounced suture drag with resultant tissue incarceration. This was not the case with 9-0 monofilament Polyglactin 910.

Fraying: No tendency to fray was noted with either suture.

Knot: With both sutures, a triple loop with a double and single throw of square knots (3-2-1) gave good knot security. Because of its braided construction the braided suture was slightly better.

Tying: A slight, but distinct, fibrillation occurred in tying 8-0 braided Polyglactin 910. 9-0 monofilament Polyglactin 910 could be tied without this suture chatter.

Because of the sutures' high tensile strength, inelasticity, and small size, care was exercised to avoid tying either suture so tightly that tissue cut-through could occur. The tissues were lightly coated when suturing, and were held in that position.

To prevent loop-throw separation, where a gap exists between the loop and the first two throws, the surgeon must take care to ensure that the triple loop is placed tangent to the first double loop.

A summary of the comparative operative observations is shown in Table 3.

COMPARATIVE OPERATIVE OBSERVATIONS

CHARACTERISTIC	8–0 BRAIDED POLYGLACTIN 910	9–0 MONOFILAMENT POLYGLACTIN 910
needle visibility	Gs–9 excellent violet dyed, easily visible	GS–9 excellent violet dyed, easily visible
strength	excellent	excellent
pliability	excellent	fair
pull-through	fair to good	excellent
knot security	excellent	good
tying	good	excellent

COMPARATIVE POSTOPERATIVE OBSERVATIONS
8–0 BRAIDED VS. 9–0 MONOFILAMENT POLYGLACTIN 910

Suture disappearance: Nearly all 8–0 braided Polyglactin 910 sutures had disappeared between 31 and 33 days. The 9–0 monofilament Polyglactin 910 sutures disappeared between 35 and 37 days.

Reaction: While reaction to 8–0 braided Polyglactin 910 was mild, reaction to 9–0 monofilament Polyglactin 910 was even less.

Wound healing: Three instances of wound dehiscence with iris prolapse occurred in my series with 8–0 braided Polyglactin 910, one with 9–0 monofilament Polyglactin 910. Of the dehiscences involving the 8–0 suture, two were believed to be surgeon-induced because they cut through the corneal side of the wound. This probably was caused by tying the sutures too tightly early in our experience with 8–0. The third instance with 8–0 was traumatic, self-inflicted by the patient.

The one case of wound dehiscence with 9–0 monofilament Polyglactin 910 could be attributed to tying the suture too tightly.

Complications: Transient corneal edema was seen occasionally with both sutures. Experiences with wound dehiscence are described above.

Recovery of function: Recovery of function following wound closure involving both 8–0 braided Polyglactin 910 and 9–0 monofilament Polyglactin 910 was generally excellent.

A summary of the comparative postoperative observations is shown in Table 4.

COMPARATIVE POSTOPERATIVE OBSERVATIONS

CHARACTERISTIC	8–0 BRAIDED POLYGLACTIN 910	9–0 MONOFILAMENT POLYGLACTIN 910
suture disappearance	31–33 days	35–37 days
reaction	minimal	minimal 8–0 braid
wound healing	generally excellent	generally excellent
complications	corneal edema, wound dehiscence	corneal edema, wound dehiscence
recovery of function	generally excellent	generally excellent

DISCUSSION

Because of my previous experience with Polyglactin 910, several aspects of 9−0 monofilament Polyglactin 910's performance were foreseeable prior to the start of this evaluation. These included the suture's high tensile strength, uniformity, predictable absorption rate, and minimal reaction.

Recalling my earlier experience with 8−0 monofilament Polyglactin 910, I was hopeful that the more pliable 9−0 monofilament would not protrude through the conjunctiva.

Because of its monofilament construction, 9−0 Polyglactin 910 was expected to provide greater ease of pull-through with less tissue incarceration. Suture chatter, evident in cinching the braid's knot, should be eliminated with the smoother monofilament. Basically, these predictions were confirmed.

Advantages of 9−0 monofilament polyglactin 910: When compared to the 8−0 braid, 9−0 monofilament Polyglactin 910 furnished sufficient tensile strength, good knot security, batch-to-batch uniformity, and absorption rate predictability. The 9−0 suture provided improved slippability and easier pull-through with less fibrillation in tying.

Precautions with 9−0 monofilament polyglactin 910: Extreme care was demanded to obtain proper tension when using the 9−0 suture to close the cataract wound. The combination of small size, inelasticity, and suture tensile strength greater than the tissue into which it was implanted made 9−0 monofilament Polyglactin 910 a threat to cut-through tissue.

To prevent suture pull-out, the following technique of tying is recommended:

Placement of the initial triple loop is most important because this established the point at which the inelastic suture will hold the wound together. The suture should be lowered into a position where the tissues are lightly, but definitely coapted. In all situations, the utmost care should be used to avoid tying the first loop too tightly.

A double throw then is placed tangent to the first triple loop. This double throw must be secured down to the loop (but not cinched) to prevent premature tie. A final throw is placed on top of the second throw in the form of a square knot, then cinched.

When a suture is tied too tightly, it tends to pull out or produce an astigmatic error.

Other operative observations: Because of their small size, both 8−0 braided Polyglactin 910 and 9−0 monofilament Polyglactin 910 sometimes required more delicate instruments and adaptation of techniques.

A loupe provided satisfactory magnification with both sutures.

Postoperative follow-up: After surgery, weekly follow-up examinations should incorporate photographing and drawing the sutures and their locations. This enables the cataract surgeon to determine both the amount of reaction to and the time of disappearance for 9−0 monofilament Polyglactin 910.

SUMMARY

This study described the operative and postoperative performances of 9—0 monofilament Polyglactin synthetic absorbable suture in cataract surgery. The evaluation represents a clinical comparison of 8—0 braided Polyglactin 910 to 9—0 monofilament Polyglactin 910 in 175 cataract surgical procedures.

9—0 monofilament Polyglactin 910 provided sufficient tensile strength, good knot security, batch-to-batch uniformity, minimal reaction, and a predictable rate of absorption that was virtually completed in 37 days.

When compared to 8—0 braided Polyglactin 910, 9—0 monofilament provided significantly improved pull-through, with less tissue drag, fibrillation, and reaction, as well as a decreased tendency toward premature tie.

The 9—0 monofilament, however, was not as pliable as the 8—0 braid. As a result, it was more difficult to handle.

Because of the suture's high tensile strength, small size, and inelasticity, extreme care was exercised to obtain proper tension when tying 9—0 monofilament Polyglactin 910.

Once case of wound dehiscence occurred in my series. It was attributed to insufficient tensioning when tying the suture.

Although a microscope was used in most instances, the sutures are easily visible in the operating field with the aid of a loupe.

The development of a pliable monofilament synthetic absorbable suture will establish a landmark in ophthalmology. It will combine the braid's handling qualities with the monofilament's ease of pull-through.

THE CATARACT WOUND: ITS CLOSURE AND HEALING

R.C. TROUTMAN

(New York, U.S.A.)

The surgeon performing microsurgical intracapsular cataract surgery currently is concerned more with the incision and its closure than with the removal of the lens.

It has become evident that with absorbable or inelastic silk sutures, the classic cataract surgical incision is better positioned at the surgical limbus and protected by a conjunctival flap. The flap serves not only to protect the patient from the irritation of the necessarily exposed suture material, but also to reinforce the wound against the inevitable wound stretch which occurs with these suture materials. Because of potential fistulization of the suture tracts induced by either absorbable or silk sutures, the suture loop never should be placed deeper than two-thirds the thickness of the cornea. Therefore the posterior aspect of the cataract incision is never closed. This results in what I have termed a lambda-shaped incision profile, often identifiable in pathologic sections 20 or 30 years later. This tendency to slippage and thinning of the wound areas has been compensated, in part, by slanting or stepping the limbal incision. The resulting broader, appositional area heals more securely. The more anterior entrance of the internal wound into the eye, together with the necessarily more shallow suture placement, avoids danger to angle structures.

In contradistinction, the microsurgical cataract incision closed with elastic monofilament suture is, ideally, in clear cornea anterior to the surgical limbus, vertical to the iris plane. The direction of the corneal flap, therefore, is the inverse of that of the traditional limbal incision and even may be deliberately slanted backward, as advocated by Charleux, for a more pronounced inverse flap effect.

The hydrodynamics of the anterior chamber closes this incision spontaneously as the aqueous reforms. The corneal flap of the limbal incision is elevated by the reformed anterior chamber. The internal aspect of the completed corneal incision is well anterior to angle structures and can be apposed precisely with through-and-through sutures so that it heals optimally from back to front.

It has been shown recently that closing the posterior lamella of the cornea with through-and-through sutures not only prevents posterior gaping, resulting in better optical as well as anatomic closure, but also prevents postoperative slippage of the posterior corneal lamella toward the angle struc-

291

tures, preventing temporary or permanent postoperative glaucoma. This effect, thought initially to be due to temporary wound leak through the through-and-through suture tracts, is primarily anatomic since suture tract leaks cannot be demonstrated postoperatively.

A second important optical aspect of corneal wound closure is to prevent slippage of the anterior corneal lamella. This is prevented by inserting two to four partially penetrating anterior lamellar sutures. These interrupted sutures are placed at one-half depth at 11 and 1 o'clock and, in a longer incision, also at 2 and 10 o'clock. Primary closing sutures are opposing continuous placed with through-and-through bites and locked at each end of the incision.

Such a precise wound closure technique requires the use of the surgical microscope, microsurgical instrumentation, and monofilament elastic sutures, either of nylon or of polypropylene. Properly inserted through-and-through suture loops will not fistulize, when properly tensioned before they are tied. Since the anterior layers of the cornea are more resistant to cheese wiring, the anterior portion of the suture loop remains on top of Bowman's membrane, easily accessible for removal, while the posterior suture loop cuts forward into corneal stroma. Our experiments on primate corneas show that through-and-through suture loops cut quickly through Descemet's into stroma postoperatively. The internal suture loop will not be exposed provided the loops have been adequately tensioned at surgery. For this reason, the continuous suture pattern is used since it can be tensioned equally along its length. Individual interrupted suture loops may loosen and internalize, inviting fistulization. When interrupted sutures are placed to prevent anterior lamella slippage, they are inserted in the middle one-third of the stroma. They should also be of monofilament nylon. Even if placed somewhat loosely, there is no danger of internalization.

The Troutman surgical keratometer should always be used to monitor for proper and exact tensioning of individual and continuous suture loops and to ensure minimal suture-induced residual meridional distortion. When the sutures are released, the incision should be healed in its full thickness, so as to assume its preoperative, essentially anastigmatic, state or a deliberate correction from preoperatively determined excessive meridional error. It should not be necessary postoperatively to release suture loops selectively to compensate suture-induced astigmatism or to leave a suture loop in place beyond three months.

Microsurgical incision and closure of the cataract wound, ensuring minimal postoperative astigmatic distortion, has assumed new importance with the increasing use of alloplastic lens substitutes. No matter the type of lens extraction selected, it is important that the cataract wound be opened sufficiently to allow the introduction of the alloplastic lens substitute, so as to inflict minimal damage to corneal endothelium. Further, it is important that, following lens implantation, the cornea be closed in such a way as to limit the development of meridional error which might necessitate postoperative overrefraction.

When either keratophakia or keratomileusis is to be performed simultaneously with the cataract procedure or is contemplated subsequently, the full-thickness closure of the incision and the absence of meridional error are essential to ensure the optimal anatomic and optical results. Even when an integral correction of aphakia is not planned, the postoperative curvature of the cornea is important to the comfortable and proper fitting of a contact lens or of an aspheric spectacle lens.

SUMMARY

The anteriorly slanted or stepped limbal cataract incision closed with absorbable or silk suture is anachronistic in the context of modern microsurgical cataract technique. Microsurgical techniques and instrumentation, combined with the use of elastic monofilament suture, are essential to ensure optical, anatomic wound healing. This, in turn, produces a regular, essentially anastigmatic, corneal curvature capable of optimal refraction whatever the correcting modality chosen.

Modern cataract surgery begins with the microsurgical incision and closure and ends when one has achieved a consecutively reproducible optical result.

Docum. Ophthal. Proc. Series, Vol. 21

SUTURING TECHNIQUES: CONTINUOUS
AND INTERRUPTED

DAVID PATON

(Houston, Texas, U.S.A.)

The goals of wound closure are: uniform apposition, wound strength, and patient comfort. Implicit is the importance of minimizing postoperative astigmatism. One cannot speak about suturing technique without alluding to the marked variations in size and configuration of incisions employed for intracapsular cataract extraction. (In the presentation of this paper I will show twelve incision-and-closure techniques and will illustrate in more detail the one I have used most often.) The method of suturing depends to some extent on the size and configuration of the incision. In regard to wound size, recall that a 160° incision in clear cornea constitutes a significantly smaller orifice for lens extraction than a 160° incision at the posterior limbus. (Paton, 1978) Some surgeons prefer corneal incisions with either vertical or shelved entry into the anterior chamber. Other surgeons make a 180° incision with a Graefe knife; others routinely employ a step or half-lap incision at the posterior limbus under a limbus-based flap. The latter has been my own preference (Paton, 1971) until recently when I have begun using the clear corneal single-plane incision at an angle that I understand is advocated by J. Charleux in France.

Needles The photomicrographs (Fig's 1 and 2) demonstrate engineering devices employed by leading needle manufacturers in the United States.* I do not intend a discussion of their comparative attributes, but I am sure that many of you who have used these needles have preferences regarding needle choice. Ophthalmologists tend to speak more about sutures than needles, but it is predictable that we will soon become conversant with such needle specifications as thickness, chord, length, radius and so on. The most significant of their differences is the contour of the needle tips. The "spatula needle" (marketed under various names) has been one of the best additions to ophthalmic surgery since the advent of the reverse cutting needle. One can only guess what the needle engineers will have to offer us in the years ahead. Looking at these illustrations it is tempting to compare the needle to the hull of a boat and to comment that needle selection just might

---

* The photomicrographs of Figures 1 through 4 have been prepared by Frank Kretzer, Ph.D., and Charlotte Levy, The Cullen Eye Institute.

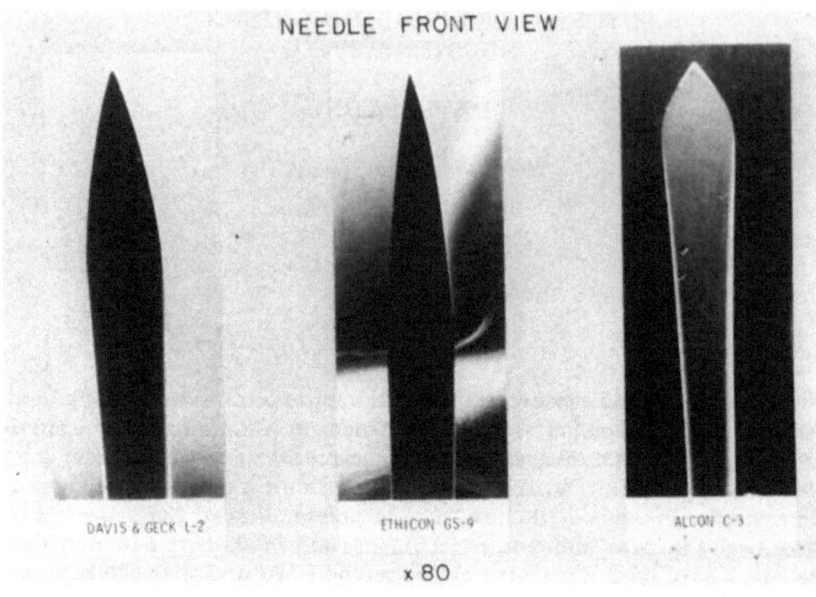

NEEDLE FRONT VIEW

DAVIS & GECK L-2   ETHICON GS-9   ALCON C-3

x 80

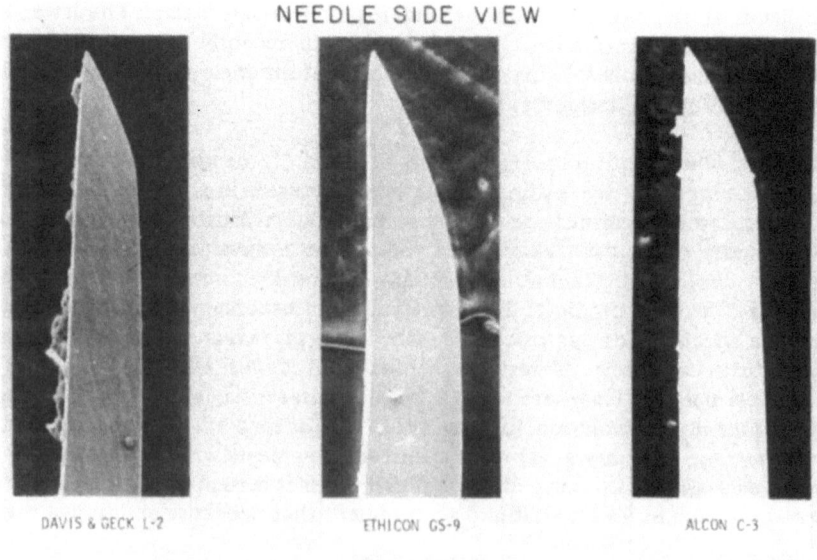

NEEDLE SIDE VIEW

DAVIS & GECK L-2   ETHICON GS-9   ALCON C-3

x 320

Fig. 1. Scanning electron photomicrographs of currently popular needles. Catalog numbers, manufacturers and magnification are indicated.

NEEDLE FRONT VIEW

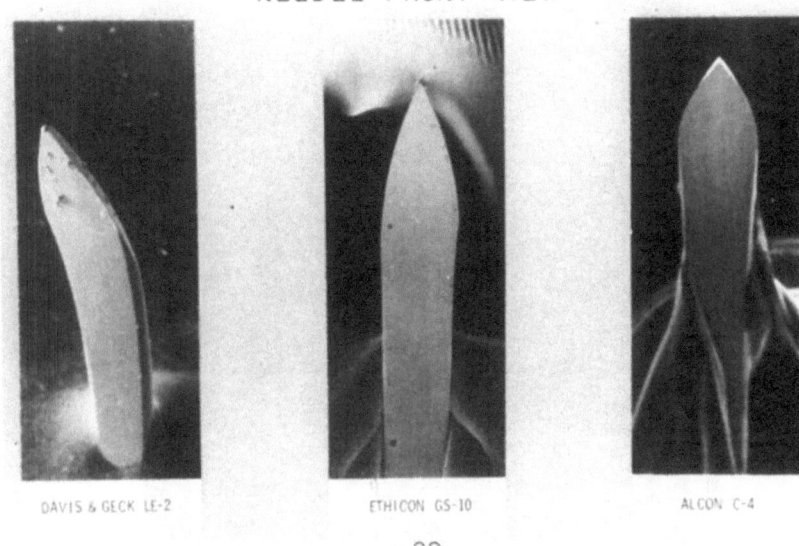

DAVIS & GECK LE-2   ETHICON GS-10   ALCON C-4

x 80

NEEDLE SIDE VIEW

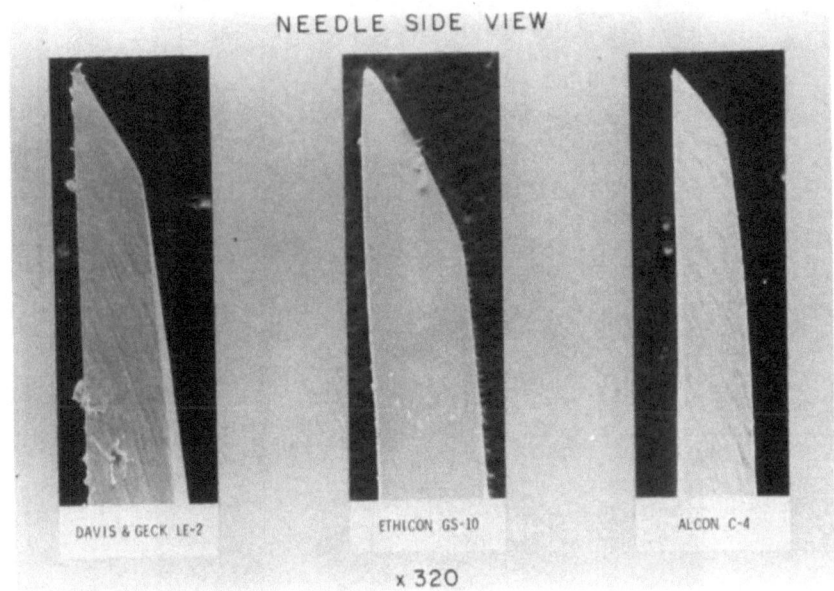

DAVIS & GECK LE-2   ETHICON GS-10   ALCON C-4

x 320

Fig. 2. Other scanning electron photomicrographs providing similar comparisons as in the preceding figure.

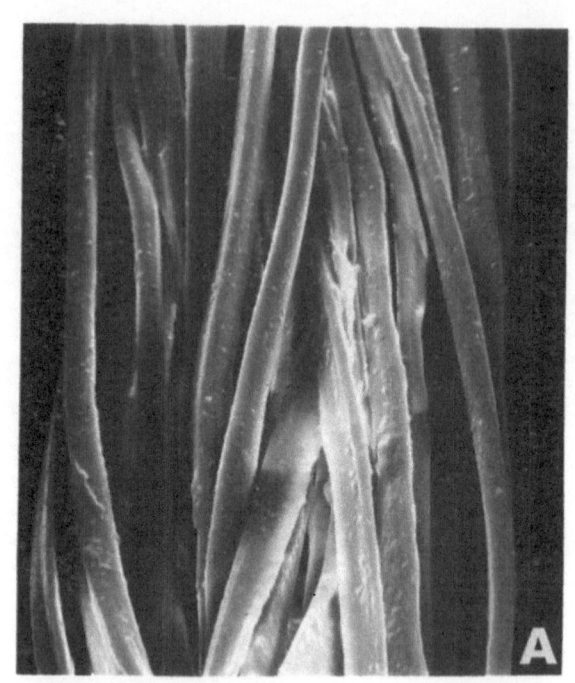

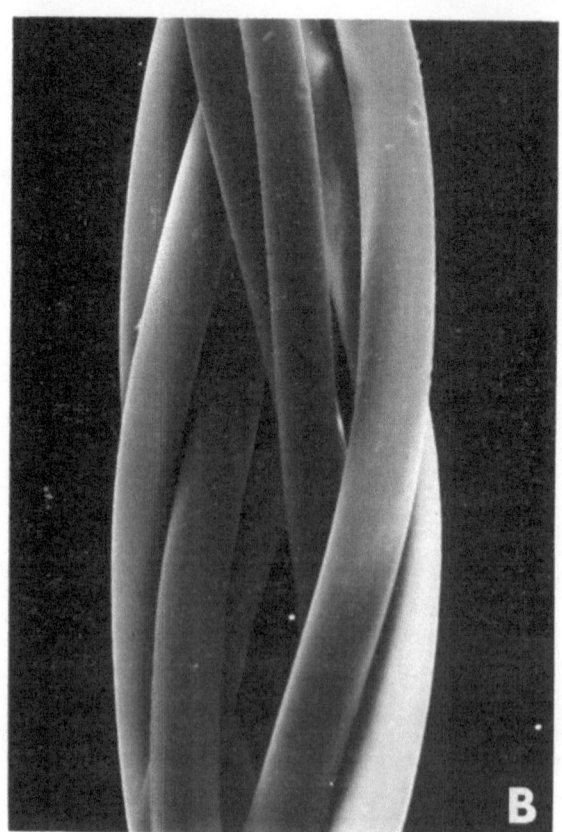

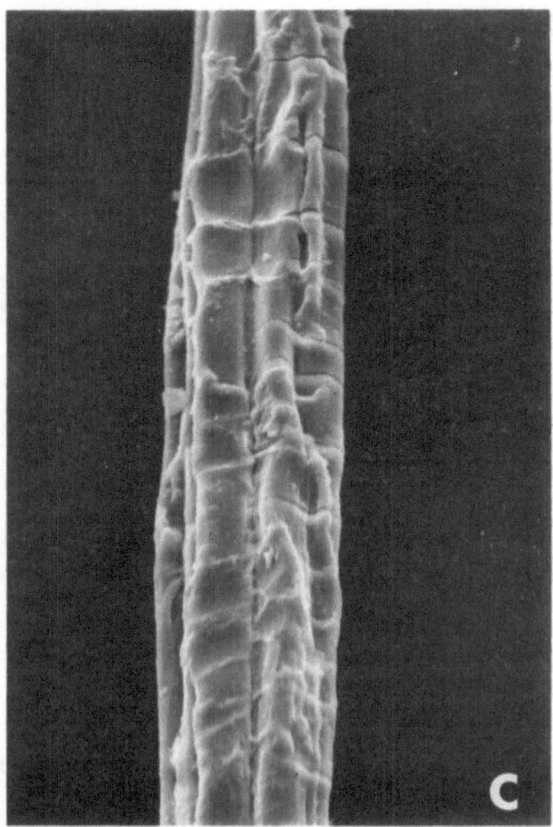

Fig. 3. Scanning electron photomicrographs showing the comparative appearances of A, 8-0 black silk; B, 8-0 vicryl (Ethicon); and C, 9-0 virgin silk. All photomicrographs are the same magnification, 600X.

be a bit like guessing the winner of a yacht race on the basis of the hull design, overlooking numerous other variables that affect performance, such as the skill of the skipper. Nevertheless, the needle design and its various qualities are important in today's world of microsurgery.

Sutures The attributes of popular suture materials have already been discussed, and I will not say more here than to indicate my own preference for the use of 9-0 nylon for closure of cataract wounds, whether continuous or interrupted suturing is employed. I admit to a possibility that I will return to interrupted 9-0 silk sutures, as discussed hereafter. (Fig's 3 and 4).

Continuous Suturing In the latter part of the 1960's I was using Maumenee's running locked nylon suture for cataract wound closure; throughout most of the 1970's I then used a single shoestring suture as a preferred routine (Fig. 5B). No interrupted sutures were employed. The shoestring's single knot is buried within the wound (see Fig. 6).

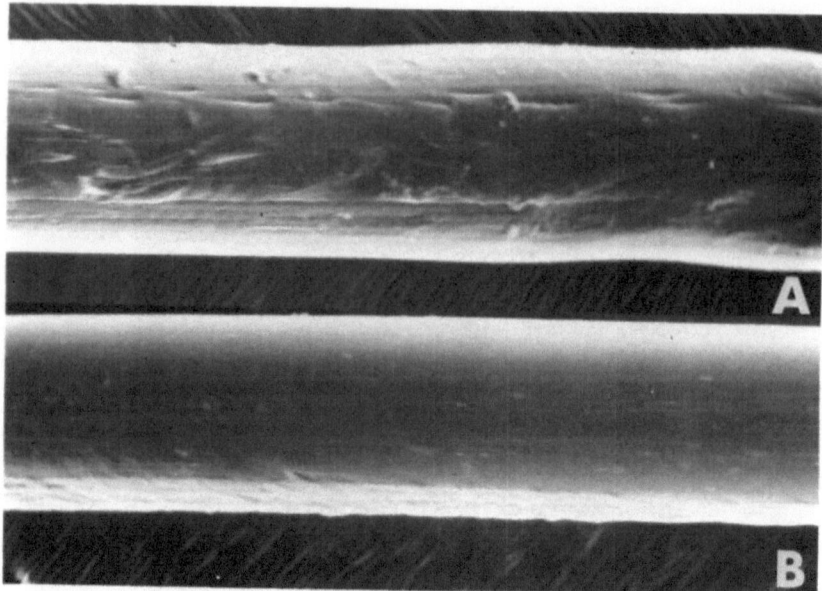

Fig. 4. Despite the considerable differences in the physical properties (such as elasticity) of A, 10-0 Prolene (Ethicon) and B, 10-0 nylon, the surface structure at the same magnification of 1600X is not markedly different.

If there is a pre-existing filtering bleb at the upper limbus, I prefer a clear corneal incision closed with a continuous nylon suture or multiple "butter-fly" (or "double-interrupted") sutures for wound repair. The butterfly suture is excellent for small wounds such as with phacoemulsification, or used in a series for larger wounds (Fig. 6).

In all suturing the tissue bites should be placed deeply, although I personally do not believe that through-and-through sutures are as desirable as merely deeply-placed tissue bites; even with nylon, and certainly with silk, one can get leakage and epithelialization of a suture tract that (at least theoretically) could lead to early chamber shallowness or late epithelial ingrowth. Whether or not this happens with nylon from through-and-through suture bites is unknown to me, for these complications can certainly occur from other wound-closure deficiencies as well.

Astigmatism It is logical that the least amount of astigmatism will occur with deep suture bites that prevent posterior wound gape and with uniform apposition of the anterior and posterior lips of the incision. Using the nylon suture as I have done routinely for more than a decade, it has been customary to obtain with-the-rule astigmatism in the early postoperative weeks (Fig. 7). Generally this subsides, but occasionally it does not. If at the eighth postoperative week there is persistence of several diopters of astigmatism (with-the-rule), I then cut the continuous suture through the overlying conjunctiva with a razor blade chip. This is done at the point of

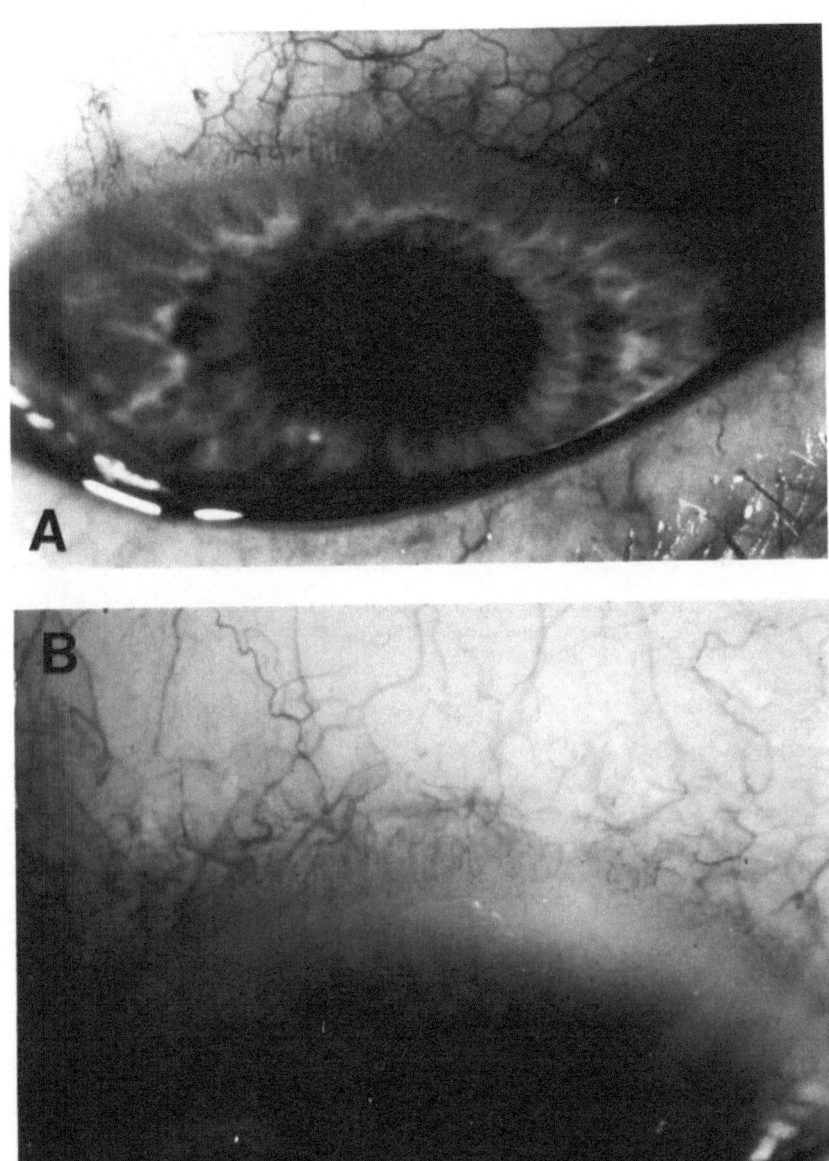

Fig. 5. A, multiple interrupted 9-0 sutures have been used to close the cataract incision; these sutures are beneath the limbus-based conjunctival flap. B, a 9-0 nylon suture has been used in shoestring configuration to close a 150° cataract incision. A single knot is buried within the wound temporarally (not seen).

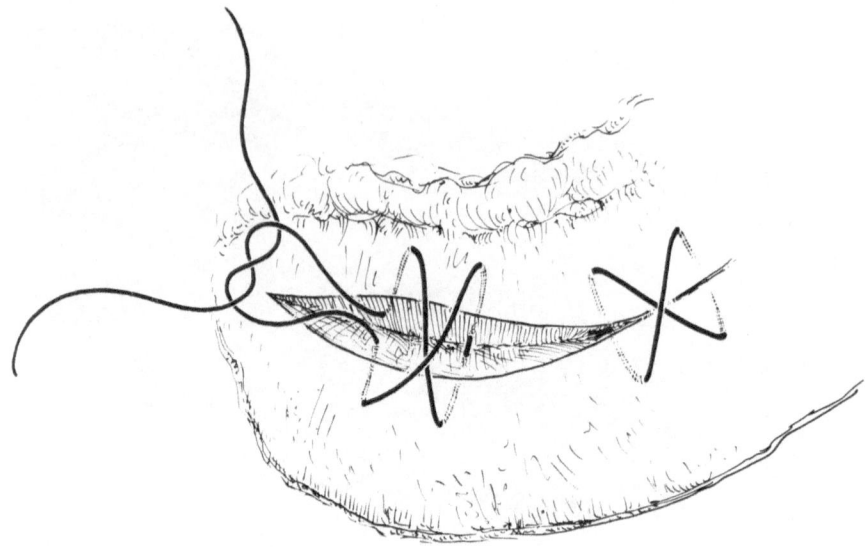

Fig. 6. The technique of a 'butterfly' suture is demonstrated, indicating how the knot of the 9−0 or 10−0 nylon can be buried within the wound. This method was taught to me by Dr. James Little of Oklahoma City.

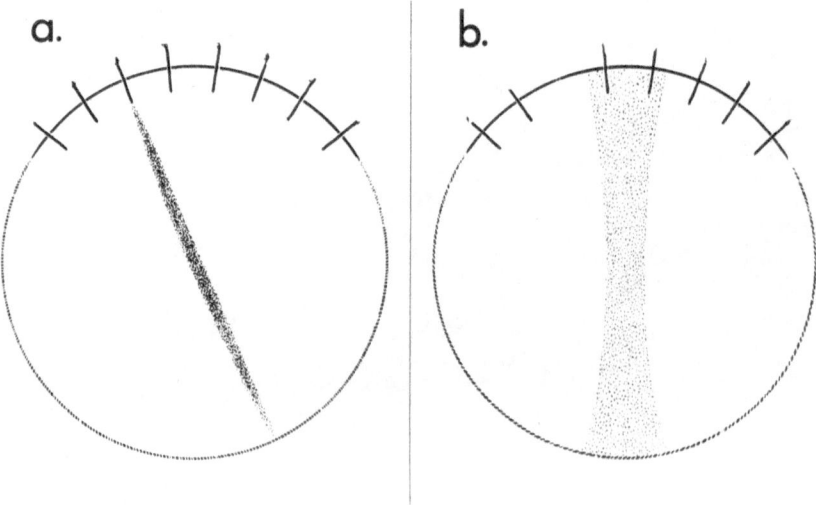

Fig. 7. The stippled linear marking indicates the retinoscopic reflex; the axis of with-the-rule astigmatism and the degree of astigmatism are indicated by a narrow line in A (high astigmatism) and a thicker line in B − one excessively tight suture has been removed.

the axis of with-the-rule astigmatism. (Paton, 1971). Almost always, this markedly reduces or totally relieves astigmatism within twenty-four to forty-eight hours. However, in two of my cases, when the suture was cut too early at four weeks and six weeks respectively, gaping of the wound occurred – with resultant against-the-rule astigmatism (Fig. 8). This necessitated resuturing.

Troutman has spoken for some years about the problem of postoperative astigmatism, and he will explain at this meeting his progress in the management of the problem following cataract surgery and keratoplasty. Several diopters of astigmatism is not uncommon after cataract surgery; at times, the surgeon is astonished to find four or even five diopters of cylinder required, despite the appearance of a well closed wound.

In very recent months, a new device has been made in prototype form for clinical testing. This is the next generation in a concept whose activator is the Troutman surgical keratometer. The Computerized Surgical Keratometer has been devised by a gifted and dedicated astigmologist (my word), Dr. Clifford Terry. Dr. Terry's instrument has a prism system interposed in the optics of the operating microscope to split the cornea's reflection of a light ring into three mires. Distortion and degree of separation of those

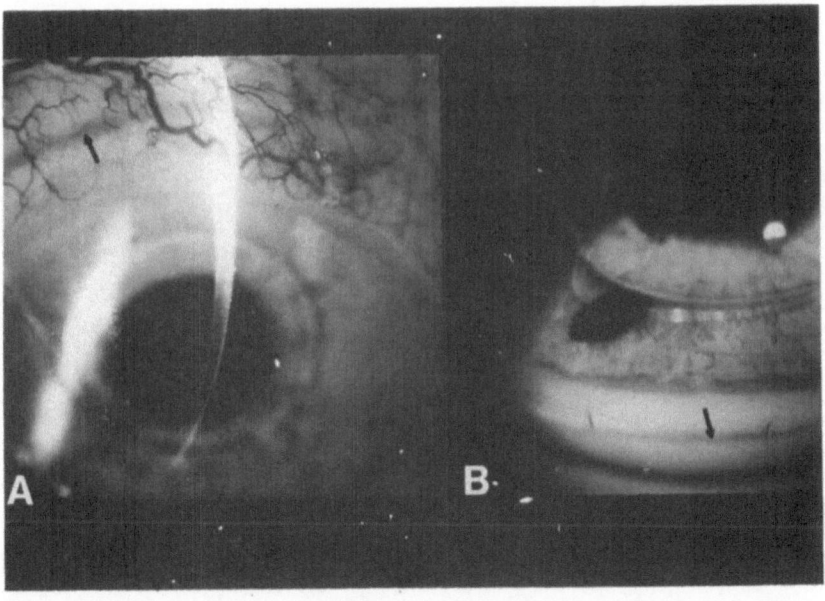

Fig. 8. Due to with-the-rule astigmatism, a 9–0 shoestring nylon suture was cut at the 12 o'clock position only one month following intracapsular cataract extraction and the placement of a 4-loop Binkhorst intraocular lens. The suture was cut too early in the postoperative course. The photograph on the left (A) demonstrates wound separation visible under the conjunctival flap. The photograph on the right (B) indicates this wound separation as viewed with the gonioprism (arrow). It was necessary to resuture the wound.

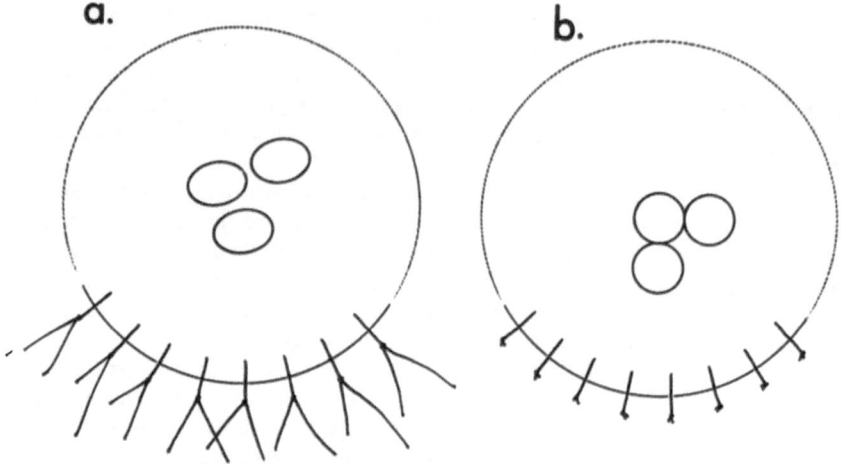

Fig. 9. The diagrams indicate the mires as viewed by the surgeon through the operating microscope while employing the Terry Quantitative Surgical Keratometer. A, separated and distorted rings determine degree and axis of corneal astigmatism. B, suture adjustments are made to bring the mires into the ideal pattern indicated here.

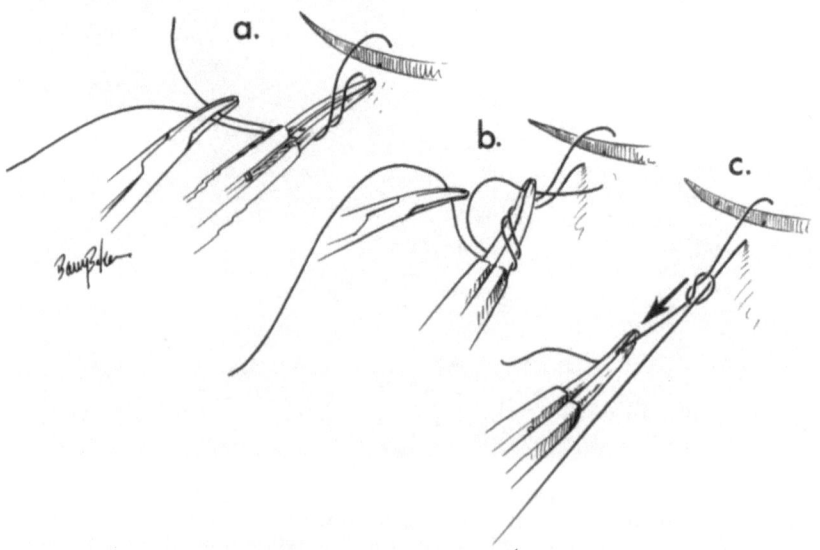

Fig. 10. Dr. Clifford Terry's technique of employing 'slip knots' for initial securing of the wound. Adjustment of the tightness of each suture is done while viewing keratometer mires through the operating microscope.

three ring images constitute guidelines for the surgeon as he closes the cataract wound (Fig. 9). Importantly, Dr. Terry advocates the use of interrupted sutures initially secured by slip knots (Fig. 8) to obtain uniformity of wound closure by modifying suture tightness before each knot is secured with the addition of the final loops of a square knot. It is not for me to be reporting Dr. Terry's prototype invention but I have obtained permission from him to show these illustrations of his method. Dr. Terry is quick to say that to date he cannot restore every eye to the same curvature measured preoperatively; but the concept of his instrument (which requires considerable explanation for completeness) is a most exciting opportunity for clinical research. I said earlier that I might well be returning to the use of interrupted 9-0 silk sutures for wound closure and that is because of my desire to participate in a cooperative clinical study with Dr. Terry. Silk sutures can be tightened to a more precise and less changeable tension than is true of the more elastic nylon suture.

In conclusion, wound closure must always conform to certain basic principles, such as uniform wound apposition, strength of wound closure, and patient comfort. Beyond that, there is an almost infinite variety of wound closure techniques. It is certain that what works best in the hands of one surgeon may not be the preferred method of the other.

REFERENCES

Paton, D.: Lens delivery in relation to cataract incision size – the preplaced continuous locked nylon suture. In Welsh, R.C. and Welsh, J. (eds.): *The Second Report on Cataract Surgery: Proceedings of the Second Biennial Cataract Surgical Congress.* Miami: Miami Educational Press, 1971, pp. 178–184.

Paton, D.: Intracapsular cataract extraction: personal technique preferences regarding cryoextraction and suturing. In Emery, J.M. (ed.): *Current Concepts in Cataract Surgery. Selected Proceedings of the Fifth Biennial Cataract Surgical Congress,* February, 1977. St. Louis: The C.V. Mosby Company, 1978. (In press)

Docum. Ophthal. Proc. Series, Vol. 21

POSTOPERATIVE ASTIGMATISM IN CATARACT SURGERY

R.C. TROUTMAN

(New York, U.S.A.)

Improved microsurgical incision and closure techniques combined with the use of the Troutman microsurgical keratometer have resulted in better control of operatively induced meridional errors. The surgical keratometer permits the ophthalmic surgeon to identify, to localize, and to quantify the intraoperatively induced meridional errors. It eliminates the "blind spot" that existed formerly between the preoperative clinical keratometry and the postoperative clinical keratometry.

Through-and-through closure of a vertical corneal incision ensures optimal anatomic tissue apposition which, in turn, results in improved postoperative corneal optics. A minimally astigmatic cornea is as essential to the optimal use of the spherical, axially correcting intraocular lens as is the A scan in determining optimal power of the IOL; combined, they obviate the necessity for an overcorrection. When a contact lens is to be used, a planned, with-the-rule direction of the astigmatism makes the wearing of the contact lens more secure and gives an improved toleration and vision result. Even when spectacle lenses are used, to maintain the maximal asphericity potential, a minimal astigmatism, less than 1 diopter, should be obtained. This is obviously true also with keratophakia and keratomileusis.

The usual physiologic astigmatism measured preoperatively is slightly with-the-rule or steeper in the vertical meridian. With increasing age, this decays toward an anastigmatic cornea or to a slightly against-the-rule direction, steeper in the horizontal meridian. In about 5% of cases, the corneal astigmatism is in excess of 2 diopters. Such excessive astigmatism is more often against-the-rule. It is important that an excessive preexisting astigmatic band be recognized and measured preoperatively so that it may be corrected by Troutman wedge resection of the cataract incision. Wound slippage also may occur as the result of defective healing when silk or absorbable closure techniques are used. The vertical meridian can become flattened to a pathological degree. The wedge resection technique, which I first proposed for retrospective correction of excessive astigmatic bands and post penetrating keratoplasty, is useful not only for correction of excessive astigmatic bands at cataract surgery but may be used also to correct excessive postoperative residual errors.

The cornea can be compared to a sector of a malleable plastic sphere contiguous to but optically isolated from a sector of a larger malleable plastic sphere, the sclera. Excision or distortion of the sclera, even when relatively extensive, such as in scleral buckling, rarely results in alterations of corneal curvature. The limbus, which delimits the cornea from the sclera, the anatomic corneal ring, delimits, as well, the posterior scleral zone from the anterior optical corneal zone. The cornea may be said to be either steep or flat, around a physiologic average of 43 diopters. A cornea less than 43 diopters is considered a flatter cornea, greater than 43 diopters, a steeper cornea. When the curvature departs from sphericity the cornea is said to be astigmatic. The resulting disparate corneal curvatures are termed the steeper meridian and the flatter meridian, and are usually at 90° to each other.

Removing a semilunar-shaped, wedge-profiled segment in depth, from the cornea peripherally, results in a decrease of the corneal radius, steepening the corresponding meridian. Because of the corneal plasticity, the radius of the opposing meridian at 90° will be increased, flattening that meridian in a ratio of approximately 1 to 2. This principle is employed to correct an against-the-rule astigmatism, where the vertical meridian of the cornea is flatter (longer radius) than the horizontal meridian. Shortening the longer radius by means of a wedge resection steepens the excessively flat vertical meridian, correcting the meridional distortion.

The semilunar shape of the wedge resection is outlined by making a partially penetrating, curvilinear, vertical, anterior cut along the line of intended incision. This is followed by a more peripheral, slightly more curved cut which is sloped so as to meet the first cut at the level of Descemet's membrane. The widest point of the crescent outlined is centered on the axis of the flatter meridian. It tapers to end 30-45° to either side of this axis. The width and length of the excision determines the amount of astigmatism corrected. Each 0.05 mm of corneal resection width corrects 1 diopter of astigmatism; therefore, a 0.5 mm resection would correct a 10-diopter error. The amount of correction obtained, however, is not necessarily linear — the narrower the width of the wedge, the less the effective correction, so that to correct smaller amounts of astigmatism may require a resection almost as wide as that required for an intermediate amount. The width of the excision at the widest point should not exceed 1 mm. Such an excision will correct 15-20 diopters of astigmatism.

In cataract surgery, the wedge resection is carried out simultaneously with the incision. Initially, the axis and the magnitude of the preoperatively determined error is identified intraoperatively with the surgical keratometer. A partially penetrating wedge resection is performed in the amount calculated to correct the preexisting measured astigmatism. When the wedge excision has been performed, the cataract incision is completed to the length necessary to remove the cataract by whatever means the surgeon chooses. Through-and-through closing sutures are placed in my opposing continuous pattern and are looped aside, the lens is removed, and other intraocular surgery is completed. The peripheral opposing continuous loops may be drawn up to reduce the width of the incision opening as required by the intracameral procedure.

The incision is closed by drawing up and tying the preplaced opposing continuous suture. Four to six interrupted anterior lamellar sutures are inserted and set temporarily with slip knots. Each loop is adjusted individually to tension the apposed wound ideally as indicated by the surgical keratometer.

The slip knot we use was suggested by Terry. After the suture is inserted, the knot is formed by grasping the short distal end of the suture with the straight tying forceps and drawing it across the wound alongside the proximal thread. The doubled suture threads are crossed using my curved tying forceps, held in the other hand. Then a loop of the double threads is formed by rotating the tip of the forceps counter-clockwise under the thread. The curved forceps are then opened to pick up the short end, which is pulled through the double thread suture loop, creating a slip knot. Pulling on the long end (attached to the needle) tightens the knot; conversely, pulling on the short distal end loosens the knot. In this way, the individual interrupted suture loops can be adjusted to equal and optimal tension.

The wedge resection excision should be done in the cornea, either alone or in combination with a vertical corneal cataract incision for an optimal, reproducible correcting effect. Should a wider resection be required, the angle structures are more easily avoided.

Postoperatively detected, operatively induced astigmatism can be corrected by using the same principle and a similar technique. In this instance, however, there is usually considerable thinning at the wound area, even ectasia, and sometimes high degrees of against-the-rule astigmatism, up to 30 diopters. In such cases, resections as wide as 1½ to 2 mm may have to be done to correct high astigmatic bands. Resection "in block" rather than as a wedge is required and may have to extend into the surgical limbus. Nevertheless the relatively few cases that warranted this approach have had uniformly satisfactory results.

In the correction of more moderate astigmatic errors, we have succeeded to correct the preexisting meridional defect (K_2) absolute, by an average of 90%, the actual correction (K_2) averaging 60%. Though the surgical conditions can vary widely, the application of the wedge resection principle to the flatter meridian has resulted, in every instance, in reducing the astigmatic band toward sphericity.

SUMMARY

The Troutman surgical keratometer is invaluable to the wedge resection technique for identification of the flattened meridian, the positioning of the correcting excision on its axis, and, finally, for optimal tensioning of the closing sutures. Full-thickness wound apposition with through-and-through sutures combine to produce an optimal reproducible optical result. Troutman wedge resection combined with properly applied surgical keratometry and use of the principles outlined can regularly correct 75% of preexisting or postoperatively occurring meridional corneal errors.

Docum. Ophthal. Proc. Series, Vol. 21

THE UVEAL VASCULAR SYSTEM: ITS IMPORTANCE AND INVOLVEMENT WITH ANTERIOR CHAMBER OPENING

L. SCULLICA

(Messina, Italy)

Circulation of the blood in the eyeball takes place as in the brain under a pressure regime conditioned by eye pressure. The two vascular systems involved in this regime are the retinal and the uveal. The retinal system, clearly of the terminal type, is devoted to the nutrition of the innermost strata of the retina. The uveal system has much more complicated functions; it is responsible, as well as for nutrition of the sensorial elements of the retina with a continous supply of Vitamin A, for the absorption of water coming from the retina and for the preservation of eye pressure. This complex of functions of the uveal system is reflected in its angiotectonics.

In the uvea, the arterial influx is dependent on the long and short posterior ciliary arteries and on the anterior ciliary arteries. The venous system is represented mainly by the venae vorticosae, while the anterior ciliary veins have negligible importance in drainage of the venous uveal blood.

Angiotectonic and functional characteristics distinguish the choroidal from the iridociliary system. In the choroid, arteries and veins run very close together, the capillary bed interposed between the pre-capillary arterioles and the venules is very short, there are no pre-capillary sphincters, the diameter of the capillaries is quite large, two or three times greater than that of the capillaries of other districts, those of the iris in particular. Moreover, contrary to what happens in the retina, the blood in both arteries and veins flows in the same direction (Fig. 1, 2, 3).

All of these special characteristics ensure that the blood flow is steady and not alternating, and that the passage of blood into the capillary bed is facilitated.

The close relationship between arteries and veins and the dimensions of the capillary bed explain why the flow is one of the most rapid in the organism. It has been measured in the monkey as 463 ± 44 ml. x 100 g. x minute, and is ten times greater than that of the brain. For this reason, the venous blood contains only 3% less O_2 than the arterial blood.

Moreover, pressure in the veins is quite high and is considerably greater than intraocular pressure. Pressure variations in the veins parallel those of the arteries, as is demonstrated in experiments performed after adminstration of acetylcholine and adrenalin (Fig. 4).

In this respect, what happens after administration of adrenalin is especially demonstrative. This substance induces a peripheral vasoconstriction due

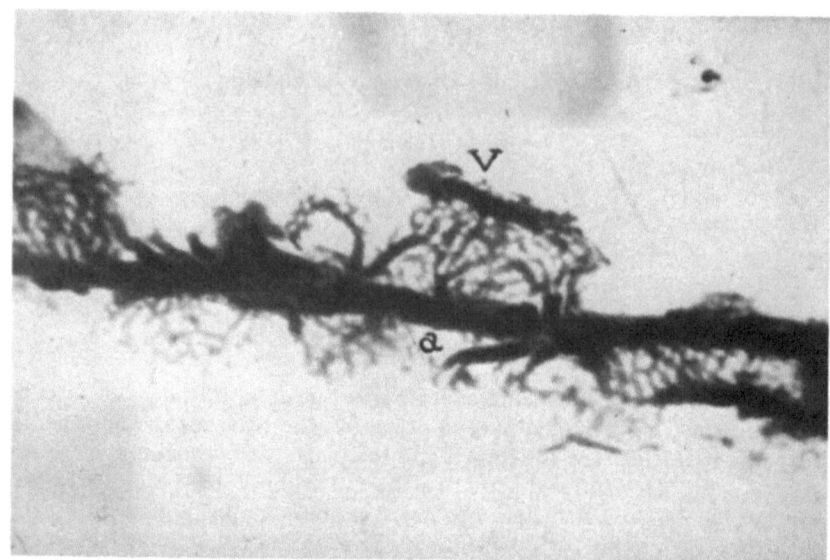

Fig. 1. The length of the capillary bed included between a choroidal arteriole and a venule is sometimes very brief (a: arteriole; v: vein). (Scullica 1957).

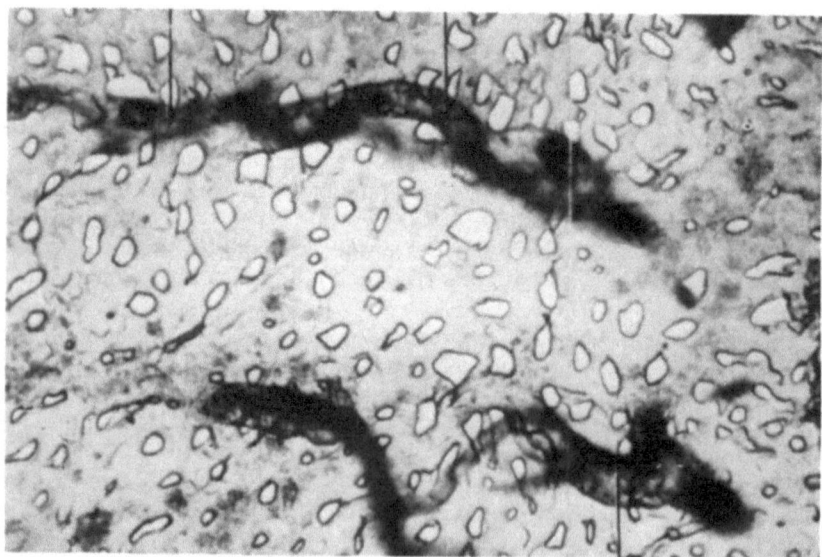

Fig. 2. Choriocapillary injected with neoprene in the zone included between two arterioles. It can be noted that the mesh of the choriocapillary network is extremely fine, and the capillaries are enormously wide. (Scullica 1957).

312

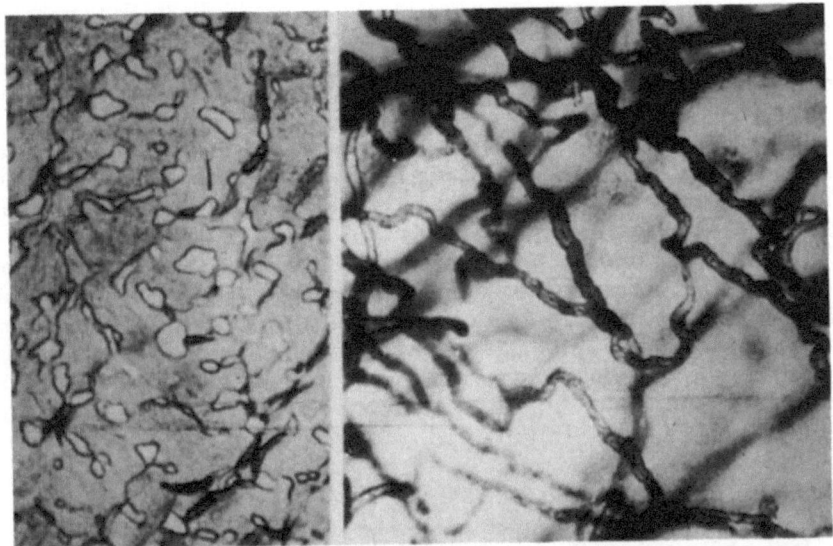

Fig. 3. Choriocapillary and iridean capillary bed injected with neoprene. While the choriocapillary bed is constituted of very wide vasa in a very close meshwork, that of the iris has a very large meshwork with very fine capillaries.

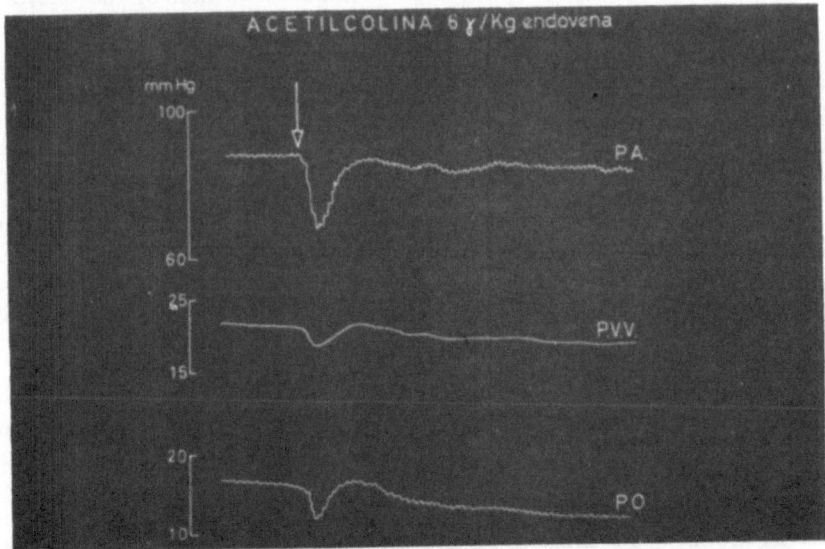

Fig. 4. Variations of the intraocular pressure, of the systemic pressure measured at the femoral artery and of choroid pressure meassured in the ampulla of vena vorticosa of a rabbit after administration of 6 g/Kg of intravenous acetylcholine. (Scullica 1971).

313

to which increase in arterial pressure is followed by reduction of venous pressure. This does not take place in the eye, where an increase of pressure in the veins of the choroid also corresponds to the increase in arterial pressure. (Fig. 5).

The modifications which take place in the posterior uvea following opening of the chamber are of great practical importance, as variations in the flow can influence the state of blood filling of the choroid which is responsible for the socalled vitreal thrust.

In normal and normocapnic conditions, the state of tension of the choroidal cushion is, given its anatomical features dependent upon arterial pressure and ocular pressure and the possibility of venous drainage. Given the great speed with which the blood flows in the choroidal system, taking for granted unimpeded venous drainage, the flow in the choroid appears to be dependent upon the difference existing between arterial pressure and ocular pressure:

$$AP - OP = F$$

It is obvious that when ocular pressure is reduced to zero as happens when the anterior chamber is opened, there is a tendency toward increase of flow in the capillaries and veins of the uvea. If the flow increase remains within limits which can be tolerated by the venous system, it will not cause stasis in the choroid and thus the eye will remain hypotonic. If, on the contrary, drainage is impeded or if the intensity of the flow is excessive, conditions of choroidal stasis may be created. This stasis will lead to capillary vasodilation and ultimately to the highly-feared congestion of the choroid.

Consequences of increased flow in the choroid

Congruous venous system (venous circulation facilitated)	Incongruous venous system (venous circulation impeded)
No statis	Choroidal congestion
No vitreal thrust	Vitreal thrust

Moreover, the higher the ocular pressure at the moment of paracentesis, the more sudden will be the variation of flow in the choroidal system and thus the greater will be the risk of choroidal congestion. If high arterial pressure with consequent overloading of the choroidal venous system is already present, even a minimum increase in flow linked to reduction of ocular pressure will be enough to determine an insufficiency of the venous system.

Another condition influencing the flow in the choroid is represented by the concentration of carbon dioxide in the aterial blood. It has been demonstrated, in fact, that if the concertation of CO_2 increases in the arterial blood there is an immediate increase of flow in the choroid, evaluated by means of Kripton 85. This may be explained by the variations of pH in the arterial blood, but it must be remembered that modifications of the arterial pressure may occur under these conditions, as has been shown by experiments made on ocular venous and arterial pressure after temporary respiratory standstill (Fig. 6).

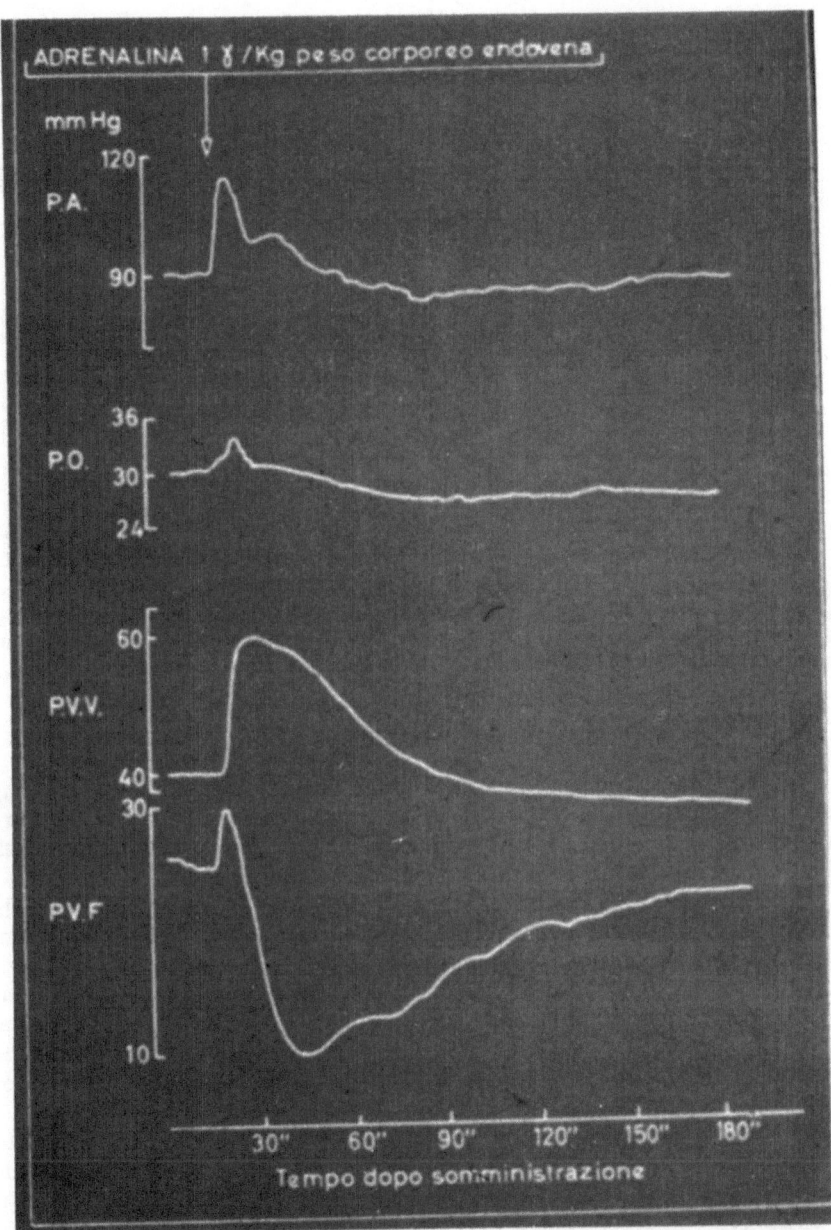

Fig. 5. Variations of arterial pressure measured in the femoral artery (A.P.), of ocular pressure measured in the anterior chamber (O.P.), of pressure in the choroidal venous network measured in the ampulla of the vorticosa (V.V.P.) and of systemic venous pressure measured in the femoral vein contralateral to the artery (P.F.V.) after injection of 0.1 g/kg of intra-venous adrenalin in a rabbit (Scullica et al 1971).

315

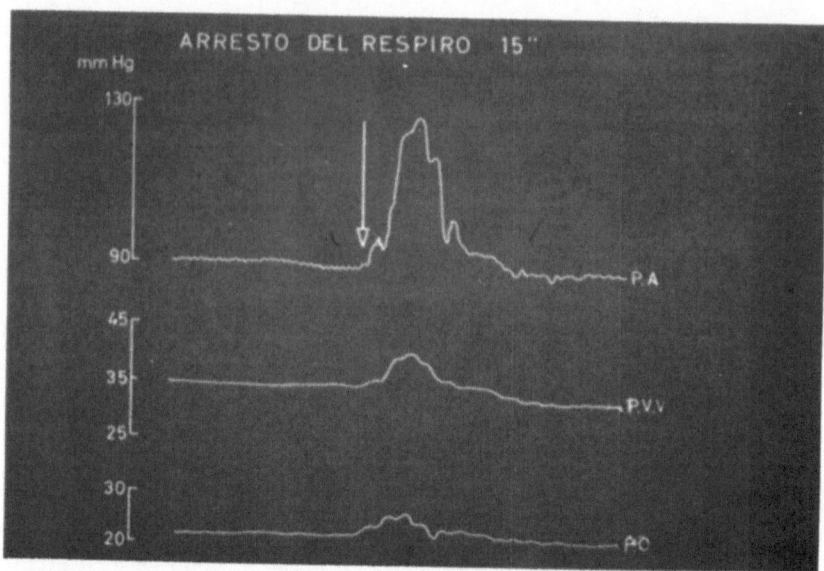

Fig. 6. **Modifications** in the systemic arterial pressure measured in the femoral artery (A.P.), in pressure in the choroid veins measured in the ampulla of the vorticosa (V.V.P.), and in ocular pressure measured in the anterior chamber (O.P.) in an anesthetized rabbit subjected to temporary respiratory standstill. (Scullica et al 1971).

In the anterior uvea, the vascular intake is largely dependent on the long ciliary arteries which consitute, in their terminal tract, the irido-ciliary arterial circle, but here too the angiotechtonic characteristics distingsuish the iridean circulation from that of the ciliary processes.

In the iris, the iridean radial arteries which derive from the arterial circle feed into a close network of slender capillaries, having a continuous basement membrane, drained by long radial veins directly or indirectly towards the venae vorticosae. In the ciliary processes, the arterial intake is represented by numerous arterioles which feed into large capillaries with a continuous but fenestrated basement membrane, drained either directly towards the venae vorticosae or indirectly with the interposition of the capillary bed of the orbiculus ciliaris.

In the irido-ciliary system, response to paracentesis is an attempt to restore ocular pressure through the production of aqueous humour. In the ciliary body after paracentesis, as has been demonstrated in numerous experiments, there is a stasis which eminently involves the anterior part of the ciliary processes (Fig. 7).

The increase in capillary permeability which follows is the expression of the breaking of the blood-aquous barrier, with the formation of the so-called 'acqueo plasmoide.' As regards this, it may be interesting to mention the effects of trigeminal stimulation. It had been noticed in the past, and recent experiments have confirmed that pre-ganglionic stimulation of the

316

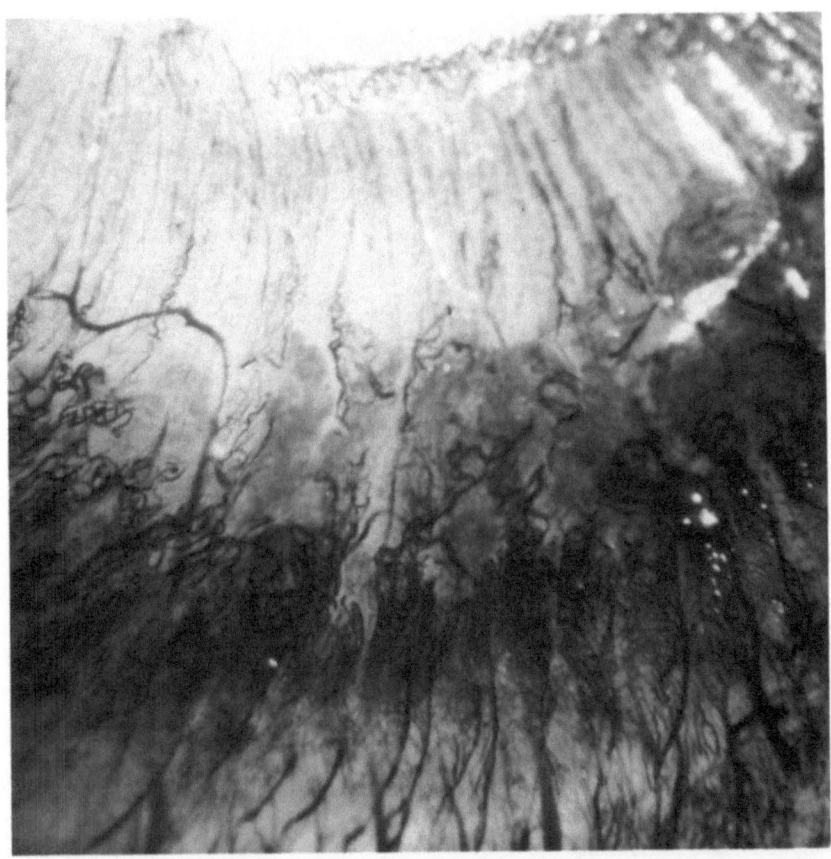

Fig. 7. Iridociliary region in an albino rabbit seen from the inner surface after paracentesis of the anterior chamber and successive injection of India ink. The stasis at the level of the anterior part of the ciliary processes is evident. (Scullica et al S.O.E. Hamburg 1976).

trigeminal determines in the experimental animal an intense miosis, the breaking of the blood-aquous barrier and a marked hypertonia in the closed eyeball (Fig. 8).

From a hemodynamic point of view, the picture is quite different from that which can be observed after paracentesis. It is, however, interesting that this effect, and above all the hypertonia, can be prevented by the addition of analgesics to the anaestehsia plan and by efficient retrobulbar blockage.

From all this, it appears obvious that the venae vorticosae represent the fulcrum of ocular hemodynamics, inasmuch as they condition the drainage of both the choroidal and the iridociliary systems, and thus have need of a continuous flow which cannot be modified without repercussions on both of these vascular systems.

317

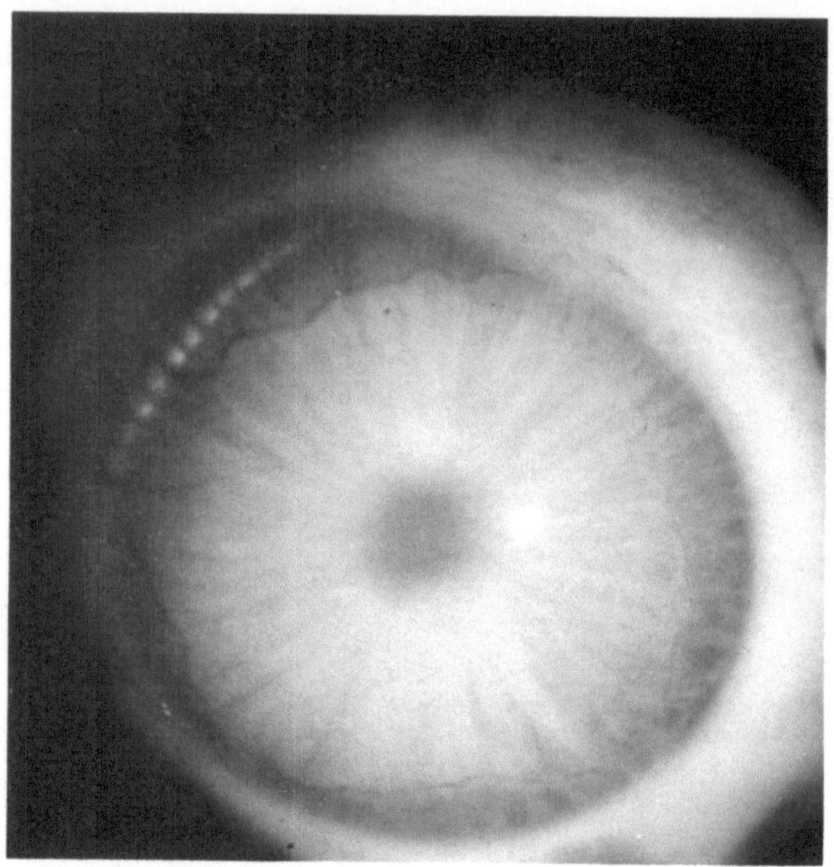

Fig. 8. Intense miosis after pre-gangliar sitmulation of the trigeminal in a rabbit. The miosis is accompanied by strong hypertonia (Scullica and co. S.O.I. 1977).

In some experimental animals, there exist regulatory systems capable of influencing venous drainage. One of these may be represented by direct anastomotic ducts which go from the arterial circle to the ampulla of the vorticosae, and act as a hydraulic suction pump (Fig. 9).

Such systems have not yet been demonstrated in man, although experimental research has been going on for more than twenty years (Scullica 1957). In man, however, the simple postural drainage provided by the antitrendelenburg position is suitable in most cases for efficient venous drainage. We have seen, moreover, the importance of the other factors, arterial pressure and ocular pressure, which must be attentively considered when operating on the eyeball.

The choice of systems most suitable for achieving the best blood flow conditions is therefore essential for obtaining complete vitreous silence.

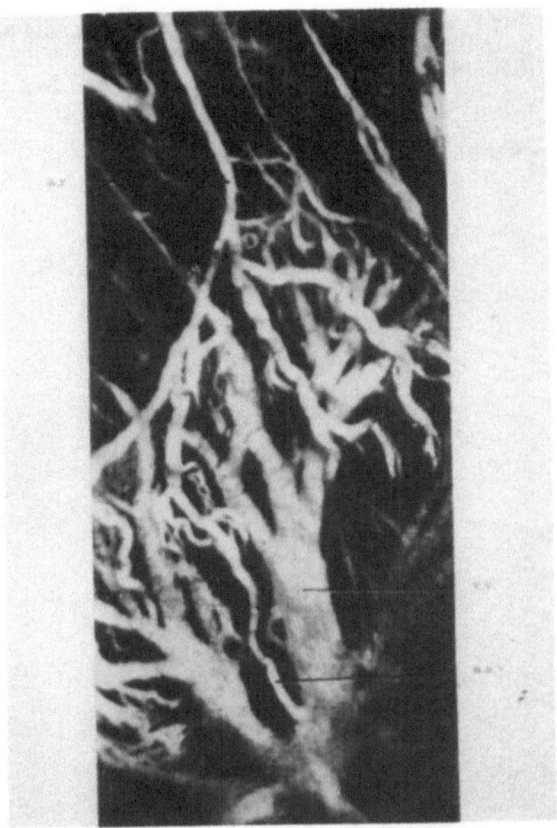

Fig. 9. Neoprene print of the choroidal vascular system in a rabbit. A brach originating from the great iridociliary arterial circle as a recurrent artery (R.A.) and entering the vena vorticosa (V.V.) directly in its ampulla (A.V.V.) can be seen. (Scullica, acta Anatomica 1958).

REFERENCES

Scullica L., Studi sull'angiotettonica della 'Tunica vasculosa bulbi'. *Biol. Lat. X Suppl.* VI, 1957.

Scullica L., Morphologische untersuchungen uber die ertirio-venosen anastomosen des Kaninchenauges. *Acta Anat.* 34: *269,* 1958.

Scullica L., Pecori Giraldi J. & Bisantis C. La registrazione della pressione nelle vene vorticose come mezzo di indagine nello studio della circolazione ematica oculare. Atti Acca. Pel. dei Pericolanti, Messina, 1971.

Scullica L., Observations of uveal blood flow pattern in excised arterially perfused rabbit eyes. *Am. J. Ophthal.* 54/6, 1962.

Scullica L., Bisantis C., Romeo G. & Candela V. The circulation in the ciliary processes and effect of rupturing of ophthalmic barrier. V. Congr. S.O.E., Amburgo, 1976.

Scullica L., Bisantis C., Romeo G. & Candela V. Circolazione del corpo ciliare e rottura della barriera ematoftalmica. LVII Congr. S.O.I., Firenze, 1976.

Strang R., Wilson T.M. & Mackenzie E.T. Choroidal and cerebral blood flow in baboons measured by the external monitoring of radioactive inert gases. *Invest. Ophth.* 16/6, 571, 1977.

Wilson T.M., Strang R. & Mackenzie E.T. The response of the choroidal and cerebral circulations to changing arterial PCO2 and acetazolamide in the baboon. *Invest. Ophth.* 16/6, 576, 1977.

Author's address:
Via 1e Reg. Margherita 61
98100 Messina
Italy

Docum. Ophthal. Proc. Series, Vol. 21

VITREOUS LOSS PREVENTION

G. VENTURI & L. BARCA

(Firenze, Italy)

In recent years, new pharmacologic protections and new operative methods have greatly reduced one of the most feared complications in cataract surgery: accidental vitreous loss during the operation. However, such a complication has not been totally averted yet. The most recent statistics in fact show that vitreous loss occurrence fluctuates between 11.8% and 1%. According to Jaffe, it takes place in 3% of the cases, on the average.

We have observed accidental vitreous loss in 12 out of 500 patients over the past two years (2.4%). Therefore, it is a rather rare complication, but when it takes place it can affect, at times even markedly, the operation's anatomic and functional results. Hence the importance of its prevention.

Among the conditions concerned in the pathogenesis of vitreous loss during an operation, one has to consider general and local situations (Tab. 1).

Table 1. Conditions likely to cause vitreous loss

General:	Local:
– Cardiovascular disorders	– Orbital
– Respiratory disorders	– Palpebral
– Metabolic disorders	– Conjunctival
– Constitutional conditions	– Bulbar
– Patient's age	– Anamnestic

Among the general ones, the patient's cardiocirculatory and respiratory conditions have primary importance, mainly for two reasons: a condition of severe circulatory and/or respiratory deficiency, may not allow for general anaesthesia, which no doubt represents, at least in our opinion, a real technical progress in cataract surgery. The second, and to our ends more important, reason is that alterated circulatory conditions may imply analogous damage to the choroidal vessels, which certainly play an important role in the pathogenesis of a possible vitreous loss. Renal emunctory conditions and some metabolic ones, first and foremost a long standing unchecked diabetes mellitus, deserve a similar evaluation.

The patient's constitutional conditions are also to be considered among the general causes. Obese patients seem to show a greater predisposition.

321

However a precise determinant, possibly a venous pressure increase, even in a supine position, has not been identified yet.

Age cannot be underrated either. In young subjects, vitreous volume is less easily influenced and modifiable, vascular reactivity at the choroidal level is greater, while the scleral tissue, being more elastic than in older subjects, is easily prone to collapse.

Among local causes the following are worth mentioning: a. Orbital conditions (oxycephaly, orbital masses, tumors in general, exophthalmos), b. Palpebral conditions (fissural narrowness), c. Conjunctival conditions (cicatricial seams and essential wrinkles), d. Bulbar conditions (outcomes of inflammatory or traumatic processes, sublocated or dislocated lenses, high myopia, hypertonia), e. Vitreous loss during cataract surgery on the other eye also represents an element to taken into the fullest account. Such an occurrence must induce a surgeon, in the event that he has to perform cataract surgery twice on the same subject, to take every precaution at his disposal.

Vitreous loss prevention can be enacted before and during the operation.

The prevention (Tab. 2) before the operation is eminently based on the use of drugs aiming at three fundamental goals: a. Improving the patient's general conditions (this must be carried out comfortably in advance of the operation), b. Performing and adequeate pre-anaesthesia, c. Creating the so called 'vitreous silence'.

Table 2. In preventing vitreous loss it is important before surgery:

- To treat all cardiovascular, respiratory, metabolic disorders
- To administer a combination of drugs inducing adequate sedation
- To use hyperosmotic agents
- To administer proper local or general anaesthesia
- To apply digital pressure

This end may be reached either through adequate pre-anaesthesia, and apt local or general anaesthesia, or by using hyperosmotic drugs.

Urea, glycerol, mannitol, and hysosorbide, generally have such properties.

These drugs' pressure-reducing action on the eye-ball seems to consist of a removal of liquid from the vitreous body and of its subsequent volume reduction.

We are now going to report seriatim on the use of these drugs, recalling their collateral effect besides their specific softening action on the eyeball.

Urea is administered intravenously in a 30% solution. The dosage is 0.5-2 grams per body weight Kilogram at a speed op 90-100 drops per minute. Maximum attention must be paid while inserting the needle, in order to avoid tissue necrosis, in case the drug spills out of the vein. Maximum pressure reduction is reached in 50-60 minutes, and return to normal values takes place in 5-6 hours.

The use of urea in hypertensive and hyperazotemic subjects is contraindicated. Among its collateral effects we recall: massive diuresis (100% of the cases); cephalalgy from dehydration (92%); arm pain (84%). nausea (31%); mental confusion (21%); phlebitis (5%); hyperthermia (2%). Even one lethal case has been reported in the literature.

Glycerol is administered orally in a 50% solution preferably with orange or lemon juice to make the potion more palatable. The dosage is 1-1.5 grams per body weight Kilogram. The drug is administered about 90 minutes before the operation, since, although an appreciable pressure reduction already manifests itself after thirty minutes, it becomes strongest after one hour, or one hour and a half. Tension tends to return to normal values in a four or five hour span. The drug is not toxic, but since it is metabolized by the organism it is contraindicated in diabetic patients. If administered orally, it may produce nausea and vomiting as negative collateral effects; if administered intravenously, it may produce hematuria, even massive, owing to glomerular artery constriction, followed by a reflex dilation.

Mannitol looks like the osmotic pressure lowering agent fittest for intravenous administration. It is administered by intravenous injection in a 20% solution. The dosage is 1.5-3 grams per body weight Kilogram, to be injected over a time span varying between 30 and 45 minutes. The lowering effect, already evident after 30 minutes, usually reaches its maximum after 50-60 minutes with a return to normal values in a five or six hour span. Since it is not absorbed by the intestine it must not be administered orally. It can be employed also in diabetic subjects because it is not metabolized by the organism and 80% of it is eliminated through urination within three hours. Collateral effects are negligible, mostly allergic in nature and easily controllable.

Occasionally, above all because of blood volume increase, ailments resembling angina episodes, which are however discounted by electrocardiological controls, may occur.

Hysosorbide is another hyperosmotic agent, which, like glycerol, can be administered orally. It can be absorbed by the intestinal tract and 95% of it can be eliminated, unmodified, through urination. In a 50% solution and with a dosage of 1.5-2 grams per body weight Kilogram it produces its maximum softening effect 60 minutes after ingestion. Its collateral effects, particularly nausea and vomiting as compared to glycerol, are practically nil.

It is evident, from the above, that urea represents the osmotic agent responsible for the greatest drawbacks.

As for ourselves, over the past two decades we have been systematically using mannitol in conjunction with general anaesthesia, in all but exceptional cases; the latter so enhances mannitol's softening effect that it reduces normal tension eye-balls' basic values by roughly 50%. This is confirmed by controls made at our Institute on 165 eye-balls with pre-operative tension varying between fourteen and eighteen mm HG (Artifoni, 1965).

Eye-ball tone, in particularly delicate cases, can be further reduced, even in narcosis, by means of a retrobulbar anaesthetic solution injection.

Eye-ball compression represents another mechanical means to induce a hypotonic condition. It is chiefly advisable in operation with local anaesthesia. It is performed after the retrobulbar anaesthetic injection by intermittently applying digital pressure on the eye-ball (with closed eye lids), for a time varying between three and ten minutes.

It is advised to interrupt digital pressure every one-two minutes, for at least 30 seconds, in order to avert vessel occlusion.

Instead of massage, constant pressure can be employed. This to the end of avoiding lens sub-dislocation or dislocation, which is possible with the former method.

Others have pointed out how hypotonicity can be enhanced by following the intermittent digital pressure with a constant one.

Summing up, eye-ball compression in conjunction with retrobulbar anaesthetic injection should induce: 1. Vitreous volume reduction, 2. Eye-ball tissue volume reduction, 3. Better anaesthetic diffusion with more effective akinesia and anaesthesia, 4. A certain degree of hemostasis at the orbital cavity level.

As for eye-ball compression induced hypotonicity, it is presently widely held that it is to be ascribed to an outflow of liquid from the vitreous body.

Considering that the anterior chamber's depth does not vary after compression, the expelled humor is probably made up for by that watery part of the vitreous body that is not linked to its macromolecular structures.

This seems to be confirmed by the lesser hypotonicity registered in young subjects whose vitreous body has not undergone any process of liquefaction.

Eye-ball tissue volume reduction, while hardly quantifiable, is clinically confirmed by the enophthalmos that usually follows a prolonged compression. It is obvious that reduced pressure by the orbital structures reduces the possibility of vitreous loss (with an open eye-ball).

The same can be said about the effect induced by a better diffusion of the anaesthetic at the level of the orbicular muscle and of the extrinsic ocular musculature.

As for ourselves, we use ocular compression very little, since we usually resort to general anaesthesia preceded by the use of osmotic drugs (mannitol), equally obtaining vitreous dehydration and relaxation of the extrinsic oculomotor muscles.

We think this is a sufficiently valid procedure, considering our, and others', statistics relative to vitreous loss cases.

On the other hand, we also are used to resorting to digital pressure, which we practice for about five minutes, in operations performed with local anaesthesia.

We choose, like others, not to resort to digital pressure in eye-balls characterized by a shallow anterior chamber and a narrow angle, because in such circumstances one could favour a complete closure of the angle with a flow of the humor towards the vitreous body with a consequent eye-ball tension increase.

Finally, how much a marked pre-operative hypotonicity may pre-empt the dangers of vitreous loss has not been established yet. We prefer to try to operate on soft or quasi-soft eye-balls, but in such eye-balls one can observe, not exceptionally, at the time of extracting the crystalline lens or immediately after, an extremely undesirable protruding of the hyaloid, and, viceversa, a perfect vitreous silence in eye-balls presenting higher pressure figures before the operations. It looks as if several authorities agree on this possibility.

The criteria for the exposure of the operating field also acquire sizable importance.

It is a good rule (Tab. 3) not to exert, whenever possible, any external pressure on the eye-ball; consequently, while some traditional blepharostats are not longer recommended, separate palpebral retractors find wider consensus.

Table 3. In preventing vitreous loss it is important during surgery:

Before corneo-scleral incision:	After corneo-scleral incision:
— To reduce external pressure on globe	— To place corneo-scleral sutures before lens delivery
— To prevent scleral collapse	— To use alpha-chymotrypsin properly
	— To deliver lens delicately
	— To rupture any capsular-hyaloidal adherences

We are used to keeping the upper and the lower eye-lid apart by means of two silk threads, the ends of which are fixed with forceps to the operating sheet. We furthermore run a vebeue thread under the upper rectus bulbar tendon. The muscle is kept minimally tense, that is to say enough to allow for the performing of all operating actions.

Sometimes, the thread through the upper eye-lid (in proximity of the free edge) may cause an eversion of the tarsus resting on the eye-ball. Trying to smooth out palpebral wrinkles in order to avoid any open eye-ball pressure on the scleral shell, is mandatory.

With local anaesthesia, it is necessary to perform correctly both akinesia and retrobulbar anaesthetic injection. This not only to avoid any small and always troublesome movement during the operation, but, above all, to obtain a complete relaxation of the palpebral and extrinsic oculomotor muscles.

The problem is different when operating with general anaesthesia, since in that case one can resort to muscle-relaxing drugs, such as curare.

Another element to be duly considered is the tendency to scleral collapse, especially if the operation is to be performed on young or pre-senile subjects, since this can exercise a compression on the vitreous body.

Flieringa's ring and all its variants have been known for over two decades.

According to Girard (Fig. 1) the rear segment's collapse is not avoided by Flieringa's ring, at least if employed as normally recommended, but it is avoided by a new model (Fig. 2) named a scleral expander by Girard. It is a metal or plastic ring with four extensions which is applied in the following fashion: after releasing the four recti, just like in a retinal detachment operation, the ring is fixed concentrically to the limbus and the four tabs are applied to the sclera in the four quadrants between two muscles. It is important not to make the four tabs adhere to the sclera, in order for them not to exert any pressure on the eye-ball. This can be obtained very easily, given that the materials employed are so ductile that the tabs themselves can be given any inclination. Such an apparatus, according to the author, should keep the scleral shell extended, and should therefore be employed in all cases in which its collapse in feared.

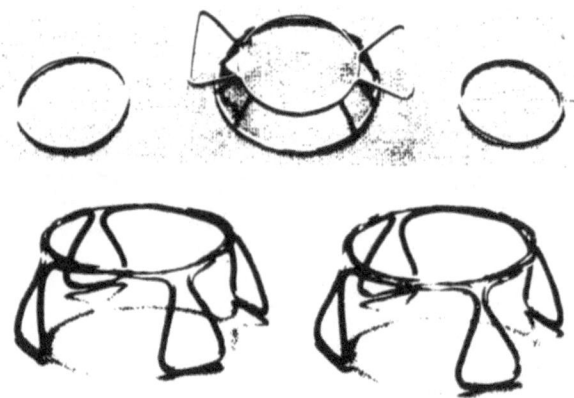

After making the incision and applying two safety corneo-scleral sutures, it is a good rule to ascertain the possible presence of posterior synechiae and, if needed, to eliminate them before proceeding with the extraction of the crystalline lens.

As for the extraction, we usually perform cryo-extraction, believing this technique to be one of the safest. We employ alphachymotrypsin (1:5000) exclusively in young subjects, usually under 50, in subjects affected by high myopia, and whenever capsule rupture is feared. In order to avoid post-operative hypertone (trypsinogen glaucoma) it is advisable to administer an inhibitor of the prostaglandines, such as indometacin, the day before the operation and for a few days after, in the dosage of 100 mg. per day (Etienne 1977).

Finally during the extraction, which must be carried out very delicately, particular attention must be paid in detecting possible adherences between the vitreous and the crystalline lens' posterior face. This is very important because such adherences must be eliminated and this can be done, without breaking the hyaloid, by means of a small brush or a spatula. On this matter, we have to recall how, not exceptionally, vitreous loss, otherwise totally unforeseen, may actually occur because such adherences were not detected.

What we have just summarized pertains to cataract extractions not presenting particular problems during the operation.

On the other hand (Tab. 4), sometimes, once the corneo-scleral incision has been performed, the iris gets incarcerated between the lips of the wound the prolapse cannot be reduced with normal techniques, the iris-cyrstalline lens plane is pushed forward, and a high ocular tone can be registered.

Table 4. Signs of impending vitreous loss during surgery before lens delivery

— Forward displacement of lens and iris with wound gaping
— Horizontal lines of tension in the cornea

Measures to adopt:
— Close wound temporarily, and wait for a few moments
— Pour cold liquid on the cornea

In case of failure:
— Close wound
— Perform extracapsular extraction
— Perform posterior sclerotomy

The incision's lips remain open, and horizontal tension lines appear on the cornea.

Such a condition may be favored, at the time the anterior chamber is open, by: scleral collapse, especially in young subjects; or by a serous or hemorrhagic choroidal detachment, probably favored by inadequate oxygenation before the incision; or by a small orbital hematoma, caused by the retrobulbar injection and slipped by undetected.

In such cases, as a first remedy, it is advisable to resort to the employment of ice water, both to favour vitreous retraction and to induce vessel constriction at the choroidal level.

If tension does not change, one may try temporarily to close the wound exerting a slight traction on the previously applied sutures and a moderate pressure on the lips of the wound itself either a spatula or wiht one's fingertips.

If the purpose is achieved, the operation can be resumed, after a few minutes' wait, and carried out; otherwise one has to: a. close up the incision and put off the operation; b. perform an extracapsular extraction; c. perform a posterior sclerotomy.

Extracapsular extraction usually allows the operation to be carried out without severe complications.

Posterior sclerotomy, as proposed by Iliff, is performed in exceptional cases, when any other remedy has proven infeasible.

The operation consists of exposing the sclera in the supero-temporal quadrant, where a cauterization of the tissue is performed at a distance of

6 mm from the limbus and for an extension of about 4 mm, parallel to the limbus itself.

The cauterized tissue is cut with a sharp Graefe knife. Once the pars plana is reached and pierced, the knife is aimed downward and backward about one centimeter deep, as to reach the vitreous body's liquid portion.

The wound is widened by rotating the knife and the liquid can flow a gain easier. The knife is then withdrawn and suturing the scleral wound is not necessary.

Intraocular tension can also be reduced by using Rizzuti's and Spirizzi's cannular needle and penetrating through the sclera and the pars plana into the posterior vitreous body; usually this is inserted in the supero-temporal sector and sucking the liquid.

The vitreous body's liquid component can be reduced (De La Vega, 1974; Kaufman, 1975) with a n 22 blunt point Gass needle, which is passed through the iridectomy and between the ciliary body and the lens to penetrate into the vitreous body and reach its liquid part.

The suction of a few drops should be enough to make the iris plane withdraw and to allow a perfectly safe lens extraction.

Antoher type of occurrence can manifest itself after the extraction (Tab. 5).

Table 5. Signs of impending vitreous loss during surgery, after lens delivery
— Vitreous bulging without hyaloid rupture

Measures to adopt:
— Avoid immediate suture tightening
— Use cold liquid and wait for a few moments
— Replace iris and use miotics

A vitreous bulging with an integral hyaloid in the anterior chamber, may force the iris between the wound's lips which remain open, with an impending danger of vitreous loss.

In such circumstances it is not advisable to rush the operation's various phases. The previously applied sutures will have to be gently pulled, without being knotted and a few minutes' wait, during which one will have to keep instilling ice water on the cornea, will be advisable.

Not rarely a spontaneous withdrawal of the vitreous bubble can be observed. In such cases the iris can be put back in place by means of a spatula.

This has to be handled very carefully and the suture can be completed after injecting acetylcholine and air into the anterior chamber.

In order to avoid operative vitreous loss, others resort to different methods or techniques, such as, for example, operating on the patient in an anti-Trendelemburg position, that is to say utilizing a particular hyperbaric chamber, where it is possible to induce atmospheric pressure modifications exclusively at the orbital level.

The expedients that have been mentioned in the context of this paper certainly do not represent the latest innovations, neither are they sophisticated procedures. But using them, it is possible, at times, to resolve very critical situations.

REFERENCES

Artifoni F.: Il mannitolo in oculistica. Aggiornamenti di terapia Oftalmologica 1965.
Barraquer J., Troutman R.C. & Rutilan J.: Surgery of the anterior segment of the eye. Mc. Graw Hill Book, 204, 281, New York 1964.
Bucci M.G.: Modificazioni ponderali del vitreo di coniglio dopo somministrazione orale di glicerolo. *Boll. d'Ocul.*, 42, *569-577*, 1963.
Bucci M.G. & Neuschüler R.: Indagini sul meccanismo d'azione ipotensiva oculare del glicerolo. *Boll. d'Ocul.*, 42, *299-315*, 1963.
Canagaratnam R.: Complications of cataract surgery. *Jap. Med. Jour.*, 12-30, (1974).
Castren J.A. & Listola J.: Results of cryo-extractions of 460 cataracts compared with 470 capsule forceps extractions. *Acta Ophthal.* 48. *468-480*, 1970.
De La Vega F.: Treatment of impending vitreous loss. In Emery J.M. and Paton D.: Current concepts in cataract surgery. The C.V. Mosby Co. 237-238, St. Louis 1974.
Etienne R.: Traitement Médical et Chirurgical des Glaucomes. 169. Diffusion Genérale de Libraire. Marseille 1977.
Flieringa H.J.: Procedure to prevent vitreous loss. *Am. J. Ophthal.* 36, *1618-1619*, 1953.
Girard L.J.: Use of the scleral expander in intraocular surgery. In Emery J.M. and Paton D.: Current concepts in cataract surgery. The C.V. Mosby Co. 231-237, St. Louis 1974.
Havener W.H.: Ocular pharmacology. The C.V. Mosby Co. 345-365 St. Louis, 1970 (Second Edition).
Iliff C.E.: A surgically soft eye by posterior sclerotomy. *Am. J. Ophthal.* 36, *1618-1619*, 1953.
Jaffe N.S.: Cataract surgery and its complications 31-40, 171-185. The C.V. Mosby Co. St. Louis 1976 (Second Edition).
Kaufman, H.E.: Vitrectomy from the anterior approach. *Ophthal. Surg.* 6, *58-65*. 1975.
Kariagin V.F. & Talenin N.I.: Prevention of vitreous prolapse in intracapsular cataract extraction. *Rec. in Ophthal.¦ Excerpt. Med.* 19, 434, 1975.
Kirsch R.E.: Preincision estimates of intraocular pressure and their relationship to anterior vitreous face during cataract surgery. In Emery J.M., Paton D.: Current concepts in cataract surgery. The C.V. Mosby Co., 41-42, St. Louis 1974.
Kirsch R.E. & Steinman W.: Digital pressure, an important safeguard in cataract surgery. *Arch. Ophthal.*, 54, *697-703*, 1955.
Maggi C.: Camera iperbarica in chirurgia oculistica. Nota preventiva. Circolo Oftalmologico Romano. Aprile 1976.
Maumenee A.E. & Meredith T.A.: A survey of 500 cases of cataract extraction. In Emery J.M., Paton D.: Current concepts in cataract surgery. The C.V. Mosby Co., 423-426. St. Louis 1974.
Schimek R.A.: Prolonged ocular compression to avoid vitreous loss: pros and cons. In Emery J.M., Paton D.: Current concepts in cataract surgery. The C.V. Mosby Co., 42-46, St. Louis 1974.
Shimizu H., Tobari I., Sato C., Uchino M. & Shibuya E.: Cataract Surgery under the microscope. Results and Problems in 300 eyes. *Jap. J. Clin. Ophthal.*, 27, *501-507*, 1973.
Süchting P.: Prophylaxis of vitreous complications and the procedure in cases of vitreous loss during cataract extraction. *Klin. Mbl. Augen.* 156, *548-551*, 1970.

Tanaka K.: The effect of intravenous injection of 500 mg. Acetazolamide (Diamox) on intracapsular lens extraction. *Folia Ophth.* 26, *474-478*, 1975.

Troutman R.C.: In Emery J.M., Paton D.: Current concepts in Cataract Surgery. The C.V. Mosby Co. 42. St. Louis 1974.

Vail D.C.: Loss of vitreous during cataract surgery. *Highlights Ophthal.*, 11, *107-119*, 1968.

Authors' address:
Università Degli Studi di Firenze
I Cattedra di Clinica Oculistica
Firenze
Italy

Docum. Ophthal. Proc. Series, Vol. 21

OPERATIVE COMPLICATIONS OF CATARACT SURGERY

B. BOLES CARENINI & G. GIROTTO

(Torino, Italy)

It is a common opinion, not to be easily refuted, that true cataract compli-cations are those occuring during surgery, the so-called operative complica-tions. These are numerous, differing in importance and consequences, but all requiring knowledge, profound experience, rapidity of decision, spirit of initiative and . . . good coranaries.

An outline of the operative complications gives an idea of the vastness of the subject.
— Complications preceding the incision.
— Complications of incision.
— Complications involving basal iridectomy.
— Complications of extraction of the cataract.
— Complications involving sutures.
— Complications of the final actions performed by the surgeon in 'refining' the procedure.

Complications preceding the incision may be summarized as follows:
— Hemorrhages coming from the canthotomy and/or from the lid stitches.
— Defective application of traction point to the superior rectus (an insuffi-cient hold on the muscle, and, very serious though extremely rare, perfo-ration of the eyeball).
— Defective application of the instrument used for holding the eyeball, the clamp or spiroclamp.
Complications of incision can be subdivided into the following groups:
— Complications of 'ab externo' incision with lancet.
— Complications of 'ab interno' incision with Graefe.
— Complications of cut incision successively enlarged with scissors.
Complications of 'ab externo' incision are as follows:
— Defective conjunctival flap due to excessive fragility of the conjunctiva or to errors made by the surgeon.
— Damage to the cornea, the iris and the lens made by the point of the instrument.
— Irregularity of the incision, such as an incision which is too corneal or too scleral or with uneven edges.
— Excessive bleeding, if the incision involves some limbar vessels.

– A too-rapid outflow of aqueous humour with abolition of the anterior chamber and possibility of iris-prolapse into the wound.

Complications of incision with Graefe may be inadequate incision (too corneal, too scleral, or irregular), or the emptying of the anterior chamber during incision, with consequent damage to the iris, to the lens (damage to integrety and to position, i.e. the possibillity of causing a subluxation of the lens itself) and excessive bleeding.

Among the complications of incision with cutting agent and scissors are found:
– Defective conjuctival flap.
– Wrong position of sclero-corneal wound
– Excessive bleeding and/or excessive cauterization with possibility of wound retraction.
– Damage to the iris and to the cornea made by the point of the instrument
– Irregularity of incision.

Complications of basal iridectomy include:
– Difficulty in grasping the root of the iris correctly, due to excessive mydriasis or to a too corneal incision.
– Incomplete section of the iris with lack of communication between anterior and posterior chamber.
– Hemorrhage of the iris.
– Lesions in the crystalline lens.

Complications which the surgeon may encounter when using alphachymotrypsin are the following:
– Myotic response to introduction of alphachymotrypsin.
– Mobilization of iris pigment.
– Hemorrhage of the iris.
– Luxation of the lens in to the vitreous, caused by mechanical action of the cannula.
– Vitreous loss due to lesions of the hyaloid produced by the cannula.
– Insufficient zonulolysis due to excessive dilution of the solution or to use of an impure solution.

Among complications common to all extractive techniques, the most important and dangerous, being such as to nullify any benefits of the operation, are:
– Rupture of the capsule.
– Luxation of the crystalline lens during extraction.
– Vitreous loss.
– Expulsive hemorrhage.

Complications peculiar to particular extractive techniques include:
In extraction by the forceps:
– Loss of grip.
– Pinching of the iris.
In extraction with ventosa:
– Loss of grip.
– Catching of iris.
– Aspiration of vitreous.

In the cryoextraction:

— Involuntary cryoadhesion with the nearest structures, such as the conjunctival flaps, the corneal endothelium, the iris, the edges of the incision, the sutures, the sponge used to dry the anterior chamber.
— Defective application of the cryode to the crystalline lens.
— Defective functioning of the cryode due to excessive cooling with the possibility that the capsule may 'explode', a defect in cooling or insufficient duration of cryoadhesion which may provoke a precarious adhesion between the point of the cryode and the lens.

Complications of suturing are:

— Incorrect apposition of the edges of the wound.
— Involvement of the iris root; the suture needle inadvertently goes through the iris.
— Too superficial suturing (the suture is weak) or bad opposition of the edges.
— Too deep suturing: the stitch, instead of bein intraparenchymal, involves the whole thickness of the cornea, creating a path for filtering of aqueous to the exterior, especially with certain suture material.
— Breaking of the thread during suturing, or detachment of thread from needle, a complication which is more frequent with atraumatic sutures.

Complications immediately following extraction may be:

— Defective re-positioning of the iris.
— Involvement complications of vitreal strands in the suturing.
— Various complications caused by introduction of air, acetylcholine or aqueous into the anterior chamber at the end of the operation.

After this brief summary of all possible complications, it is well to discuss further those complications common to all extractive techniques, as they are the most serious, the most difficult to remedy, and the most disstressing for the surgeon. They are:

— Rupture of the capsule.
— Luxation of the crystalline lens.
— Vitreous loss.

As for hemorrhage, and expulsive hemorrhage in particular, this subject has been treated in an other chapter.

RUPTURE OF THE CAPSULE OF THE LENS

Although the incidence of this complication is much less frequent since the introduction of the technique of cryoextraction, rupture of the capsule may occur in any phase of extraction, from the moment of applying the forceps, ventouse or cryoextractor up to the actual extraction. Causes for rupture of the capsule may be subdivided as follows:

a. Causes due to mistakes made by the surgeon.
b. Causes due to characteristics of the lens itself.

Among the causes due to the surgeon's mistakes we may note:

1. Insufficient width of incision.
2. Inadequate mydriasis.
3. Wrong application of the instrument.

4. Too hasty extraction.

Among those due to lens characteristics, the most important are:
1. Intumescent cataract.
2. Hypermature cataract.
3. Particularly resistant zonule.
4. Adherence between capsule and hyaloid and/or iris.

PREVENTION

To prevent rupture of the capsule, it is necessary first of all to make a sufficiently large incision. The surgeon may, after having made the incision, lift the corneal flap in order to check visually that the width of the opening is sufficient. To be absolutely proscribed are maneuvesrs turning over the corneal flap in a forward direction, as this can damage the corneal endothelium and thus provoke striated keratopathies in the post-operative period.

Although the recent tendency is towards the smaller poosible corneal incisions, it must be remembered that in this matter, too much is better than too little. Obviously, the size of the incision will vary according to the type of instrument used to extract the lens; a wider opening is necessary with forceps and with the erysiphake while a smaller incision is sufficient with the cryoextractor. It is obvious too that a scleral incision will be larger than a corneal incision.

Adequate preventive mydriasis is very important. This can be obtained with drops of cocaine or of a light mydriatic or with retrobulbar injection of anesthetic, with epinephine if necessary. If, notwihtstanding these measures, the pupil remains narrowly closed, it may be that the sphincter of the iris is rigid. In this case, sphincterotomies or a sectorial iridectomy are advisable.

Wrong application of the instrument (cyroetractor, forceps, erysiphake or ventouse).

The point of the cryoextractor is applied to the surface of the lens, which has been previously dried with a cellulose sponge, halfway between the 'stella lentis iridica' and the upper edge of the lens.

If the point is applied too close to the edge, it can cause freezing of the zonule which produces excessive traction on the ciliary body. If the point is applied on the 'stella lentis iridica', traction is made on the whole zonule at the same time, making initial rupture of a part of the zonule more difficult. For correct application, the point of the cryode must be perfectly clean and dry. For this purpose, the surgeon generally uses a sterile gauze pad, taking care to remove even the slightest trace of humidity. It is also very important that the point of the cryode touches the anterior surface of the cornea without the interposition of a liquid film. Immediately prior to application of the cryofixer it is necessary to dry the anterior chamber and the capsule of the lens of any liquid which may be present, including aqueous humour, vitreous or buffered washing solution.

As regards application of the forceps, it should be remembered that this differs according to the type of extraction to be performed: in proximity to the lower edge of the lens for the up-turning method and in proximity to the upper edge for the sliding method. This blades of the corceps are opened for acout 3-4 mm. Wider opening could in itself provoke the rupture of the capsule at the moment of tightening the hold.

Erysiphake or ventouse: For correct functioning of the device, the cup must be placed on the superior pole of the lens in order to get the right hold. In this way, moreover, the suction exerted on the lens will cause a uniform reduction of volume thus facilitating the tearing away of the zonular fibers. The exact point of placement will vary, being lower when the up-turning technique is used and higher when the sliding method is adopted.

Too hasty extraction: The extraction of the lens is the culminating act of the operation, in which the surgeon makes use of all his experience and manual ability. The extraction must be performed in a manner which is both extremely delicate and decided; the extracting action is accompanied by small lateral movements which facilitate the rupture of the zonular fibers.

Instrumescent or hypermature cataract: The use of cryoextraction, universally advisable for avoiding rupture of the capsule, is the method to be preferred whenever the surgeon suspects the presence of a fragile lens, as happens especially with intumescent or hyper mature cataract. In these cases, it is advisable to prolong the cryopexic action up to ten seconds so as to have a larger frozen area to work with; in this way, the extracting force is distrubuted more uniformly over the structure of the crystalline lens. Some authors advise the use of alpha-chymotrypsin in these cases, even when the patient is old, in order to facilitate to the macimum extraction of the cataract.

Particularly resistant zonule: It is advisable to extend the use of zonulolysis to alle patients under 55-60 years of age; in these subject, the zonule fibers are probably still resistant and the capsular-hyaloidal adherences are stronger. It must also be considered whether the patient's general state is still youthful or not. It is probable, in fact, that in patients of advanced age who still maintain a youthful aspect the zonule is more resistant than expected.

Adherences between capsule and hyaloid and/or iris: The presence of adherences between the capsule and the hyaloid represent even today one of the uncertain elements in cataract surgery. These adherences, which are due, according to most writers, to the persistence of Berger's hyaloideocapsular ligament, are not detectable during preliminary examinations. Although in older subjects their presence is reduced to quite a low percentage, these capsulo-hyaloidal synechiae, expecially when tenacious, may be responsible for accidents such as the rupture of the capsule and the loss of vitreous.

Irido-capsular adherences, instead, show up during examination with the slit lamp and while controlling pupillar mobility by the use of mydriatic substance during preparatory examinations. If small synechiae are present, they may be eliminated, after corneal incision, by means of a cyclodialysis spatula. If the synechiae are larger, it is advisable, after a synechiotomy performed passing with the spatula behind the iris through the basal iridectomy, to perform two or more iridotomies at the level of the sphincter so as to facilitate lens extraction. In some cases, synechiae may be such as to make intracapsular extraction inadvisable.

If the rupture of the capsule is of limited extension, the surgeon may attempt extraction with the cryoextractor again, applying it on an area of the capsula which has remained intact and prolonging the freezing time up to ten seconds so as to obtain a larger than usual frozen zone. As an alternative to the cryoextractor, the surgeon may try to remove the lens by grasping it with one or two slender capsular forceps (Arruga's forceps or the like) or with.

A third method consists of attempting extraction by applying external pressure at the six o'clock position and at the same time depressing the posterior edge of the incision.

If, in spite of such precautions, complete rupture of the capsule occurs and part of the lens remains in loco, particular attention must be given to the extraction of the lenticular residue, remembering that the retention of cortical material is less serious than the retention of fragments of the nucleus. Therefore these fragments must be extracted, as the nuclear substance does not tend to re-absorb spontaneously and may cause serious problems in the eye, such as hypertonia and reactive phenomena of the phacoanaphylactic type. The operation may be performed with one or two slender forceps or with a syringe equipped with a cannula for suction of masses, according to the consistency of the material to be extracted, or even by means of prolonged irrigation, appropriately directed and graduated.

The retention of cortical material is less serious as it does not usually provoke post-operatory reactions. For removal of this material too, the surgeon may use one, or better two, forceps while an assistant lifts the corneal flap slightly; always, however, after having first attempted to remove capsular residue with irrigation of the anterior chamber with a buffered saline solution. To see retained capsular residue clearly, some writers advise the use of an ultraviolet lamp (Hague's lamp). The introduction of an air bubble into the anterior chamber can also help the surgeon to distinguish lenticular fragments from the vitreous.

The use of the microscope makes these manoeuvres, which may meet with serious complications, much easier and safer. Possible complications are:

a. damage to corneal endothelium.
b. damage to the iris.
c. rupture of the hyaloid with possible vitreous loss.

a. Special care must be taken to avoid damages to corneal endothelium. It is well-known that this extremely delicate structure plays a fundamental part in the reparative processes of the cornea and in the good post-operative recovery of the cornea itself. It is advisable to perform manoeuvres for extraction of capsular residue after having closed one of the pre-placed stitches and after having injected a buffered saline solution into the anterior chamber in order to reform the chamber so as to give the surgeon a larger field of action and make less probable any contact, always darmful, of instruments with the endothelium.

b. The iris too may be involved in these manoeuvres, and, as well as suffering various lesions or bleeding, may be pinched or pulled during attempts to grasp the lenticular residues; this dislocations of the iris should be treated using either a sable brush or a fine spatula for re-positioning the iris.

c. The possibility of rupturing the hyaloid is always present: but this complications becomes even more serious when lenticular material mixes with the vitreous. When this happens, it is better to give up and abandon the residue inside the eye rather than run the risk of vitreous loss. It is however necessary that the lenticular residue does not remain incarcerated in the corneal wound where it would hinder healing and would expose the eye to the danger of a fibrous transformation, to inflammatory processes and to severe post-operative astigmatism. A carefully performed irrigation can eliminate all residue from the wound. As for vitreous loss, this subject will be discussed more fully later.

LUXATION OF THE LENS

This complication may occur either in one of the phases preceding extraction of the lens or during the extraction itself. The present discussion will deal only with luxation during extraction, as the other cases have already been covered.

PREVENTION

Possible causes of luxation of the lens are:
1. extreme fragility of the zonule.
2. incorrect use of extraction instruments.

Extreme fragility of the zonule condition may be pre-existant (constitutional fragility of the zonule or fragility due to age) or induced by the surgeon (by small accidental traumas to the crystalline lens prior to extraction, and/ or by the use of zonulysis). Usually in these cases dislocation of the lens toward the outside of the eye takes place spontaneously, provoked by a state of ocular hypertonia or by pressure exerted on the eyeball by lid contraction due to insufficient akinesia. This type of luxation can be avoided by correct use of pre-anesthesia, of akinesia and of hypotonizing agents.

Incorrect use of extraction instruments

Luxation may occur the moment the instrument (forceps, erysiphake or cryode) touches the eye, if this contact is not made with the necessary delicacy. When this happens, the lens is dislocated backwards into the vitreous, where, especially in subjects with fluid vitreous, it may sink.

Luxation can also take place consequent to a inefficient grasp of the instrument on the capsule; for example, in an intumescent cataract, the capsule may be so tightly-stretched that the forceps cannot get a good hold. A wrinkled capsule may make adhesion between capsule and erysiphake precarious.

337

Other factors which may make it difficult to grasp the capsule correctly are:

- Defects in instruments, such as bad closing of the blades of the forceps, inadequate cup size in the erysiphake, a cryode point which is not perfectly dry.
- Involuntary movement of the surgeon's hand when applying the instrument.
- Insufficient or insufficiently long cryoadhesion, inadequate suction force of the ventouse, inadequate force in closing the forceps.

TREATMENT

When vitreous loss occurs in spite of all precautions taken, the surgeon must first distinguish whether this loss in progressive or non-progressive. To do this, he must close the eye by drawing tight the pre-placed sutures, and wait to see what happens. If the eye remains soft and the vitreous loss stops, the eye can be re-opened and the operation can continue. If, instead, the eye becomes progressively harder and the vitreous continues to flow out copiously, the wound must be closed by suturing as quickly as possible without attempting other manoeuvres.

As for the portion of vitreous which has escaped, there are different techniques for treatment, among them: a. Reduction of the prolapsed vitreous, b. Resection of the prolapsed vitreous, c. Anterior vitrectomy ('open sky') method, d. Aspiration of vitreous, e. Instrumental vitrectomy.

REDUCTION OF PROLAPSED VITREOUS WITHOUT RESECTION

In this technique, some of the pre-placed sutures are first closed. Then the surgeon penetrates the anterior chamber with a very fine angled spatula, frees the wound from the vitreous with a movement parallel to the iris plane, closes the remaining pre-placed sutures, injects a solution of acetylcoline into the anterior chamber and, having obtained pupillar myosis, introduces an air bubble into the anterior chamber.

It is a good rule to keep the patient in bed without a pillow in order to keep the vitrous pushed back behind the plane of the iris by the air bubble as long as possible. This method has the disadvantage that often the vitreous even when correctly reduced, flows back into the anterior chamber, teaching the wound and drawing up the pupil.

RESECTION OF PROLAPSED VITREOUS

Classic resection is performed as follows: the wound is tightly closed with the pre-placed sutures, except in the temporal sector; a cellulose sponge is used to show clearly the driblets of vitreous coming out of the wound; the driblets are resectioned as close as possible to the wound. Then an air bubble is introduced into the anterior chamber, after which a very fine angled iris spatula is passed from within under the corneo-scleral lips all along the incision, to liberate the surgical wound from the vitreous dirplets which

338

have remained incarcerated in it.

This operation is very important for maintaining a round pupil. Vitreal driblets remaining in the anterior chamber, incarcerated in the wound, can rapidly develop fibrosis and thus cause deformation of the pupil, which is stretched upward. To prevent this, the surgeon can perform an ample sectorial iridectomy and an inferior sphincterotomy; if he prefers to avoid these procedures and to keep an integral pupillary sphincter, he can attempt the use of myotics (acetylcoline) in the anterior chamber, which, by their action on the pupil, may free the wound of vitreal residue.

When the vitreal prolapse shows no progressive tendency and the eyeball is sufficiently hypotonic without any further thrust toward prolapse, the surgeon may proceed to an 'open sky' vitrectomy, lifting the cornea, holding the vitreous jelly with an absorbent sponge and cutting it off at the level of the iris plane with long-bladed forceps scissors. The vitreous jelly should not be pulled outside the eyeball in order to excise as much vitreous as possible, as this could exert unnecessary traction on the retina causing detachment or a vitreous hemorrhage. When the excaped vitreous has been resected, the iris tends to become concave, thus freeing the irido-corneal angle. The edges of the incision and the angle must then be cleaned with the cellulose sponge; special care must be taken that vitreous residue does not block the angle exactly at the point of the basal iridectomy.

To avoid possible scleral collapse following vitrectomy, it is advisable to use Flerings'a ring (or a similar expander) in all cases in which vitreous loss may be anticipated. If this occurs when the ring is not already in place, and it seem useful to place it, the surgeon must close the pre-places sutures and put the ring in place with four sutures. After this the wound is re-opened and the incision enlarged up to 180° or more so as to facilitate removal of vitreous and avoid damage the corneal endothelium. The surgeon's assistants lifts the cornea and the vitrectomy can be performed by the 'open sky' method as discussed above.

ANTERIOR VITRECTOMY

This procedure attempts to avoid the complications of vitreous loss linked to the presence of vitreous in the anterior chamber by removing a rather large portion of vitreous. With this 'open sky' method too, the corneal incision must be enlarged up to approximately 180°-200°. To avoid unnecessary damage to the cornea, it is advisable to turn it up once only and to keep it in position during the entire vitrectomy. A small, narrow cellulose sponge (it may be crimmed at the edges to make it narrower) is then introduced into the pupillary opening. The sponge is gently rotated and pulled out of the pupil; the vitreous pulled out with it is cut of at the level of the iris plane. This operation is repeated several times until about half of the vitreous has been removed. The iris then falls backward assuming the form of a frustum of cone. When enough vitreous has been removed, the surgeon introduces a balanced saline solution into the vitreous cavity, cleans with the sponge the anterior chamber, the angle and the wound of possible vitreous residue, and then instils a myotic.

A few observations on this procedure should be made: 1. The operation is rather long and there is the danger that the aneasthetic, if local, may cease to be effective, 2. This method is traumatizing to the ocular structures: when the sponge reaches a zone of liquid vitreous it swells considerably, remaining entrepped in the pupil were it can cause trauma to the iris and its sphincter. If we think that 30-50 sponges are used to obtain the desired effect, it is easy to understand why post-operative iritis is so frequent in eyes subjected to this treatment. Moreover the sponges are in themselves a source of inflammation in the eye. They can fray or be accidentally cut and the small pieces of cellulose remaining in the vitreous can cause granulomas or induce chronic eye inflammation, 3. When the sponge, soaked with vitreous, is pulled out, there is inevitable traction which can contribute toward causing detachment of the retina, retinal hemorrhages or macular edema.

Kasner has published an investigation of 105 case histories of anterior vitrectomy, with the following results:

- Cystoid macular edema: 13%
- Detached retina: 5%
- Transitory corneal edema: 3%
- Vitritis: 2%
- Chronic iritis: 2%
- Excessive astigmatism: 1%
- Bullous keratopathy + glaucoma 1%

ASPIRATION OF VITREOUS

This method is bases on the observation that often in the eyes of elderly patients, vitreous does not remain in a jelly-like state (already-dormed vitreous) but passes into a fluid state. After a certain age, moreover, a retro-vitreal space located supero-posterially, containing only the liquid part of the vitreous, may form. The procedure consists of introducing a cannula needle into the vitreal cavity possibly through the basal iridectomy, and gently drawing out the fluid within; at this point the prolapsed vitreous tends to fall backwards freeing the anterior chamber and the incision. This technique also is not risk-free. When the surgeon introduces the needle into the vitreous and applies suction, dangerous traction of the vitreous on the retina may be created.

INSTRUMENTAL VITRECTOMY

There is no doubt that, for performing 'open sky' vitrectomy, the perfecting of an instrument such as the vitrectome is an important step forward in comparision with the method using sponges. Greater sterility is coupled with lesser danger of damaging corneal endothelium and provoking dangerous vitreal traction on internal ocular structures. Moreover, the procedure takes much less time.

This instrument works on a simple principle: the vitreous is drawn into a small opening at the extremity of the instrument where the vitreal fibrillae are cut by rotating blade. To these advantages must be weighed the following defects: the vitrectome must be used with great caution and precision lest the iris may be partially sucked in and cut. This sophisticated instrument is costly and delicate. Its correct use requires the microscope, which necessarily lengthens the time of the operation, partially neutralizing the advantage of greater speed in performing the vitrectomy.

Authors' address:
Corso Vittorio Emanuele 18
Torino
Italy

Docum. Ophthal. Proc. Series, Vol. 21

OPERATIVE COMPLICATIONS OF CATARACT SURGERY

R.M. FASANELLA, M.D.

(New Haven, Connecticut, U.S.A.)

One thing that I would like to say is that I am very, very happy to be here among my Italian countrymen. It's a real pleasure. In terms of the incision, since we are talking about complications and their prevention, may I pass on to you what I consider a 'pearl'. Every time you open any eye, whether it be for a corneal transplant or a cataract, you should at the time take a culture. You will be surprised at what you will get back on that culture. In the last 100 cases that I have done, I have got among organisms, E. coli, Streptococci, etc., yet fortunately no infection resulted. What happened? Did the person who brought that to the lab make a mistake or did I make a mistake? Every time you open an eye, especially in the United States, take a culture. It will save you many headaches and many lawsuits.

Now as to sutures, some years ago, in the Archives of Ophthalmology, with Dr. David Freeman, I wrote about the ideal suture, a wire suture. We performed this operation on some 30 rabbits and there was no finer suture, no failure in any case. In removing the suture in one human, everything happened. We have never used a wire suture again. Keep that in mind. It was described in the Archives of Ophthalmology, about 10 or 15 years ago. Now I shall limit my talk to bleeding and I shall try to tell you some practical points about the prevention and management of bleeding. I shall not go into the details of bleeding as related to intraocular lenses, but I shall cover the broader points. Retrobulbar hemorrhages can follow even if one uses a blunted Atkinson needle. For re-operation if surgery cannot be done under general anaesthesia, and if the patient has bilateral cataracts, get two operative permits, two separate operative permits to do either the right or the left eye if the cataracts warrant that. Next, as to the superior rectus, you don't have to use a superior rectus, stabilizing suture. Use a cardiovascular needle. You will not get any hemorrhage with that needle, I can almost guarantee you. I haven't seen it in the last 10 years. But if you should get hemorrhage, a very simple little trick is just to tie that superior rectus suture. It will stop the bleeding. You can evacuate it and proceed. Now as to the incision, and in terms of bleeding — today you heard beautifully described for you the fact that using a corneal incision is the best way to prevent bleeding. If you choose to use the more standard corneal-scleral incision, don't forget that in the 9 to the 3 o'clock position, go more corneal and you can help avoid some bleeding at that stage. With your incision, as a rule, if you do

343

have some bleeding, usually waiting will suffice. Of course, if it is not at the wound edge, apply mild diathermy. A bi-polar is the ideal type. If bleeding persists despite this, I have on occasion used a Mira unit, about 3 to 4 mm. in back of the incision to stop bleeding. It's also a very excellent little trick for trauma. If you know where that bleeding is coming, use a Mira unit set at 0.5, 3 or 4 mm. back from the limbus and it will usually stop bleeding. Now as to bleeding with the iridectomy, if you want no bleeding, do no iridectomy. I have done that on several occasions and I've gotten away with it.

There are other things that you can do. If you do want an iridectomy, you can simply crush the area that you want to cut. Or you can use a bipolar diathermy set at 10 or 15. By using a bipolar diathermy you may make your cut and you will not get any bleeding, nor will you involve the capsule or any other portion of the eye. The bipolar cautery or the laser can also be used pre-operatively for doing your iridotomies or your iridectomies. Bipolar cautery may be used to get blood vessels that are in the angle. Now my subject was so beautifully covered by the previous speakers that I have very little to do other than review for you what Drs. Scullica and Ventrui said. In the literature there are about eleven cases of spontaneous hemorrhage that have been reported. About one third are operative. Post-operatively it can occur from about three hours or in 3 to 9 days.

What are causes? Included are the subchoroidal hemorrhage usually due to the ciliary arteries, the short and the long ones, the valsalva effect, bucking, vomiting, and very important the arterial CO_2. If you have a good anaesthetist, he can control.

Many of these causes have been outlined previously, so I just need only mention as to preventative measures diamox, mannitol and blood pressure for the use of control. I remember a very wonderful older lady, an alcoholic who had been referred to me from another city because she had moved into our area. I had done the first eye on her under local anaesthesia and got away with it. But during the operation on the second eye, the blood-pressure at the time she had the expulsive hemorrhage went sky-high and I lost that eye. Now venous pressure — we have ways of treating this; elevate the head of the bed. On occasion I have operated, actually, on people with asthma at a 90° angle. It's a little bit difficult, but it can be done. I've done it actually with the patient sitting upright in the bed. In Russia, when a patient has had one expulsive hemorrhage, they make a trephine opening in one portion of the other eye prior to opening that eye. They do not take out the plug completely unless there is an expulsive hemorrhage. Perhaps, maybe, rather than the upper temporal quandrant, it might be better to make this scleral opening down in the lower temporal quandrant, because this is where most of them occur. But if you want to actually tell where you should tap, if you are going to tap, you should look in with an ophthalmoscope, a reverse Trendelenburg. A good anaesthetist can help prevent some expulsive hemorrhage. Now what are we going to do when this happens? We'll need wound clusore. And this is what I'm going to talk about a bit later. Your sclerotomy — I mentioned what they do in Russia. Anticipate detachments and treat the area of sclerotomy. — And in our country, because of malpractice, bring in a consultant immediately. Now which of these eyes do we save with expulsive hemorrhage? Perhaps the ones that we save are those that have a choroidal effusion rather than those with a real expulsive hemorrhage. I asked Donald Praeger, who speaks on complications for Kelman in all his courses, how many choroidal hemorrhages he has seen during or following phacoemulsification. He had sent a question to all of his colleagues throughout the United States and two months ago, he had found only one. So perhaps in some cases where everything else indicates it might be used, the second eye might be done with phacoemulsification because the whole trick is to try to close the wound. And if you close a 3-mm. incision, the size used in phacoemulsification, perhaps it will be much easier to save that eye. Thank you very much.

Author's address:
24 Rolling Royle Rd
Orange, Connecticut 06477
U.S.A.

EYE SURGERY IN A NEW HYPERBARIC ROOM
(VITREOUS LOSS PREVENTION)

C. MAGGI*

(Roma, Italy)

Two years ago, in April 1976, there was a first report to the Rome section of the Italian Ophthalmological Society on a small number of cases operated in a hyperbaric room of my own design. This hyperbaric room consists of a cubic airproof cabin inside in which the operating team is placed. (Fig. 1). The patient, lying on the operating table outside the cabin has his head only apparently inside the operating room. In fact on the front wall of the cabin there is a hole fitting round the patient's eye, to which the borders of his orbit are sealed. In this way the patient's eye only is exposed to the hyperbaric pressure to be produced in the operating room.

Today a second model of this operating room is presented, much wider then the previous one, being 2 x 2 metre cubic cabin with enough space to contain the operating microscope and all the routine equipment of an operating theatre, yet allowing comfortable movement to the surgeon and his two assistants. (Figs. 2, 3, 4, 5, 6, 7, 8, 9.)

Few slides demonstrating the main steps in an intracapsular extraction

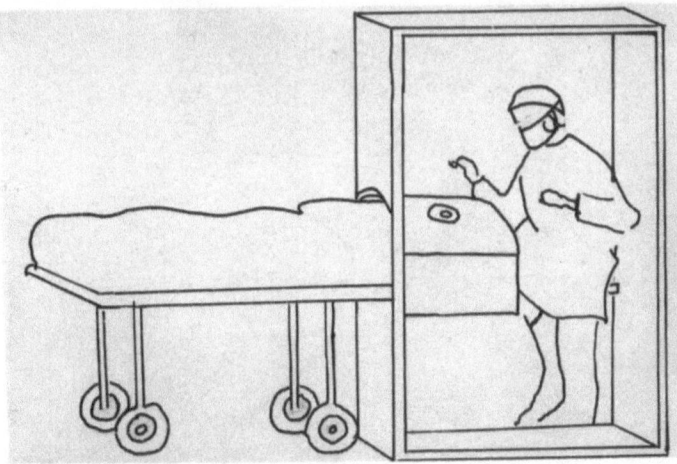

Fig. 1. Sketch of hyperbaric operating room. The anterior wall has a cubic recess in which the superior part of the patient's body is contained.

* This article was not in the program and it has been included as special discussion on vitreous loss prevention.

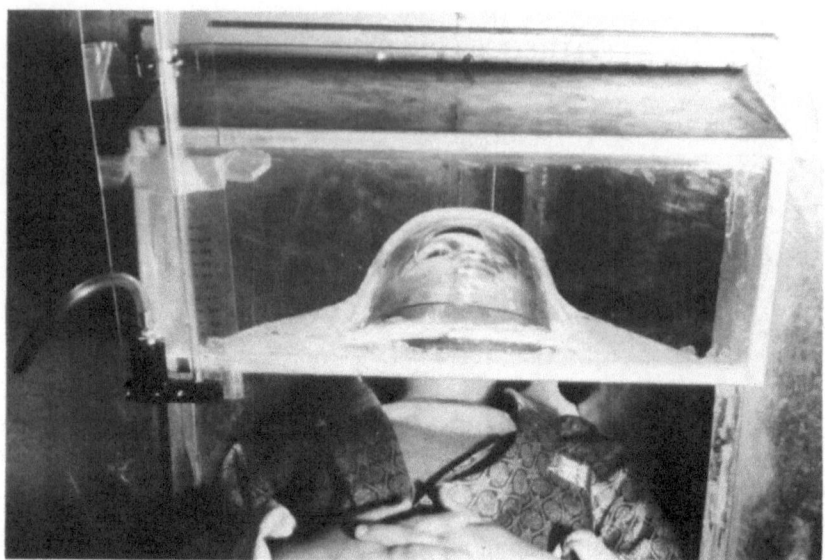

Fig. 2. **Detail from first** type of cabin to show the patient lying externally; his face is seen from the outside through the glass of the frontal wall of the cabin. This has a glassed box protruding from the inside of the frontal wall to allow more room for the surgeon's hands.

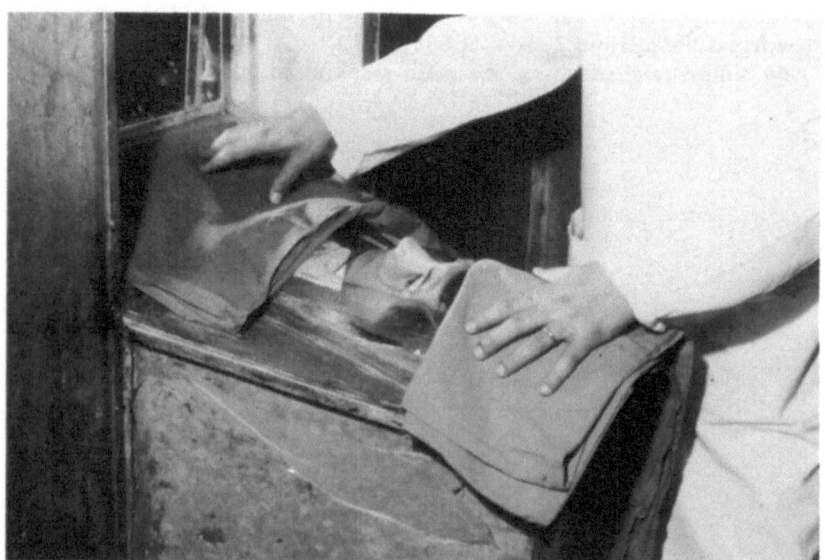

Fig. 3. **Same situation seen** from inside the cabin. The patient's face is seen through the transparent recess in the anterior wall of the cabin, which like a square funnel protrudes into the inside of the cabin. The patient's nose and left eye are engaged in the hole visible at the top of the funnel.

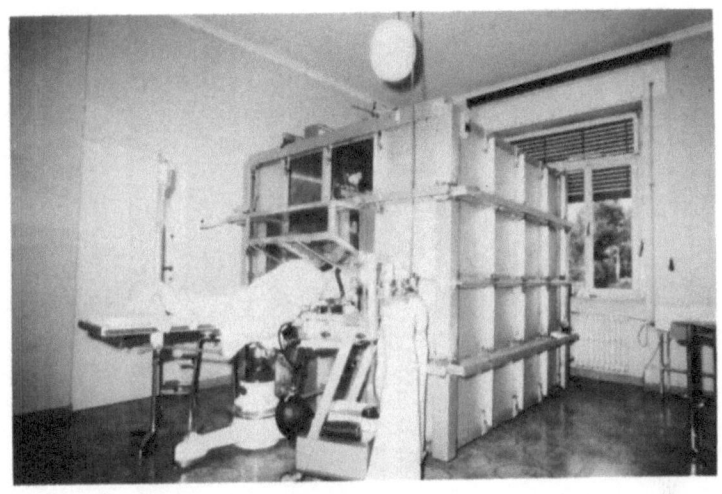

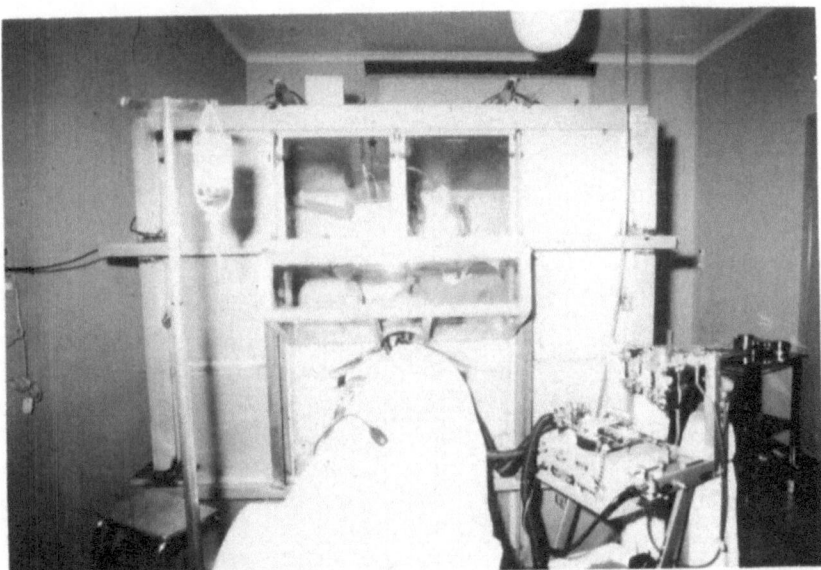

Fig. 4, 5. **Different** views of present type cabin, with the superior part of the anaesis-thetized patient in the funnel. The patient's face, with the breathing tube, is visible to the anaesthetist from the outside, and he has easy access to it.

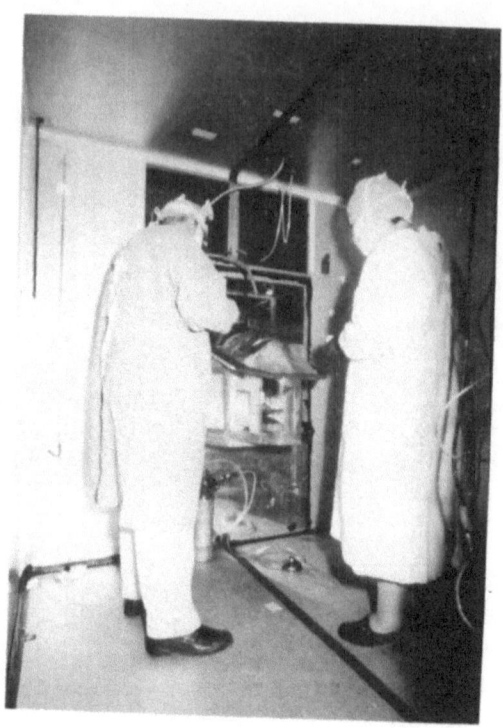

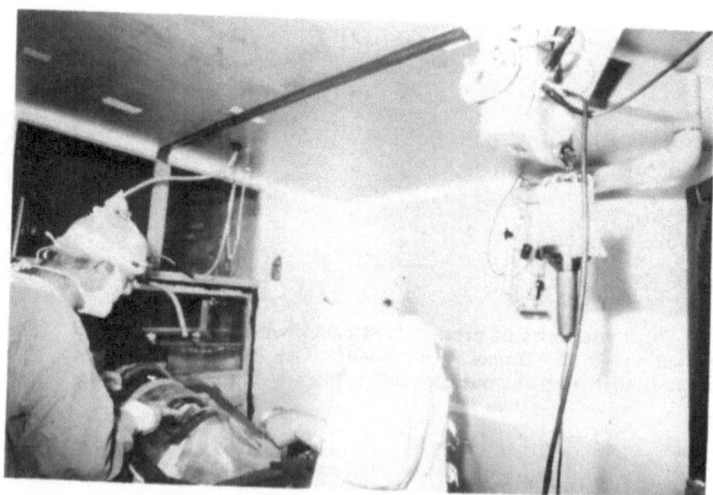

Fig. 6, 7. **Inside view. The transparent funnel and its superior wall with airproof plastic cover. The surgeon is sealing the rim of the patient's orbit to the hole in the cylindrical roof of the funnel.**

350

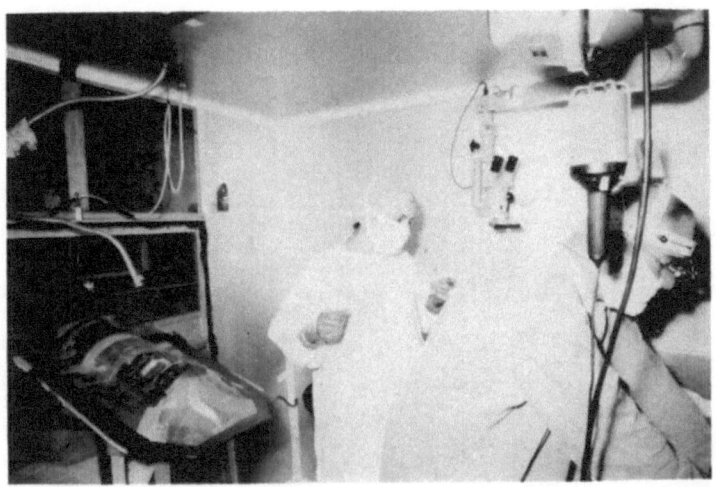

Fig. 8. Only the well-sealed orbit of the patient is exposed to the interior of the operating room. The surgeon has washed and wears gloves.

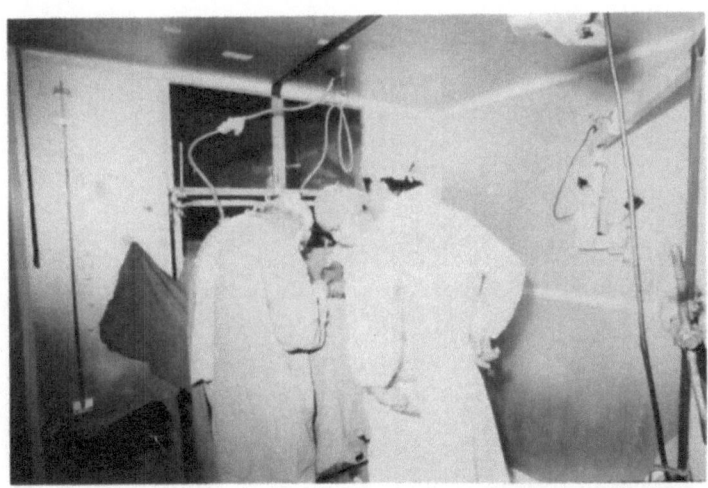

Fig. 9. The funnel is covered with a sterile cloth and the operation can begin.

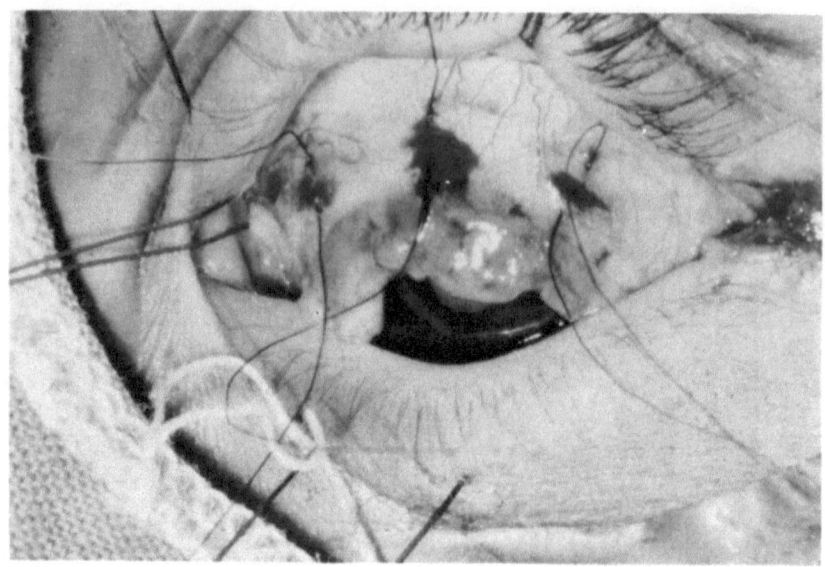

Fig. 10. Intracapsular cataract extraction in a baby of seven months. Three pre-placed stitches to ensure a perfect juxtaposition.

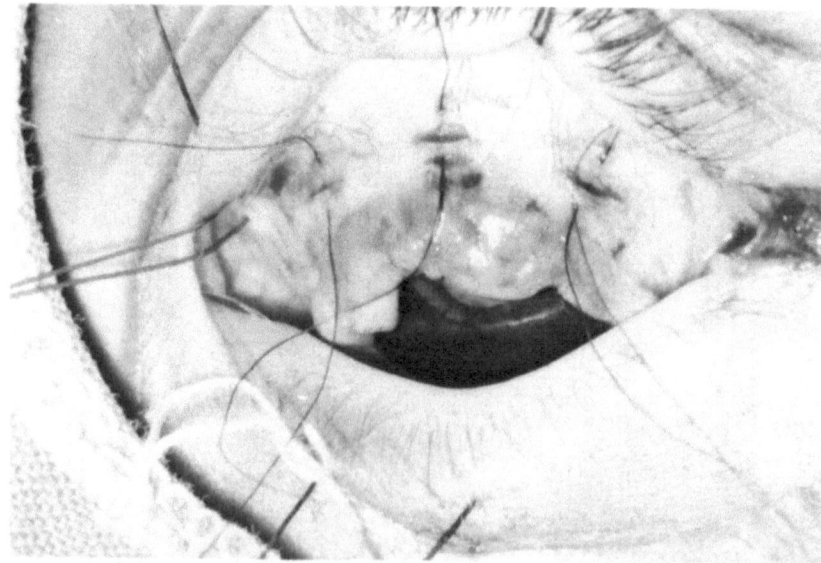

Fig. 11. Pressurisation has begun. Note the narrowing of the vessels: any bleeding is now impeded.

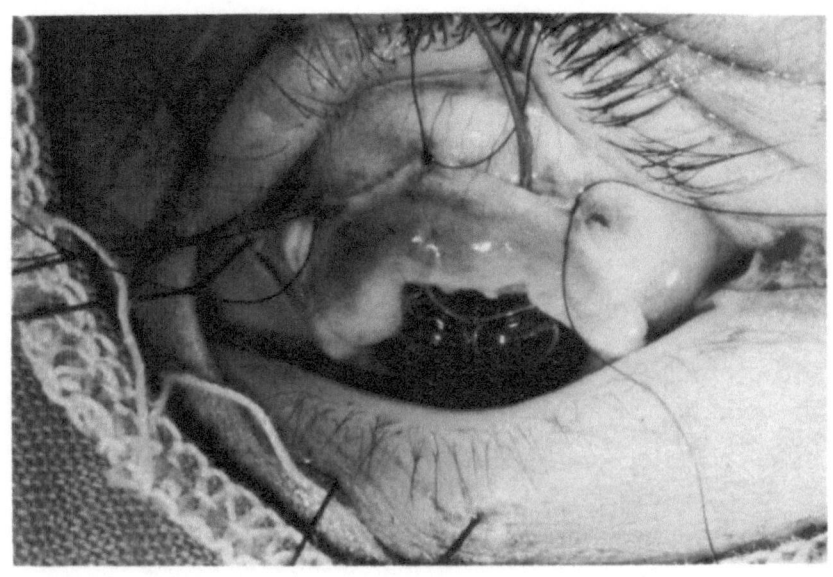

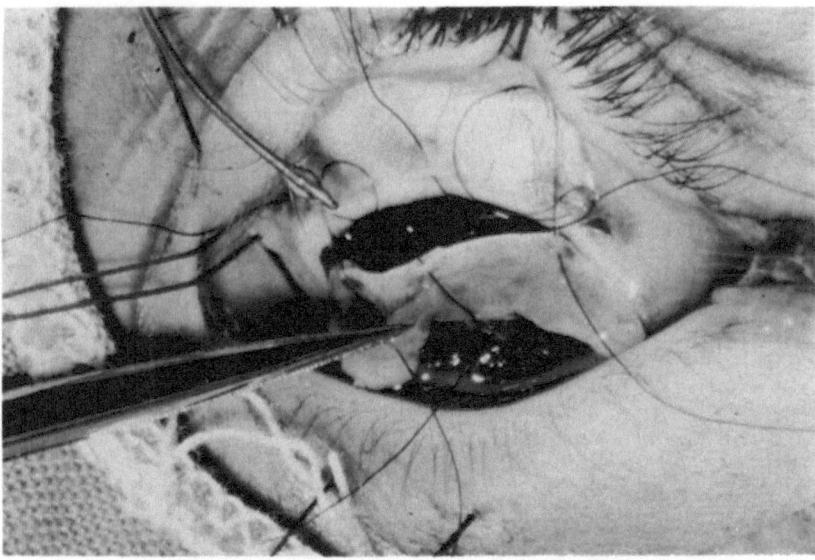

Fig. 12, 13. Opening of anterior chamber started and completed. Irrigation with enzyme. Note collapse of the eye.

353

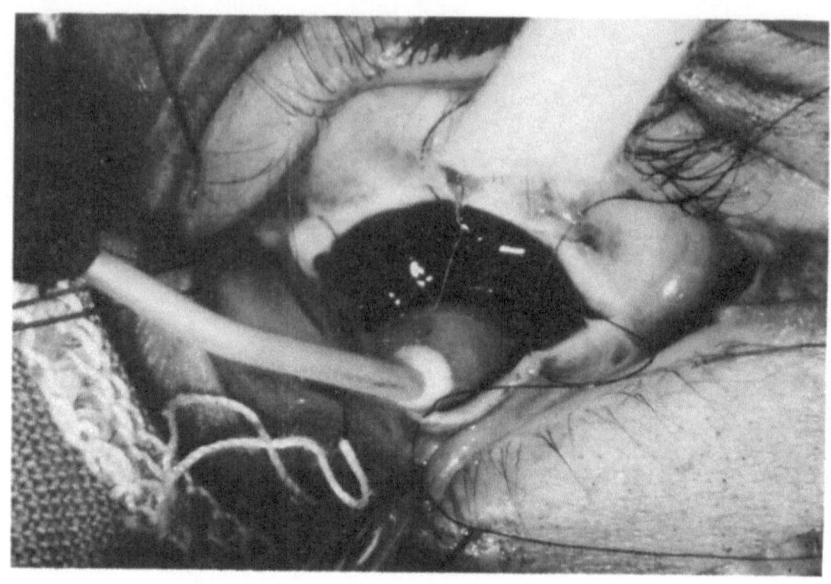

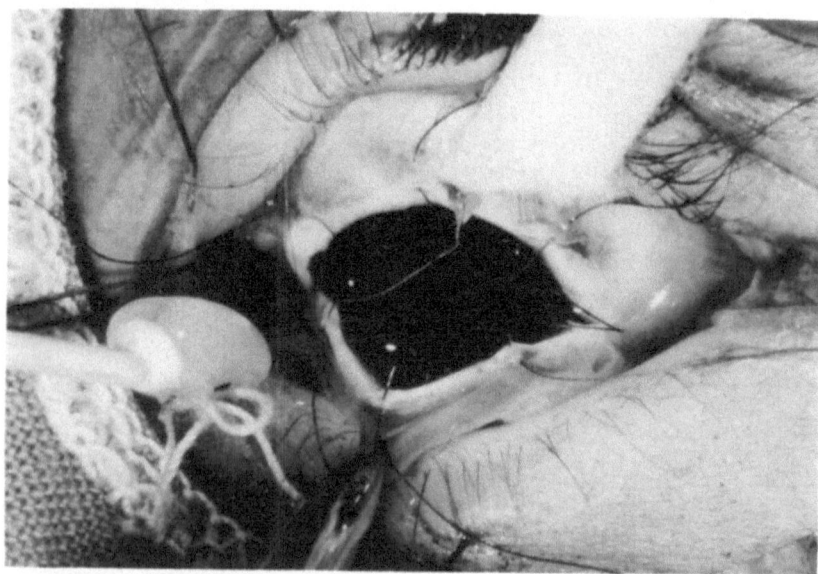

Fig. 14, 15. Unhurried cryo-extraction.

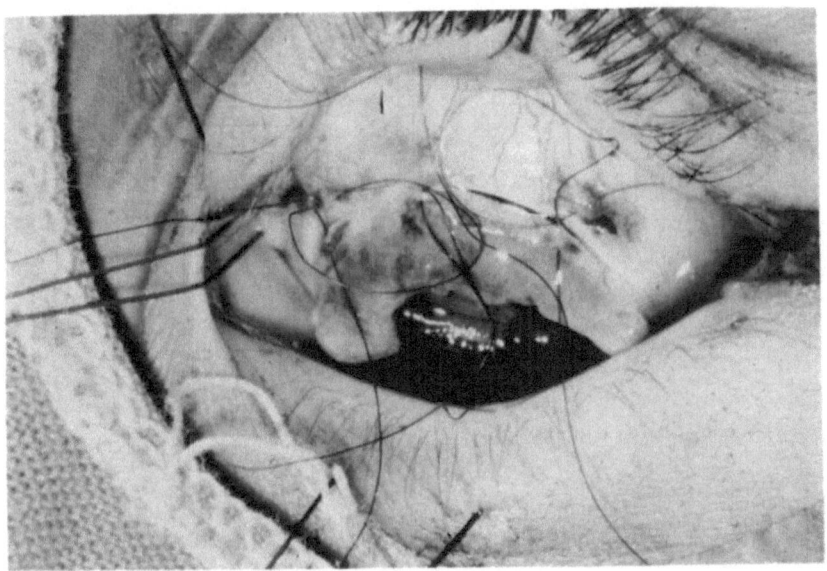

Fig. 16. Sutures tied and air injected into A.C.

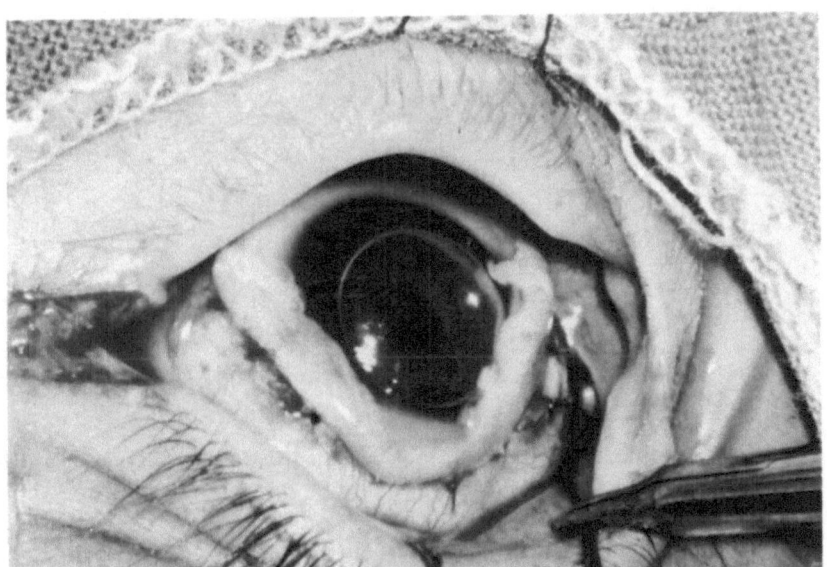

Fig. 17. Pressurisation stopped. Note immediate congestion of eye.

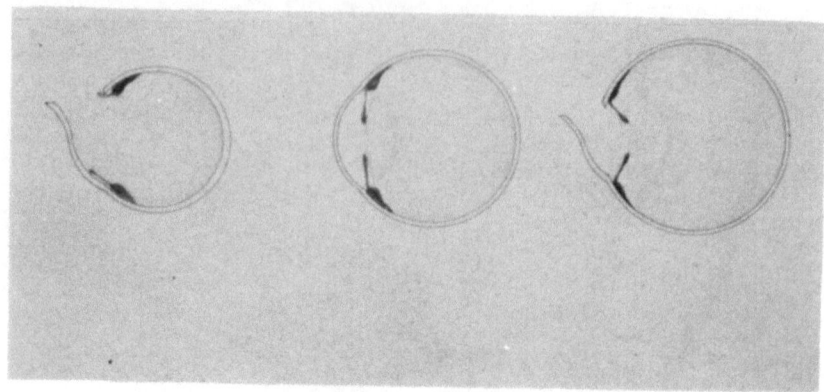

Fig. 18. The eye after lens extraction.

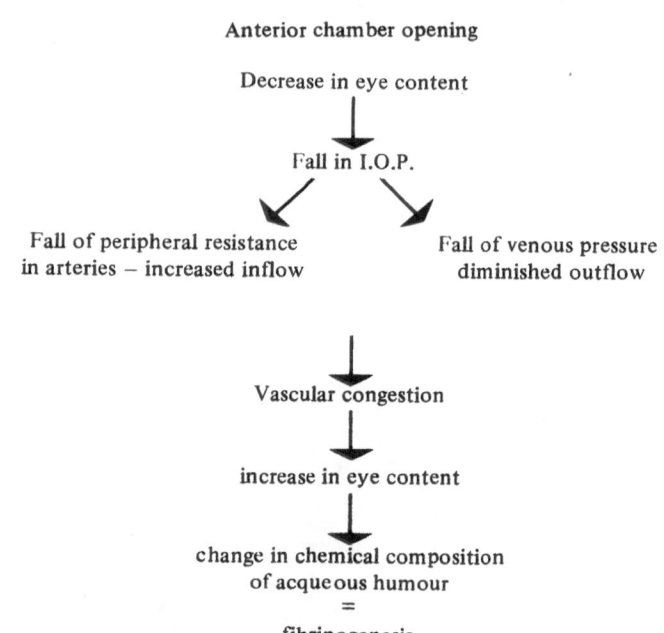

Anterior chamber opening

Decrease in eye content

Fall in I.O.P.

Fall of peripheral resistance
in arteries – increased inflow

Fall of venous pressure –
diminished outflow

Vascular congestion

increase in eye content

change in chemical composition
of acqueous humour
=
fibrinogenesis

Fig. 19. Consequences in the ocular blood circulation, when the eyeball is opened as in intraocular surgery.

356

performed in a baby of seven months. Previously, or during the operation, nothing is done to soften the eye or prevent vitreous loss. The pre-placed sutures only aim at a better juxtaposition of the wound margin and a cantotomy can be useful in small-sized patients.

This method offers two main advantages: a. Vitreous loss is rendered impossible; b. The opened eye will keep soft for any desired length of time.

I will briefly discuss these two points: a. Fig. 18 shows the eye after lens extraction. On the left the size of the eye is diminished at normal atmospheric pressure after the loss of A.C. content. On the right the size is increased at hyperbaric pressure.

In both cases the volume of the vitreous remains unchanged. Hyperbarism means a flow of air against the orbit and through the opened A.C. into the inside of the globe. Under this pressure the elastic scleral walls of a very young patient will expand leaving more room for the compact vitreous body. While the aqueous leaves the A.C. by capillarity the vitreous body, owing to its high superficial tension, will be pushed toward the 'cul de sac' of the enlarged scleral cavity.

In an elderly patient the inelastic sclera hardly feels the air pressure, but nevertheless more room is left for the comparatively smaller vitreous body. In fact, in the adult or myopic patient owing to some liquefaction of the vitreous, the balance of its two components (colloid gel and aqueous content) as a rule is altered and more aqueous will leave the eye under the air inflow. As a result the behaviour of the eye in hyperbarism will not show any significant difference with the age of the patient.

b. Fig. 19. Shows the consequences in the ocular blood circulation when the eyeball is opened as in intraocular surgery. The eyeball is already a miniature hyperbaric chamber and the intraocular tension is the gauge of this physiological hyperbarism. The blood vessels entering the eyeball have to balance the increased external pressure. As a consequence there is an increase in peripheral resistance in the arteries and an increased facility in the blood outflow through the very thin-walled intraocular veins. The sudden fall of I.O.P. at the operating table inverts the balance between intraocular pressure and blood pressure in both arteries and veins. As a consequence the arterial pressure will be too high for the decreased eye pressure and the pressure in the veins is too low to force the blood out of the eye. The final result is an increase in the blood content of the eye.

On the contrary, when surgery is performed in the hyperbaric room, the intraocular blood pressure seems unaffected by the opening of the eye (which shows no vascular congestion whatever) even in long-lasting procedures. It seems as if the intraocular vascular pressure remains constant in a leaking eye.

Two and a half years' eperience has convinced us to use the hyperbaric room routinely with great benefit to the patient and also to the surgeon'.

Author's address:
8 V. Latina
Rome
Italy

Docum. Ophthal. Proc. Series, Vol. 21

GENERAL AND LOCAL POST-OPERATIVE TREATMENT

F. PINTUCCI

(Rome, Italy)

In aphakic patients after operation, post-operative care varies with the *operating technique used, the conditions at the end of the operation* and *the patient's general condition.* Therapeutic possibilities are many; to limit the discussion, the author will describe only the treatment used on his own patients.

Before the operation in all the patients, an injection of 20 mg. of gentamycine is made into the inferior fornix.

At the end of the operation, the possibilities which may occur most frequently are:

1. miotic pupil
2. mydriatic pupil
3. blood in anterior chamber
4. cataract residue in anterior chamber
5. results of vitrectomy
6. air in anterior chamber

1. Miotic pupil.— If the pupil is miotic, the only treatment is an ointment with an association of antibiotics (tetracycline, chloramphenicol, colimycine, gentamycine), which is introduced into the conjunctival sac.

2. Mydriatic pupil.— If, in spite of the intra-operational introduction of acetylcoline the pupil is not in miosis, a 2% pilocarpine ointment is added to the antibiotics.

3. Blood in anterior chamber.— If at the end of the operation a hyphema remains in the anterior chamber, it is advisable to keep the patient in bed with the head in a raised position.

4. Cataract residue in anterior chamber.— Cataract residue increases post-operatory ciliary reaction, also because the surgeon has probably often performed various manoeuvres in the anterior chamber.

In these cases, intense miosis is avoided; an ointment with cortisone is added to the antibiotics.

5. Results of vitrectomy.— If during the operation a vitrectomy has been performed and it has been necessary to introduce air into the anterior chamber for diagnostic purposes or to keep the vitreous away from the cornea,

the patient's head is kept in a lowered position in order to avoid pupil blockage, and an attempt is made to obtain maximum miosis, adding, if necessary, 3% pilocarpine.

6. Air in anterior chamber.— It is usually advisable to avoid the introduction of air, since any foreign substance must be avoided as far as possible, and since it may cause pupil blockage. If the bubble is no greater than 3 mm. in diameter and is surrounded by aqueous humour, pupil blockage does not usually occur but it must be remembered that the diameter of the bubble varies with ocular pressure and that a small bubble, due to the forward displacement of the iris diaphragm, takes on the form of a meniscus with a much greater diameter (Fig. 1). Thus if there is a post-operative hypertension, if the coloboma of the iridectomy is small and if the patient is kept in a sitting position, there is flattening and upward displacement of the bubble, blockage of the pupil and of the iris coloboma. For this reason, on the patient's clinical chart must be indicated the positions in which the head and body are to be kept (Fig. 2). Four positions may be distinguished:

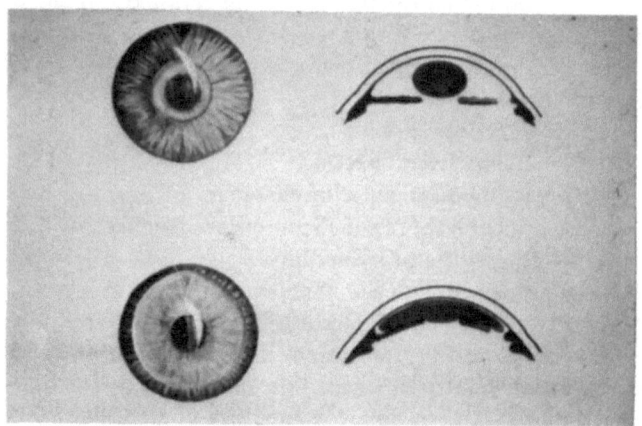

Fig. 1. See text.

Position 1   R.L.
Position 2   R.L.
Position 3   R.L.
Any position

DRESSING AND PATCHING

After having applied the ointment in the conjunctival sac and having closed the eye, a damp sterile patch, some cotton-tufts and a plastic (Fig. 3) shell attached with adhesive tape are placed on the eye. The unoperated eye is left unpatched but if the patient has been operated in both eyes, a bilateral occlusion is performed.

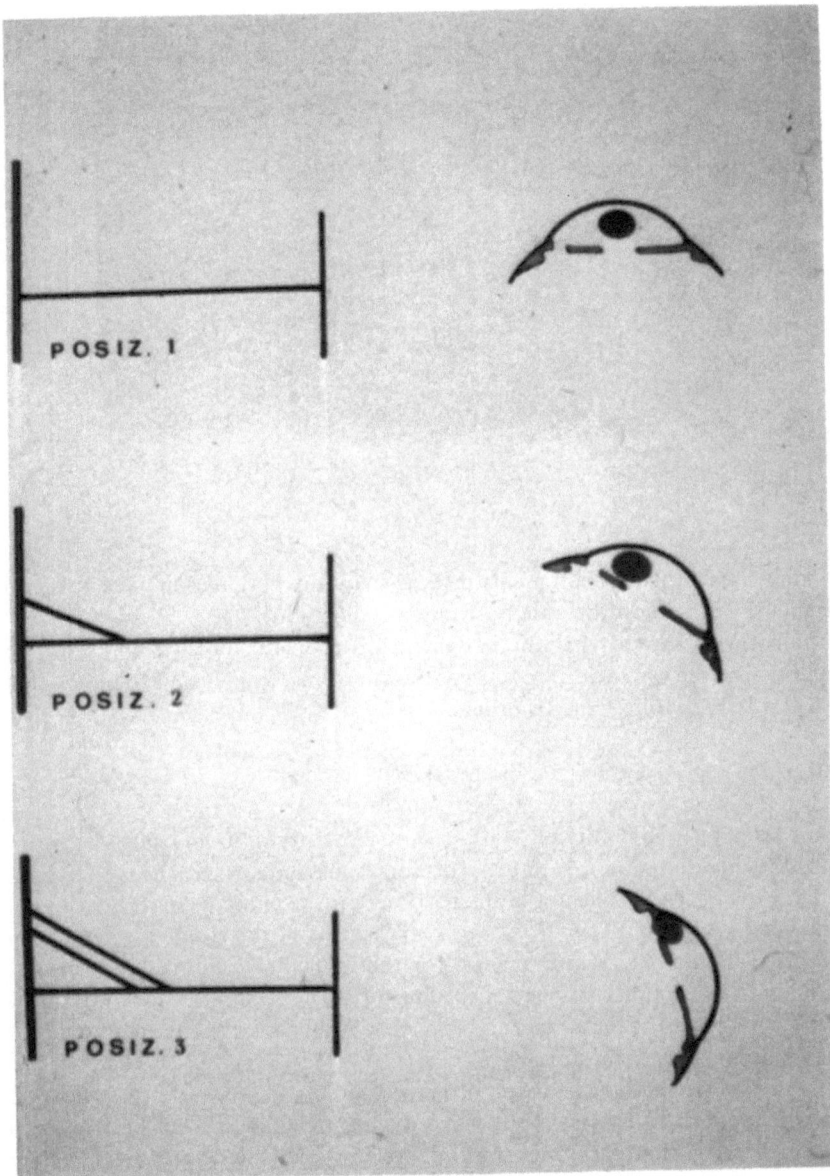

POSIZ. 1

POSIZ. 2

POSIZ. 3

Fig. 2. See text.

TRANSFERRAL TO BED

For transferral of the patient to bed, a canvas with handles may be used. The patient must be moved from the operating table by trained staff. The head must always be supported. The positions in which the head and body should

361

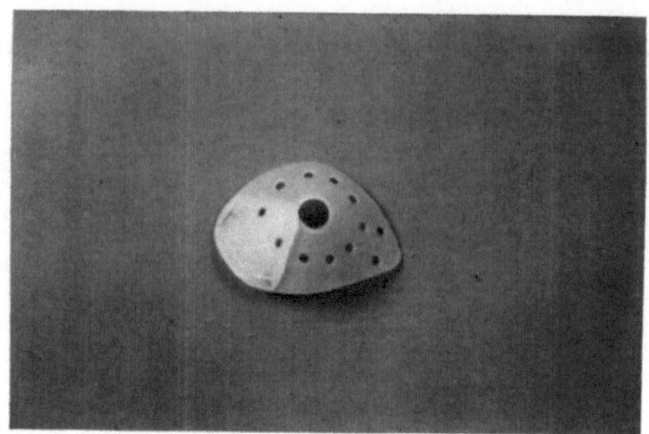

Fig. 3. See text.

be kept have already been mentioned. Usually the patient can be left free to assume the most comfortable position (any position).

The surgeon should visit the patient in his room to reassure him as to the outcome of the operation, to answer his questions, to give and to check that hospital staff is following his orders.

NURSING

The role played by nursing staff is quite important in the post-operative period. Once the patient is in bed, the nurse must remain until he is completely awake and must follow the instructions on the clinical chart. She should attach a bell to the patients pillow, keep lighting in the room dim, and keep out visitors so as to assure, at least for the first twelve hours, a useful rest.

Under these conditions, and also due to the continuing effects of aneasthesia, the patient falls asleep and spontaneously closes the unoperated eye, guaranteeing greater immobility.

As long as the patient is in bed, urination and defecation must be checked and the patient must be kept awake during the day so that he will sleep better at night. Patients with varicose veins should be given massage, dyspnoeics must receive oxygen and must be kept in a raised position, those with both eyes patched must be carefully aided during meals. The choice of diet must be made considering the patient's general conditions and must in any case be easily digestible food.

Before getting up, patients, especially older ones, should be kept in a sitting position for about one hour, then with the help of the nurse they may leave the bed and sit up in a chair. After 24—28 hours, if there are no complications, nursing assistance becomes less intense.

362

DRESSINGS

The first dressing is made after 24 hours. After instillation of anaesthetic drops, the eyeball is washed with a physiological solution, conjunctival secretion is removed with a damp, sterile cotton pad, and after examination of the anterior segment, a short examination of the fundus is made to see at least whether it illuminates in the various sectors. Ocular pressure is digitally carefully tested. Then an antibiotic ointment is used and, according to pupil diameter, atropine. The gauze, some cotton-tufts and the plastic shell are again applied and, if there are no complications, the patient is helped by a nurse to get up.

After 48 hours, for patients operated in both eyes, the shells are replaced by others (fig. 4) which are supplied with lenses for aphakia: in the rare cases of delirium due to occlusion, this may be anticipated. Once the eye is unpatched, of course, dressing is made with drops only, and is repeated in the evening if necessary.

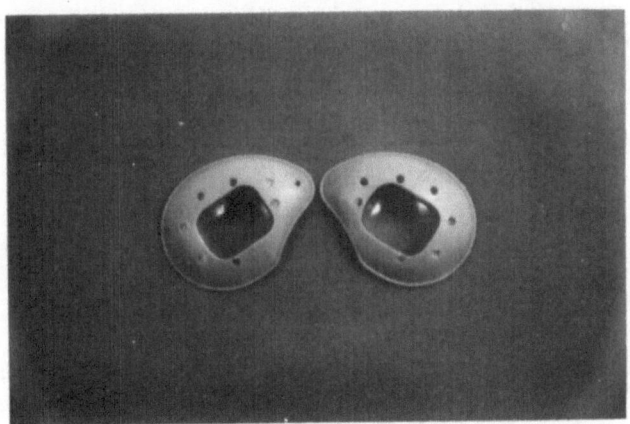

Fig. 4. See text.

GENERAL THERAPEUTICS

	Anaesthetic
General therapeutics	Internal
	Ocular

The general treatment must meet the needs of the anaesthesist, the internist and the surgeon; it should be decided by them together and should, as far as possible, bring together the various necessities in a polyvalent treatment in order to reduce drugs.

363

Anaesthetist	Intravenous physiological serum
	Intravenous glucose solution
	Antiemetics etc.

Immediately after the operation, the anaesthetist, in order to make up for loss of liquids caused by diuretics, may give intravenous physiological or glucose serums, or, if there is a tendency to vomit, anti-emetics.

Internist	Respiratory drugs
	Cardiocirculatory drugs
	Antidysmetabolic drugs
	Analgesics, tranquillizers, soporifics.

The internist, according to the patient's general condition and the therapeutics given before the operation, will continue those treatments which are suitable to the case or decide any new treatment which may be necessary.

Usually, treatment is composed by drugs for respiratory apparatus, cardiocirculatory apparatus and for metabolic diseases. In anxious patients or those suffering from insomnia, analgesics, tranquillizers and soporifics may be added.

Ophthalmologist	Diuretics
	Vasoprotectors, coagulants

The general treatment of strictly ocular relevance regards Diamox, vasoprotectors and coagulants. Diuretics: in patients operated for cataract, a dosage electrolytes (Na and K) is made, as this is useful for the aneasthesia and for the dosage of diuretics to be given before and after the operation. In normal conditions, oral supply of Diamox should be continued for 3—4 days and, if there have been oscillations in pressure, should be continued also at home. Vasoprotectors-coagulants: if the haemogenic tests are normal, coagulants and vasoprotectors are not usually given pre-and post-operatively.

Using the keratotome, the vertical incision affects only slightly the vascularized tissues of the limbus and in any case, as the anterior chamber is closed, the blood cannot penetrate and there is plenty of time to perform a careful haemostasis (fig. 5). The horizontal part of the incision is parallel to the iris, well within the corneal tissue. For this reason, hyphaemas dependant on the opening of the anterior chamber are usually not present.

Great importance must be given to the iris, which should be studied carefully. As a general rule, coagulants and vasoprotectors should be given pre- and postoperatively to diabetic patients, those with heterochromic cataracts or with post-inflammatory cataracts or post-operative hyphema.

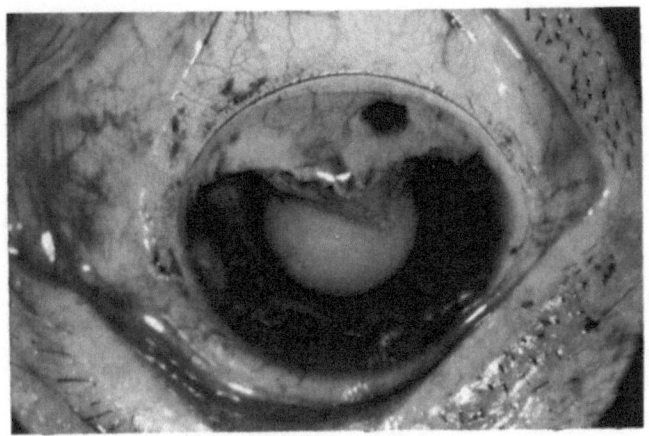

Fig. 5.

DISMISSION FROM HOSPITAL: CLINICAL CHECK-UP, LENS PRESCRIPTION

The safety offered by new suturing materials and the precision of manoeuvre made possible by the use of the microscope allow progressive reduction of hospitalization; however, it must be remembered that several weeks are necessary to obtain wound closure. Thus it is essential to respect a few basic rules, such as leading a very quiet life for ten or twelve days, avoiding strain and any trauma to the eyeball. If the patient is well aware of these necessities, does not live far from the hospital and has a good nursing care at home, hospitalization may be reduced to a minimum; but as all these conditions are only rarely present, patients are usually dismissed on the third or fourth day, or in the lack of assistance at home, even on the seventh or eight day.

After biomicroscopic examination of the anterior segment, of the ocular pressure, of the fundus and visual acuity, the patient is dismissed with prescriptions of atropine and an association of antibiotics and cortisone drops and of any drugs needed by his general health, as well as some instructions written on the dismissal form. If ocular pressure is at the limits of normality, also diamox is prescribed.

It is advisable to use the plastic shell for the first seven days, and at night only, for another seven days. Patients operated bilaterally for cataract are dismissed with shells with lenses and are advised to use them for 10—15 days until temporary glasses are prescribed.

Author's address:
Primario Ospedale Oftalmico
Via Bertoloni, 37
Rome
Italy

Docum. Ophthal. Proc. Series, Vol. 21

INFLAMMATORY COMPLICATION

FUMIO KOGURE

(Tokyo, Japan)

INTRODUCTION

Frequency of severe postoperative intraocular inflammation is diminishing owing to the application of the operation-microscope, improvement of operative apparatus and suturing materials, the progress of operative technique, sterilization and disinfection, and the development of antibiotics and steroids. However, if severe intraocular inflammation occurs, it is hardly controlled today even with antibiotics or steroids, and sometimes brings forth a miserable result: thus, postoperative complications continue, against which surgeons cannot be off their guard.

MATERIAL AND METHODS

We have experienced 9 cases of remarkable postoperative inflammation out of 1606 eyes subjected to cataract surgery during 5 years (1971—1975) in our clinic.

Prophylaxis and postoperative cares

In cases having inflammation in the anterior segment prior to operation, they were of course treated beforehand. The culture for bacteria from the conjunctival cul-de-sac was not performed in all cases generally, but performed in the cases in which it seemed to be necessary. For 4 or 5 days before the operation antibiotic eyedrops were instilled 5 times a day; from the day before the operation antibiotics were given systemically, routinely 5 days. Immediately after the operation antibiotics and steroids were injected subconjunctivally. From the next day after the operation, antibiotics and steroid ointment or eyedrops were instilled successively for about 2 weeks, 5 times a day.

Case 1: A 65-year-old female. One month after the operation, she complained of eye pain; increase of flare and cells in the anterior chamber were seen. An opaque mass which indicated proliferation of yellowish white spherical fungi having projections in the vitreous body was observed. The aqueous humor was taken and examined bacteriologically, but the result was negative. The patient was treated with antibiotics and steroids, but it was ineffective. During the open-sky vitrectomy expulsive hemmorrhage occurred, then ex-

367

centeration bulbi was performed. In the vitreous body resected during the operation, fungi were observed.

Case 2: A 67-year-old female. Extracapsular extraction was done as the capsule was ruptured. After the operation iridocyclitis appeared and she was diagnosed to have phacoanaphylactic endophthalmitis and treated with antibiotics and steroids, but recurrent hypopyon and eye pain appeared repeatedly. From the appearance of the process, the presence of the fungi was doubted, 3 months after the operation the aqueous humor was cultured, but fungi were not proven. However, one year later fungi were detected from keratic precipitates in another hospital.

Case 3: A 67-year-old female. Two days after the operation circumcorneal flush was remarkable, corneal abscess with hypopyon occured. Four days after the operation, the anterior chamber was irrigated with Sulbenicillin and Gentamycin. After this, the inflammation was improved, but the visual acuity was very poor.

Case 4: A 74-year-old female. Seven days after the operation eye pain and hypopyon appeared, and a yellowish white membrous mass was observed in the vitreous body. The anterior chamber was irrigated with Sulbenicillin and Gentamycin, the result of the bacteriological examination performed simultaneously was negative. The tendency of phthisis bulbi remained.

Case 5: A 73-year-old female. 3 months after extracapsular extraction, she had severe circumcorneal flush and elevated intraocular tension. Simultaneously, flare and cells in the anterior chamber were observed in the contralateral eye. Systemic and local administration of steroids improved the inflammation of the operated eye, but inflammation of the other eye was severe and intraocular tension remained high. The intraocular tension was controlled by trabeculectomy and iridocycloretraction.

Case 6. 7, and 8: A 68-year-old male, a 62-year-old female, and a 63-year-old female. In these cases the postoperative inflammation was very severe, and 6 days after the operation, a white thread-like material which seemed to be gauze fiber was found in the pupil zone by slit lamp examination. In all cases, the inflammatory condition could be controlled by systemic and local treatment with steroids. The thread-like material did not change.

Case 9: A 62-year-old female. Intracapsular extraction was performed in both eyes, immediately after removal of the sutures blurred vision appeared in left eye. The circumcorneal flush was remarkable, and the fibreous anterior opacities were observed, the fundus could not be seen. Then, iridocyclitis appeared recurrently, and white mass was found to be produced on the iris surface. In the vitreous body, bead-like opacities which seemed to be connected to the white mass were observed (through the iris). Systemic steroids therapy produced no response. The serum of this patient reacted on the specimen of a normal human retina by the indirect fluorescent antibody technique, and a specific fluorescence was seen in the outer segment of visual cells.

The pathogenesis of the above-described 9 cases was attributed as follows: fungi in Case 1 and 2, bacteria in Case 3 and 4, sympathetic ophthalmia in Case 5, and foreign bodies in Case 6, 7 and 8. In case 9 a severe destruction of retina and uvea resulted from severe recurrent inflammation and vitreous opacities.

TABLE 1. Nine cases of remarkable postoperative inflammation.

Case	Complication	Onset	Cause
1	(−)	31 days	Fungus
2	Capsule rupture	3 months	Fungus
3	(−)	2 days	Bacteria?
4	Capsule rupture	7 days	Bacteria?
5	(−)	3 months	Exciting eye (Sympathetic ophthalmia)
6	(−)	6 days	Foreign body
7	Vitreous loss	6 days	Foreign body
8	(−)	6 days	Foreign body
9	(−)	2 months	Unknown

DISCUSSION

Endophthalmitis after cataract operation was seen in about 10% at the end of the 19th century. It was reduced to about 1% due to the development of sterilization, and due to development of antibiotics the rate was further reduced by 0.2% on an average, from 0.079% reported by Locather-Khorazo (1956) to 0.7% by Neveu (1972). In Japan, Inatomi and Shimizu (1973) reported 0.5%, 0.3% respectively. In our study the patients attacked by bacteria and fungi were 0.25%.

Antibiotics have been playing a great role in the reduction of the post-operative infection rate, but in these days the side effects and the reduction of effect of antibiotics bring forth some problems because of widespread administration of various antibiotics.

According to Fujii et al. (1972), the annual consumption of the main antibiotics such as chloramphenicol, penicillin and tetracycline in Japan was about 50 tons respectively in 1966. In 1974 the consumption greatly increased to 190 tons of chloramphenicol, about 185 tons of tetracycline, and 145 tons of penicillin: cephalosporin also tends to be used more. As the result of this large consumption of antibiotics, there occur some problems such as drug resistance and colonization. However, the surgeons have to use antibiotics and steroids for prevention of postoperative inflammation and control of inflammation, and in fact, reduction of the infection rate is proved as described previously. It is recommended to perform multi-drug systemic and local therapies with high concentrations of the drugs which have wide antibacterial spectra and are transferred well into eyes, since inflammation may not be controlled by some drugs, if they are given after identifying the pathogenic germs. However, antibiotics are not always completely effective and it is very difficult to control completely the intraocular germs. It is more important to kill the germs so as to prevent entrance to eyes before operation than to treat them after they have entered eyes, as Allen (1975) states. For this purpose, care must be taken to sterilize well the operation field, the operation devices and the fingers and hands of surgeons before the operation, as well as preoperative administration of antibiotics. Though Allen states that 48-hours eyedrops and ointment treatment before the operation is adequate, in our clinic we only use eyedrops 5 days before the operation. It is also recommended to give antibiotics systemically before the operation so as to get an effective blood level of antibiotics prior to the time when germs can enter the eye.

Myotic endophthalmitis is an important problem at present when large amounts of antibiotics and steroids are used. The features of fungal infections after cataract surgery are: (1961) (1) long latent period to the onset, (2) eye pain and scleral hyperaemia, (3) cells in the anterior chamber, (4) hypopyon, (5) grayish white cells in the anterior vitreous adjacent to the pupillary edge, and (6) good light perception. In Case 1 and 2 the result of culturing the aqueous humor was negative, but germs were detected from the focus in the vitreous body and deposits on the posterior surface of corcea. This indicates that for early diagnosis and early therapy detection of fungi by resection of the vitreous body as well as the examination of aqueous humor serves to achieve a high fungus detection rate and effective therapy.

In Case 1 and 2 the latent period of the onset of the fungal infection was as long as 31 days and 3 months, and thus it is a question whether infection occurred during the operation or after it. According to Miura's (1973) report the term ranged from 2 days to 1 year. Though there is a possibility of postoperative infection, infection occurs during the operation in most cases.

The possible infecting causes are: (1) air-infection (splashes from breathing of surgeons and patients, air conditioning), (2) contamination of drugs used (saline for anterior chamber irrigation, α-chymotrypsin and eyedrops), (3) incomplete sterilization of instruments and suturing materials, and (4) incomplete sterilization of fingers and hands of surgeons and the operation field. In the cases reported here, as factors increasing the infection rate can be mentioned vitreous loss, prolongation of the operation time, and poor operation technique, though the infection causes are unknown.

For preventing introduction of foreign matter into the anterior chamber during the operation, it is important to take care in handling gauze, medical absorber, and suture threads, and to use millipore filtration for saline injection into the anterior chamber. For preventing postoperative intraocular inflammation, sufficient and adequate preoperative administration of antibiotics, the clean environment in the operation room, asepsis of drugs to be used in the operation, exact and atraumatic operation technique and methods are effective. For adequate therapy for the postoperative intraocular inflammation, daily and careful observation through a slit lamp is necessary from an early stage after the operation.

Case 9 showed severe recurrent inflammation and vitreous opacities, and the indirect fluorescent antibody technique suggested the presence of anti-retina antibody. Matsuo (1978) reported that he recognized outer segment visual cells in the aqueous humor in severe uveitis resistant to steroids, the cause of which was unknown. It is supposed that cataract surgery or rapid physical change in an eye affects the retina to cause immunological response to the retinal outer segment haveing strong antigenicity. It is reasonably supposed form Nakayama's (1978) report that anti outer segment antibody was observed in Guinea pigs in which autoimmune uveo-retinitis was experimentally induced by their own retinal antigen. In this case in our study the anti-outer-segment antibody was seen by the indirect fluorescent antibody technique, but the genetic mechanism was not revealed.

As other pathogenetic factors for postoperative inflammation there may be considered secondary glaucoma, vitreous loss, epithelial downgrowth and the like, but in this study the intraocular inflammation caused by these factors were excluded because it was induced by complications during the operation.

CONCLUSION

Nine cases of severe postoperative intraocular inflammation are reported here out of 1606 eyes subjected to cataract surgery during 5 years. The pathogenetic cause was fungi in 2 cases, bacteria in 2 cases, foreign matter in 3 cases, and exciting eye of sympathetic ophthalmia in 1 case. It was unknown in 1 case in which immune response to retina was observed and it was supposed to be a cause for inflammation: it will have to be considered in the future study.

REFERENCES

Allen, H.F.: Highlights of ophthalmology, Vol. XIV: 136–144, 1975.

Fujii, Y.: Chemotherapy., 25: 418–423, 1977.

Inatomi, M., et al: Complications following cataract surgery a nine-year survey. Jpn. J. Clin. Ophthalmol., 26: 563–570, 1972.

Locather-Khorazo, D., and Gutierrex, E.: Eye infections following cataract extraction, with special reference to the role of staphylococcus aureus. Amer. J. Ophthal., 41: 981–987, 1956.

Matuo, N.: Personal communication. Folia Ophthalmologica Japonica., 29: 464, 1978.

Miura, O.: On the ocular mycosis. Ophthalmology., 15: 101–112, 1973.

Nakayama, S.: Studies on auto-antibody of experimental autoimmune uveo-retinitis in guinea pig sensitized with autologous retinal extract. Folia Ophthalmologica Japonica. 29: 456–464, 1978.

Neveu, M., and Elliot, A.J.: Prophylaxis and treatment of endophthalmitis. Amer. J. Ophthal., 48: 368–373, 1959.

Shimizu, H., et al: Cataract surgery under the microscope. Results and problems in 300 eyes. Jpn. J. Clin. Ophthalmol., 27: 501–507, 1973.

Theodore, F.H.,: The diagnosis and management of fungus endophthalmitis following cataract extraction. Arch. Ophthal., 66: 163–175, 1961.

Author's address:
Tokyo Medical College Hospital
6–7–1 Nishishinjuku, Shinjuku-ku
Tokyo, Japan

Docum. Ophthal. Proc. Series, Vol. 21

BLEEDING AND ITS CONTROL

W. POCKLEY

(Sydney, Australia)

Bleeding is generally not a serious problem during routine cataract surgery. It may, however, range from being little more than a transitory nuisance, to the ultimate calamity of expulsive haemorrhage, and the latent potential of bleeding should never be forgotten.

It is not common practice in Australia to carry out routine pre-operative haematological investigations, but of course such should be done if there is anything to suggest an haemorrhagic diathesis. We rely more on the attendant physician to assess the patient and to report upon the general cardio-vascular state, but one would always be happier to have reassurance as to the blood picture where the history or clinical appraisement suggests the abnormal. In such circumstances, and as far as is practical, prudence dictates that surgery should wait until an acceptable blood picture has been confirmed. In this regard the widespread use of anti-coagulant therapy in coronary disease has created a situation where extreme care should be exercised.

If local anaesthesia is used, sooner or later the frustration of an immediate orbital haematoma from retrobulbar injection will arise. There is no way of avoiding this occasional mishap, but gentle insertion of a fine needle, with not too sharp a tip, together with slow delivery of the anaesthetic solution, is important in minimising the risk. If it occurs, operation should be postponed, since the extravasated blood raises intra-ocular pressure and makes it dangerous to open the eye. I was once an observer when it was decided to proceed with the contemplated surgery on the assumption that the orbital haemorrhage was not excessive. The consequences were unfortunate indeed. Vitreous presented as the section was made. The lens dislocated spontaneously and then fell back, necessitating vectis removal. The eye was subsequently, but unsuccessfully operated for detachment. Therefore, if ever frank or even suspected retro-bulbar haemorrhage ensues, surgery should be deferred.

If one is forced to operate in the presence of a blood disorder, a purely corneal section at least eliminates the hazard of bleeding from conjunctiva or sclera. Blood from a conventional corneo-scleral section in the average case can always be controlled by cautery or alternative means, and it is highly desirable that it should not ooze into the anterior chamber. When it does so in any quantity, details are obscured, and this in turn necessitates the minor, but preferably avoidable, and otherwise probably unnecessary insult of lavage.

Haemorrhage from the iris is always a contingency, and especially so in diabetics, where there may be rubeosis. Gonioscopy prior to admission is important in prevention (and therefore in control), because, if there are obvious vessels at or near the iris root, it may be possible to site the iridectomy so as to avoid them. If blood does flow into the anterior chamber from either of these routes, and if details are obscured, it should be washed out. This is always preferable to a poor view, for, as Amsler once remarked to me when just this situation arose, "ophthalmic surgery can be difficult enough when you can see what you are doing, and it should never be allowed to become more so by blood which can be removed". It is only rarely that haemorrhage from the iris persists at this surgical stage, but when it does, irrigation is the only course to pursue.

This brings me to the major catastrophe of expulsive haemorrhage. There is no certain way to eliminate this ultimate calamity, which happily is rare — and becoming more so, I believe, through improved pre-operative management and better surgical techniques. But the potential for disaster is always present. The crisis usually occurs at an early stage of extraction, soon after the anterior chamber has been opened, but it may happen at any time, and it has been known to commence towards the end of a long operation. It is generally thought to stem from rupture of a diseased choroidal or retinal vessel. The long posterior ciliary artery has also been implicated, as have the proliferating vessels of glycosuric retinopathy. The bleed is thought to be a response to the sudden loss of supporting intra-ocular pressure consequent upon opening the anterior chamber, and whilst this must be the usual precipitating factor, sudden haemorrhage after prolonged surgery suggests that it is not the only one. Be that as it may, if intra-ocular pressure could be maintained throughout operation, the risk of disaster would, without doubt, be enormously reduced. But I suggest that after aqueous escapes, another material consideration is that movement anteriorly of lens and vitreous may well be instrumental in leading to tearing of vitreo-retinal adhesions, with consequent free and sometimes massive haemorrhage. Prevention (and again, in consequence, control) of this whole complex of factors should involve the pre-operative reduction of high blood pressure, and avoidance of anoxia during general anaesthesia, which latter leads to a rise in intra-ocular pressure, associated with a dangerous, bounding pulse. In suspect cases the use of Diamox, and of mannitol or urea, in order to lessen the pressure differential, which inevitably ensues as the A.C. is opened, is also a rational and worth while prophylactic expedient. The risk is also diminished by very gradual commencement of the section, so that escape of aqueous is slow rather than abrupt. As well, gentle extraction of the lens, desirable on all counts, lessens the risk of vessel rupture from precipitous drag on vitreous adhesions and retinal vessels. All these measures, single or together, assist in prevention, and lessen, but never entirely eliminate the basic hazard.

A massive bleed may present suddenly and without warning, but more commonly is foreshadowed by a gradual and sinister sequence of events

374

— e.g. change of corneal reflex, often due to fine, horizontal folds; forward movement of the iris; slow, but relentless gaping of the section; copious vitreous loss; spontaneous dislocation of the lens, if this has not already been delivered; and finally by profuse, and generally bright arterial blood. In the worst cases the retina and uveal tissue may also present, avulsed from their natural positions by the vis a tergo of excaping blood.

In the even, prompt action is mandatory if the eye is to be saved. Immediate stab incisions in one or both inferior quadrants of the globe should be made with a Graefe knife or alternate instrument, in order to allow blood to escape from where it has collected near the point of haemorrhage, and before there is extrusion of the entire contents of the globe. This emergency action, followed in proper time by meticulous wound toilet, offers the only chance of saving the eye as a useful organ of sight.

Expulsive haemorrhage has been known to occur, even as long as several days after surgery, but this is extremely rare. The most frequent problem subsequent to surgery is hyphema, which may present at the first dressing, or not until some days later. Firm and accurate wound closure with multiple sutures is certainly the most effective single factor in the prevention of solitary or repeated post-operative bleeding. The blood usually absorbs, sometimes rapidly, sometimes gradually, but progressively. Provided the vitreous face has remained intact, it need not cause real concern, except when it is accompanied by a rise in intra-ocular tension. The worry then is that it may lead to bloodstaining of the cornea. This is relatively infrequent, and unless it threatens, the right initial approach is an expectant one to allow the blood to clear spontaneously. However, if the cornea is at risk from haematic infiltration, or if there is fear that the wound may give way, evacuation through one or more limbal incisions should be undertaken. If the blood is fluid it may be washed out; if it has clotted, it is often possible to remove it dramatically, and more or less intact, by sliding it out on a vectis or wire loop, or with the aid of small clot forceps. It should be borne in mind, nevertheless, that whenever there is blood in the anterior chamber, the integrity of the hyaloid face is critical, since absorption of intra-vitreal blood is likely to be slow, and may take many weeks or months, or even be delayed indefinitely.

Recurrent haemorrhage into the anterior chamber is a much more challenging situation. The site of the leak usually remains hypothetical, but it probably comes from the posterior lip of the section, and less often from the iris. It can prove to be a most frustrating complication both for patient and surgeon; to the former because it necessitates prolonged hospitalisation, and to the latter because there is little really positive that can be done to relieve the condition. The picture is that of an anterior chamber, partially or even completely full of blood, fluid or semi-solid, which may clear to a greater or lesser extent, showing varying blood levels from day to day, due to fresh bleeds at irregular intervals. Although some advise early, active intervention to evacuate the blood, I incline to be more conservative. If there is concern because of raised tensions, Diamox should be given. High doses of Vitamins C and K are also held by some to be helpful. Premarin, a preparation of conjugated oestrogenic substances, is claimed to be useful in the control of bleeding from various sites, including hyphaema. It may be given intravenously at operation and continued afterwards by mouth. I was inclined to try this therapy for recurrent hyphaema not so long ago, but was discouraged by comment from the Haematology Department, and I would be interested to know if others here have had experience with this drug. Opinion is often divided about the use of mydriatics or miotics, but there is more unanimity as to the value of bed rest and double padding, and of course, the blood picture should be thoroughly assessed. Although it is tempting when all else fails to try tapping the A.C., with or without lavage, unless the problem of an high intra-ocular tension arises, in just about all these cases the bleeding will ultimately cease spontaneously, and the blood will absorb without having caused permanent damage.

The last complication to be canvassed is that of persistent, organized blood clot on the vitreous face or in the vitreous substance. The degree and rate of resolution of such blood is always unpredictable, but again emphasis should be towards conservatism. I recall one case in which there was a massive bleed early in the post-operative period, which reduced vision to little more than light perception for upwards of two years, but then, within a period of a few weeks, the blood absorbed entirely, and the eye regained and has retained normal vision. The patient attributed this dramatic cure to an high intake of raw carrot juice, but a similar diet has not, I am sorry to say, confirmed this as an effective form of therapy. If vitreous blood persists, in the absence of other evident or presumed pathology, and if it is sufficient to preclude useful sight, vitrectomy, either through the anterior or pars plana approach, carried out by someone with the necessary skill and experience, is now a viable procedure, which may restore sight otherwise irretrievably lost.

Author's address:
187 Macquarie Street
Sydney 2000
Australia

TREATMENT OF LIMBIC FISTULE AND EPITHELIAL INVASION OF ANTERIOR CHAMBER AFTER CATARACT EXTRACTION

M. BONNET

(Lyon, France)

Twenty years ago, limbic fistule were a frequent complication of cataract extraction and epithelial invasion, which was rarer but by no means exceptional, was the most serious complication.

Use of virgin silk, introduced by Joaquim Barraquer, was followed by dramatic improvement of post-surgical course.

Use of perlon monofilament, whose perfect biological tolerance allows for deep sutures, has probably led to the disappearance of limbic fistules and epithelial invasion of the anterior chamber as well.

The few therapeutic notions which will be discussed here only concern, therefore, eyes operated in accordance with techniques and materials which are no longer performed.

TREATMENT OF LIMBIC FISTULES WITHOUT EPITHELIAL INVASION

This treatment varies according to whether the fistule is recognized at an early stage or at a late one.

Fistules recognized at an early stage

These may be characterized by the following two aspects:
— cystoid wound
— external fistule
a. Cystoid wound
Such cystoid wounds modify very little, or not at all, the depth of the anterior chamber. In the majority of the cases these cystoid wounds disappear spontaneously in less than 10 days after the operation and leave no sequel. Their disappearance can be facilitated by systemic ocular hypotensive drugs (acetazolamide and/or glycerol) and by eye patching. Only rarely do they turn into a permanent cystoid wound.
b. Treatment of external fistules with Seidel sign.
— ablation of the defective suture;
— placing of a fibrin film;

377

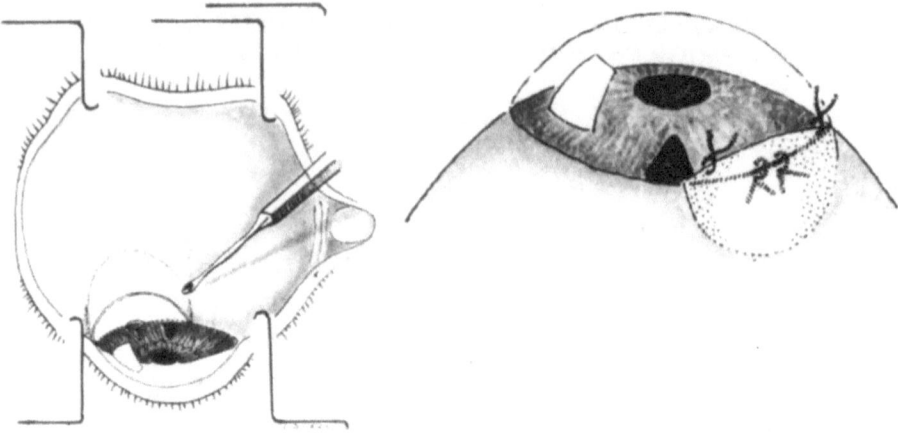

Fig. 1. Surgical treatment of recent external fistule; a. Scraping of the fistule; b. Suture of the scraped region and partial temporary conjunctival flap.

— binocular compressive patching for 48 ours;
— acetazolamide.

Such treatment is usually effective within 48 hours. In case of failure, the treatment must not be kept up for more than four days and must give way to surgical reconstruction of the wound under general anaesthesia and with microscope.

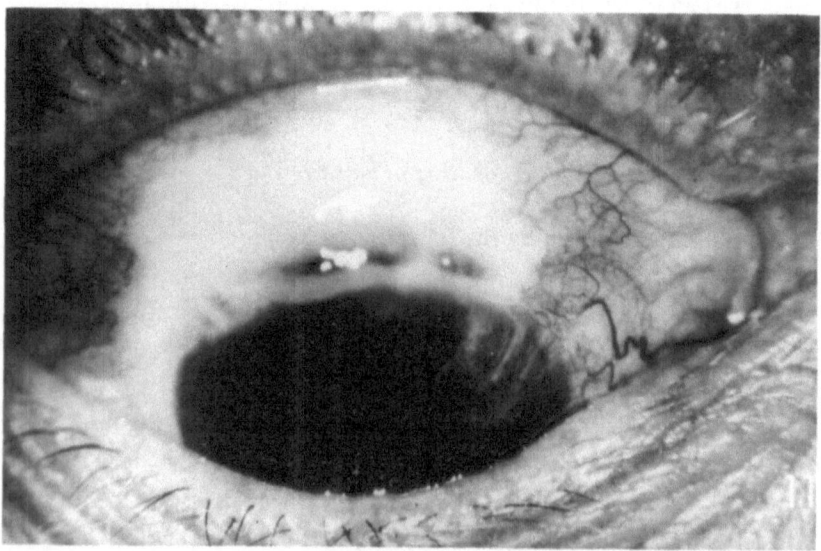

Fig. 2. Cystoid wound after cataract operation. In this case the extension and fragility of the wound lead to an indication for surgery.

Fistules recognized at a late stage

Fistulus recognized at a late stage are also characterized by two aspects:
— cystoïd wounds
— external fistules

CYSTOID WOUNDS

These are an indication for surgery only in the following cases:
— a cystoid wound which is very spread out
— visual discomfort connected to watering of the eyes, the feeling of the presence of a foreign body and to the rupture of the pre-corneal lacrimal film;
— hypotony with signs of decompensation.
— desire on the part of the patient to wear corneal lenses.

The proposed therapeutic means are varied; the best treatment remains the surgical treatment, for example in accordance with the technique of Scheie. Whatever the variations of the technique used may be, the results are good. The proportion of success varies from 92.5% of the cases (Scheie, Pitts & Martin, 1977) to 100% of the cases (Christensen & Rundle 1970; Fitzgerald & McCarthy 1962). However, it should be born in mind that the risks of such cystoid wounds are not very serious and that, therefore, an indication for surgery need not be taken as obligatory in all cases, nor as urgent.

b. Chronic external fistules (Seidel's sign +).

In such fistules in contrast with the above, need for surgery is both mandatory and urgent in all cases because of the risk of Epithelial Downgrowth into the Anterior Chamber.

Two surgical procedures can be used.

The plug graft of L. Paufique gives excellent results where cure of the fistula is concerned. But this operation is almost always followed by secondary glaucoma.

It is for this reason that the autor prefers to adopt the technique of the permanent conjunctival flap; this technique transforms the external fistula into a filtering bleb, thereby avoiding the risk of secondary glaucoma.

A keratectomy of the superficial third of the cornea is made 2 mm. in front of the fistula. The external fistula is transformed into a filtering bleb. There is no secondary glaucoma. Results are constant.

TREATMENT OF EPITHELIAL DOWNGROWTH OF THE ANTERIOR CHAMBER

Prophylaxis is based on the following

— rigorous surgery with microscope
— sutures buried under a conjunctival flap

379

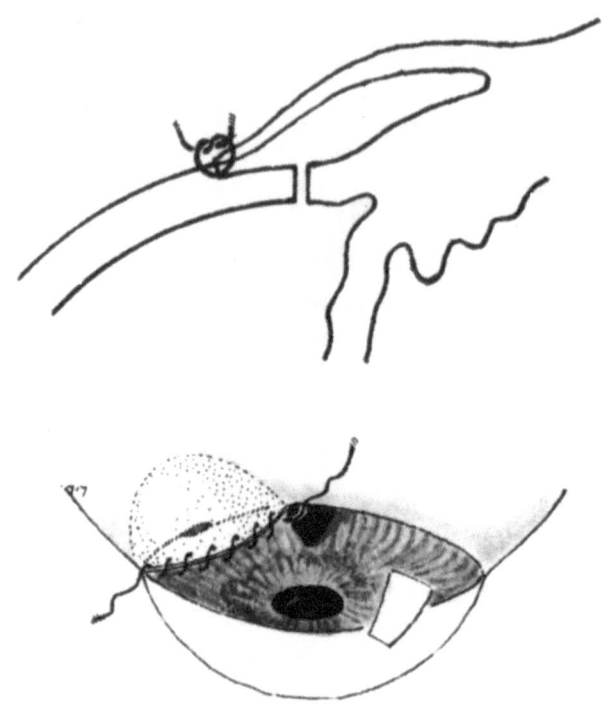

Fig. 3. Surgical treatment of chronic external fistule; a. A partial definitive conjunctival flap has been fastened with perlon monofilament at the edge of the fistule; b. Cut showing the fastening of the conjunctival flap at the edge of the keratectomy.

— use of perlon monofilament
If such rules are not abided by, an E.I.A.C. can be the result.

Curative treatment

a. Cyst

Therapeutic indications must be clearly distinguished. The only indications for operating are as follows:
— enlarging of the cyst
— association of an external fistule
— secondary glaucoma

Surgical treatment

The only surgical treatment which one can advise is the complete ablation of the cyst, followed by radiotherapy with antitumoral doses.

b. Membranous form

In contrast to the cystis form, the membranous form of the E.I.A.C. has always a poor prognosis. The chances of durable success of treatment are directly linked to how early one begins such. Therapeutic indications are, therefore, urgent in all cases.

Treatment is based on two methods: surgery and radiotherapy.

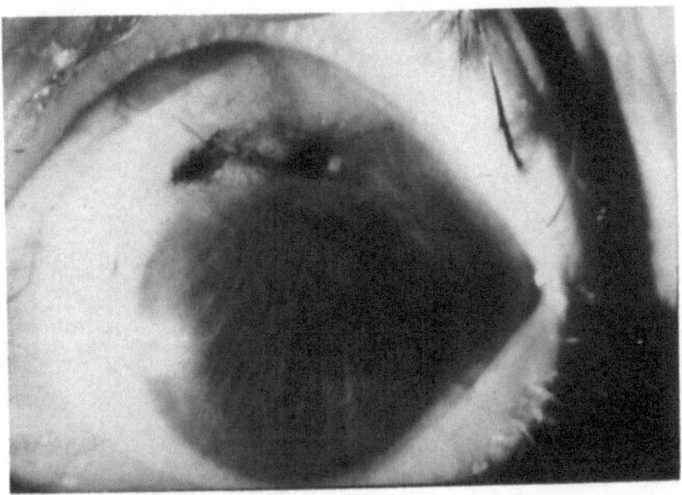

a. Before operation

Fig. 4. Chronic fistula with complete pupillary ascension after cataract extraction; a. Before surgical treatment; b. After surgical treatment; (permanent conjunctival flap and hook corepraxis).

b. After surgical treatment

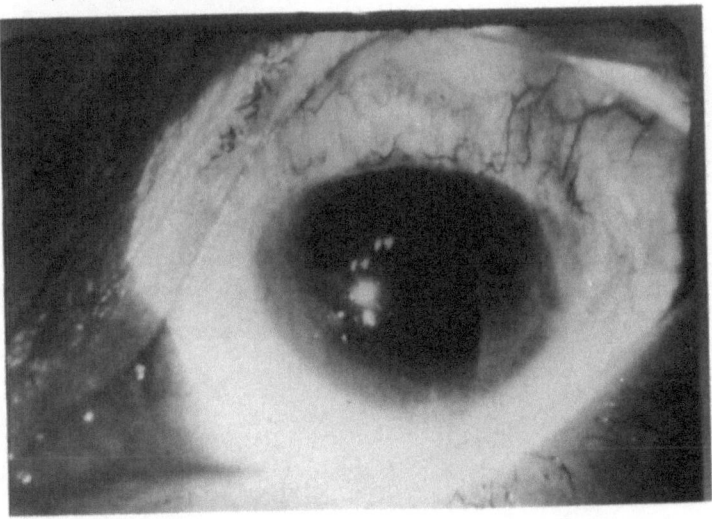

381

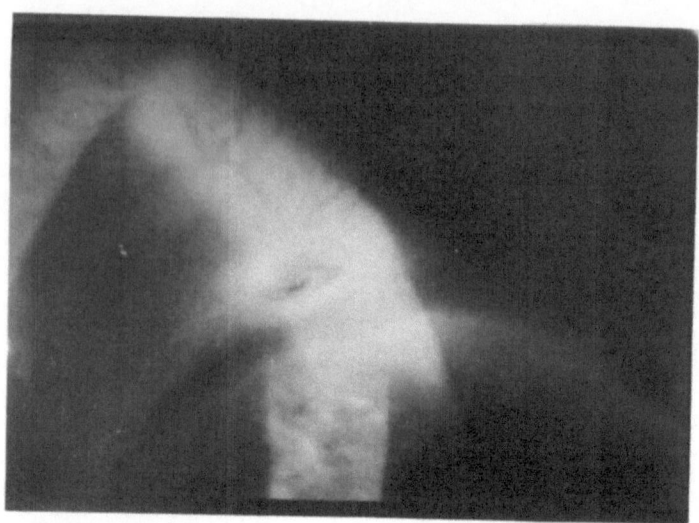

a. Before treatment

Fig. 5. Chronic fistule after cataract operation; a. The fistule before treatment O.P. = 5 mm. Hg. Seidel; b. The fistule after treatment (permanent conjunctival flap P.O. 15 mm. Hg. Seidel negative.

b. After treatment

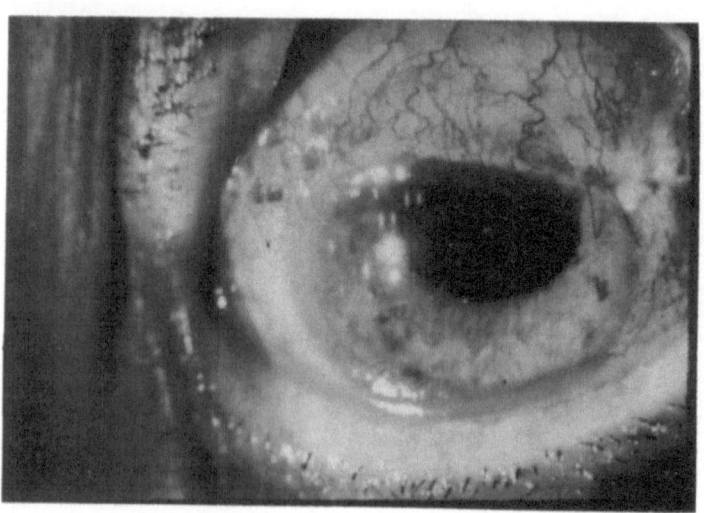

Surgery

The 'en block' resection followed by a kerâtoplasty is in fact rather illusory for the control of posterior extension is so to speak impossible. It is, therefore, better to associate it, or replace it completely, with radiotherapy.

Results are poor. In the author's experience, in only 2 cases out of 15 (approx. 13%) did the progression of the epithelial downgrowth appear to have been arrested, while the patient retained a usefull visual acuity.

CONCLUSION

As a conclusion, one cannot but express a wish; the present discussion should soon come to find its place in the history of cataract extraction.

REFERENCES

Allen J.C. Epithelial and stromal ingrowths. *Amer. J. Ophthal.*, 65, *179-182*, (1968).
Allen J.C. & Duehr P.A. Sutures and epithelial Downgrowth. *Amer. J. Ophthal.*, 65, 2, *293-294*, (1968).
Ballereau L.P. L'invasion épithéliale de la chambre antérieure, Thèse Médecine Nantes 1974.
Barraquer J. Invasion épithéliale de la chambre antérieure, Kératoplastie reconstructive. *Soc. Franc. Ophthl.*, Paris, 3-7 Mai 1970. Film.
Barraquer J. El colapso de la camara anterior en la cirurgia de la catarata y del glaucoma. *An. Inst. Barraquer*, 10, 1-2, 77-79, (1971-72).
Bernardino V.B., Kim J.C. & Smith T.R. Epithelialization of the anterior chamber after cataract extraction. *Arch. Ophthal.*, Chicago, 82, 6, *742-750*, (1969).
Bonnet M. Les fistules externes de la cornée et de la région limbique. Thèse Lyon 1962.
Bronner A., Brini A., Payeur G., Flament J. & Gerhard J.P. Les kystes carulaires par invasion épithéliale. *Bull. Soc. Ophthl. Fr.*, 70, 1, *125-130*, (1970).
Christensen R.E. & Rundle H.L. Repari of filtering blebs following cataract surgery. *Arch. Ophthal.*, 84, *8-11*, (1970).
De Laage P. Prévention et cure chirurgicales de l'invasion épithéliale de la chambre antérieure. *Ann. Oculist.*, 209, 4, *287-292*, (1976).
Dohlman C.H., Finlay J.R., McDonald P.R., Karakashian N.A. Epithelial ingrowth. In Emery J.M. & Paton D. 'Current concept in cataract surgery'. The C.V. Mosby Co. Publ., Saint-Louis, 309-314, 1974.
Douvas N.G. Cystoïd bleb cryotherapy. *Amer. J. Ophthal.*, 74, *69-71*, (1972).
Fitzgerald J.R., McCarthy J.L. Surgery of the filtering bleb. *Arch. Ophthal.*, 68, *453-457*, (1962).
Gehring J.R., Ciccarelli E.C. Trichloroacetic acid treatment of filtering blebs following cataracte extraction. *Amer. J. Ophthal.*, 74, *622-624*, (1972).
Harbin T.S. Maumenee A.E. Epithelial Downgrowth after surgery for epithelial cyst. *Amer. J. Ophthal.*, 78, 1, *1-4*, (1974).
Haye C., Jammet H & Dollfus M.A. L'oeil et les radioations ionisantes. Masson Paris 9165.
Jensen P., Minckler D.S. & Chandler J.W. Epithelial ingrwoth. *Arch. Ophthal.*, 95, 5, *837-842*, (1977).
Kirk H. Cauterization of filtering blebs following cataract extraction. *Trans. Amer. Acad. Ophthal. Otolaryngol.*, 77, *573-579*, (1973).
La Flamme M.Y. L'invasion épithéliale de la chambre antérieure. A propos de 8 cas opérés selon la technique de Maumenee. *Canad. J. Ophthal.*, 11, 1, *17-20*, (1976).
Maumenee A.E., Paton D., Morse P. & Butner R. Review of histologically proven cases of Epithelial Downgrowth following cataract extraction and suggested surgical management. *Amer. J. Ophthal.*, 69, 4, *598-603*, (1970).
Moreau P.G. & Haut J. Cryo-ophtalmologie Masson Paris 1971.

383

Rabault M.P. & Durand L. Technique d'exérèse chirugicale des kystes épithéliaux de la chambre antérieure. *Bull. Mem. Soc. Franc. Ophthal.*, 84, *310-314*, (1971).

Saracco J.B. & Arneodo J. Traitement physique de l'invasion épithéliale de la chambre antérieure. *Ann. Ther. Clin. Ophthal.*, 23, *107-113*, (1972).

Scheie H.G., Pitts E. & Martin F.J. Management of persistent filtering cicatrix following cataract extraction. *Arch. Ophthal.*, 95, *1835-1838*, (1977).

Swan K.C. & Campbeel L. Unintentional filtration following cataract surgery. *Arch. Ophthal.*, 71, *43-49*, (1964).

Swan K.C. & Christensen L. The half lap incision and closure in cataract surgery. *Amer. J. Ophthal.*, 61, *1330-1338*, (1966).

Theobladg. D. & Haas J.S. Epithelial invasion of the anterior chamber following cataract extraction. *Tr. Amer. Acad. Ophthal. Otolaryng.*, 52, 470, 1948.

Witmer R. Therapie der epithelinvasion der vorderkammer nach staroperation. *Ophthalmologica, Basel*, 161, 2-3, *286-291*, (1970).

Yannuzzi L.A. & Theodore F.H. Cryotherapy of post-cataract blebs. *Amer. J. Ophthal.*, 76, *217-222*, (1973).

Author's address
Clinique Ophtalmologique Universitaire
B. de Lyon
Lyon
France

PUPILLARY COMPLICATIONS AFTER CATARACT EXTRACTION

M. BONNET

(Lyon, France)

Four pupillary complications can be observed after cataract extraction: a. pupillary block; b. synechiae on the hyaloid and pupillary pseudo-dilation without block; c. pupillary deformation; d. up drawn pupil.

Pupillary block is dealt with by J. Barraquer within the framework of the post-operative flat anterior chamber. Therefore only the other three complications will be discussed here.

SYNECHIAE ON THE HYALOID AND PUPILLARY PSEUDO-DILATION

Etiology

Synechiae between the iris and the hyaloid are the consequence of an untreated or unsufficiently treated post-operative inflammation. Their formation is induced by injection into the anterior chamber of an over-concentrated solution of acethylcholine and, above all, by intra- and post-operative complications, among which delay of cicatrisation and hyphema are particular causes.

Iris synechiae to the hyaloid must all the more specifically be expected and prevented in the case of cataracts associated with an abnormal iris. They include the cataract in diabetic patients, previous anterior uveitis, and cataract after filtering operations.

Clinical aspects

Iris synechiae to the hyaloid are usually a benign complication, not having a visual consequence. They often are not recognized except in the late or even remote sequels. All clinical aspects are possible, ranging from the unique synechiae to pupillary seclusion. The latter does not give rise to complications when the iridectomy is patent. It can even be not recognized due to the pseudo-dilation related to the traction of the iris on the anterior elastic hyaloid. The pseude-dilation is, however, limited. It can, therefore, be an obstacle to the examination and the treatment of the ocular fundus when retinal detachtment occurs or when a diabetic retinopathy is associated to the cataract.

In very few cases, the iris adherence to the hyaloid is associated with densification and pigmentary deposition on the hyaloid in the pupillary area. This can be opaque enough to prevent vision (tertiary cataracts).

Treatment

Prophylaxis, carried out in order to be able to examine and treat the ocular fundus in case of need, is the very basis of treatment of synechiae on the hyaloid. Such treatment consists in topical corticoids and mydriatics postoperatively by as long as a tyndall of the anterior chamber persists. Duration of the treatment must, therefore, be adapted and prolonged in the specific circumstances favourable to the formation of synechiae, i.e., intra- or postoperative complications, diabetes, uveitis, or previous antiglaucomatous operations.

A late curative treatment is recommended in exceptional cases. Indications for surgery are limited to the following two cases:
— insufficient pupillary pseude-dilation to treat lesions of the retina. The treatment consists in enlarging the pupil by photocoagulation of the pupillary margin or in completing the iridectomy either by photocoagulation or by surgery.
— tertiary cataract. Needling of the anterior hyaloid membrane is the most effective treatment.

PUPILLARY DEFORMATIONS

Etiology

The causes for pupillary deformation after surgery are as follows:
— persistence of capsular fragments in the wound, poor cleaning of the wound and iris incarceration in the wound.
— rupture of the anterior hyaloid membrane at the end of the operation or post-operatively;
— delay of cricatrization with anterior synechia, embedding or prolapse of the iris.

Clinical aspects

Pupillary deformation due to persistence of a capsular fragment

Pupillary deformation due to the persistence of a capsular fragment embedded in the incision is visible at the end of surgery. Such deformation is immediately reversible by means of extraction of the capsular fragment. If not treated, it does not increase assuming that there is no other associated complication.

Pupillary deformation due to rupture of the anterior hyaloid membrane: the peaked pupil syndrome

Pupillary deformation due to rupture of the anterior hyaloid membrane is a much more serious complication precisely because it may increase and lead to other complications. It may occur in the two following circumstances:
— during surgery: after extraction of the lens the anterior chamber is filled with vitreous and the pupil is not round.
— post-operatively: this case is more frequent. Pupillary deformation follows a secondary rupture of the anterior hyaloid membrane. This rupture is favoured by an excessive and over-prolonged pupillary dilation. It is more frequent in old patients. A particular local predisposition probably explains the bilateral and symmetrical nature of the syndrome even when the two eyes have not been operated with the same technique and by the same surgeon.

Fortunately pupillary deformation does not occur in all secondary ruptures of the hyaloid membrane. It occurs only in cases where the vitreous fibrils adhere to the corneal wound. And it is just this adherence to the wound which can lead to further complications.

The syndrome almost always occurs before the fourth month, for after this delay the deep layers of the wound are healed. It is rare with perlon predescemetic sutures which ensure a more rapid and better coaptation of the deep layers of the wound. It is more frequent in corneal endothelial dystrophies. On the other hand, there is no significant difference in frequency related to the type of iridectomy (Jaffe, 1969).

The diagnosis is made from the biomicroscopic examination; a vitreous strand passes through the pupil and adheres to the deep layers of the wound. The vitreous strand condenses and retracts progressively. It gradually leads to a horsetail condensation which dips into the posterior vitreous. The syndrome is associated to irritative signs as redness and photophobia. After intra-venous injection of fluorescein, an abnormal fluorescence of the anterior chamber can be observed, and a yet more intense and lasting fluorescence of the vitreous strand.

This syndrome, identified by Irvine, is a serious complication, not only due to the progressive pupillary deformation which it brings with it, but also and above all due to the complications involving the ocular fundus which it can bring about or at least *favour:* macular edema (Irvine-Gass' syndrome). The existence of a previous Anterior Vitreous Syndrome of Irvine is the most important prognostic factor of macular edema following cataract extraction. Macular oedema associated to a normal pupil spontaneously disappears and leaves no sequel in 91% of cases. If, on the other

387

hand, the pupil is deformed by a vitreous strand, macular edema remains and leads to macular degeneration in 2/3 of cases. Macular prognosis is the more uncertain the more pronounced the anterior vitreous syndrome is (6).

Macular retraction syndrome. In this case this syndrome is always associated with macular edema. Prognosis is always poor (6).

Retinal detachment. Tears are often found on the same meridian as the vitreous adherence to the wound. Prognosis is poor.

Pupillary deformation due to anterior Synechiae, embedding, or hernia of the iris

Pupillary de-centering due to anterior Synechia, embedding, or hernia of the iris is only a secondary aspect of the problems arising as the result of an imperfect wound. The problem has not to do with the pupil, but rather with the wound. This problem, which has been treated in other papers, will not be discussed here.

Treatment

Pupillary deformation due to capsular embedding

Pupillary decentration due to capsular enbedding occurs during surgery and as such must be treated during the operation. The treatment is simple: it consists of taking hold of the capsular fragment by means of a pair of Bonn Forceps and extracting it. Such extraction is simple because the free end of the capsular fragment is close to the incision. This end is grasped, being careful of the iris so as not to risk wounding the anterior hyaloid membrane.

Washing of the anterior chamber with acetylcholine makes it possible to ascertain whether the pupil has been satisfactorily freed.

Pupillary deformation due to rupture of the anterior hyaloid

Treatment of pupillary deformation due to rupture of the anterior hyaloid membrane must be considered in two distinct ways, according to whether it occurs during surgery or post-operatively.

Rupture of the hyaloid during surgery

Different methods have been proposed. The choice for each depends on the severity of the rupture of the hyaloid, of the consistency of the protruding vitreous and of operatory *calmness,* which is the function of the anesthesia. When the rupture of the hyaloid is of a limited nature and when the vitreous humour does not go into the incision, an attempt can be made to re-establish the position of the pupil by means of a number of simple manoeuvres of reduction of the vitreous. The sutures being tied, the anterior chamber is filled with air. Then the closed eyeball is plentifully washed with iced serum so as to induce retraction of the vitreous. A Barraquer's Vitreous Spatula is introduced into one of the lateral ends of the incision. The tip of the spatula is then directed into the angle of the twelve o'clock meridian. Then the spatula is given a rotating movement of $180°$ which follows the camerular angle to six o'clock. This semi-circular movement is necessary because of the elasticity of the vitreous strands. At the end of this manoeuvre the air must take up the entire camerular angle, which means that there is a corresponding absence of vitreous humour. When a rupture of the hyaloid membrane is associated with a protrusion of the cohesive vitreous in the wound, an anterior vitrectomy becomes necessary. The discussion emphasizes the importance which it is well to ascribe to this vitrectomy.

The most judicious attitude would seem to be situated halfway between the resection solely of the vitreous protuding into the wound, practiced in the past and most certainly insufficient, and the 'savage' vitrectomy advised between 1970 and 1972 by a variety of different surgeons, especially J.D. Gas (1970) on the one hand, and the Parisian school of J. Haut & S. Limon (1972) on the other, after a series of publications of Kasner (1968). The resection of the vitreous must be pursued in such a manner as to obtain the formation of the future neo-hyaloid behind the iris. But most probably it is not necessary for the above purpose to go so far with the vitrectomy that the anterior face of the iris has concave plane. In all cases it would seem preferable to complete the iridectomy and, when necessary, to carry out an inferior sphincterotomy.

Post-operatory rupture of the hyaloid

Surgical indications in pupillary deformation due to secondary rupture of the hyaloid are rare. This disadvantages, risks and failures of surgery must, in effect, be evaluated warning regard to the complications given rise to by the syndrome itself. Hence an indication is to be considered only in the case of major, evolutive and complicated anterior vitreous syndromes with macular edema and visual impairment. The surgery consists of carrying out a total section of the vitreous strand adhering to the wound in the course of a vitrectomy made through either the anterior ot the posterior approach.

There is no significant recent statistic which allows us to be sure of the value of these techniques.

UPDRAWN PUPIL

Etiology

Major updrawn pupil has become very rare thanks to the prophylaxis of

389

the loss of vitreous and also to an immediate and more adequate treatment of the later (see above).

Clinical aspects

In contrast to simple pupillary deformation in which the optical axis still passes through the pupil despite deformation of the latter, updrawn pupil is characterized by a complete obstruction of the visual axis by the displaced iris.

It is necessary to distinguish between a variety of clinical forms which condition more or less complex therapeutic problems. It is, in fact, worthwhile to distinguish between the forms which are associated to the persistence of lens residue and the forms in which the extraction of the lens has been total. It is advisable to distinguish between those cases in which there is no longer a pupil and the cases in which a very de-centered pupillary orifice persists.

Treatment

Due to the fact that they always constitute a total obstacle to vision, the up-drawn pupil must always be treated, (assuming, of course, that the light projections, the E.R.G. and the P.E.V. lead to think that the retina and the optical nerve still have a functional capacity). The purpose of the treatment is to enlarge the pupillary orifice so as to re-center it or to create a neo-pupil in an entirely ascended iris. Two different therapeutic means are possible: photocoagulation and surgery. The one and the other both have their advantages and disadvantages.

a) Surgery

Various surgical techniques make it possible effectively to treat the various clinical forms of pupillary ascension.

Updrawn-pupil with persistence of a small, decentered pupil are treated by corepraxis with a hook;

Updrawn-pupil with total disappearance of pupil requires a more complex technique. The Franceschetti's technique, and above all, the Seymour-Philips technique remain the most satisfactory;

Updrawn-pupil associated with lens remmants can be treated either with iridocapsulectomy with the Elsching's technique or with corepraxis followed by needling of the secondary cataract (Guillaumat, Paufique, de Saint-Martin, Schiff-Wertheimer & Sourdille, 1957).

It would go beyond our purpose to describe the details of the technical variations of these operations. It should, however be emphasized that the precision and the results of this surgery have largely benefited from the use of the surgical microscope and from the security afforded by general anaesthesia and dehydratation of the vitreous body by means of osmotic drugs.

Surgical treatment of updrawn-pupil offers the following numerous advantages over photocoagulation:
— the result is immediate and permanent.
— the complications are exceptional.
— the treatment is efficient even in case of a secondary associated cataract.

On the other hand, surgical treatment does have some disadvantages which are the following in particular:
— the need for surgery
— the difficulty of judging the precise size of the resection of the iris.

b) Photocoagulation

Photocoagulation can be carried out with a xenon photocoagulator (Burns 1965; Charamis 1964; Charleux 1965; Cleasby 1970; Weekers, Watillon, Lavergne 1960), a ruby laser (Zweng, Vassiliades, Paris, Rose & Hayse, 1970) or with an argon laser (Hager 1973; Massin & Gernet 1973; Zweng & Little 1977). The technique varies according to the degree of pupillary ascension. Moderate ascensions are treated with a photocoagulation of the lower edge of the pupil. The more pronounced ascensions are treated with a photocoagulation of the entire lower pupillary edge from 3 o'clock to 9 o'clock. With an argon laser the constants advised by Zweng and Little are as follows: 500 microns, 0,2 s. 500 mW. A double row of coagulations is placed at 1 mm from the pupillary edge.

In the case of total ascensions a neo-pupil is made at the center of the iris curtain. In this case, photocoagulation can be combined with surgery (Burns 1965; Meyer-Schwickerath 1960; Pischel 1962). A central photocoagulation of weak intensity is carried out in the first stage with the purpose of bringing about an atrophy of the iris without pigmentary dispersion. Some months later a needling of the atrophic iris can be made without running the risk of hemorrhage.

Excellent results of photocoagulation have been published. Photocoagulation has a number of unquestionable advantages over surgery, and in particular the following:
— it does not require surgery
— the treatment can be carried out on out-patients

Yet photocoagulation of the iris has also its disadvantages, which are as follows:
— its possibilities of action depend on the degree of pigmentation of the iris;
— its results are delayed. At times it takes several months to be complete. Delayed progressive atrophy of the iris can, therefore, lead to a result going too far, beyond the purpose desired. Cleasby (1970) has published a case in which 4,5 years after photocoagulation the pupil had become immense

391

due to extensive atrophy of the iris. This late complication is probably linked to an overtreatment.

– inversely, the results might be unsufficient or even temporary, with a return to the previous state after several months (Corral & Landres, 1975).
– complications have been observed, inflammatory reaction, pigmentary dispersion, burning the cornea leading to permanent opacity (Weekers quoted by Charamis, 1964). The latter complications is to be feared in the case of a shallow anterior chamber. Carral (Carrik & Landers, 1975) has also brought attention to a case of rubeosis iridis brought about, or rather precipitated by photocoagulation of the iris with argon laser on an eye affected by an old detachment of the retina.

In truth, serious complications are rare. They are usually the result of a mistake in the technique or an overtreatment.
– Finally, photocoagulation is not sufficient in case of a secondary associated cataract. Complementary surgical treatment is necessary.

CONCLUSION

Pupillary complications of cataract extraction show up today under a quite different aspect from that of 20 years ago. Thanks to an effective and well codified prophylaxis, the major pupillary ascensions have practically disappeared and, therefore, indications for corepraxis and isidocapsulectomy have become quite exceptional. On the other hand, peaked pupil due to a secondary rupture of the hyaloid membrane remains a worrisome problem. The prophylaxis remains to be discovered. Treatment is not entirely satisfactory and the complications arising in the ocular fundus continue to darken the visual prognosis of some uneventfull cataract extractions.

SUMMARY

Pupillary complications after cataract extraction are subdivided into 4 groups: pupillary block, synechiae on the hyaloid with pseudodilation without block, pupillary deformation and updrawn-pupil. The causes, prophylaxis and treatment of these four complications are here briefly discussed.

REFERENCES

Burns R.P. Improvements in technique of photocoagulation of the iris. 1 - Higher magnification as an aid in focusin the light beam. 2 - Combiantion of photocoagulation with discussion. *Arch. Ophthal.*, Chicago, 74, 3, *306-309*, 1965.
Carroll R.P. & Landers M.B. Pin wheel rubeosis iridis following argon laser coreoplasty. *Ann. Ophthal.*, 7, 3, *357-360*, 1975.
Charamis J. Corépraxie par photocoagulation. Soc. Franc. Ophtal., Paris 10-15 Mai 1964. *Bull. Mem Soc. Franc. Ophthal.*, 77, *449-456*, 1964.
Charleux J. Dilatation pupillaire articifielle par photocoagulation. Soc. Ophthal. Lyon, 13 Decembre 1964. *Bull. Soc. Ophthal. Fr.*, 65, 5, *495-498*, 1965.
Cleasby G.W. Photocoagulation coreplasty. *Arch. Ophthal.*, Chicago, 83, 2, *145-151*, 1970.

Francois P. & Bonnet N. La macula, Edit, Masson Paris 1976.
Gass J.D. Management of vitreous loss after cataract extraction. *Arch. Ophthal. (Chicago)*, 83, 3, *319-323*, (1970).
Guilaumat L., Paufique L., de Saint-Martin R., Schiff-Wertheimer S. & Sourdille G.P. Traitement chirurgical des affections oculaires. Vol. 1 - Doin Paris 1957.
Hager H. Besondre mikrochirurgische eingriffe. 2. Teil: Erste erfahrunge mit dem argon-laser-gerät 800. *Klin. Mbl. Auge-Heilk.*, 162, 4, *437-450*, (1973).
Haut J. & Limon S. Chirurgie pratique du vitré. Masson Paris 1972.
Jaffe N.S. The vitreous in clinical ophthalmology. Moshy St. Louis 1969, p. 99-145.
Kasner D. Vitrectomy: a new approach to the management of vitreous. *Highlights ophthal.*, 11, *303-309*, (1968).
Massin M. & Gernet H. Der Argon-Laser in der chirurgie des vorderen augenabschinittes. *Klin. Mbl. Augenheilk.*, 162, 3, *369-373*, (1973).
Meyer-Schickerath G. Light coagulation. Drance St. Louis Moshy 1960.
Pischel D.K. Symposium on photocoagulation IV - Further therapeutic indications. Trans. Amer. Acad. Ophthal. Otolaryngol., 66, *56-71*, (1962).
Weekers R., Watillon N. & Lavergne G. Corépracie par photocoagulation. *Arch. Ophthal. (Paris)*, 20/6, *581-587* (1960).
Zweng C., Vassiliadis A., Paris Q., Rose H. & Hayes J. Laser photocoagulation of the iris. *Arch. Ophthal.*, 84, *193-199*, (1970).
Zweng H.C., Little H.L. Argon Laser photocoagulation. Moshy St. Louis 1977.

Author's address:
Clinique Ophtalmologique Universitaire B
Hôpital de la Croix Rousse – 93 Grande
Rue de la Croix Rousse
Lyon
France

Docum. Ophthal. Proc. Series, Vol. 21

WOUND LEAK, COLLAPSE OF THE ANTERIOR CHAMBER CHOROIDAL DETACHMENT

JOAQUIN BARRAQUER

(Barcelona, Spain)

WOUND LEAK

The causes of wound leak are the following: 1. A perforating suture. Edema of the wound lips may initially prevent the escape of aqueous. 2. A deep suture, which may become perforating due to necrosis (Fig. 1). 3. A superficial suture which may cause posterior gaping (Fig. 2). 4. Deficient coaptation of the wound edges. 5. Incarcerations of extraneous material in the wound e.g. lint, fragments of glass or rubber, suture material, lens capsule, iris, vitreous, conjunctiva, and eyelashes. This may cause excessive granulation tissue or a filtering cicatrix. 6. Excessive cauterization of the wound edges. 7. An irregular incision and undue trauma to the wound lips by unsuitable or defective instruments (1). 8. Accidental trauma, which ruptures a suture. 9. Increased intraocular pressure. Its effect may be similar to that of trauma. An abrupt increase in ocular tension is usually due to pupillary block. The wound may reopen and the iris may prolapse (Fig. 3). 10. Delayed wound healing, which may be responsible for prolonged filtration or fistulization due to any of the above mechanical factors.

Wound leak is usually an early complication and may be responsible for delayed re-formation of the anterior chamber, collapse of the anterior chamber, endophthalmitis, epithelial invasion of the anterior chamber, anterior synechiae, and secondary glaucoma. Intermittent minimal wound filtration may develop, however, as late as several months postoperatively. The patient experiences episodes of blurred vision. Usually some cells appear in the vitreous as evidence of a mild iridocyclitis, which may subsequently take a severe course.

Prophylaxis. The incision should be sclerocorneal and must be correctly made and sutured, with meticulous toilet of the wound. External fistulas may be prevented by placing the sutures subconjunctivally. If there is any fistulization, a filtration bleb will form beneath the conjunctiva. The anterior chamber may be retained, and the bled usually disappears within a few days. A plastic shield and postoperative sedation offer the best protection against accidental trauma.

Management: With the help of the Seidel fluorescein test the area of the

(1) Davis observed a greater incidence of wound leak in a group of cases operated on with keratome and scissors than in a group of cases in which a Graefe knife had been used. The other factors in both groups were the same.

395

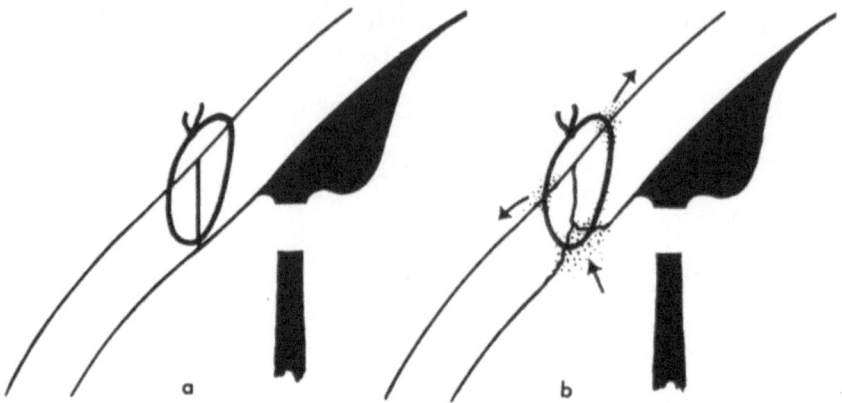

Fig. 1. Deep suture. a. Initially the incision may be closed. b. Late necrosis and wound leak.

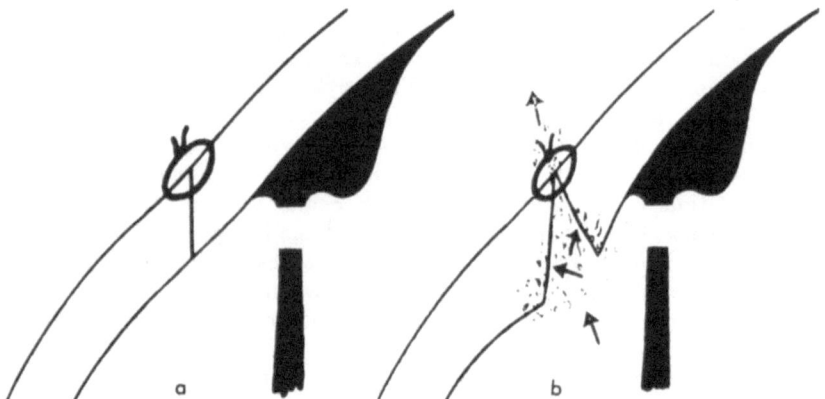

Fig. 2. Superficial suture. a. Initially the incision may be closed. Posterior gaping, edema, and wound leak.

wound leak can be determined. If a perforating suture is responsible for the wound leak it is removed and generally after 24 hours of binocular occlusion the anterior chamber will be reformed.

If there is slight gaping of the wound which does not resolve in two days, a new suture is applied. If these measures are not sufficient it will be best to check the incision and cover it by a conjunctival flap. The anterior chamber should not remain absent for more than 7 days. The procedure for recovering the incision with a conjunctival flap is extremely delicate and will effectively seal the wound only when it is carried out correctly. The technique in the case of a previous limbus-based flap is as follows: 1. The conjuntival incision is re-opened. 2. The conjunctiva is dissected toward the upper fornix to obtain a fornix-based flap large enough to reach to 2 mm.

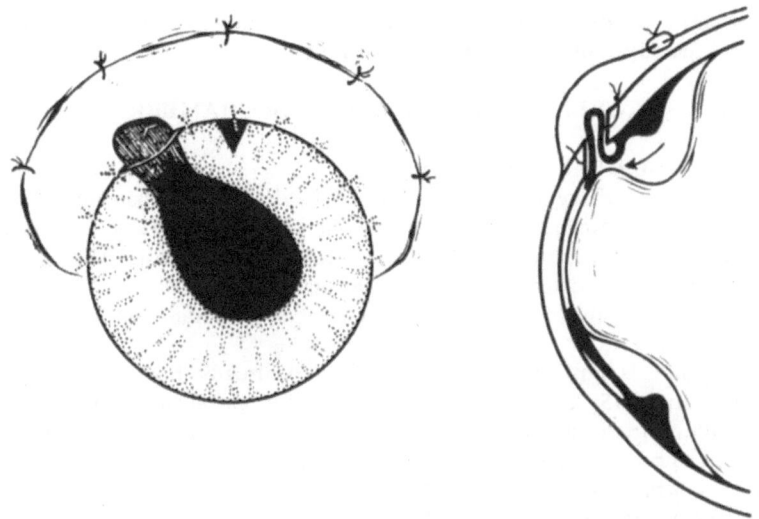

Fig. 3. Iris prolapse due to pupillary block. The increased tension ruptures the wound.

inside the limbus. If necessary, a relaxing incision is made in the upper fornix. 3. The limbus-based flap is resected from the limbus, and any incorrectly placed sutures are removed. 4. A superficial keratectomy is performed superiorly, on the wound edges to create a surface to which the fornix-based flap can adhere. 5. If necessary, the wound is resutured. Previous suture sites are avoided. 6. The fornix-based flap is anchored to the cornea (Fig. 4). 7. Air is injected into the anterior chamber through a small paracentesis inferiorly.

The technique is relatively simple in the case of a previous fornix-based flap. The flap is dissected, and about 1 mm. of conjunctiva is trimmed along the free border. The rest of the procedure is the same.

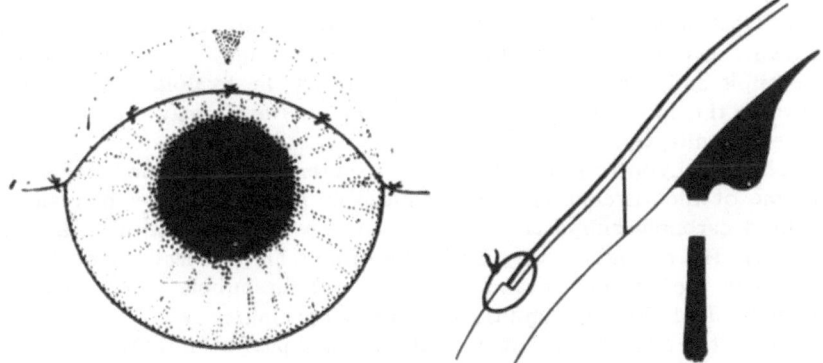

Fig. 4. Fornix-based flap anchored to the cornea after superficial keratectomy in the area adjacent to the incision.

397

Traumatic wound rupture, which may be followed by iris or vitreous prolapse, usually requires this method of repair.

COLLAPSE OF THE ANTERIOR CHAMBER

Causes: 1. Wound leak; 2. Pupillary block.

The term **pupillary block** is employed to denote an obstruction to the flow of aqueous from the posterior to the anterior chamber. This implies the absence or simultaneous block of an iridectomy opening. The retention of aqueous in the posterior chamber may lead to angel closure, causing the intraocular pressure to rise, unless there is a simultaneous inhibition of aqueous secretion.

Although this important complication had already been recognized by Bowmann in 1865, it was not until 1946 that it was again brought to light, by Chandler and Johnson, later followed by Shaffer and Sugar. Nevertheless, ignorance about the pathogenesis of pupillary block is still responsible for the loss of some eyes after cataract surgery.

The mechanism of pupillary block may or may not be of inflammatory origin. **Early pupillary block** is usually noninflammatory and due to obstruction by vitreous or air. Late pupillary block is usually caused by inflammatory adhesion of the iris to the vitreous. Early as well as late pupillary block may occur not only after lens extraction with peripheral iridectomy, but also, though less frequently, after lens extraction with sector iridectomy.

Early pupillary block (noninflammatory). This form of pupillary block may appear within hours after surgery and be due to the following mechanical causes: 1. Obstruction of the pupil and the iridectomy opening by vitreous (Fig. 5). Low ocular rigidity in young patients and myopes, or due to thyrotropic exophthalmos or recent surgery, may contribute to the occurence of pupillary block. The flaccid or elastic sclera tends to exert pressure on the vitreous.

Loss of the anterior chamber as a result of inadequate wound closure or accidental trauma may cause the vitreous to prolapse and establish a pupillary block. On the other hand pupillary block may cause the anterior chamber to collapse.

2. Obstruction of the pupil and the iridectomy opening by air. An excessive amount of air in the anterior chamber may press the border of the pupil and the iridectomy opening against the hyaloid and may thus obstruct the flow of aqueous (figs. 6 and 7). The air may even block the trabeculae directly.

Extreme hypotony facilitates the occurence of air block. When the volume of the vitreous has been reduced by intravenous urea or mannitol or by a carbonic anhydrase inhibitor, an excessive amount of air is easily injected. The air bubble may initially assume a more or less spherical form, but when the vitreous regains its volume the air bubble will be flattened and may block the pupil and the iridectomy opening.

When it is excessive in amount, the air may pass behind the iris. The air bubble may either assume the form of an hourglass and obstruct the flow of aqueous (fig. 8 A) or it may pass completely behind the iris, pushing

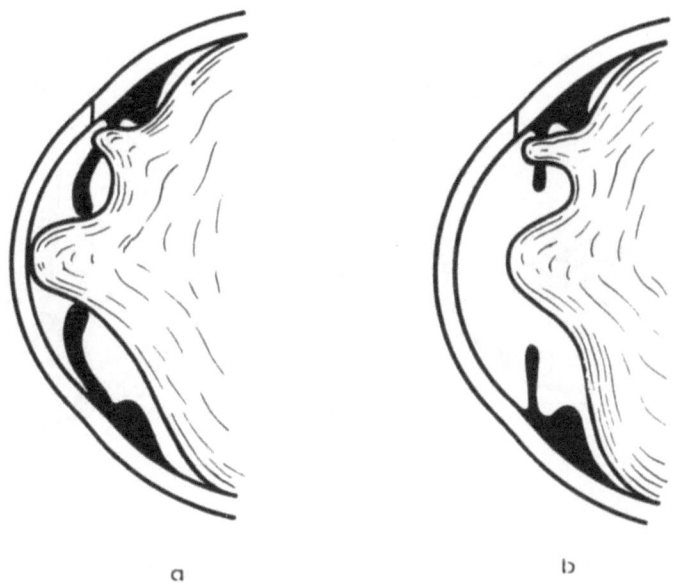

Fig. 5. a. Obstruction of pupil and iridectomy opening by vitreous with intact hyaloid. b. Dilatation of the pupil relieves block.

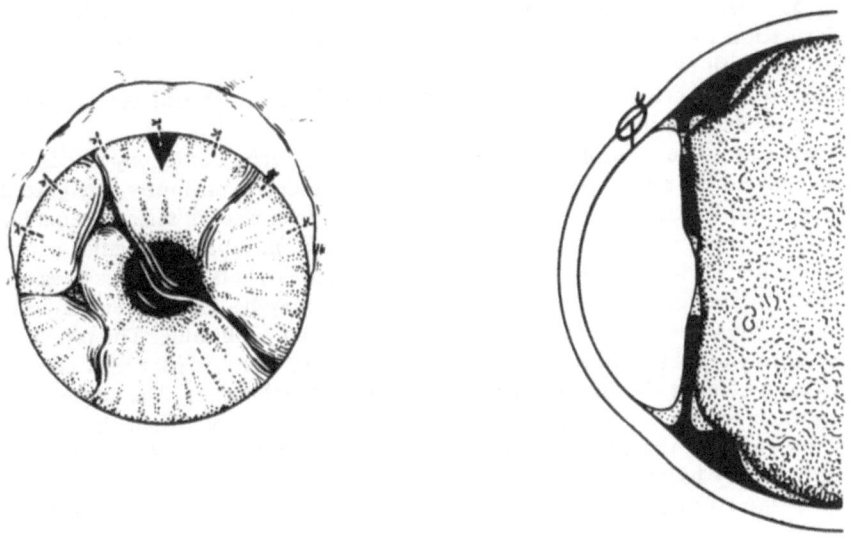

Fig. 6. Obstruction of pupil and iridectomy opening by air. Initial phase.

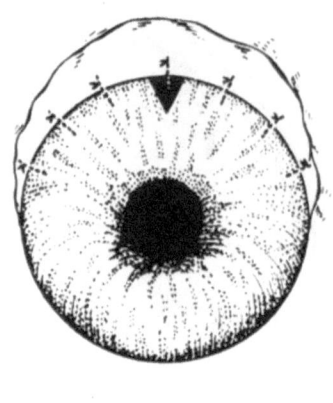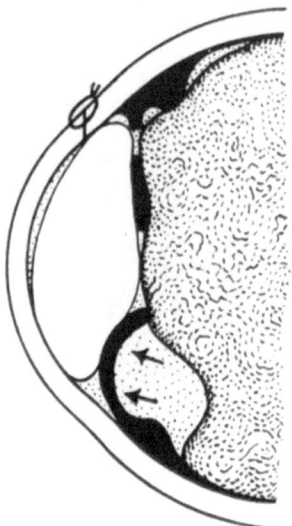

Fig. 7. Obstruction of pupil and iridectomy opening by air. Iris bombé.

the latter against the cornea and causing a fulminating glaucoma (fig. 8 B).

3. Obstruction of the iridectomy opening by clotted blood or lens remnants, with a simultaneous block of the pupil by vitreous or air.

4. Vitreous loss, which may be responsible for pupillary block, if the vitreous has not been reposited behind the iris or if an excessive amount of air has been injected.

5. Obstruction of a peripheral iridectomy opening, as a result of the formation of an anterior synechia of its borders, with a simultaneous block of the pupil by vitreous or air.

6. A nonperforating iridectomy or the omission of an iridectomy, which greatly increase the risk of pupillary block.

Diagnosis: The complaint of pain in the eye, accompanied by headache, should always arouse suspicion of pupillary block. If promptly recognized, this complication can be corrected before the onset of serious sequelae.

The anterior chamber is usually shallow and may be of irregular depth. The aqueous may accumulate behind the iris, in pockets of various sizes and push the iris forward(1). The anterior chamber may be deepest centrally due to the presence of a mushroom of vitreous or an air bubble. The retention of aqueous in the posterior chamber may bring the iris root into contact with the trabeculae, the incision, and the peripheral cornea. The cornea may appear edematous, due to increased intraocular pressure. When the hyaloid is broken and the anterior chamber is filled with free vitreous, the diagnosis of pupillary block may be difficult (Fig. 9).

If the free communication between the chambers is not restored prompt-

(1) In Spanish, an irregular iris bombé is called 'iris en tomate'.

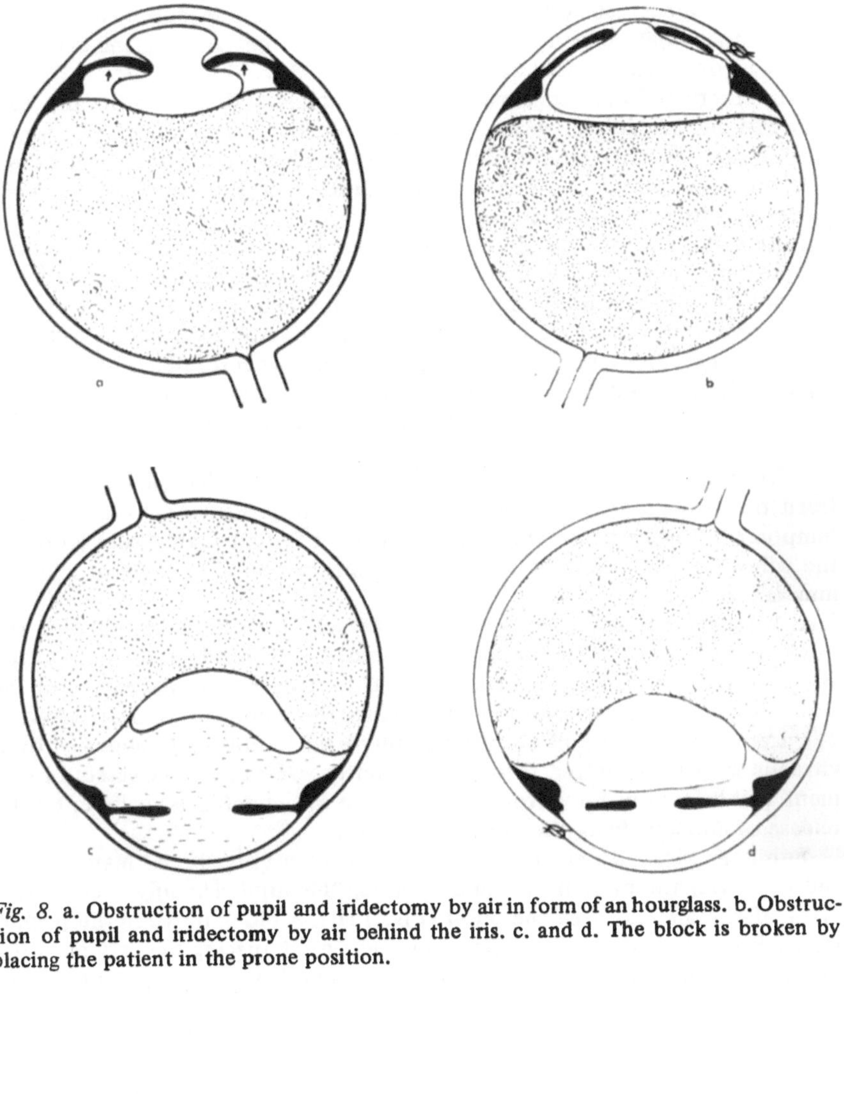

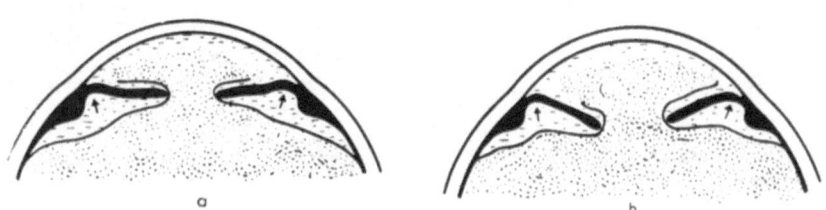

Fig. 8. a. Obstruction of pupil and iridectomy by air in form of an hourglass. b. Obstruction of pupil and iridectomy by air behind the iris. c. and d. The block is broken by placing the patient in the prone position.

Fig. 9. Pupillary block with free vitreous in the anterior chamber. a. Initial phase, wich may be recognized only on gonioscopy. b. Peripheral anterior synechiae established.

ly, anterior synechiae and irreversible damage to the trabeculae will develop. Usually the pupil becomes distorted. The wound may rupture and allow the iris to become incarcerated or to prolapse (Fig. 3).

The increased ocular tension may produce a dull pain in the eye, followed by ipsilateral fronto-occipital headache and vomiting. The ocular tension may be only moderately increased or it may remain normal if there is hyposecreation of aqueous or if the block is not absolute. This is rare, however, with early pupillary block.

Prophylaxis: The iridectomy opening must be sufficiently peripheral and its patency must be verified, especially following hemorrhage into the anterior chamber, capsule rupture or vitreous loss. Secure wound closure may prevent the mechanism of collapse of the anterior chamber followed by pupillary block. The anterior chamber must be reformed with artificial aqueous humor and, if necessary, air (2). Care must be taken not to leave an excessive amount of air in the anterior chamber. The air bubble should remain surrounded by a ring of aqueous.

After vitreous loss the incision, the pupil, and the iridectomy opening are freed of vitreous adhesions with a spatula. An excessive amount of air is temporarily injected into the anterior chamber for adequate visualization of the adhesions. Some of the air is withdrawn, and an air bubble of about 7 mm. is retained.

Management: Pupillary block by vitreous may be relieved by dilating the pupil (Fig. 5), even if the tension is elevated. Another iridectomy is indicated when mydriasis is ineffective (Fig. 10). The situation may also be approached by dehydrating the vitreous by the administration of intravenous urea or mannitol and a carbonic anhydrase inhibitor. Aqueous or fluid vitreous may be aspirated through a posterior sclerotomy. Successfull treatment will be followed by prompt restoration of the anterior chamber by the release of aqueous from the posterior chamber.

Pupillary block by air in the anterior chamber (Fig. 11 A) may be relieved by sitting the patient up and by dilating the pupil. The upward displacement of the air may free the pupil (Fig. 11B). A block by air in the posterior chamber may be treated effectively by simply placing the patient in the prone position, so that the air may move away from the pupil (Fig. 8 D).

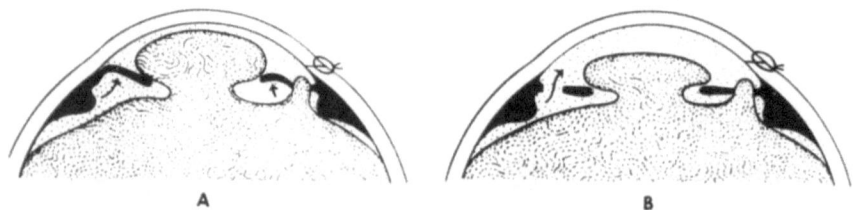

Fig. 10. a. Pupillary block unrelieved by mydriasis. b. The block is relieved by another iridectomy.

(2) Air injection is indicated when the aqueous tends to escape in spite of careful wound closure, when vitreous has been lost, when the iris or the incision tends to bleed, when there is corneal dystrophy, and after penetrating keratoplasty.

When the air assumes the form of an hourglass (Fig. 8 A), either the pupil is dilated or the patient is placed in the prone position (Fig. 8 C), depending on whether the greater part of the air is in the anterior or in the posterior chamber. Once the block has been relieved the patient is kept in a sitting position or lying on either side until the air has been absorbed. The pupil is kept dilated. Rarely is it necessary to withdraw part of the air through a paracentesis or a posterior sclerotomy.

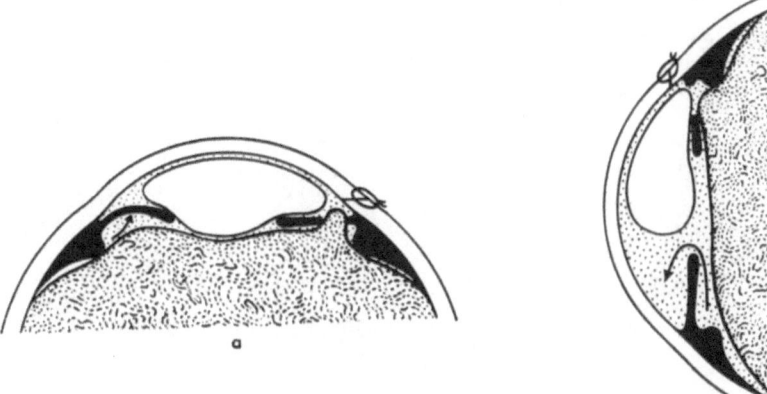

Fig. 11. a. Obstruction of the pupil by air in the anterior chamber and obstruction of the iridectomy opening by vitreous. b. The block is relieved by sitting the patient up.

Unrecognized and incorrectly treated pupillary block, e.g. when the increased tension has induced the use of pilocarpine, is probably the most frequent cause of iris prolapse and secondary glaucoma. These complications often can be prevented by such simple measures as the opportune instillation of a drop of mydriatic and adequate positioning of the patient.

The **surgical treatment** of pupillary block consists in an iridectomy inferiorly. Since the eye has recently been operated on and may be irritated, reopening the wound for another iridectomy superiorly may cause profuse bleeding. The technique is as follows:

1. Dissection of a small fornix-based conjunctival flap.
2. Vertical or somewhat slanting limbal incision ab externo.
3. If general anesthesia, intravenous urea or mannitol, and a carbonic anhydrase inhibitor have not lowered the ocular tension sufficiently, a posterior sclerotomy is done before the limbal incision is completed. Aqueous or fluid vitreous is then aspirated. It may be necessary to search for a pocket of fluid vitreous (Fig. 12).
4. Synechiae between the iris and the incision are separated with a spatula introduced inferiorly through the limbal incision after the anterior chamber has been filled with air (Fig. 13). Resistant synechiae are left alone to avoid the risk of hemorrhage.

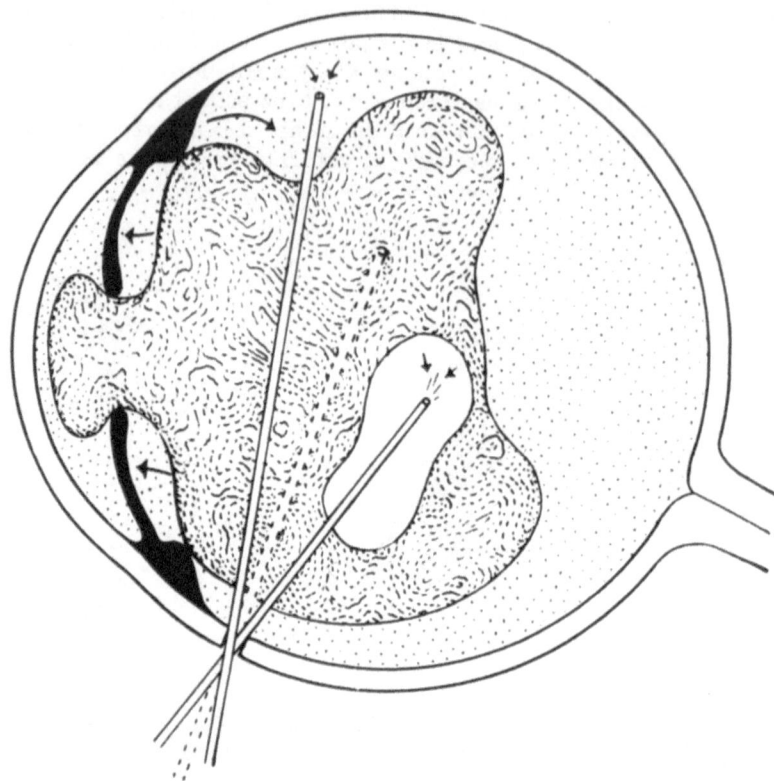

Fig. 12. Aspiration of aqueous or fluid vitreous through a posterior sclerotomy.

5. The iris is grasped carefully, to avoid damaging the hyaloid and a peripheral iridectomy is done.

6. The anterior chamber is filled with 1 per cent acetylcholine and a moderate amount of air.

If necessary, this procedure must be done without delay. Permanent peripheral anterior synechiae will form if the anterior chamber remains absent or shallow for some time. An iridectomy may then be ineffective, and a cyclodialysis may be required (Fig. 14).

Late pupillary block (inflammatory). This form of pupillary block may occur 10 to 20 days postoperatively, and, sometimes, later. Postoperative iridocyclitis may cause late pupillary block or it may be a contributing factor. Severe iridocyclitis with pupillary block may be mistaken for hypertensive iridocyclitis. The following **mechanisms** may lead to late pupillary block;

1. Formation of posterior synechiae, completely surrounding the pupil and the iridectomy opening. The pupillary block may be relative when a minute communication between the chambers remains.

2. Thickening of the anterior hyaloid with occlusion of the pupil and the

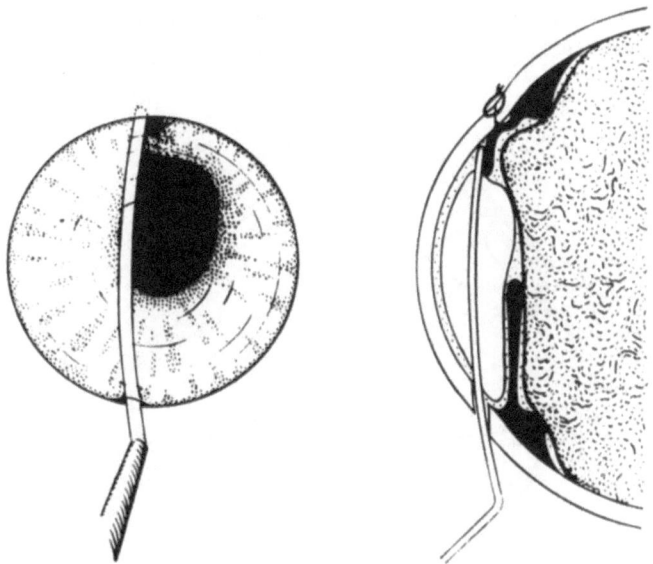

Fig. 13. Separation of recent anterior synechiae.

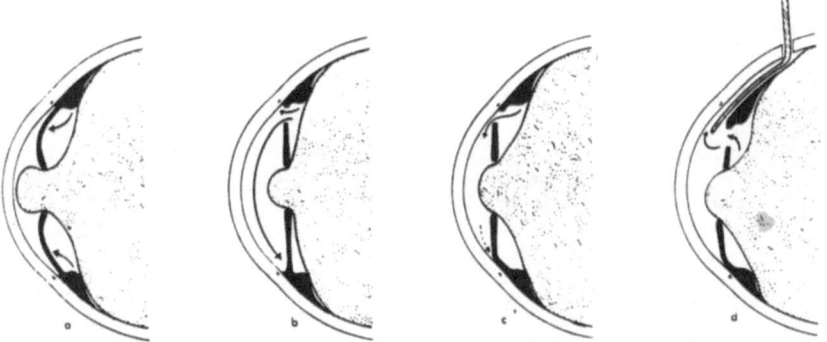

Fig. 14. Pupillary block. a. The aqueous accumulates in the posterior chamber, and the iris bombé may block the angle. b. A peripheral iridectomy relieves the pupillary block and, if performed in time, also an angle block. c. The iridectomy may not be effective in relieving the glaucoma when extensive peripheral anterior synechiae have formed. d. A cyclodialysis is indicated when the angle is irreversibly closed.

iridectomy opening by synechiae (Fig. 15). Condensation of the vitreous may accompany iridocyclitis, especially if vitreous is incarcerated in the incision (Fig. 16). Also, a sector coloboma may thus become obstructed. A variation of this mechanism is the condensation and retraction of the entire vitreous with thickening of the posterior hyaloid. The aqueous accumulates behind the vitreous (Fig. 16). The pathogenesis resembles that of malignant glaucoma. The vitreous acts in the former as the lens does in the later condition.

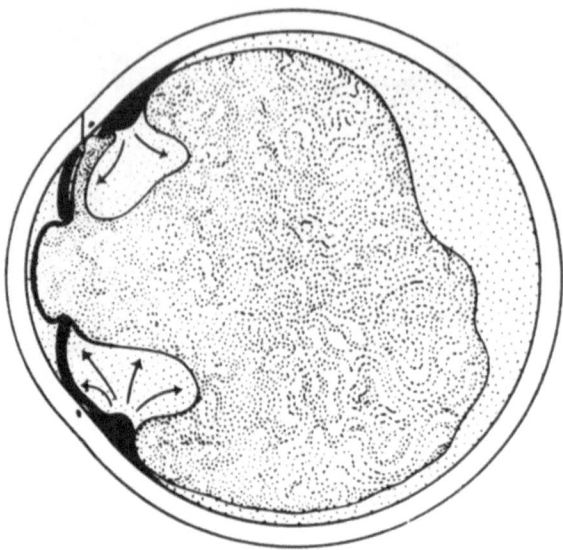

Fig. 15. Late pupillary block with thickening of the anterior hyaloid and occlusion of the pupil and the iridectomy opening by synechiae.

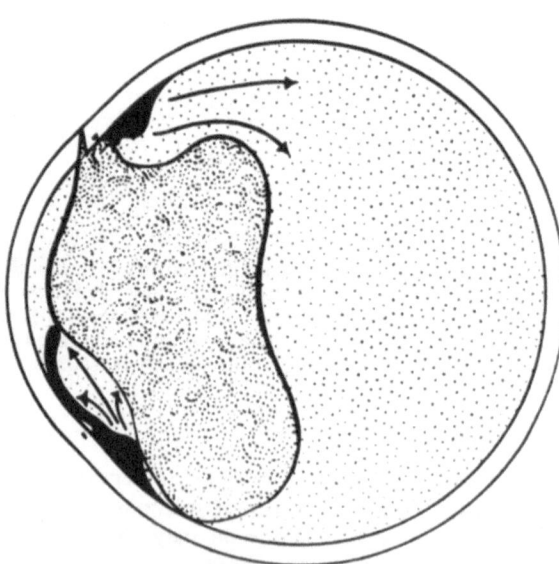

Fig. 16. Pupillary block with retraction of the vitreous, thickening of the hyaloid, and incarceration of vitreous in the incision.

406

3. Delayed reformation and late collapse of the anterior chamber. When the anterior chamber is empty, the iris is in contact with the cornea and the hyaloid, and synechiae form easily. Excessive dilatation of the pupil and subsequent contraction may cause pupillary block by strangulation of the vitreous.

4. Choroidal detachment. This is frequently associated with a shallow anterior chamber. There is a separation of the ciliary body, which may be responsible for hyposecretion of aqueous. Pupillary block may thus occur without elevated tension.

Diagnosis: The clinical picture of late pupillary block may be similar to that of early pupillary block, but the onset is insidious. The signs of inflammation may be minimal. The tension may be elevated, normal, or even low. A relative pupillary block may decrease the depth of the anterior chamber. On becoming absolute the block may further reduce the depth of the anterior chamber, and the tension may rise. However, a relative block may cause repeated contact between the iris root and the trabeculae, as in angle-closure glaucoma, and result in permanent damage to the trabeculae.

Prophylaxis: Systemic steroid therapy has proved extremely effective in reducing the inflammatory reaction to surgery. The pupil is dilated with atropine 1 to 4%. Complicated cataract secondary to uveitis should not be treated surgically until the inflammation has subsided, and then only under the protection of intensive steroid therapy. A sector iridectomy is indicated. If surgery has to be performed in the presence of an active inflammation, an intravenous drip of corticotropin is indicated.

Management: Late pupillary block requires essentially the same therapeutic measures as early pupillary block. Mydriatics are effective only if used early, however, when they may still be able to break the synechiae.

Chandler recommends the incision of the hyaloid. This would relieve the pupillary block by releasing fluid from the vitreous; it would be indicated especially when a pupillary membrane is responsible for the block.

Becker and Shaffer recommend a complete incision through a detached vitreous body when the latter blocks the flow of aqueous. The aqueous accumulates behind the posterior hyaloid, which may be thickened, and incision of the anterior as well as the posterior hyaloid may be neceesary to restore the flow of aqueous to the anterior chamber (Fig. 17). An iridectomy would not be effective, since the obstacle to the flow of aqueous is the entire vitreous body.

CHOROIDAL DETACHMENT

Choroidal detachment is probably a consequence of collapse of the anterior chamber. The volume of the ocular contents is reduced and the tension is low. The choroidal vessels form a transudate to restore the intraocular volume. Choroidal detachment is more frequent in eyes with formed than with fluid vitreous. On being displaced forward the vitreous pulls on the retina and the choroid, especially at the base of the vitreous, and creates a decrease in the pressure in the potential suprachoroidal space, which will become

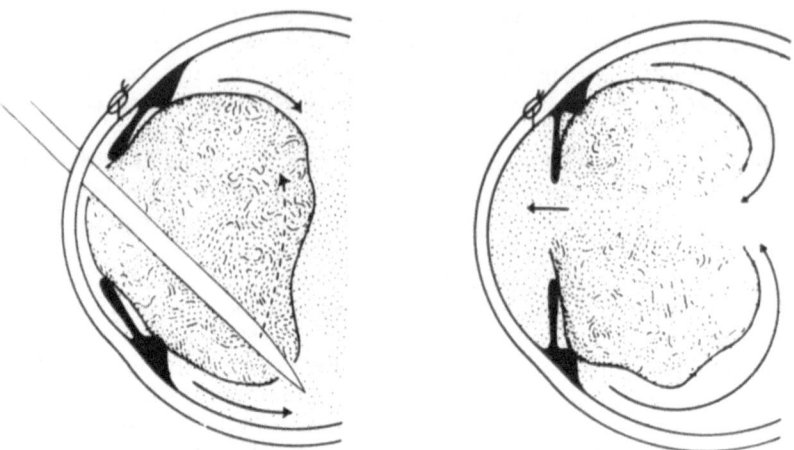

Fig. 17. 'Malignant' pupillary block relieved by incision through the detached vitreous body.

filled with a transudate. A posterior vitreous detachment may prevent the formation of a choroidal detachment.

Detachment of the ciliary body may be responsible for continued hypotony due to hyposecretion and subsequently flat anterior chamber.

Management: Carbonic anhydrase inhibitors, intravenous urea or mannitol, and pressure dressings are usually ineffective. Rest by the patient and patience on the part of the surgeon are indicated when there is no obvious wound leak or pupillary block. When the anterior chamber has been very shallow or absent for 7 days a posterior sclerotomy is indicated, to release the suprachoroidal fluid. Often a flat detachment of the ciliary body and the choroid, which may not be detected on ophthalmoscopic examination, is present. The sclerotomy is done in the inferior temporal quadrant, and if no fluid is obtained, the procedure is repeated in the inferior nasal quadrant. Air is injected into the anterior chmaber, and an iridectomy inferiorly is done. All factors that may be responsible for the collapse of the anterior chamber — hyposecretion, pupillary block, and small wound leaks — are thus taken care of.

Author's address:
Instituto Barraquer
Barcelona
Spain

Docum. Ophthal. Proc. Series, Vol. 21

MEMBRANE FORMATION FOLLOWING CATARACT SURGERY

R.A. D'AMICO

(New York, U.S.A.)

The great advances in instrumentation and technique of cataract surgery in the last 50 years have not only improved the quality of the resulting vision but have reduced the incidence of complications. Nevertheless, no surgical procedure is free of complications and the surgeon's efforts are continually directed toward early recognition and therapy when complications occur.

Membrane formation behind the cornea following cataract extraction presents a problem both of diagnosis and treatment. The most dreaded of these abnormalities is epithelial downgrowth.

Considering the relentless progression of this ingrowth once it gains access to the anterior chamber, it is remarkable that it occurs so infrequently.

Epithelial implantation cysts offer slightly better prognosis since they may remain isolated and allow complete excision.

Stromal overgrowth into the anterior chamber is usually limited to the region of the surgical wound but may progress where inflammation and endothelial cell damage is extensive.

Descemet's Membrane detachment usually results from improper manipulation of the corneo-scleral scissors, while Descemet's Membrane reduplications are usually fixed folds associated with endothelial disfunction and corneal edema.

Occasionally, chronic low grade endothelial cell disease may lead to new layers of Descemet's membrane material being laid down as hyalin-like tubules on the endothelial surface or iris face.

The vitreous will adhere to the surgical wound or an inflamed endothelium if it comes into direct contact with it and its zone of condensation may be membrane-like, offering some difficulty in differential diagnosis.

Factors influencing retrocorneal membrane formation are:
1. Poor wound apposition — allowing ingrowth of tissues.
2. Iris or vitreous incarceration interfering with posterior wound closure

409

and encouraging connective tissue overgrowth. (Fig. 1)
3. Inflammation — damaging the endothelium and encouraging connective tissue overgrowth and epithelial cell proliferation.
4. Direct contamination of the anterior chamber with epithelial cells at the time of surgery.

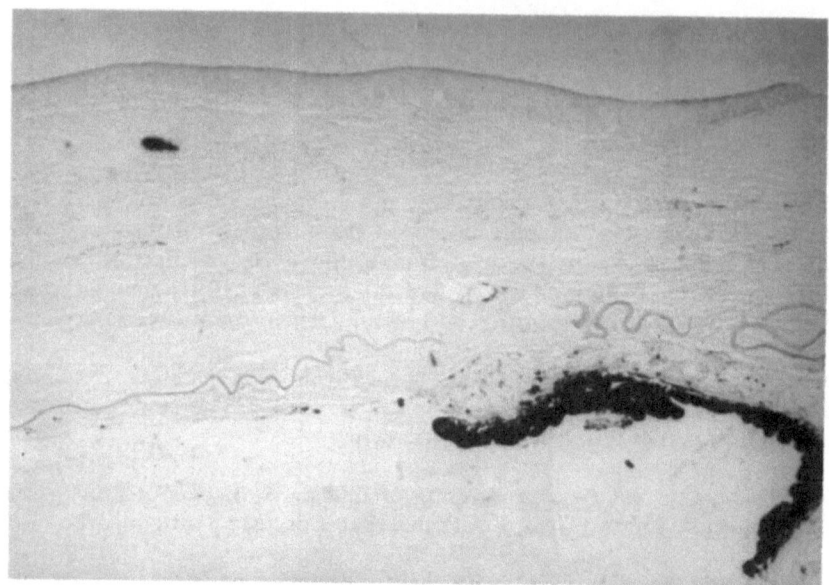

Fig. 1.

Since the prognosis and therapy of the various kinds of retrocorneal membranes is vastly different, their diagnosis is of great importance.

The Clinical Signs of Epithelial Downgrowth are:
1. Wound leak — as demonstrated with fluorescein dye.
2. A cystoid cicatrix — indicating defective wound healing. (fig. 2)
3. Descending corneal edema — indicating progressive endothelial cell disfunction. (fig. 3)
4. Interstitial corneal vascularization.
5. Presence and progression of a delicate retrocorneal membrane with a scalloped border. (fig. 4 — see arrow)
6. Presence of a membrane on the iris surface or vitreous face.
7. Secondary glaucoma due to involvement of the angle.
Biopsy may be necessary to confirm the diagnosis prior to definitive therapy.

The Clinical Signs of Stromal overgrowth are:
1. A Semi-opaque membrane with folds.

410

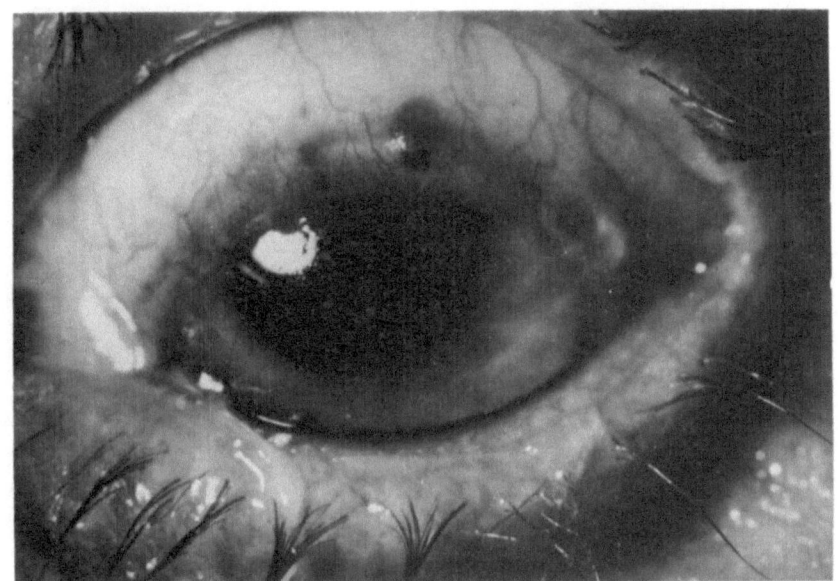

Fig. 2.

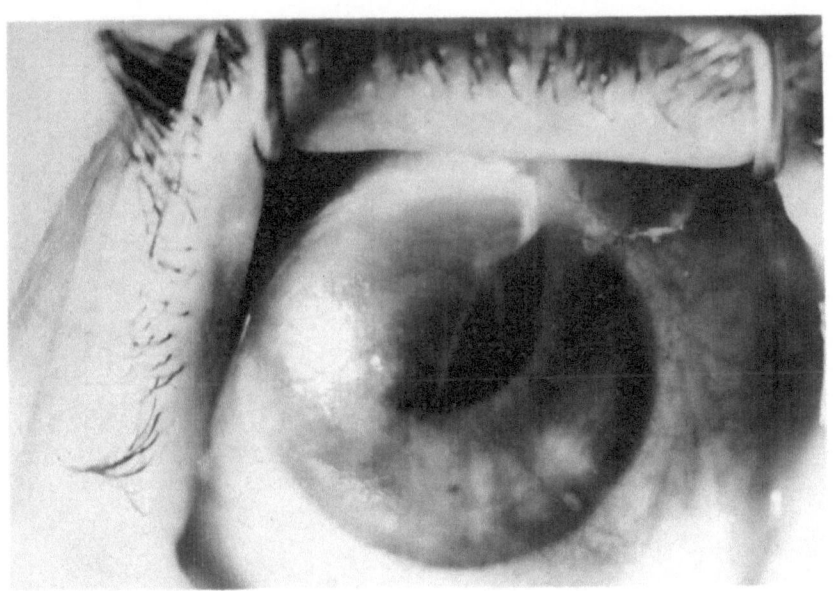

Fig. 3.

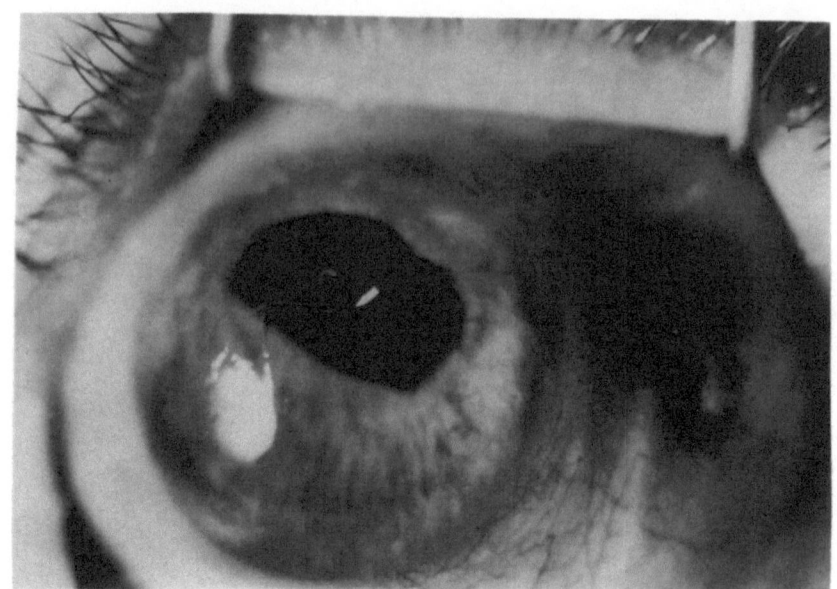

Fig. 4.

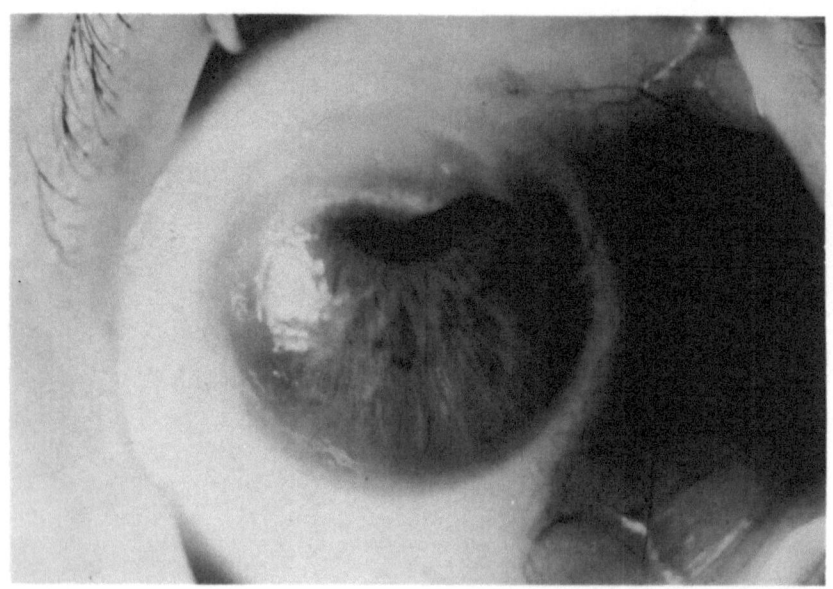

Fig. 5.

412

2. A concave advancing edge — usually limited to the region near the surgical wound. (fig. 5)
3. While vascularization of the membrane may occur if iris adhesion is present, interstitial corneal vascularization is uncommon.

The Clinical Signs of Descemet's membrane separation are:
1. A distinct linear edge.
2. Evident projection of the membrane into the anterior chamber. (fig. 6)
3. Absence of vascularization.

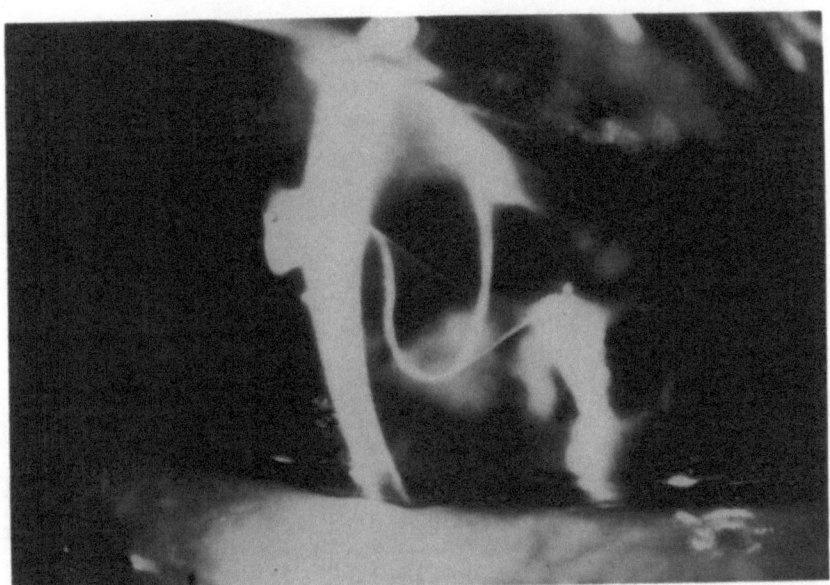

Fig. 6.

The Signs of Retrocorneal vitreous condensation are:
1. A "Membrane" of indistinct borders.
2. Stromal edema prominent to the edge of the "membrane". (fig. 7)
3. Interstitial vascularization uncommon.
4. Pupillary displacement due to vitreous strands likely.
5. Vitreous evident in the anterior chamber.

The treatment of Epithelial Downgrowth will require firstly, excision of the tract or route of epithelial ingrowth. (fig. 8)
In the removal of evident epithelial invasion, the manner in which this is best undertaken varies with the tissue involved.
Corneal-cryoprobe method as described by Maumenee and Paton allows epithelial removal without unnecessary stromal injury.

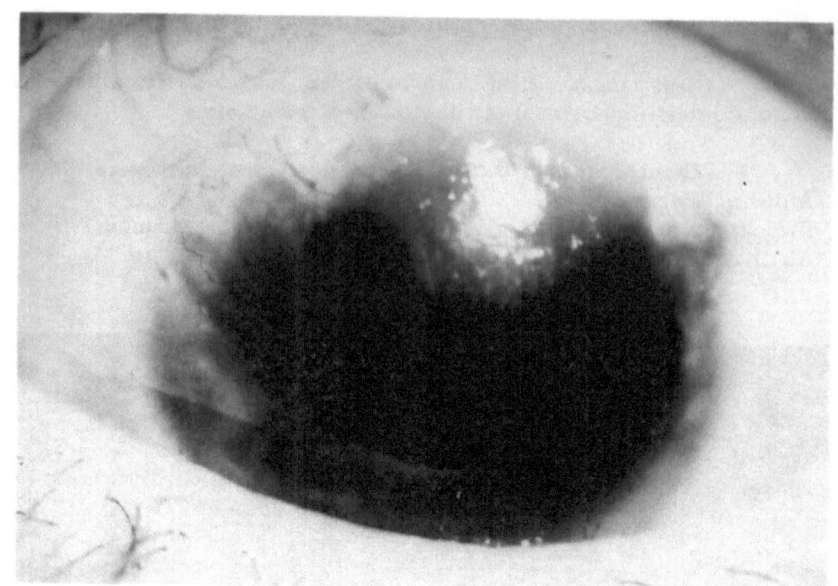

Fig. 7.

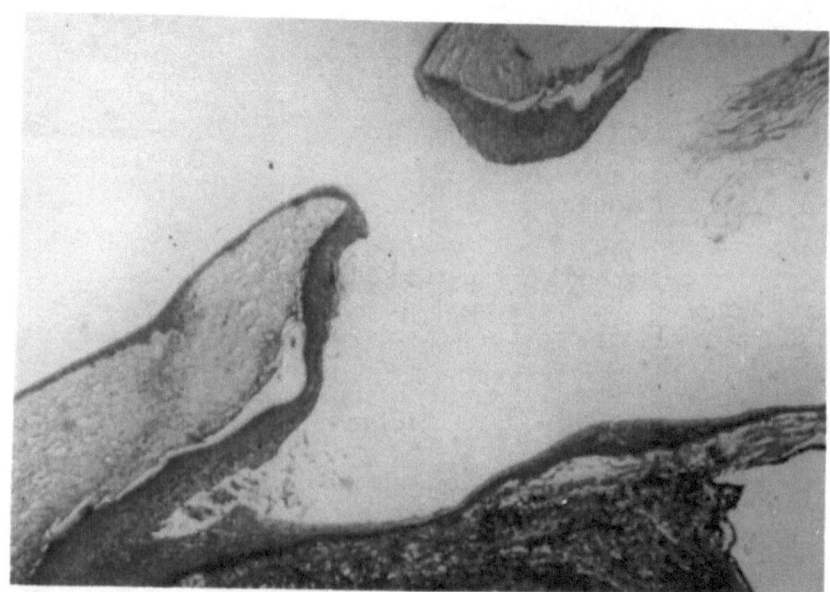

Fig. 8.

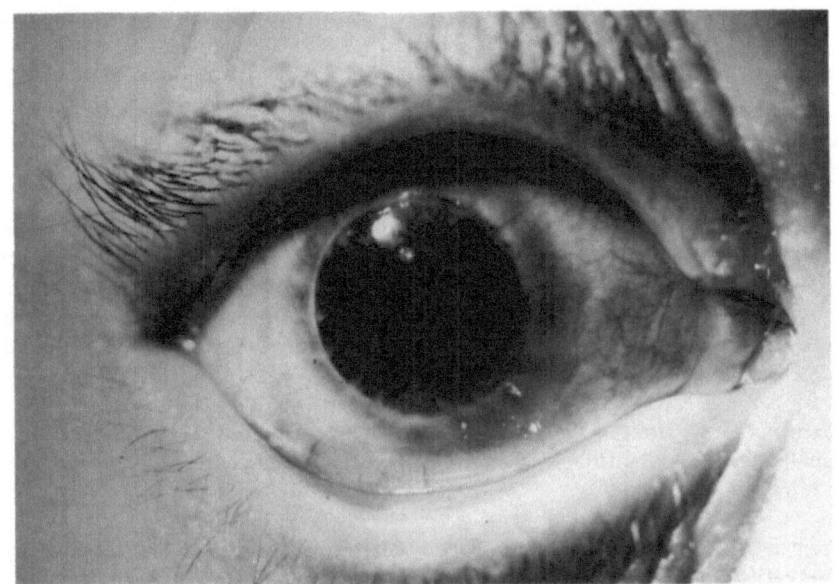

Fig. 9.

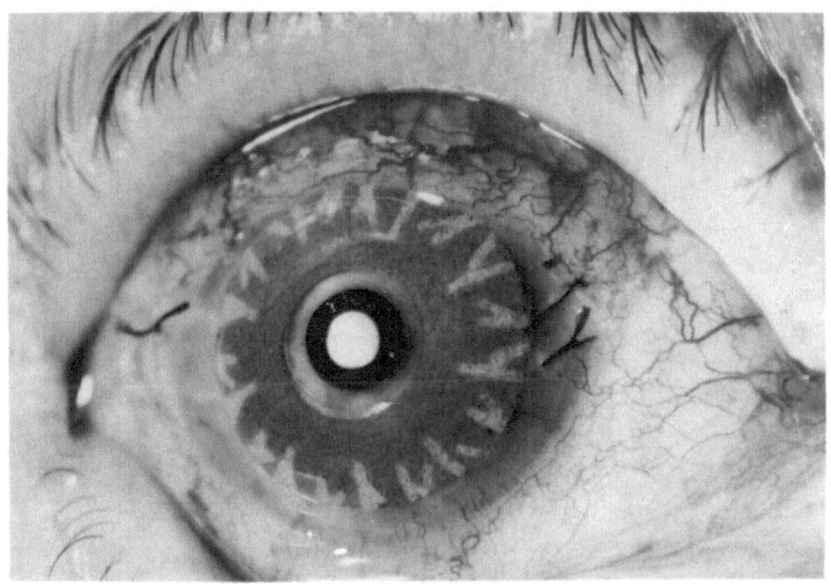

Fig. 10.

Iris-excise. The extent of iris involvement can often be delineated pre-operatively by its response to photocoagulation.

Ciliary Body involvement may be treated by either cryoprobe or diathermic coagulation with a wet-field coagulator. We prefer the latter because of less likelihood of hemorrhage.

Vitreous-when involved, should be excised by 'open-sky' technique.

Keratoplasty may be undertaken later for visual rehabilitation if there is no evidence of regrowth of epithelium. This may be occasionally successful (fig. 9) but more often epithelial or stromal membrane formation behind the graft will occur. Prosthokeratoplasty (fig. 10) may also be used for visual rehabilitation but membrane formation behind teh optical cylinder will occur if epithelial removal is not complete.

Treatment of stromal overgrowth or Descemet's membrane reduplication is usually unnecessary unless it compromises the visual axis, then keratoplasty may be necessary.

Treatment of Descemet's membrane detachment may be carried out by re-positioning with a spatula inserted through a small libal incision. (fig. 11). The membrane may be maintained in position by air or by a penetrating nylon suture until normal anterior chamber hydrodynamic forces take over.

Treatment of vitreous condensation into the cornea may be spatulation combined with pars plana vitrectomy or opensky vitrectomy. Keratoplasty may be necessary for visual rehabilitation.

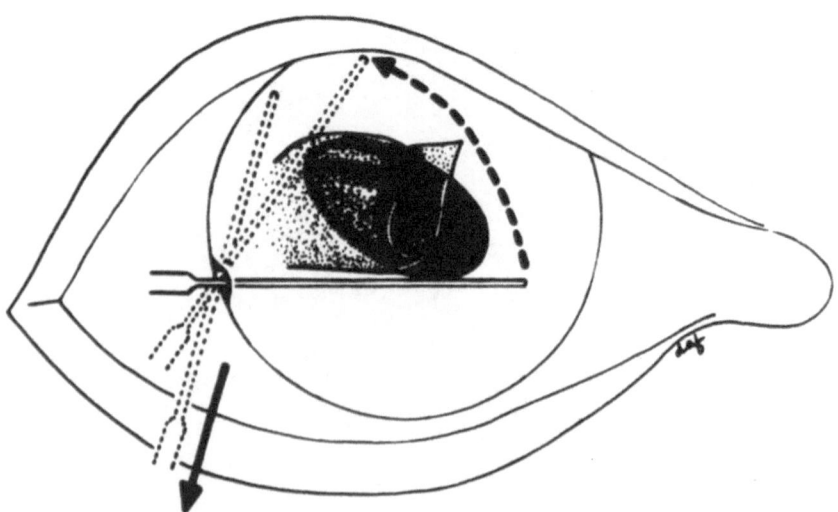

Fig. 11.

PREVENTION OF EPITHELIAL INVASION
OF THE ANTERIOR CHAMBER

The possibility of contamination of the anterior chamber structures by instruments should be considered and forceps or scissors used for external should not be used within the anterior chamber.

Secure would closure is probably the most important factor in the prevention of epithelial downgrowth and multiple sutures and accurate apposition of wound edges are essential.

The type of flap-fornix or limbus based or section without flap is probably unimportant as long as accurate, secure wound apposition is achieved.

Late wound disruption by elevated intraocular pressure due to pupillary block may occur in cases where secure wound closure was initially achieved and may result in late retrocorneal membrane formation.

Docum. Ophthal. Proc. Series, Vol. 21

MANAGEMENT OF ADVANCED BULLOUS KERATOPATHY PAST—PRESENT—FUTURE (PROSTHOKERATOPLASTY RESULTS)

A.B. RIZZUTI

(New York, U.S.A.)

Primary bullous keratopathy is most commonly seen in Fuch's dystrophy. Secondary bullous keratopathy frequently follows complicated cataract extraction particularly after vitreous loss. It has been reported that in 450,000 cataract extractions performed annually in the United States, 25,000 cases (6%) resulted in bullous keratopathy.

Medical therapy is of limited use in the management of bullous keratopathy. Osmotherapy including hypertonic solutions of 5% sodium chloride or ointment, 40% glucose ointment and surface-active agents such as ophthasilozane, instilled several times a day may prove clinically useful in lessening epithelial edema, but has little or no effect in clearing stromal or endothelial edema.

Conjunctival flaps, diathermy of Bowman's membrane, full thickness lamellar grafts and soft contact lenses often alleviates pain, but seldom results in visual improvement and surgery is usually indicated.

Penetrating Keratoplasty is the operation of choice in the treatment of advanced bullous keratopathy. With our present methods of refined surgical techniques and improved instrumentations, approximately 80% of clear grafts may be expected.

When penetrating keratoplasty fails, a prosthokeratoplasty procedure should then be considered. Prosthokeratoplasty is a surgical procedure in which a corneal prosthesis usually consisting of a special polymer of plastic material, is inserted in an eye to replace a diseased or scarred cornea.

Within the past decade significant technological advances have been made in methods of refining keratoprosthesis. Following the pioneering experiments in animals by Stone et al., an enthusiastic group of clinical and research investigators persisted in their endeavors to replace diseased corneas with a variety of synthetic materials.

A clinical study was undertaken by the author in performing prosthokeratoplasty procedures in patients afflicted with advanced bullous keratopathy in eyes that were considered hopeless by other means of surgery. In this series of cases, the Cardona 'nut and bolt' keratoprosthesis was implanted in all of the damaged corneas.

PATIENTS AND METHODS

From April 1969 to January 1977, the author operated on 72 eyes of 69

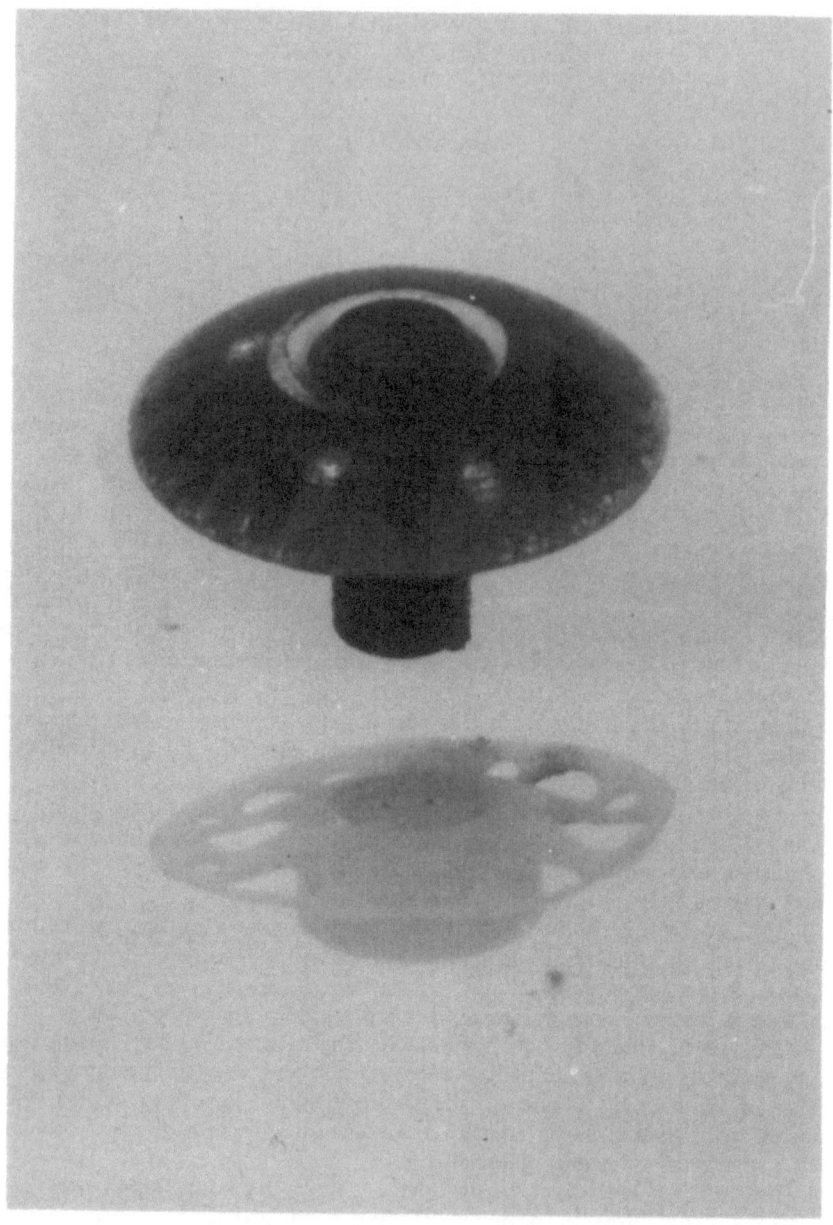

Fig. 1. Cardona 'nut and bolt' keratoprosthesis contact lens fused to optical cylinder. Perforated flexible teflon plate.

patients with severely damaged corneas. The study group consisted of 44 females and 25 males with an age range of 8 to 82 years (mean 65). Twenty-nine eyes underwent previous cataract extractions and 43 eyes were phakic. Prosthokeratoplasty was performed as the primary procedure in 9 eyes. In the remaining 63 eyes, multiple surgical procedures had been previously performed prior to attempting prosthokeratoplasty. The preoperative visual acuity in all eyes ranged from light projection to counting fingers at a few feet.

Table 1. ,Prosthokeratoplasty — 'Nut and Bolt' prosthesis post operative complications (72 eyes)
1

Clinical diagnosis	No. of Eyes	Pre-Op Vision
Bullous Keratopathy (Advanced)	4	H/M
Bullous Keratopathy (Advanced)	2	to
Corneal dystrophy	3	C/F
Badly diseased corneas and graft failures	63	H/M C/F
TOTAL	72 Eyes (69 patients)	

NUT-AND-BOLT KERATOPROSTHESIS

The keratoprosthesis used in all eyes was the Cardona transcorneal penetrating type (nut and bolt). It was made of purified methyl methacrylate and consisted of three integrated parts: 1. Anterior contact lens surface 8.5 mm in diameter; 2. Central optical cylinder 3.5 mm in diameter: 5.5 mm in height; 3. Posterior (screw type) perforated teflon skirt 5.5 mm in diameter.

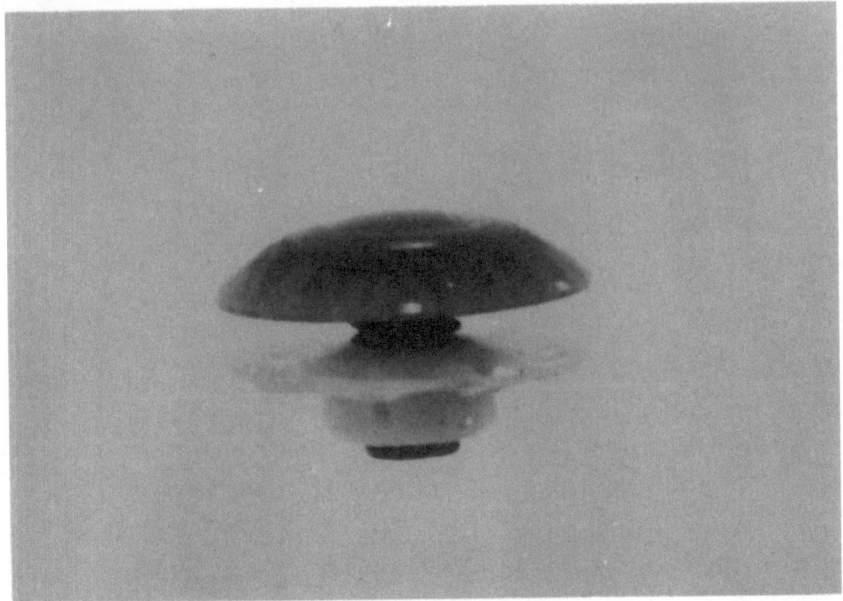

Fig. 2. Keratoprosthesis viewed as a single optical unit.

The anterior contact lens surface is painted to match the color of the iris of the fellow eye. The optical cylinder contains 3 lenses with an average dioptric power of +66. The prosthesis is sterilized with ultraviolet light and ethylene oxide after which it is immersed in a small receptacle containing 1:750 Zephiran chloride.

PRE-REQUISITES FOR PROSTHOKERATOPLASTY

It was mandatory that all eyes showed satisfactory light projection and normal intraocular pressure. The MacKay—Marg tonometer which has a small foot plate was the preferred tonometer and gave more accurate intraocular pressure readings. In severely altered corneas, finger palpation was the only means of estimating the ocular tension. A and B scan ultrasonography proved valuable in recording the axial diameter of the globe in calculating the dioptric power of the prosthesis and in ruling out vitreous hemorrhage or intraocular neoplasm.

The keratoprosthesis was not imbedded in corneas with less than 1.3 mm thickness. The corneas were reconstituted with a full thickness lamellar or penetrating graft. The prosthokeratoplasty procedure was performed either at the time of the keratoplasty procedure, or after a waiting period of several months. Corneal thickness was determined with the pachyometer attached to the slitlamp. When the anterior radius of curvature of the cornea could not be calculated with the ophthalmometer, an estimate was obtained with the author's keratoguide.

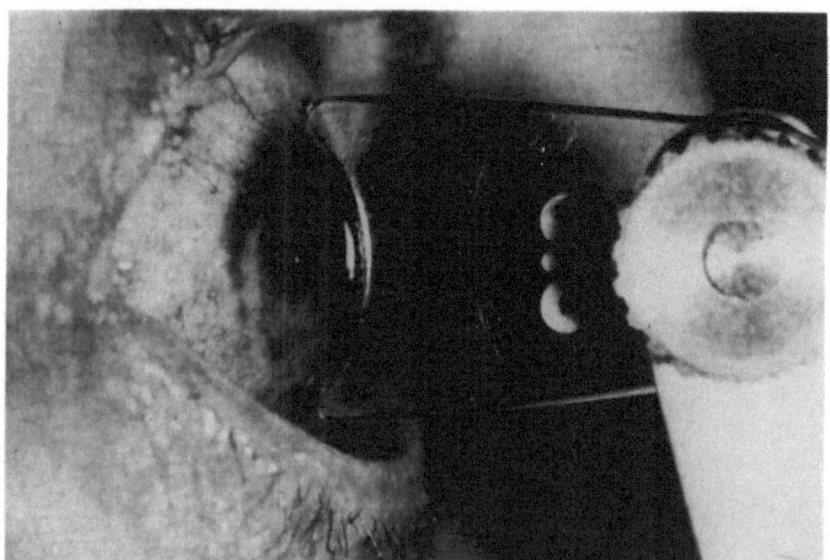

Fig. 3. Author's keratoguide used to estimate radius of corneal curvature from 6.4mm to 8.4mm.

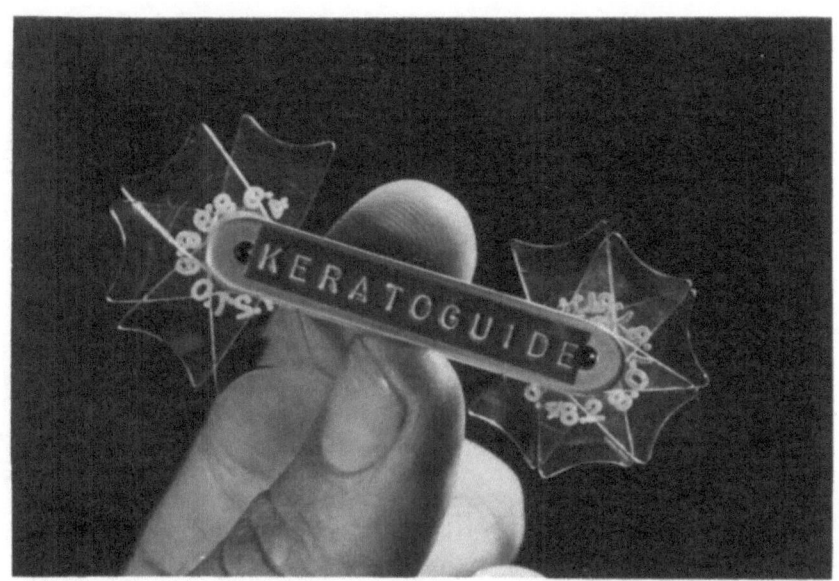

SURGICAL TECHNIQUES

Description of the surgical technique has been previously reported. The main points of the surgery consist of making a central corneal opening with a 3.5 mm trephine.

The opening is temporarily occluded with a plastic insert to prevent excessive vitreous loss. A 150° corneo-scleral incision is made and the lens is extracted regardless whether it is clear or opaque. Cryosurgical extraction of the lens was found to be the method of choice. The central opening must be cleared of any aberrant iris tissue, secondary membranes or remnants of lens material. The corneal portion of the keratoprosthesis with its optical cylinder is held firmly with a small rubber suction tip. The optical cylinder is then passed through the corneal opening and by rotating the suction tip, the cylinder is slowly and firmly screwed to the retaining teflon plate held against the posterior corneal surface by means of a special fixation forceps.

RESULTS

In this series of 72 eyes, there was an improvement in 26 eyes (36%). Twenty-seven eyes (37%) ended in failure and 15 eyes (21%) remained unchanged. Four patients were unaccountable. See table 2.

Total extrusion of the prosthesis occurred in 5 eyes (7%) and sterile necrosis or partial extrusion was noted in 4 eyes (5%) with an overall extrusion problem of 9 eyes (11%).

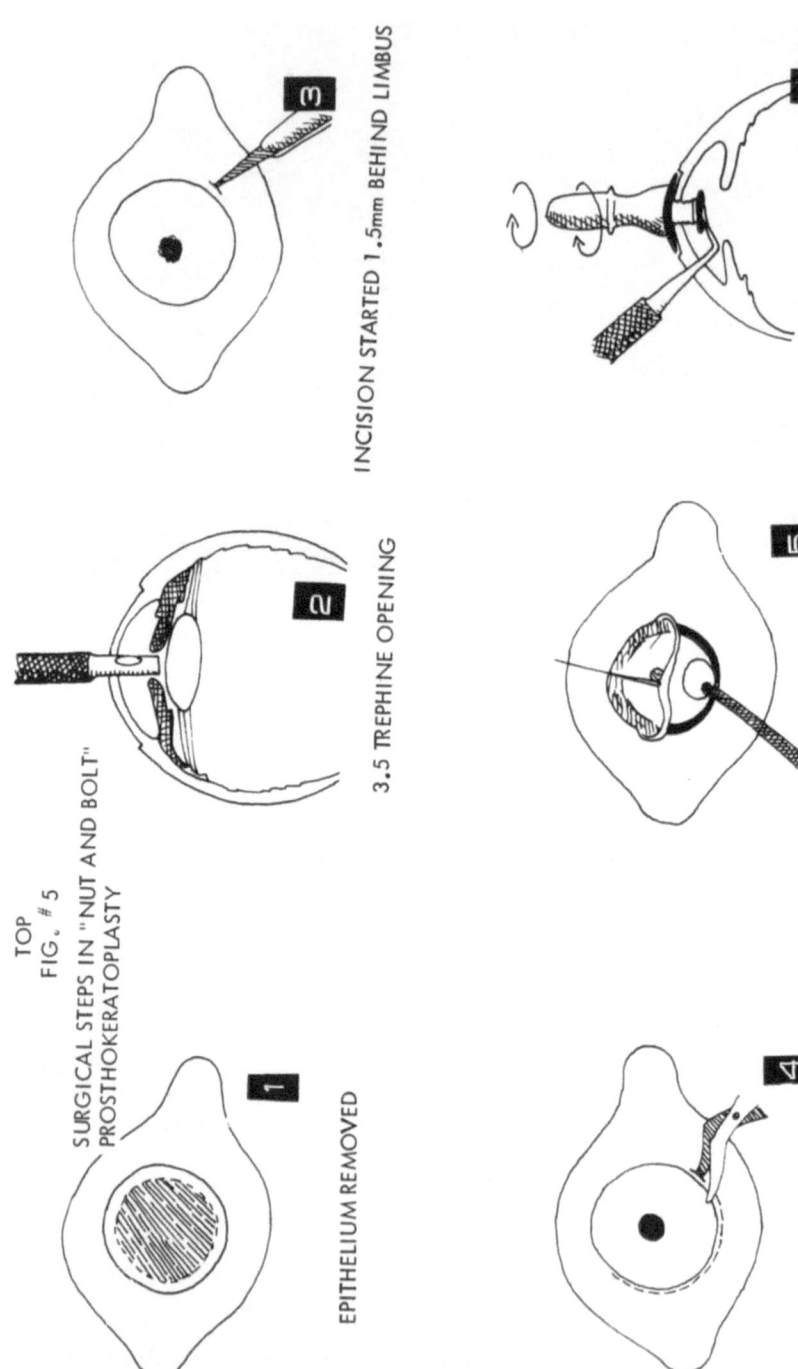

TOP
FIG. #5

SURGICAL STEPS IN "NUT AND BOLT"
PROSTHOKERATOPLASTY

EPITHELIUM REMOVED

3.5 TREPHINE OPENING

INCISION STARTED 1.5mm BEHIND LIMBUS

CORNEA–SCLERAL SECTION ENLARGED 150°

LENS EXTRACTED WITH CRYO UNIT

NUT & BOLT KERATOPROSTHESIS POSITIONED

Fig. 5. Surgical steps in 'nut and bolt' prosthekeratoplasty.

424

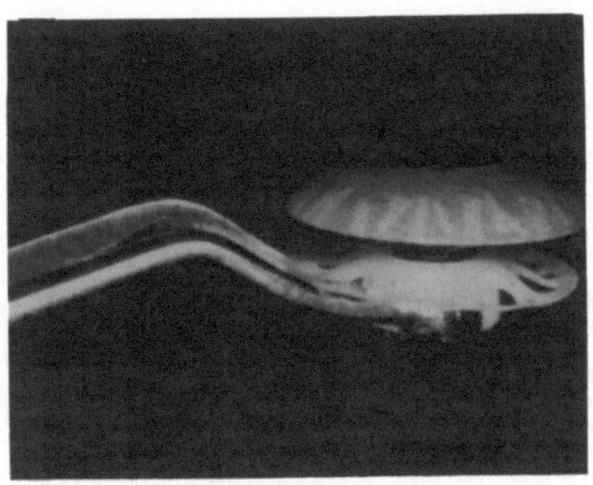

Fig. 6. Keratoprosthesis held with special forceps.

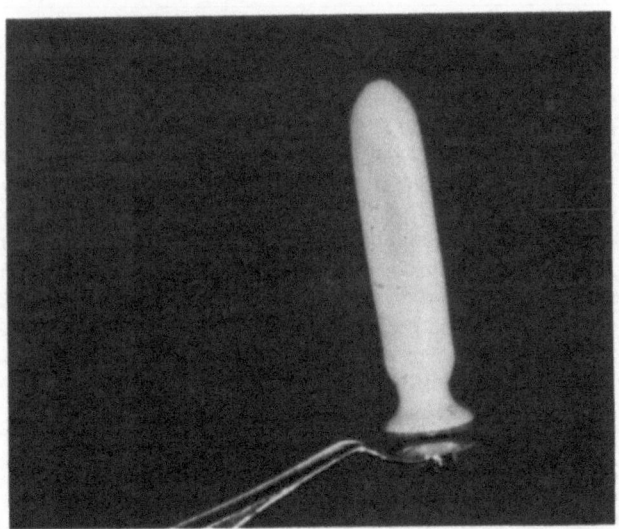

Fig. 7. Rubber bulb tip used to rotate contact face of prosthesis to optical cylinder.

Table 2. Prosthokeratoplasty – 'Nut and Bolt' prosthesis final post operative results (72 eyes)

Results	No. of Eyes
Successes	26 (36%)
Failures	27 (37%)
Unchanged	15 (21%)
Unaccounted	4 (6%)

COMPLICATIONS

Glaucoma, phthisis bulbi and retroprosthetic membrane or varying degrees of condensation of the vitreous face comprised the large majority of the post operative complications. The total number of complications that occurred are listed on table 2.

Table 3. Prosthokeratoplasty – 'Nut and Bolt' prosthesis post operative complications (72 eyes).

Complications	Number of Eyes	Improved with treatment
Glaucoma	12	8
Phthisis bulbi	15	0
Extrusion Prosthesis	5	0
Partial extrusion prosthesis	4	3
Retroprosthetic membrane	5	2
Condensation vitreous face	7	2
Vitreous hemorrhage	3	0
Iris prolapse	1	1
Infection	2	0
	54 Eyes (75%)	16 (22%)

Complications 75%
Treated successfully 22%

Glaucoma resulted in 12 eyes. This complication responded poorly to medical or surgical therapy. In 6 of these eyes, the tension was controlled after performing one or several cyclodiathermy, cyclocryotherapy or a combination of both procedures. Two glaucomatous eyes responded favorably to maximum miotic and systemic therapy. Four eyes ended in blindness.

Fifteen eyes progressed to phthisis bulbi which in the large majority was secondary to vitreous hemorrhage, retinal detachment or from leakage along the cylinder of the prosthesis. This complication occurred with greater frequency in eyes that were previously subjected to multiple operative procedures which is illustrated in table 4.

Table 4. Prosthokeratoplasty – 'Nut and Bolt' Posthesis Incidence of Phthisis Bulbi (15 eyes) 20%

No. of Eyes	No. of Operations that Preceded Prosthokeratoplasty	Onset of Phthisis
12	1 to 7	4 Mos. to 24 Mos.
1	7	5th Year
1	3	6th Year
1	5	6th Year

15 Eyes – 20% Unimprovable

Retinal detachment was diagnosed by ultrasonography in 6 eyes. Most of the detachments were of the 'morning glory' type and were considered beyond surgical repair. A mild condensation of the anterior vitreous face was noted by slitlamp biomicroscopy in 7 eyes. Five eyes showed a dense white retroprosthetic membrane. Two eyes were improved by removal of the anterior face of the prosthesis and excising the retrocorneal membrane.

Vitreous hemorrhage occurred in 3 eyes. In 1 eye, this complication followed trauma to the globe and in another eye bleeding occurred soon after the removal of sutures. The incidence of infection was surprisingly low and occurred in only 2 eyes. Endophthalmitis was confirmed by ultrasonography which demonstrated marked vitreous debris. Both of these eyes were eviscerated. The total failure in 27 eyes (37%) is illustrated in table 5.

The reasons for total extrusion which occured in 5 eyes (7%) are illustrated in table 5.

Table 5. Prosthokeratoplasty – 'Nut and Bolt' Prosthesis causes of extrusion of Prosthesis (5 Eyes) 7%

Clinical diagnosis	No. of surgical procedures Prior to Prosthokeratoplasty	Onset of Extrusion
Mooren's Ulcer	5	16 Months
alkali burn of cornea	3	24 Months
Malignant Glaucoma (Bullous Keratopathy)	3	23 Months
Keratoglobus with Cataract	2	3 Months
Aphakic Epithelial downgrowth	1	60 Months

VISUAL RESULTS

The pre-operative vision in this series of 72 eyes, ranged from hand motion to finger counting with satisfactory light projection. The visual improvement obtained following prosthokeratoplasty showed the highest percent of success in eyes in which prosthokeratoplasty was performed as the initial surgical procedure. See table 1.

In 26 eyes (36%), vision pre-operatively of hand motion or finger counting was improved to 20/25 to 20/200 over a general follow-up period of 6 years. In 16 of these eyes (21%), the visual acuity ranged to 20/25 to 20/70, as illustrated in table 6.

Table 6. Prosthokeratoplasty – 'Nut and Bolt' Prosthesis post-operative visual results (72 Eyes)

Pre-operative vision	Post-operative vision	No. of Eyes	Follow-up period
In all cases vision	20/25	4	1 To 3 Years
Ranged from:	20/30	2	1 Year: 6 Years
Hand motion	20/40	2	4 Years: 6 Years
Counting Fingers	20/50	6	1 To 6 Years
Light projection	20/70	2	1 Year: 2 Years
	20/100	4	1 To 5 Years
	20/200	4	1 To 5 Years
	20/200	2	7 Mos.: 5 Years
	Visual improvement		26 Eyes (36%) Ranging from 1 TO 6 Years

427

DISCUSSION

Donn reported on 34 eyes with advanced aphakic bullous keratopathy treated with the Cardona 'Nut and Bolt' keratoprosthesis as a primary procedure. He obtained visual improvement in 28 eyes (82%) over a follow-up period of 6 to 72 months. There were 3 extrusions (5%) and an overall failure rate of 15%.

In the author's series of the 6 eyes with advanced aphakic bullous keratopathy and in 3 leucomatous eyes in which prosthokeratoplasty was performed as the primary procedure, visual improvement was obtained in all cases over a follow-up period of 8 months to 5 years. All of the eyes in this series were free of postoperative complications except for one eye that showed a retroprosthetic membrane. The membrane was excised and vision of 20/70 finally resulted.

One can conclude from these studies that the relatively low rate of extrusion in bullous keratopathy is probably related to the fact that the corneal stroma has not been severely damaged and that it contains a fairly high collagen content.

If the corneal stroma is of sufficient thickness to retain a 'nut and bolt' keratoprosthesis, prosthokeratoplasty may then be performed for cosmetic improvement.

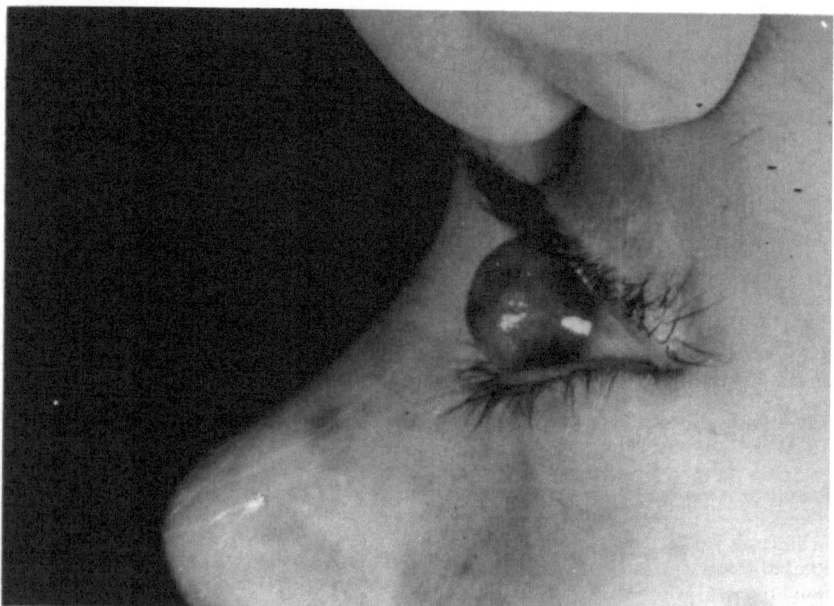

Fig. 8. Opaque cornea in 10 year old female following several graft failures.

In a clinical analysis of 159 eyes in which a 'nut and bolt' keratoprosthesis was implanted, Cardona et al. reported an overall extrusion rate of 12 percent with a follow-up period of 4 years. Forty seven eyes (30%) showed

428

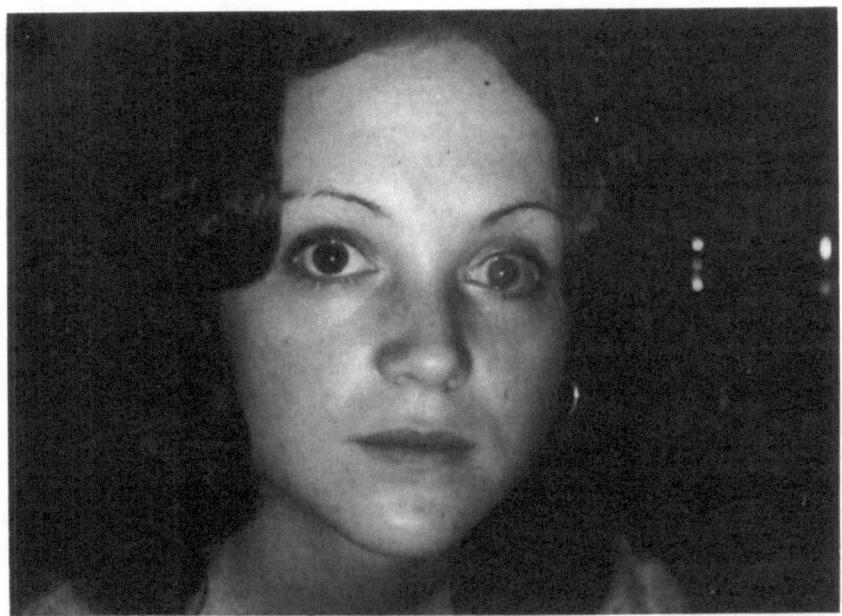

Fig. 9. Keratoprosthesis 'nut and bolt' has been retained over a 4 year follow-up with preservation light perception.

no improvement. In 60 eyes (37%) vision improved from light perception and projection pre-operatively to 20/15−20/60. They concluded that prosthokeratoplasty with implantation of the 'nut and bolt' prosthesis is contraindicated in highly vascularized eyes which resulted from severe chemical burns or badly diseased eyes included in the dry eyed syndromes. In the latter group encouraging and successful results were obtained when the corneal stroma was reconstituted with autogenous periosteum from the patient's tibia and covered with a sliding conjunctival flap or a free mucous membrane graft obtained from the lip.

De Voe, Cardona et al, in a study of 186 eyes afflicted with bullous kerato-pathy obtained a 26% improvement in visual acuity with a 30% failure and a 13% extrusion rate (personal communication).

The more severe or repeated trauma to the cornea, the less likely the success of prosthokeratoplasty. In the final analysis, the improvement of vision obtained regardless of the type of corneal surgery performed is entirely dependent upon retinal function.

Prosthokeratoplasty is not a difficult procedure to master by the average experienced ophthalmic surgeon. The time required for the procedure is comparable to that required for the usual cataract extraction. The postoperative course is smooth and is not unusual for a patient to show considerable visual improvement on the day following surgery. The use of local or systemic steroids in high or continued doses is not required. The patient may be discharged from the hospital after 5 days and is given instructions in the manner in which the prosthesis should be cleansed to remove any accummu-

429

lation of mucous on its anterior surface. The patient seldom complains of any foreign body sensation unless there is evidence of corneal erosion or impending extrusion. Following surgery the visual field is constricted to about the 30 degree isopter but this does not present any real problem to the patient nor does it interfere with carrying out his daily duties or from enjoying watching television.

SUMMARY

A clinical analysis is presented in a study of 72 eyes in 69 patients who underwent prosthokeratoplasty with an imbedded Cardona 'nut and bolt' prosthesis, between 1969 and 1976. All eyes of this series showed marked pathologic changes and the majority of the eyes had been previously subjected to multiple surgical procedures. Prosthokeratoplasty was performed as a primary procedure in only 9 eyes. In the remaining 63 eyes, prosthokeratoplasty was done as a secondary and final procedure. Visual improvement was obtained in 26 eyes (36%) with vision ranging from 20/25 to 20/70 in 16 eyes from a 1 to 6 year follow-up period. Vision was 10/200 to 20/100 in

Table 7. Prosthokeratoplasty – 'Nut and Bolt' prosthesis post operative visual results (72 Eyes) (Pre-op vision ranged from – H/M – C/F or L/P)

Follow up period	NO. OF EYES	Visual range
1 Year	10	20/20 to 20/200
2 Years	6	20/25 to 20/200
3 Years	1	20/25
4 Years	2	20/70 : 20/200
5 Years	4	10/200 to 20/50
6 Years	3	20/30 to 20/40
	26 Eyes (36%) – Vision improved	

the remaining 10 eyes. The most common complications were formation of retroprosthetic membrane, glaucoma, and phthisis bulbi. The overall extrusion problem was 12% with total extrusion occuring in 5 eyes (7%). There was a total failure in 27 eyes (37%) and 15 eyes (21%) were unchanged.

Table 8. Prosthokeratoplasty – 'Nut and Bolt' prosthesis post operative failures (72 Eyes) Six year follow-up

Type of Complications	No. of Eyes
Phthisis Bulbi	15 (20%)
Extrusion Prosthesis	5 (7%)
Glaucoma	3 (4%)
Infection	2 (3%)
Vitreous Hemorrhage	2 (3%)
	27 (37%)

Not withstanding, the post-operative complications and other intrinsic factors associated with prosthokeratoplasty, this surgical procedure has shown promising results in a sufficient number of eyes with advanced bullous keratopathy to warrant further research and clinical investigation. The surgery is not difficult to perform, and it seems to offer the only hope in eyes that were previously doomed to complete blindness or enucleation.

REFERENCES

Barraquer, Joaquin: Optical corneal prosthesis, acrylic corneas, and the keratoprosthesis, *Ann Inst Barraquer,* 1:243, 1960.

Cardona, Hernando: Keratoprosthesis: Acrylic optical cylinder with supporting intralamellar plate, *Amer. J. Ophthal.,* 54:284–294 (Aug) 1962.

Cardona, Hernando; Castroviejo, Ramon & deVoe, A. Gerard: The Cardona keratoprosthesis, the first clinical evaluation. Acta XIX Concilium Ophthalmologicum, 2:1211–1229, 1962.

Cardona, Hernando et al: Corneal grafting. Edited by T.A. Casey, Appleton-Century-Crofts, New York, pp 313–329, 1972.

Choyce, D.P.: The present status of intra-cameral and intra-corneal implants, *Canad. J. Ophthal.,* Vol. 3 (April) 1968.

Dohlman, Claes H.: Refojo, Miguel F. & Rose, Jeannette: Synthetic polymers in corneal surgery, *Arch. Ophthal.,* 77:252–257 (Feb) 1967.

Donn, Anthony: Aphakic bullous keratopathy treated with prosthokeratoplasty. *Arch. Ophthalmol.* 94:270–273, 1976.

Girard, Louis J.: Personal interviews: A new keratoprosthesis, *Highlights Ophthal.,* 10:226–234, 1967.

Rizzuti, A. Benedict: Prosthokeratoplasty procedures for advanced corneal disease. *Ophthalmology Digest,* 36:20–26 (August) 1974.

Stone, William, Jr., & Herbert, E.: Experimental study of plastic material as replacement for the cornea. *Amer. J. Ophthal.,* 36:168–173 (June, Pt. II) 1953.

Strampelli, B.: Keratoprosthesis with osteodontal tissue, *Amer. J. Ophthal.* 89:1039, 1963.

Thomas, T.: Prognosis in lamellar keratoplasty and the possible use of buried acrylic mushroom in keratoplasty, *Ann Inst. Barraquer,* 3:776, 1963.

Torres, Manuel Alamillo & Ruiz, Rafael Alamillo: Implantation of an artificial cornea. *Amer. J. Ophthal.* 56:937–941 (Dec.) 1963.

De Voe, A.G.: By personal communication.

Wind, Chiel A. & Kaufman, Herbert E.: Validity of MacKay-Marg applanation tonometry following penetrating keratoplasty in man. *Amer. J. Ophthal.* 72:117–118 (July) 1971.

APHAKIC GLAUCOMA

G. CRISTINI

(Bologna, Italy)

In speaking of glaucoma in aphakia it is necessary first of all to establish whether the glaucoma has developed together with the cataract, all the more prior to the cataract or was caused by the cataract, or whether it is a secondary glaucoma which has developed as a consequence of the cataract operation.

Primary glaucoma
— pre-existent to the cataract
— developed together with the cataract
— appearing after the cataract operation
Secondary glaucoma
— after extra-capsular extraction
— after intra-capsular extraction

PRIMARY GLAUCOMA IN THE APHAKIC EYE

As a general rule, glaucomas present before the cataract operation, with to-day's improved means of diagnostic investigation, rarely escape the attention of the ophthalmologist, especially if he is accustomed to performing a careful pre-operative examination. It may be more difficult to establish whether the glaucoma has developed together with the cataract, all the more so as the mechanism by which development of a cataract may favour the appearance of glaucoma is not fully understood; it is easier to verify the inverse relationship, i.e. that a glaucoma favours the development of a cataract.

Glaucoma may develop in nuclear cataracts with a large nucleus, or in intumescent cortical cataracts, which reduce the space within the anterior chamber and partially block the anterior drainage. Every good ophthalmologist should take to heart Ellnett's words, 'a mature cataract should be extracted in any case, since its real danger is that of causing a glaucoma'.

It is more difficult to recognize or interpret pathogenetically a so-called primary glaucoma which appears some time after cataract extraction performed by either the intra- or the extra-capsular method in the absence of those alterations found in secondary glaucomas in aphakics. These are glaucomas which develop in aphakia in highly myopic eyes; they are generally underestimated, as they are of the 'perimetric' rather than 'tensional'

433

type where, for the perimetric damage, it remains uncertain what part is due to myopia and how much depends, instead, on ischaemic damage of the optic nerve caused by alteration in circulation. In these cases a thorough semiological examination, including the most sophisticated tests, among them the rheographic test with amyl nitrate, and repeated ophthalmodynamographic examinations are essential. Already from this summary analysis it is clear which therapy is to be used in these different types of glaucoma.

SECONDARY GLAUCOMA

Here without doubt a causal connection with the cataract operation can be recognized; if the operation had not been performed, the glaucoma would not have appeared. The glaucoma must thus be considered a complication of the cataract operation. According to Weekers' 1958 statistics, secondary glaucoma occurs in 2-4% of cases; in children, after operation for congenital cataract, the frequency rises to 7.8%.

According to Kirby, the frequency of secondary glaucoma is greater by 0.6% after extracapsular extraction. Recent statistics of Cernea and coll. (1976) report the occurrence of glaucoma in 1.77% of aphakics.

From an etiological point of view, the following outline may be given:
1. retarded formation of anterior chamber
2. epithelialization in anterior chamber
3. pupil and ciliary blockage
4. intra-ocular hemorrhage
5. post-operative iridocyclitis including also phacoanaphylactic inflammation and inflammation with progressive iris atrophy due to intra-ocular lens implant.

SECONDARY GLAUCOMA FROM RETARDED DEVELOPMENT OF ANTERIOR CHAMBER

A retarded formation of the anterior chamber or a loss in its depth caused either by filtration through wound stitches or by a detachment of the choroid, or due to incarceration of the iris or to lenticular residue in the corneal wound, gives rise to the formation of peripheral anterior synechiae. The hypertension is not always in relationship to the existence itself of the goniosynechiae, but rather to their line of coalescence, i.e. whether or not they block the chamber angle.

SECONDARY GLAUCOMA FROM EPITHELIALIZATION IN ANTERIOR CHAMBER

When penetration of epithelium from the corneal or conjunctival surface into the anterior chamber occurs, either from an incorrectly performed incision or introduced into the anterior chamber by the surgical instrument, an epithelial invasion, which may be either simple or cystic, develops. This is a complication in occurring in 0.5-0.11% of cases.

434

Secondary glaucoma from ciliary and pupil blockage

This is a complication occurring in about 12.5% of all cases. The hypertension is caused by an impediment to the circulation of aqueous between the posterior and anterior chambers due to adherence between the iris and the vitreous or to an actual iridovitreal pupil blockage. In fewer cases, the hyaloidal membrane in the pupillary space may be so thin that the aqueous into the anterior chamber. This produces a deep anterior chamber filled with vitreous.

Ciliary blockage, caused by vitreous adhesions to the secreting part of the ciliary body, is an even more serious occurrence; the aqueous which is secreted into the vitreous pushes it together with the iris against the cornea, creating a total peripheral synechia with abolition of the anterior chamber.

Secondary glaucoma from hemorrhage

Much more rarely, a glaucoma may develop as a consequence of an extensive hemorrhage in the anterior chamber in the vitreous; the organization of the fibrin blocks the anterior chamber angle. This complication is generally found in subjects affected by senile purpura.

Secondary glaucoma from iridocyclitis

An iridocyclitis may become hypertensive when it blocks the anterior chamber angle. It occurs in about 0.66% of cases operated on for cataract, and in about 37,5% of secondary glaucomas in aphakia. It is more frequent with extracapsular extraction and in the presence of crystalline masses and extraneous proteins in the anterior chamber, which produce a state of chronic inflammation with alteration of the trabecular permeability and the development of goniosynechiae. A form of inflammation which accompanies iris atrophy is found especially in diabetics and often as a complication of an intraocular lensimplant.

Author's address:
Direttore Clinica Oculistica Universitarià
Ospedale S. Orsola
Via Massarenti 9
Bologna
Italy

Docum. Ophthal. Proc. Series, Vol. 21

SURGICAL MANAGEMENT OF APHAKIC GLAUCOMA

M. H. LUNTZ

(Johannesburg, South Africa)

Aphakic glaucoma is not a single entity — there are a number of differing mechanisms that cause glaucoma in the aphakic patient. It is more accurate to speak of glaucoma in the aphakic rather than aphakic glaucoma. The choice of treatment will therefore depend in part on the pathogenesis of the raised pressure, but there are also other factors related to the aphakic state, for example, the association of epinephrine with macular disease in aphakics and the possibility of displacement of vitreous into the anterior chamber which influences the choice of surgical method.

Not every eye with persistently raised intraocular pressure after cataract surgery needs to be treated. The decision to treat an eye whether medically or surgically is based on the following:

1. All eyes with pathological cupping and glaucomatous field loss.
2. Eyes with normal discs and fields with intraocular pressure persistently over 25mmHg in patients of 60 years or over, because of the higher incidence of retinal vein occlusion (David et al).
3. In eyes with normal discs and visual fields where surgical intervention is necessary for other reasons for example, vitreous strands adherent to the cataract section, corneo-vitreous touch with decompensation of corneal endothelium.

To adequately discuss the surgical management of glaucoma in aphakia requires knowledge of the mechanisms which are causing the glaucoma. This has been comprehensively reviewed by Francois (1974). At that time trabeculectomy with vitrectomy was not being used in the treatment of aphakic glaucoma.

The purpose of this communication is to report on the incidence of aphakic glaucoma in this Department and its' causes and the results of surgical treatment, where indicated, with a combined operation of trabeculectomy with partial anterior vitrectomy.

MATERIALS AND METHODS

A retrospective study was done on all cataract operations performed in 1976 and followed in a clinic for at least 12 months, excluding patients with intraocular lens implants. There were 752 patients, 1014 eyes and of these 27 (2.6%) developed a level of raised intraocular pressure that required treatment — this point is elaborated in the discussion. Follow-up of the aphakic eyes included a full ocular examination with regular intraocular pressure measurement, examination of the optic disc and in selected cases visual field examinations. The 27 eyes with raised intraocular pressures were evaluated in the glaucoma clinics, the investigations including careful slit lamp examination of the anterior chamber, tonometry, optic disc evaluation, gonioscopy, measurement of the anterior chamber depth and visual fields.

Eyes with acute pupil block glaucoma were treated by mydriasis. If this did not control the pressure and in chronic cases that developed angle closure glaucoma, peripheral iridectomy was performed. (O.Idy)

In eyes with secondary angle closure the pathogenesis was usually not obvious and they were treated with maximum glaucoma therapy. If the angle remained closed on medical therapy, peripheral iridectomy was done at 6 o'clock and if this did not control the intraocular pressure a trabeculectomy combined with vitrectomy was performed. (Trab./Vit.)

The 3 cases with primary open angle glaucoma (diagnosed pre-operatively and the angle remained open post-operatively) were treated with medication except in one eye in which the intraocular pressure was uncontrolled and trabeculectomy combined with vitrectomy was done.

RESULTS

The pathogenesis for raised intraocular pressure in our cases fall into three major groups:
1. Pupil Block (12 eyes).
2. Secondary Angle Closure Glaucoma, some of these probably superimposed on a pupil block mechanism (12 eyes).

Table 1. Pathogenesis, Management & Result.

Pupil Block	Eyes	Treatment	Vision (Ave.)
Acute	8	Mydriasis	6/18 – 6/9
Acute & vitreous Loss	4	Mydriasis	Cf – 6/12
Total	12		

Table 2. Pathogenesis, Management & Result

2° Angle Closure Glaucoma	Eyes	Medical Treatment	Surgery	Vision.
25% closed	3	3	–	6/6
50% closed	7	5	2 (P.Idy)	LP – 6/6
50% closed & vitreous	1	–	Trab/Vit	6/6
100% closed	1	–	Trab/Vit	CF
Total	12	8	4	

Table 3. Pathogenesis, Management & Result

Primary Open Angle Glaucoma			
EYES	MEDICAL TREATMENT	SURGERY	VISION.
3	2	1 (Trab/Vit)	6/9

3. Primary Open Angle Glaucoma (3 eyes).
The results of treating these eyes are documented in Tables 1, 2 and 3.

Acute Pupil Block

All eyes with an acute pupil block mechanism responded to pupil dilatation
with Mydriacyl, including those with vitreous loss and anterior vitrectomy
at the time of surgery (Table 4). No further treatment was required to
maintain normal intraocular pressure. The final visual result was good
ranging from 6/18 to 6/9 in eleven eyes and one eye with CF vision.

Table 4. Treatment

Mechanism	Eyes	Medical	P. Idy.	Trab/Vit.
Pupil Block	12	12 (100%)	—	—
2° A.C.GI.*	12	8 (66.6%)	2 (16.7%)	2 (16.7%)
1° O.A.GI.**	3	2 (66.6%)	—	1 (33.3%)
Total	27	22 (81.5%)	2 (7.5%)	3 (11.0%)

*Secondary Angle Closure Glaucoma.
**Primary Open Angle Glaucoma.

Secondary Angle Closure Glaucoma

The management and results are closely related to the extent of angle
closure (Table 2). Eyes with 25% of the angle closed were controlled on
medication only and retained good vision. Those with 50% angle closure
required peripheral iridectomy together with medication in two eyes but
were controlled medically without surgery in five eyes. However, the final
visual result was poor (LP − 6/60) as these patients neglected to report for
adequate follow up after the initial cataract surgery and had deeply cupped
and atrophic discs when first seen with aphakic glaucoma.

One eye with 50% angle closure which had suffered vitreous loss and
undergone vitrectomy at surgery and another eye with 100% angle closure
were not controlled on medication alone or on medication with peripheral
iridectomy and were finally brought under control with combined trabeculectomy and vitrectomy.

439

Two of the three eyes (Table 3) were controlled with medication alone, one required combined trabeculectomy and vitrectomy with medication. Good vision (6/9) was retained in all three eyes.

In summary, the majority of eyes (81.5%) were controlled by medication alone, 18.5% requiring surgery either peripheral iridectomy or combined trabeculectomy with vitrectomy (Table 4).

DISCUSSION

Francois (1974) in his review of aphakic glaucoma quotes an incidence between 1% and 7% following cataract operation, depending on the author. He also mentions a higher incidence when chymotrypsin is used, which is similar to our experience. In most cases aphakic glaucoma is the result of technical problems during the original cataract surgery and can be prevented by detailed attention to the surgical technique at that time.

In this retrospective study of 1014 eyes operated on for cataracts (752 patients) and followed for a minimum of 12 months, 27 or 2.6% were considered to require treatment for raised intraocular pressure. In 11 of these eyes the optic discs are not pathologically cupped and visual fields are normal; in the remaining 16 there is disc pathology and visual field deficit.

Younger patients with pressures over 21mmHg, normal discs and visual fields and patients over 60 years of age with normal discs and fields in whom intraocular pressures were less than 25mmHg were carefully watched but not treated. In the majority of these the intraocular pressures have gradually subsided to normal levels without therapy.

A transitory rise of intraocular pressure is seen in eyes following cataract surgery in which chymotrypsin is not used (8% of eyes operated on in this Department) with no defineable cause and in 12% of eyes in which chymotrypsin is used. However this pressure rise is transitory, seen from the 2nd or 3rd day to the 5th day and resolves spontaneously. If the intraocular pressure is too high it can be controlled with acetazolamide. These eyes have not been included in this discussion.

The major lesson from this study is that most aphakes with glaucoma (81.5%) are successfully treated by medication alone (Table 4).

Surgery is indicated if medical treatment fails to control the disease or if surgery is required for another reason, for example, reconstruction of the anterior chamber after trauma. An impressive variety of operations have been tried and reported on, mainly with disappointing or conflicting results. Cyclodialysis, once a popular operation for aphakic glaucoma or cyclodialysis with angiodiathermy rarely give a good long-term result, only one third or fewer of the operated eyes remaining under control (Sugar, 1977, Paufique & Sourdille 1969). D'Ermo (1975) claims good results with the iridocycloretraction operation of Krasnov but Chavand, Clay, Poulsen & Offret (1976) and Sugar (1977) using the same operation report very poor results. Villon (1976) suggests cyclocryotherapy in aphakic glaucoma but does not give detailed supportive results.

Our experience confirms the unsatisfactory results with these operations in aphakic glaucomas. It has been difficult to obtain long-term control of intraocular pressure with any of these procedures, while after cyclocryotherapy permanent peripheral corneal oedema has been noted and one eye developed phthisis bulbi after repeated cyclocryotherapy. In 1976 Haut suggested a combined trabeculectomy and vitrectomy and claimed 'average success.'

Consequent on our poor results with these procedures I have used, when surgery is indicated, trabeculectomy combined with partial anterior vitrectomy as the primary operation in aphakic eyes with glaucoma, except those due to pupil block. The vitrectomy is mandatory in aphakic glaucomas. The operation has few complications (David et al. 1977) and gives good results (Tables 1, 2, 3). A standard trabeculectomy technique (Luntz 1974) modified from the Cairns' method is used with a fornixbased conjunctival flap and an opening in the deep sclera measuring 2mm square. The vitrectomy is performed via the trabeculectomy opening using either Weck swabs or a vitreous suction and cutter.

Cyclocryotherapy is useful as an adjunct to combined trabeculectomy and vitrectomy either before the operation if intraocular pressure is very high (over 45mmHg) to reduce the pressure and present a less congested eye for intraocular surgery or after surgery if the pressure has not fallen to an acceptable level.

The operation was necessary in 3 eyes with angle closure of greater than 50% of the angle circumference and in one eye with open angle glaucoma. Eyes with secondary angle closure in which less than 50% of the angle circumference was closed responded well to medication alone. Anterior vitrectomy at the time of the cataract operation (1 eye) did not preclude the presence of vitreous in the anterior chamber and a vitrectomy was still necessary at the time of the trabeculectomy procedure. Of the four eyes with secondary angle closure that required surgery, 2 were controlled with peripheral iridectomy and did not require a more extensive procedure.

SUMMARY

A retrospective survey of 1014 eyes operated on for cataract over a one year period yielded 27 eyes (2.6%) with raised intraocular pressure considered sufficiently serious to require hypotensive therapy. Not all aphakic eyes with raised intraocular pressure require therapy.

Of the 27 eyes, 12 had pupil block, 12 were found to have secondary angle closure glaucoma and 3 had primary open angle glaucoma. The majority could be controlled by medication alone (81.5%). Two eyes with secondary angle closure glaucoma were controlled by medication and peripheral iridectomy. In another 2 eyes with secondary angle closure glaucoma peripheral iridectomy did not provide adequate control and further surgery became necessary. In both these eyes more than 50% of the circumference of the angle was closed. These 2 eyes and a third eye with uncontrolled primary open angle glaucoma did well with the combined operation of trabeculectomy and partial anterior vitrectomy. This procedure was selected because of our previously unsatisfactory results with other procedures particularly cyclodialysis and cyclocryotherapy. It is important in aphakic eyes that trabeculectomy be combined with vitrectomy as there is always vitreous in the anterior chamber before or after the trabeculectomy.

ACKNOWLEDGEMENTS

My thanks are due to the Medical Superintendents of the Johannesburg Hospital and the Baragwanath Hospital for allowing me access to case records and for permission to publish.

REFERENCES

Chavand, D., Clay, C.I., Pouliquen, Y. Offret, G. (1976) Iridocyclorectraction in the Surgical Treatment of Aphakic Glaucoma. *Archives Ophtalmologie* (Paris) 36: 829—824.

David, R., Freedman, J. & Luntz, M.H. (1977) Comparative study of Watson's and Cairn's trabeculectomies in a Black population with open angle glaucoma. *British Journal of Ophthalmology* 61:117—119.

D'Ermo, F. (1975) Modified Iridocyclorectraction in the Surgery of Aphakic Glaucoma. *Albrecht von Graefe's Archives Klinische Ophtalmologie* 197:229—231.

Francois, J. (1974) Aphakic Glaucoma. *Annals of Ophthalmology* 6:429—432.

Haut, J. (1976) Value of the combined trabeculectomy-vitrectomy operation in the treatment of secondary glaucoma by closure of the angle in aphakia. *Bulletin des Societes d'Ophtalmologie de France* 76:233—234.

Luntz, M.H. (1974) Primarbuphthalmos (kindlisches glaukom) behandelt durch trabekulotomie ab externo. *Klinische Monattsblatter fur Augenheilkunde.* 165:554.

Paufique, L. & Sourdille, Ph. (1969) La cyclodialyse diathermique dans les hypertonies oculaires de l'aphaque. *Archives Ophtalmologie* (Paris) 79:551—554.

Sugar, H.S. (1977) Experiences with some modifications of cyclodialysis for aphakic glaucoma. *Annals of Ophthalmology* 9:1045—1052.

Villon, J.C. (1976) The place of cyclo-cryotherapy in the treatment of glaucoma. *Bulletin des Societes d'Ophtalmologie de France* 76: 693—696.

Author's address:
University of Witwatersrand
Johannesburg
South Africa

MACULOPATHY AFTER INTRACAPSULAR
CATARACT EXTRACTION

R. BRANCATO

(Trieste, Italy)

Introduction

In recent years technical progress has diminished post-operative complications of cataract surgery. However, cystoid macular edema following intracapsular cataract extraction has on the contrary, due to its frequency, taken on a leading role among complications of this type of surgery. This affection, already observed by Vogt in 1918, was described by Irvine in 1953, who connected it with vitreous lesions resulting from the cataract operation. In 1966 Gass & Norton made other important contributions to knowledge about this disease, in particular with a description of the fluoroangiographic characteristics.

Definition

Macular edema in the aphakic, also known as the Irvine-Gass syndrome, is a late-appearing complication which occurs after a certain period of time in an eye operated for cataract extraction; it consists of a microcystic edema of the macular area, frequently associated with papilledema.

Clinical characteristics

It is characteristic of this disease to appear after a certain asymptomatic 'free period'. During this period there is no alternation or symptom to arouse the suspicion that this complication may occur. The operation seems to be perfectly successful, to the complete satisfaction of the surgeon and the patient. Instead, after a certain time the first symptoms appear. The time interval may vary from a few weeks up to, in rare cases, several years. In our observations made on 34 cases of true cystoid macular edema, the average free period was three months, with a minimum of one month and a maximum of one year.

The term 'true' or 'persistent' cystoid macular edema is understood to exclude all of those practically asymptomatic cases which show, upon angiographic examination in the first few weeks or even after a month or two, a modest diffusion of fluorescien form the perifoveal capillary bed. These alterations, though they must be considered as initial edema, do not assume the characteristic and unmistakeable aspect of cystoid edema. The incidence of this leakage from the perifoveal vascular network in the

443

first and second months after the operation is truly conspicuous. Irvine and Coll have found a leakage of the contrast medium in the macular area in 40% of the angiograms performed on patients 4 to 16 weeks after operation (with maximum incidence around the fourth to sixth week). Hitchings has observed an even greater incidence of 50%, six weeks after the operation.

M. Bonnet has reported an incidence of 18% two months after the operation. In another angiographic survey conducted on a sample of forty subjects chosen at random, leakage from the perifoveal capillary bed was found in 43% of the cases. Leakage was slight and practically asymptomatic in the great majority of cases (Fig. 1). In three cases it assumed the aspect of cystoid edema.

These very frequent cases, characterized by a slight diffusion of the stain from the perifoveal capillaries should not be included in the category of the Irvine-Gass syndrome. The majority of them, in fact, tend to regress spontaneously or remain unchanged without determining any notable functional alteration. Only a much smaller percentage of cases shows development of the typical characteristics of cystoid macular edema, with evident and lasting functional disturbance. The case material of the true Irvine-Gass syndrome as reported in the literature dealing with the subject shows a frequency of from 1 to 5% (J. Francois and collaborators) and even 7.6% (Gehring), but the actual frequency may be much higher, since only a part of the subjects affected consults the physician as to the cause of the diminishing of visual acuity in the months following the operation. To determine the incidence of the syndrome in the 3 to 5-month period after the operation by us was chosen at random a group of 80 patients (whose case histories showed no particular ocular affection), for functional and angiographic examination.

In this group, cystoid macular edema with more or less accentuated functional disturbance was found in 11.6% of the cases examined. In a previous statistic, the incidence of maculopathy found in a group of subjects over 60 who spontaneously consulted a physician for visual disturbances

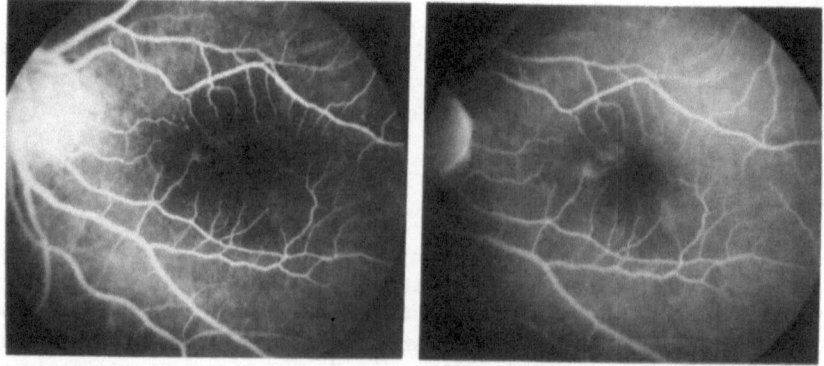

Fig. 1. Leakage of fluorescein from the peri-foveal capillaries one month after cataract operation. Retinal angiography.

was of 2.43%. All of the patients in this second group had undergone intracapsular cryoextraction with peripheral iridectomy and sclero-corneal suturing in virgin silk under a conjunctival flap. In both of these statistics, the sex of the patient was irrelevant to the frequency of the disease. Of course, in this last, systematically conducted statistic, the incidence of the disease is destined to regress as time passes due to the spontaneous improvements which may occur. As regards age, cases of the disease were found in subjects ranging in age from 45 to 90 years, although the incidence appears to be higher among older subjects. In the second group the average age was 67. **Subjective symptomatology** is characterized by an alteration of central vision, almost always accompanied by irritative ocular symptoms. After the operation, the patient, following a certain period of time (free period) becomes aware of a more or less marked diminishing of visual acuity, with difficulty especially in short-focus vision. Frequently metamorphoses can be found, although their presence is difficult to detect due to the particular optical conditions of the aphakic. A perimetrical examination may reveal peripheral reduction of the field of vision. The intensity of irritative symptomatology varies from case to case; it consists mainly of photophobia.

Objective findings include several different alterations varying in frequency.

a. **Perikeratic injection** and sometimes slight **conjunctival chemosis.**

b. The occurrence of **rupture of the anterior hyaloid membrane** is not constant: always present according to some writers (Irvine), quite frequent according to others (Gass), rare for still others (Tolentino & Schepens). In the series reported here, rupture of the hyaloid was present in 50% of the cases. This type of lesion does not seem to be a determining factor in provoking the syndrome, but its presence has a negative influence on its evolution.

c. **Modifications in vitreous body:** these are of three main types: 1. prolapse or vitreous swelling with integral hyaloid; 2. presence of free vitreous in the anterior chamber with laceration of the membrane; 3. incarceration of the escaped vitreous in the operation wound.

In the case of simple prolapse, the surface of the integral hyaloid may touch the endothelial surface of the cornea or may remain at the level of the pupillar foramen. In time, the prolapse may withdraw behind the pupil; it may remain stationary; or it may evolve into a late-occuring rupture of the hyaloid. It should be noted that when there is a small solution of continuity of the hyaloid, there is never a tendency to vitreous prolapse: the vitreous thus remains behind the pupillary plane even though a certain quantity of it may penetrate into the anterior chamber through the foramen.

If instead there is an escape of vitreous after rupture of the hyaloid, various possibilities may occur. The first is that the vitreous may liquefy. This tendency toward liquefaction may be determined by hyaluronidase. Hyaluronidase may be set free by the tissue damage connected with surgical incision or by the rupture of the hyaloid itself. The second possibility is that the vitreous may tend to conglomerate in a globose formation which limits itself by forming a membrane and which remains united to the vitreous body by a shaft. This eventuality is related to the organization of hyaluronic acid and free proteins with a certain quantity of collagen. It should be pointed out that vitreous organized in this manner easily becomes opaque; if this phenomenon involves the pupillary space, it can interfere considerably with vision. It has also been observed that the possibility of self-delimination is more frequent for vitreous which has been lost during the surgical operation than for vitreous which escapes when a later rupture the hyaloid occurs.

The third and last possibility, and certainly the most important, is that the escaped vitreous becomes incarcerated in the margins of the operation wound.

d. **Modification of the posterior hyaloid**: it has been demonstrated with certainty that all aphakic eyes show the posterior vitreous considerably separated from the surface of the retina. Though it is true that we never observe a decollement on the level of the ora serrata, different writers are instead in disagreement as to whether or not vitreo-macular adherences are present; these, if present, would constitute a justification of the mechanical theory in the pathogenesis of the Irvine-Gass syndrome.

It is important too to note the presence of inflammatory haematic cells and of fibrillary residue of vitreous material in the space between the retina and the posterior hyaloid. On this fact, among others, the pathogenetic theory of inflammatory type is based.

e. **Alterations of the macula**: these are certainly the most important and the most characteristic. Conventional ophthalmoscopy rarely reveals the presence of macular lesions. Greater objectivity may be had by observing the macula with a biomicroscope, applying Goldmann's lens; in this way we can observe microcysts occupying the macular area, frequently leaving untouched the foveal zone, which stands out with its bright red colouring (it is true). These microcysts are not real cysts, as they do not have walls of their own; in fact, we speak of cystoid edema and not of cystic edema. The microcysts in the center are bigger, while those at the periphery have a smaller diameter. Dimensions of macular lesions can be as much as two disc diameters.

f. **Angiographic patterns**: fluorescein angiography of the retina is an essential examination both for diagnosis and for evaluation of the evolution of the disease. The fluoroangiographic aspect is unmistakeable, altough it is not typical only of cystoid edema in the aphakic, but is common to cystoid macular edemas of other origin also. During the early arterial and venous time, no particular alternations can be observed, with the exception of a lack of definition of the perimacular vascular ramifications within the context of a central zone which appears darker and wider than the normal fluoroangiographic picture.

During the late venous phase, the perimacular capillaries show up more clearly. It is, in fact, by means of these capillaries that fluorescein is diffused after some time: thus there is the formation of small fluorescent points arranged more or less regularly around the foveola. The progressive confluence of these points gives the macular region a flower-petal aspect in the late phases of retention (Fig. 2). The dimensions and regularity of this fluorescent area vary from case to case. The limitation of the fluorescent

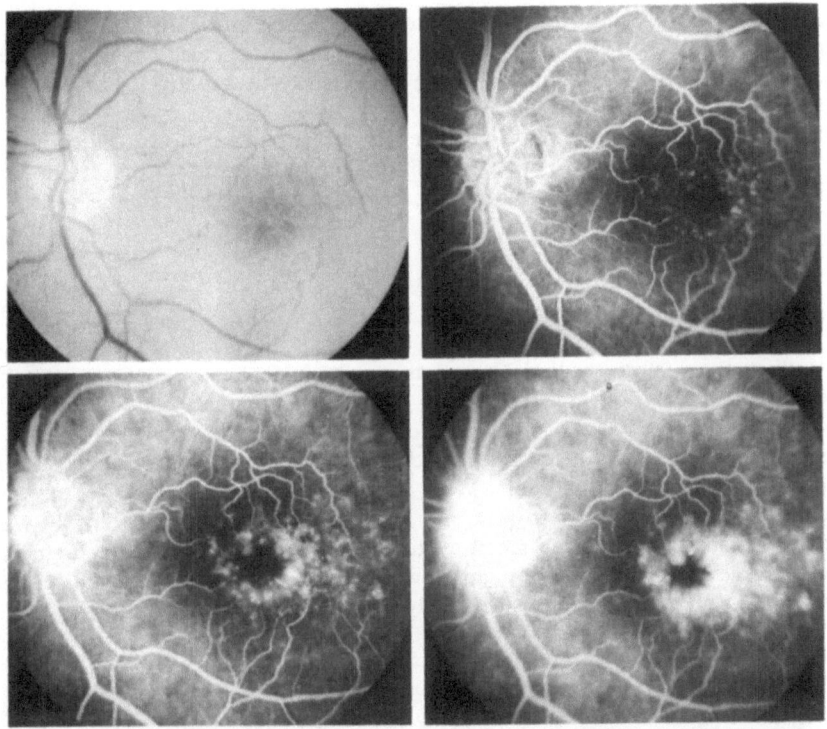

Fig. 2. Cystoid macular edema four months after intracapsular cataract extraction. Various angiographic phases.

spot is variable too, in some cases reaching its greatest degree of extension even after thirty minutes.

This fluoroangiographic pattern, so characteristic, is due in part to the alteration of the perimacular capillaries, in part to the particular histological characteristics of this area. The stain issuing from the capillaries accumulates in small cystoid formations formed by dissociation of Henle's fibers, and circumscribes a dark area, that of the fovea. Frequently, however, in the very late phase, it can be observed that the small dark central area too takes on a slight colouration (Brancato and collaborators). It should be noted that the quality of the late fluororetinographic shots is often mediocre due to fluoresceinic diffusion in the vitreous.

g. **Alterations in the optic disk:** In about half of the cases studied, a slight papilloedema, characterized by a slight blurring of the margins of the optic disk, was found. In the late angiographic phases, in practically all of the cases studied by the author, a more or less marked hyperfluorescence of the optic papilla has been found, testifying to the participation of the capillaries of the optic disk in the disease process.

h. **Modification of the retinal vessels:** This can be observed especially in the veins, which are turgid, gyrate and enlarged. The capillaries, as can be evidenced only by fluoroangiography, are dilated and show an increase in permeability, as revealed by the escape of stain, especially in the macular region; in fact, the macular pseudocysts seem to be exactly in continuation with the surrounding capillaries.

i. **Modifications of the vessels of the iris and the ciliary body**: Fluoroangiographic examination of the iris in patients affected by the Irvine-Gass syndrome shows an abnormal fluoresceinic diffusion through the vessels of the iris (Fig. 3).

Pathology

There is very little to be found in the literature on this subject. We have studied the histopathological reports on the macular area of ten aphakic eyes, but without establishing precise clinico-anatomo-pathological correlations. A careful search for the possible existence of vitreal adhesions involving the macula has not detected them in any case. In five observations, intra- and infra-retinal edema was found: in one of these cases, a large central pseudo-cystic formation with a still-integral internal wall, surrounded by numerous small cystoid cavities, could be observed. In one case, large accumulations of pigment were found. Two cases showed disciform degeneration with numerous drusen lying upon Bruch's membrane.

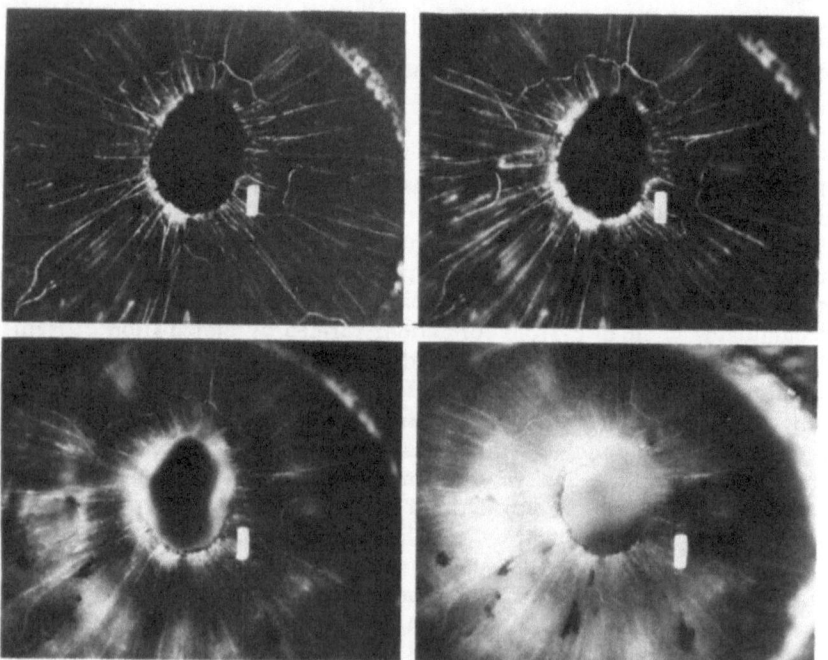

Fig. 3. Angiography of the iris in a case of cystoid macular edema after cataract extraction.

1. **General pathological predisposing factors**: the diseases which are most frequently blamed are logically those which have repercussions on the posterior pole of the retina, i.e., hypertension, diabetes and vascular diseases such as arteriosclerosis.
2. **Local pathological predisposing factors**: as previously mentioned, in some cases there is the concomitance of chronic glaucoma, but without significant frequency from the statistical point of view.
3. **Factors linked to the operation and the post-operative period**: it might be thought that the cause of the Irvine-Gass syndrome is an unsuccessful operation. Instead, this syndrome may appear even after a successful operation with no complications whatsoever. It has been shown, however, that certain operative and post-operative 'accidents' increase the frequency or the severity of the maculopathy significantly. The following elements must be kept in consideration:

a. **Incision**: according to some writers on the subject, the corneal cut increases the incidence and the severity of the syndrome; therefore the sclero-corneal cut should be preferred.

b. **Type of iridectomy**: correlation between the incidence of the syndrome and the type of iridectomy performed has never been demonstrated irrefutably. In patients showing predisposition to the disease, a sectorial iridectomy may be preferable.

c. **The use of enzymatic zonulolisis**: it has been observed that its use can increase the frequency of this complication by two pathogenetic mechanisms: the first is the delay in healing, the second the weakening, provoked by the enzyme, of the anterior hyaloid.

d. **Type of cataract extraction**: almost all of the cases published have been observed after intracapsular extraction, as this is still the more widely used operation. But cases found after extracapsular extraction, also performed by phacoemulsification, have also been described.

e. **Escape of vitreous during the operation**: we have seen that this operative complication increases the incidence of the syndrome.

f. **Later rupture of the hyaloid and prolapse of vitreous**: in numerous cases it has been observed that the hyaloid, at first integral, after several weeks may rupture with consequent invasion of vitreous into the anterior chamber. This occurrence too increases the incidence of the disease.

g. **Prolonged use of mydriatics in the post-operative period**: the use of mydriatics undoubtedly favours vitreous prolapse through the pupillary foramen, and consequently increases the possibility of a rupture of the hyaloid later. It can therefore be sustained that a good prophylatic rule to follow is that of abandoning indiscriminate and prolonged use of mydriatics after cataract operation.

h. **Instillation of epinephrine**: maculopathy from epinephrine, considered by Kohler & Becker to be a cystoid maculopathy with its own individuality in aphakic subjects, should be re-examined for a possible aggravating role which adrenalin derivates may have on macular capillaries. The lens, in fact, constitutes a physiological barrier; its removal allows adrenergical substances instilled in the conjunctival sac to act directly on retinal vessels.

All of the factors discussed above are, however, only predisposing elements. It must be maintained, in fact, that the only certain and constant etiological factor is aphakia.

Pathogenesis

The pathogenesis of this disease is still widely discussed. There are theories founded on the action of the vitreous and on the anatomo-functional modifications brought about by extraction 'in toto' of the lens, an inflammatory theory and a vascular theory. The following is a brief survey of these theories.

1. **Theory of traction of the anterior vitreous**: this is the mechanical theory sustained by Irvine in his first description. The rupture of the anterior hyaloid with the involvement of vitreous in the anterior chamber and the incarceration of a vitreous bridle in the operation wound may provoke, during pupillary movements, a stretching action on the vitreous and on the macula.

2. **Theory of traction of the posterior vitreous**: the forward displacement of the vitreal mass after extraction of the lens may provoke alterations due to traction on the macular and disc level where adherences between vitreous and retina exist (Tolentino & Schepens, 1969).

3. **Theory of modifications induced by aqueous humour after lens removal**: according to this theory suggested by Worst (1975), the formation of macular edema may depend upon biotoxic action carried out by enzymes (the prostaglandins among others) contained in the aqueous humour (aqueous biotoxic complex) which, facilitated by the total removal of the lens, appears to act on the macular area, concentrating in the 'bursa premacularis'. The harmful action takes place when the 'pars patellaris' is affected by the posterior detachment of the vitreous. This theory could also explain a possible effect of adrenalintype drugs on perimacular vessels in the absence of the physiological barrier constituted by the lens.

4. **Vascular theory**: this theory sees in vascular alterations the primary cause of macular alterations. The type of vasculopathy responsible has not, however, been defined with certainty. It may be that there exists a generic pre-existing vasculopathic predisposition. Vascular lesions might, however, be determined also by the mechanical or enzymatic stimuli mentioned previously, or might be affected by inflammation provoked by these.

5. **Inflammatory theory**: This theory considers inflammation as a proces which is not necessarily of an infective type, but also and more probably, of the post-traumatic type. Numerous considerations sustain this pathogenetic hypothesis:

a. The cellular components present in the retro-vitreal space.

b. Vitreous opacity and the frequent concordance of irido-cyclitic or uveitic processes in general, as evidenced by perikeratic injection.

c. Similarity of the angiographic pattern to that of other diseases of certain inflammatory nature.

d. The leakage of fluorescein present both at the level of the vessels of the posterior pole and of the retina and ciliary body may be interpreted as an alteration determined by an inflammatory stimulation.

As can be seen from the above, the pathogenic interpretations are numerous but not mutually irreconcilable. It may be sustained that there is a torbid inflammatory reaction which determines an alternation in the vasal permeability on the macular and the irido-ciliary levels. Anterior and posterior vitreous trauma, rather than an essential element, may be considered as valid reasons for worsening the prognosis, especially perhaps on a particularly predisposed vascular terrain.

Differential diagnosis

Differential diagnosis from other maculopathies which can be found in aphakic subjects is usually easy. Biomicroscopic examination of the fundus and angiography are essential for proper diagnosis. Other maculopathies following cataract operation are macular folds and papillary edema from hypotonia. There are also maculopathies which are independent of the cataract operation and which may be pre-existent or may appear some time afterwards.

Evolution

The evolution of the disease may be almost stationary or may even trend toward spontaneous improvement. Many cases, however, show progressive worsening, arriving at macular degeneration a with macular hole (Fig. 4).

Prophylaxis

In consideration of the uncertain etiopathogenesis, prophylactic measures must take into account all of the factors which seem to increase the incidence of this type of complication.
1. The surgeon should tend to use a sectorial rather than a peripheral iridectomy, especially in those cases where the syndrome has already appeared in the other eye.

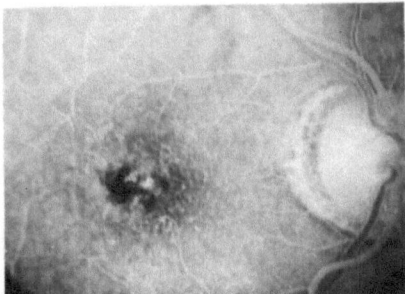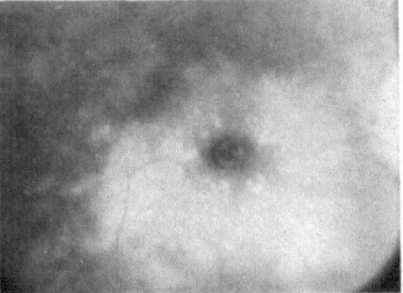

Fig. 4. Evolution of cystoid macular edema after cataract extraction in a retinal macular hole. Retinal angiography.

451

2. Sclero-corneal rather than corneal incision should be preferred.

3. The use of enzymatic zonulolysis should be limited to those extractions in which it is considered particularly desirable.

4. In the post-operative period, mydriatics should not be over-used, especially in eyes which show little inflammatory reaction.

5. Collyriums containing adrenalin derivates, especially epinephrine, should not be used. Local corticotherapy may be used to relieve post-operative inflammation.

6. The utility of extracapsular extraction (there are no well-documented statistics on the subject) must be evaluated.

Therapy

There is no well-codified therapy with which to combat this complication once it has developed. The possible types of therapy may be divided into three main groups: the first includes medical treatment, the second surgical, and the third treatment by physical methods.

1. **Medical treatment**: vaso-protectors and vaso-actives agents are used in consideration of a possible vascular pathogenesis. Widely used is a therapy based on cortisone given both locally and generally (Fig. 5): in this way, both its anti-edema and its anti-inflammatory effects are used. A therapy using prostaglandin inhibitors (indomethacin or enzymatic inactivators, via the retro-bulbar spaces, has also been used.

2. **Surgical treatment**: this consists of a section of the vitreous bridle incarcerated in the surgical wound, if such a bridle is present. It is a good rule to try medical therapy first, and to resort to surgery only if this fails.

3. **Treatment by physical methods**: these methods are without doubt the least used, and results are uncertain. Anti-inflammatory radiotherapy may be used, or, as a means of destroying a possible vitreo-macular adherence on the posterior pole, applications of ultra-sound. Finally, laser photocoagulation should be mentioned: this technique (in a horseshoe shape temporally to the macula) may be attempted when medical therapy has been unsuccess-

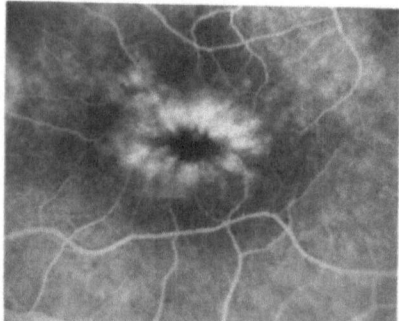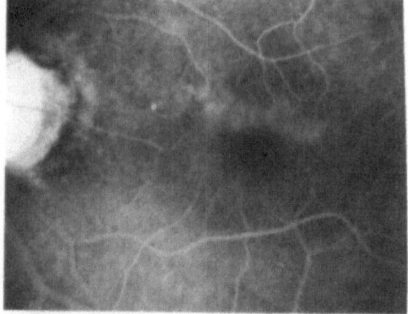

Fig. 5. Cystoid macular edema after intracapsular cataract extraction (at left). At right, regression of cystoid edema after two months of treatment with cortocosteroids. Late retinal angiography.

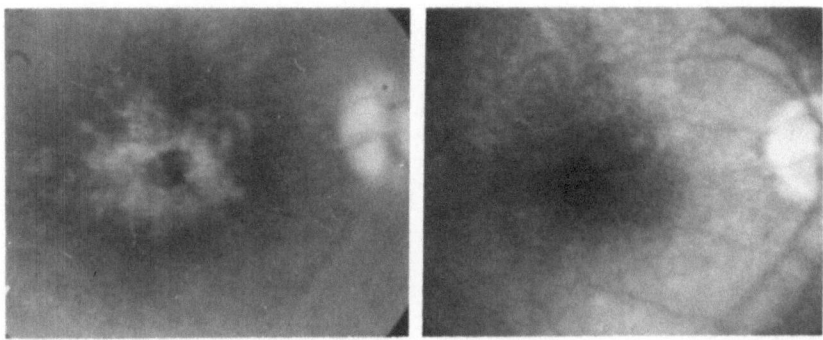

Fig. 6. Cystoid macular edema after cataract extraction (at left). At right, regression after treatment with laser photocoagulation.

ful and the affection has been present for a long time, with evolution for the worse. Although this type of treatment may seem illogical, it has sometimes given good results. The hypothesis that the post-coagulative necrosis may liberate substances active in limiting macular edema must not be excluded.

In evaluating the results of both medical and surgical therapy, we must always keep in mind the possibility of spontaneous regression of cystoid edema.

Author's address:
Istituto di Clinica Oculistica
dell' Universitá degli Studi di Trieste
Trieste
Italy

RETINAL DETACHMENT IN APHAKIA

MORTON L. ROSENTHAL

(New York, U.S.A.)

As a retinal surgeon at a meeting where recent technical changes in cataract surgery are being enthusiastically discussed, I feel somewhat like a guest at a wedding who notices in a loud voice that the bride is somewhat pregnant.

The increasing use of intraocular lenses and the resurrection of the extracapsular operation have not made life easier for retinal surgeons.

Retinal detachment has been estimated to occur in the general population of the United States at a rate of 18 cases per 100,000 population. One third of these cases occur in aphakic eyes. Retinal detachment occurs in 1% to 3% of eyes operated on for cataract. The occurrence retinal detachment in aphakia is 80 to 250 times more common than in nonaphakic eyes.

There is no evidence that retinal detachment occurs less often with any particular type of cataract technique. Vitreous loss, however, markedly increases the incidence of retinal detachment.

What still remains uncertain is the absolute incidence of retinal detachment in aphakia. The figure that I gave, namely 1% to 3%, is almost certainly too low. Published reports of large series of cataract extractions that attempt to establish the incidence of retinal detachment as a complication necessarily must err on the low side. This is true for a number of reasons.

No matter how long the followup following cataract surgery is, some cases will always develop after the report has been published. Furthermore, many patients do not return to their original cataract surgeon when the retina detaches and he may be quite unaware of these cases.

However, whatever the absolute incidence of retinal detachment in aphakia may be, the rate of successful reattachment of these cases has been steadily improving over the past 15 to 20 years. In the hands of experienced retinal detachment surgeons, the reattachment rate for aphakic retinal detachments is only slightly below the 90% rate that we achieve for nonaphakic eyes. Modern scleral buckling techniques have certainly been instrumental in achieving this excellent cure rate but by far the most important factor has been good ophthalmoscopy and our ability to detect the tiny, multiple, peripheral retinal breaks that are so characteristic of this disease. The intracapsular cataract extraction and binocular indirect ophthalmoscopy have been two positive factors in the modern success rate.

Lorimer Fison has stated 'The retinal surgeon hates extracapsular cataract surgery'. Yet we have heard at this meeting many thoughtful surgeons advocate this procedure. What are the reasons for the differences in attitude in this situation?

455

Let us contrast the experiences of two ophthalmic surgeons. In Figs. 1 and 2, the first performs 400 cataract extractions per year and the other performs 400 retinal detachment operations. If the cataract surgeon has a rate of retinal detachment in his patients of 3%, he will see approximately 12 retinal detachments a year generated out of his population of aphakic eyes. If we assume a 90% cure rate in these retinal detachment cases, in all likelihood somewhere between 10 and 11 of these patients will have successful reattachments. If the cure rate in these 12 eyes was to drop by 10% to an 80% rate it would be very difficult for the cataract surgeon to notice the difference in the small number of the retinal detachment cases that he encounters.

400 CATARACT EXTRACTIONS ANNUALLY
3% = 12 RETINAL DETACHMENTS
IF 90% ARE SUCCESSFULLY REATTACHED ONLY ONE
OR TWO EYES LOST THROUGH RETINAL DETACHMENT
IF 80% REATTACHED THEN TWO OR THREE EYES LOST

Fig. 1

400 RETINAL DETACHMENTS ANNUALLY
1/3 APHAKIC = 133 CASES
IF 90% REATTACHED = 13 BLIND EYES ANNUALLY
IF 80% REATTACHED = 27 BLIND EYES ANNUALLY

Fig. 2

On the other hand, the surgeon performing 400 retinal detachment operations a year will be treating 133 aphakic eyes because, as you know, 1/3 of all retinal detachments occur in aphakic eyes. If 90% of these 133 eyes undergo successful retinal surgery, 119 eyes will be salvaged but 13 will not. If the surgeon's cure rate drops to 80%, a 10% decline, then 106 of these 133 eyes will be salvaged. There will be 27 eyes blind as a result of unsuccessful retinal detachment surgery.

The difference between 13 eyes and 27 eyes in a single practice is quite obvious, and accounts for the sensitivity of retinal surgeons to anything that reduces their cure rate by even 5%.

Extracapsular cataract surgery by reducing the visibility of the peripheral retina probably reduces the cure rate in retinal detachment, in such eyes, by at least 10%. The use of an intraocular lens has a similar effect. The combination of an extracapsular cataract extraction plus an intraocular lens has the most serious effects on the visibility of the peripheral fundus.

What direct evidence do we have that the retinal detachment cure rate is significantly affected by these newer modalities, aside from the anguished cries of retinal surgeons?

The American Academy of Ophthalmology recently sponsored a study of complications of intraocular lens implantation. Retinal detachment was one of the complications considered. The retinal detachments of 252 patients were studied out of a population of intraocular implant cases from all over the U.S. Dr. Hal Freeman who organized this aspect of the study has permitted me to use his data.

Some of the findings are summarized below: The reattachment rate was 5% less than in the control group.

A functional result of 20/40 or better was achieved in 5% fewer cases than in the control group.

71% of cases had undergone extracapsular extraction and 16% had undergone phakoemulsification.

Iris supported lenses were used in 73 % of cases. Capsular supported lenses were used in 19%. 8% were angle supported.

78% of the retinal breaks were tears.

18% were retinal holes.

2% were dialyses.

1% were giant retinal breaks.

38% of eyes had a poorly dilatable pupil.

Retinal breaks could not be found in 18% of eyes.

In those eyes in which vitreous was lost only 17% obtained 20/40 or better compared to 39% of eyes without vitreous loss.

FACTORS IN PSEUDOPHAKIA THAT MAKE OPHTHALMOSCOPY DIFFICULT
1. LIGHT REFLEXES FROM LENS SURFACES
2. LIGHT REFLEXES FROM CAPSULE REMNANTS
3. POOR MYDRIASIS
4. CAPSULE CLOUDING
5. SECONDARY MEMBRANES
6. LENS PRECIPITATES
7. KERATOPATHY

Fig. 3

Most of these lenses were implanted following intracapsular cataract surgery. It seems probable that if more of these cases had been done with an extracapsular technique the reattachment rate would have been significantly lower because of even greater ophthalmoscopic problems. It must be emphasized that we are discussing only retinal detachment as a complication of intraocular lens implantation and that the increase in the failure rate from 10% to 15% or 20% in this group is due only to this single factor, namely, intraocular lens implantation.

What if lens implantation and extracapsular extraction were accepted as standard procedures in most or all patients? In the light of the figures cited what could we expect with respect to the overall cure rate of retinal detachment cases in the United States for example?

There are approximately 400,000 cataracts removed annually in the United States. What would be the difference in the number of blind eyes as a result of aphakic retinal detachment if these eyes were operated on with intraocular lenses or without them?

If there is a 3% retinal detachment incidence, then approximately 12,000 retinal detachments will develop in these 400,000 eyes. (Figure 4). This figure corresponds well with the known incidence of aphakic retinal detachment in the U.S. population which is six cases per 100,000 population- or 12,000 cases annually. (Figure 5).

400,000 CATARACT EXTRACTIONS ANNUALLY IN U.S.
3% RETINAL DETACHMENT RATE = 12,000 CASES

Fig. 4

RETINAL DETACHMENT

18 PER 100,000 = 36,000 RETINAL DETACHMENTS IN POPULATION
OF 200,000,000 U.S. ANNUALLY
1/3 OR 12,000 APHAKIC DETACHMENTS PER ANNUM

Fig. 5

If 90% of these 12,000 cases are successfully reattached, then 1,200 eyes will remain blind following our unsuccessful surgery. If, on the other hand, only 80% of these cases are reattached then 2,400 eyes will be blind following unsuccessful retinal detachment surgery.

This difference of 1,200 blind eyes would be due solely to the single factor, the use of an intraocular lens.

It should also be clear that if 400,000 eyes be operated on annually for cataract, this 5% or 10% difference in cure rate would represent somewhere between 600 and 1,200 eyes per annum lost from retinal detachment as a complication, aside from any other. Each reduction of 5% in our reattachment rate represents 600 lost eyes. (Figure 6).

As the use of these devices becomes more widespread these data will inevitably come to the attention of public health agencies and the public at large.

Intraocular lenses offer the promise of early recovery of good vision following cataract extraction and the freedom from distortion, field defects and the other problems of aphakic spectacles.

12,000 APHAKIC RETINAL DETACHMENTS

CURE RATE	FAILURE RATE	NO. OF FAILURES	LOST EYES DUE TO PSEUDOPHAKIA (EXCESS FAILURES)
90%	10%	1200 CASES	
85%	15%	1800 CASES	600
80%	20%	2400 CASES	1200

Fig. 6

Phacoemulsification offers the promise of early ambulation in many cases.

We as ophthalmologists must ask ourselves if these rewards are worth the long term risks of severe functional loss in many eyes.

If we are not critical in our judgement now, our patients may be asking us in future years why we did not better advise them.

Docum. Ophthal. Proc. Series, Vol. 21

TREATMENT OF RETINAL DETACHMENT IN THE APHAKIC

F.M. GRIGNOLO

(Torino, Italy)

Detachment of the retina in the aphakic has a multiple genesis, the common denominator of which is constituted by the extraction of the cyrstalline lens and by the anterior dislocation of the vitreous body. We can distinguish on the one hand an idiopathic detachment, in which extraction of the lens acts to trigger a phenomenon which was already 'in fieri' due to retino-vitreal 'meyoprofic' (retino-vitreal degenerations of the myopic or senile type). On the other hand, a secondary retinal detachment, in which the pathogenesis of the cataract (trauma, perforating wound) or its extraction (vitreous loss, presence of posterior synechiae) leads to pre-, or post-operative complications such as to constitute the direct cause of the retinal detachment. In particular, we can distinguish between 'aphakic type' detachments where numerous small holes at the base of the vitreous are found, anterior to the ora serrata, with circumferential traction on the retina in several quadrants, and 'phakic type' detachments, with continuous ruptures of greater dimensions and varied forms, localized more posteriorly than the first, on the equatorial level; and, yet again, retinal detachments complicated by inflammatory and/or traumatic reactions with bands of vitreo-retinal traction responsible for the retinal lesion.

In consideration of the gravity of retinal detachment, its greater frequency whenever the above-mentioned pre-disposing conditions are present, as well as the difficulty of treating it (60-80% of successful operations in comparison to 80-90% of success whith phakic patients), it is well to remember first of all the possibilities of prevention.

PROPHYLAXIS

Prophylaxis of detached retina in the aphakic, or better, in the subject who must undergo cataract operation, may be distinguished as preoperative, peroperative and post-operative.

Examination of the retina is impossible in a high percentage of cases of cataract, in which only part of the periphery is explorable, where those solutions of continuity which can lead to lifting are more apt to form. An examination of the retinal periphery, opacity of the lens permitting, allows the surgeon to identify possible rhegmatogenous areas, tears which can

461

be treated preventively. When the opacity of the lens does not permit such examination, indications for prophylactic treatment are given by the presence of myopia, medium-grade or severe, by the conditions of the other eye and by its behaviour during a previous cataract operation, if such has been performed.

Peroperative prophylaxis consists of respect for those measures and precautions which can limit the occurrence of complications (type of anesthesia, hypotonia of eyeball, choice of type of operation, zonulolysis, vitreous silence, use of miotics, suture of the wound, etc.)

Post-operative prophylaxis, as well as aiming at the least traumatizing recovery possible, makes use of systematic examination of the fundus oculi so as to be able to recognise in good time the appearance of degenerative areas or of tears. The frequency of such lesions during the first year after the operation makes frequent repetition of ophthalmoscopic examination necessary. Examination of the retina in aphakic subjects shows peculiarities. From the optical point of view, the absence of the crystalline lens allows less enlargement of the image of the fundus oculi, but the lack of the prismatic effect, makes possible complete examination up to the ora serrata without having to recur to indentation. This is possible in the ideal aphakic, where perfect extraction of the lens has been followed by no complications, thus making possible a good mydriasis, and where no alterations of the vireous have occured. Therefore in the overwhelming majority of cases, examination of the fundus oculi by indirect ophthalmoscopy and biomicroscopy present no difficulty at all and is even easier than in the phakic patient; the same is true for post-operative prophylaxis (search for possible rhegmatogenous areas and/or zones of rupture) and treatment of lesions

Greater difficulties are encountered in examining the fundus oculi in aphakic patients in whom, owing to complications or to the type of operation performed, posterior membranes remain, or where synechiae have formed, with consequent difficulty or impossibility of mydriasis. In case of necessity, indirect methods of examination may be used (visual field, transillumination and ecography) or chorepractic methods (surgical or photocoagulative) may be used to permit easier exploration of the fundus oculi.

Photocoagulation

This technique in the treatment of detached retina is indicated only for prophylaxis and for treating special cases in which spontaneous re-attachment is obtained by rest or in which it is impossible to operate due to the patient's general state of health or local contraindications (giant rupture with retinal eversion). In these cases, photocoagulation is used to create a 'barrage' along the edges of the tear or of the detachment in such a way as to create a chorio-retinal adhesion which hinders the progress of the lesion and limits its effects. Moreover, in giant ruptures where surgical treatment could present complications and uncertain success, 'barrage' along the edges of the detached area, constituting a valid barrier to the progression of the lesion, may be useful.

Cryotherapy

The use of cryopexia, like photocoagulation, is indicated for prevention of detachment: in the treatment of rhegmatogenous areas, tears in flat retina, and in cases where, consequent to pre-operative immobilization of the patient, the retina spontaneously re-attaches to the choroid, restoring the situation to the case of rupture in adhering or partially detached retina. The possibility of transconjunctival application makes cryopexia the ideal technique for pre-operative prophylaxis, which will be focal and aimed whenever the opacity of the lens still permits examination of the ocular periphery, and circumferential, involving the whole periphery and the retinal equator in cases where examination of the fundus oculi is impossible and there are anamnestic and objective data (medium-grade or severe myopia, peripheral degenerations or previous detachment in the contralateral eye) which indicate the possibility of a retinal lesion during the cataract operation or successive to it.

Transcleral diathermy

This method, which when used alone has practically the same indications as photocoagulation and cryotherapy, has been replaced by the latter methods because of their greater innocuity; they do not cause the scleral damage which diathermy provokes, and surgical exposure of the scleral wall is not needed.

TREATMENT

Treatment of retinal detachment in the aphakic obviously requires a complete and thorough examination of the patient so as to be able to recognise every characteristic of the vitreo-retinal situation (importance and extension of the detached area, conditions of the retina, localization of the tears, relationship between tears and vitreous, state of the subretinal fluid, its mobility, visual function), all of which is entered on a chart, the evaluation of which can establish the best method of treatment.

Pre-operative immobilization must be maintained for the time necessary (two or three days) for evaluation of the possibility of a spontaneous re-attachment of the retina to the choroid; it can be prolonged whenever there seems to be the possibility of a total re-attachment. In this case, the retinal rupture is treated by bordering its edges by means of photocoagulation and/or cryotherapy. The patient is then kept at rest until an initial pigmentary mobilization testifies to the establishment of a chorioretinal cicatrix.

Scleral introflexion

The choice of this type of surgical approach is dictated by the presence of a retinal detachment limited to one or two quadrants with a single tear or

463

localized and adjacent tears. As for the choice of technique (episcleral implant and cryotherapy or scleral resection with or without silicon inclusion, and diathermy), the first type or treatment is preferable when the object is that of obtaining a less intense introflexion and when the thickness of the sclera is not such as to permit its resection. The application of an implant of this type provokes an introflexion of lesser degree and of greater extension than the second technique. These implants fixed to the sclera by sutures tend with the passage of time to shrink and become externalized due to the cutting out of the suturing material in the sclera. For obtaining good introflexion, repeated cryopexic applications are necessary to distend the sclera and obtain hypotonia. If at the end of the operation the rupture is well-contained in the treated area and is in the upper quadrants, evacuative puncture may not be necessary.

The choice of the second technique is dictated by the presence of a detachment which is likewise localized with one or more adjacent solutions of continuity, in which an introflexion of considerable degree and stability is desired, either for the size of the raised area or from the presence of strings of vitreal traction. The use of diathermy in the resection bed, because of its coarctating action on the sclera, makes evacuative puncture necessary, so as to establish a hypotonia which permits indentation without compromising retinal-choroidal circulation.

Circling

Circling is the operation chosen in the overwhelming majority of cases of detached retina in the aphakic. It permits extensive treatment of the whole peripherial retina in cases of 'typical' detachment where the dimensions and the localization of holes do not always make total visualization easy, and it achieves the object of 'creating a new ora serrata'. The circling with a silicon band is positioned on the level of the posterior border, and in the case of lesions at the Ora spread over several quadrants, these are treated with aimed or circumferential cryopexic applications, and in the case of equatorial lesions ('atypical') this can be associated with scleral resection with or without implant according to the degree of introflexion desired. Extensive cryopexic application may avoid evacuative puncture in the first case; this is, however, necessary with diathermy and scleral resection.

Circling is without doubt the most effective operation. Since it permits treatment of the tradition exerted on the retina by retinal membranes, it is permanent, and it allows treatment of the whole peripheral retina. It permits releasing of any fixed retinal folds, vitreous membranes, or preretinal retractions when it is associated with evacuative puncture and with intravitreal injection of gas or liquids, which, in the aphakic subject, can easily be introduced into the anterior chamber by paracentesis. Its action can be extended in an anterior-posterior sense through the association of a localized implant.

Circling is indicated, moreover, in all of those cases of detached retina in aphakics when exploration of the fundus is made difficult by the persistence of lens membranes and posterior synachiae which limit mydriasis.

SPECIAL CASES

Treatment of special cases of retinal detachment in the aphakic must also be mentioned. These cases include: co-existence of detached retina and cataract, detachment of the retina consequent to congenital cataract and in Marfan's syndrome, detachment consequent to traumatic cataract with or without retention of an intrabulbar foreign body, and finally, detachment consequent to complicated cataract extraction with involvement of vitreous in the wound.

The *co-existence of detached retina and cataract* puts before the surgeon the choice of a 'blind-fold' operation for detachment or an operation for cataract extraction which risks compromising the retinal situation. In the first case, after ecographic study of the detachment, using as a basis statistical clinical data as to the equatoral or pre-equatoral location of the retinal ruptures, the surgeon proceeds to equatoral circling with circumferential cryotreatment and, if necessary, evacuation a fluid in the inferior temporal quadrant. The cataract operation may then be performed after at least six months' interval, taking care to loosen the circling band in order to avoid peroperative complications. In the second case, the surgeon proceeds to extraction of the lens with ample sector iridectomy so as to facilitate later examination of the fundus oculi, and sutures the sclerocorneal wound with a large number of stitches. Examination of the fundus at this point allows the surgeon a determine the operation to be chosen, which, even in the case of a circling, may be performed after only one month.

The author's experience leads him to advise the second technique, which is certainly the more precise.

A very serious surgical problem is represented by *Marfan's syndrome:* here we find collected all the possible complications of surgery of the lens and of the retina. Considering the frequent occurrence of detached retina, a circumferential prophylactic treatment seems advisable before proceeding to extraction of the lens, or when the lens is luxated in the vitreous chamber. The problems of treatment in the absence of vitreous complications goes back, as in detachment consequent to congenital or juvenile cataract, to the localization of the zone of rupture. Whenever there is mobility of the subretinal liquid, a circling is performed, if necessary reinforced at the level of the tear by a resection or scleral implant so as to obtain perfect sealing.

Post-traumatic aphakia is frequently complicated by posterior synechiae, lens membranes, and especially when there has been extraction of an intrabulbar foreign body, by the presence of vitreous membranes, responsible, for the most part, for the genesis of detachment. The treatment, in addition to requiring a sufficient mydriasis (which can be obtained surgically or with photocoagulation), may present the necessity of removing during the operation any vitreal traction band which is hindering re-attachment of the retina. Circling, which due to the frequent impossibility of complete examination of the fundus, is the preferred method of operation, is therefore frequently associated with vitrectomy, or in the more favourable cases, with the injection of air, gas or saline.

465

Lastly, we must discuss treatment of *detachment consequent to vitreous involvement in the surgical wound*. Faced with this classic example of detachment due to traction, the surgeon's behaviour will be analogous to the procedure as regards retinal surgery; preceded by removal of the vitreous involved, with re-opening of the wound and pupilloplasty, if necessary.

Therefore, with the exception of minor cases where the detachment is limited in extension and shows localized solutions of continuity, the ideal operation is represented by circling, either simple or associated with indentation, evacuation, vitrectomy in the more serious cases. Only this operation, in fact, assures, in the absence of posterior lesions, sealing with certainty each retinal rupture 'closing the globe with a new Ora'.

Author's address:
Instituto di Clinica Oculista
dell' Universita di Torino
Torino
Italy.

Docum. Ophthal. Proc. Series, Vol. 21

COMBINED OPERATION FOR CATARACT AND GLAUCOMA

J. FRANCOIS

(Ghent, Belgium)

The association of cataract with glaucoma confronts the ophthalmologist with a difficult problem. Should the eye be operated upon for glaucoma first and later for cataract? Should the eye be operated upon for cataract and the glaucoma treated afterwards medically? Would it be possible to operate for both diseases at the same time?

1. CATARACT EXTRACTION, FOLLOWED BY A MEDICAL TREATMENT FOR GLAUCOMA.

This medical treatment is not always efficacious. Diamox cannot be taken for very long periods of time. Epinephrine may produce a maculopathy in aphakic patients of older age. Phospholine iodide may cause a retinal detachment in the case of peripheral degeneration of the retina. If an operation becomes necessary for the glaucoma, cyclodialysis is still the best one, but the results are not always good, even when the cyclodialysis is performed in an area without goniosynechiae.

2. GLAUCOMA OPERATION, FOLLOWED BY CATARACT EXTRACTION.

The incision for the cataract has to be corneal, 1½ or 2 mm in front of the filtering bleb, in order to maintain the filtration. The cataract can also be removed below with a peripheral iridectomy at 6 o'clock. When doing so, the filtering bleb may, nevertheless, disappear from time to time, particularly the small ones, the disappearance being due to an inflammatory reaction, a postoperative hypotony or a fibrous reaction in the trepanation canal.

3. COMBINED OPERATION FOR CATARACT AND GLAUCOMA.

This solution is clearly the best one, because it avoids two consecutive operations. Although there have been a few earlier trials (Wright, 1937), the vast majority of the combined techniques for the simultaneous operation of cataract and glaucoma have been published since 1945. More than 125 publications on the subject are now available: Guyton, 1945; O'Brien, 1947; Mc Millan, 1950; Lee & Weilh, 1950; Wolfe, 1952; Birge, 1953; Wenaas & Stertzbach, 1955; Gill, 1959; Hughes, 1959; Sakic, 1960; Hauer, 1960; Kudogarov & Chemodanova, 1961; Verzella, 1961; Küchle, 1962; Bessiière & Pelegris, 1962; Cordero-Moreno, 1962; Di Tizio & Leonardi, 1963; Verzella, 1963; Offret & Pouliquen, 1963; Hughes et al., 1963; Bangerter, 1963;

Scuderi & Schillaci, 1964; Boberg-Ans, 1964; Nectoux et al., 1964; Stocker & Young, 1965; Simon, 1965; Bell, 1965; Menezo, 1965; Zuccoli, 1965–1966; Harrington, 1966; Preste, 1966; Pittar, 1966; Jebejian, 1966; Nagpaul et al., 1966; Nath & Shukla, 1966; Streiff, 1967; Marchi, 1967; Galeazzi & Vozza, 1967; Brancato & Campana, 1967; Elie, 1967; Mawas et al., 1967; Mc Donald, 1967; Sambursky et al., 1967; Scuderi, 1967; Zuccoli, 1968; Sarda et al., 1968; Legrand, 1968; Corbel et al., 1968; Scuderi & Cardia, 1968; Vörösmarthy & Ballschuh, 1968; Boyd & Fink, 1968; Leydhecker & Knapp, 1969; Loh, 1969; François, 1969; Corrado, 1969; Boyd, 1969; Mandras et al., 1969; Bessière et al., 1969; Demailly et al., 1969; Klouman, 1969; Benedikt, 1969; Colombi, 1969; Stocker, 1969; Maumenee & Wilkinson, 1970; Naval & Dizon, 1970; Ismail, 1970; Spaeth, 1970; Protonotarios, 1970; Ershkovich, 1971; Jaffe, 1971; Veirs & Tate, 1971; Golovine, 1971; Johnson, 1971; Verin et al., 1971; Ferreira, 1971; Suga & Nagata, 1971; David et al., 1971; King, 1971; Dellaporta, 1971; Bietti, 1971; Takats & Pinter, 1971; Castelli, 1971; Eggers, 1971; Barreau & Perez, 1971; Borellini & Bellomio, 1971; Sbordone et al., 1971; Dellaporta, 1972; Shmeleva & Mukhina, 1972; Thyer & Wilson, 1972; Hommer, 1972; Roveda, 1972; Shmedeva, 1972; Bessière et al., 1972; O'Donoghue, 1972; Ferreira, 1972; Vasilev, 1972; Kliachko, 1973; Labib et al., 1973; Emarah, 1973; Fougères-d'Esperey, 1973; Yigitsubay, 1973, Sautter et al., 1974; Hilsdorf, 1974; Vancea & Schwartzenberg, 1974; Frankelson & Schaffer, 1974; Stelzer, 1974; Palimeris et al., 1974; Rich, 1974; Boudet et al., 1974; Eustace & Harun, 1974; Brégeat et al., 1974; Diotallevi et al., 1974; Mukhina, 1975; Neetens, 1975; Rodriquez Gonzalez, 1975; Khasanova & Fedorova, 1975; Coudere, 1975; Grom et al., 1975; Brégeat, 1975; Lugossy, 1977, etc.

This great number of papers and techniques shows how much ophthalmologists are interested in a combined operation for cataract and glaucoma. All the proposed techniques combine a cataract extraction with a basal iridectomy, an inverse cyclodialysis, an iridencleisis with one or two pillars, a Lagrange sclerectomy or a sclero-iridectomy, a Scheie's cauterization or since a few years, a trabeculectomy, or even a trabeculotomy. Protonotarios (1970) performs a cyclodialysis as well as a sclerotomy with inclusion of a silicone sheet. Some authors, such as Veirs & Tate (1971), obtain a permanent filtering bleb by dissecting a large limbal based conjunctival flap and placing only a few corneoscleral sutures.

The positive results with permanent normalization of the intraocular pressure are variable and according to the various surgeons lie between 33 and 80%. It is certain that the skill and the experience of the operator have a great importance, as was shown by Brégeat et al., (1974). Moreover, for some authors, the results are better with an iridencleisis or a trabeculectomy than with an Elliot, a Lagrange or a Scheie (Table I).

Besides the usual complications of cataract extraction, the complications of the combined operation for cataract and glaucoma are; 1. Heavy hopotony, 2. Flat anterior chamber, 3. Hyphaema, which should be rather frequent, 4. Vitreous haemorrhage, 5. Vitreous prolaps or loss, 6. Subchoroidal haemorrhage in arteriosclerotic or hypertensive patients, 7. Post-

Table 1. Comparative study of the intraocular pressure normalization after various combined operations for cataract and glaucoma (after Brégeat, 1975).

Ocular pressure	Miotics	Elliot	Lagrange	Scheie	Iridencleisis	Trabeculectomy
normalized	without	33%	50 %	54,5%	66,6%	76 %
	with	33%	12,5%	27,2%	16,6%	22,5%
not normalized		33%	37,5%	18,1%	16,6%	1,5%

operative increase of the intraocular pressure, 8. Uveitis, Expulsive haemorrhages have been mentioned, but are exceptional.

The two most important complications are: (1) hypotony, which may produce goniosynechiae and secondary ocular hypertension, (2) flat anterior chamber, due to a too heavy filtration and often to a choroidal detachment. Cyclodialysis may cause an anterior chamber haemorrhage. It necessitates a miotic instillation, what increases the difficulties of cataract extraction. Its results are, moreover, very variable and rather not good. On the other hand, trabeculectomy, which consists in dissecting a protective scleral flap, diminishes the postoperative hypotony and avoids the flat anterior chamber.

We have performed three different techniques for combined operation of cataract and glaucoma: (1) cataract extraction combined with Scheie's cauterization, (2) cataract extraction combined with Lagrange sclerectomy and (3) cataract extraction with trabeculectomy. All our operated cases were open angle glaucomas.

I. CATARACT EXTRACTION COMBINED WITH SCHEIE'S CAUTE-RIZATION (FIG. 1)

After classical local anesthesia, we massage the eye ball for 1 to 1½ minute. This massage always gives us good hypotonia and in no case has it been necessary to give an intravenous injection of urea or mannitol. We never observed an intraocular haemorrhage, which some authors attributed to the massage.

Then we dissect a triangular conjunctival flap by cutting the conjunctiva from the level of the insertion of the superior rectus muscle, with complete denudation of the sclera. The dissection of the flap is continued right up to the limbus from 11 o'clock to 1 o'clock.

Subsequently, with a bistoury we make a superficial incision into the sclera precisely at the level of the posterior edge of the limbus over a distance of 5 mm. Using a strabismus hook heated to red, we cauterize the bed of this incision which then widens to approximately 1,5−2 mm. At this moment we make another incision, also superficial, but nearer to the anterior than to the posterior lip, so that we incise in the direction of the iridocorneal angle. We repeat the cauterization with the strabismus hook in the same way. Finally, with successive repetitions of superficial incisions and cauterizations, we open the anterior chamber.

469

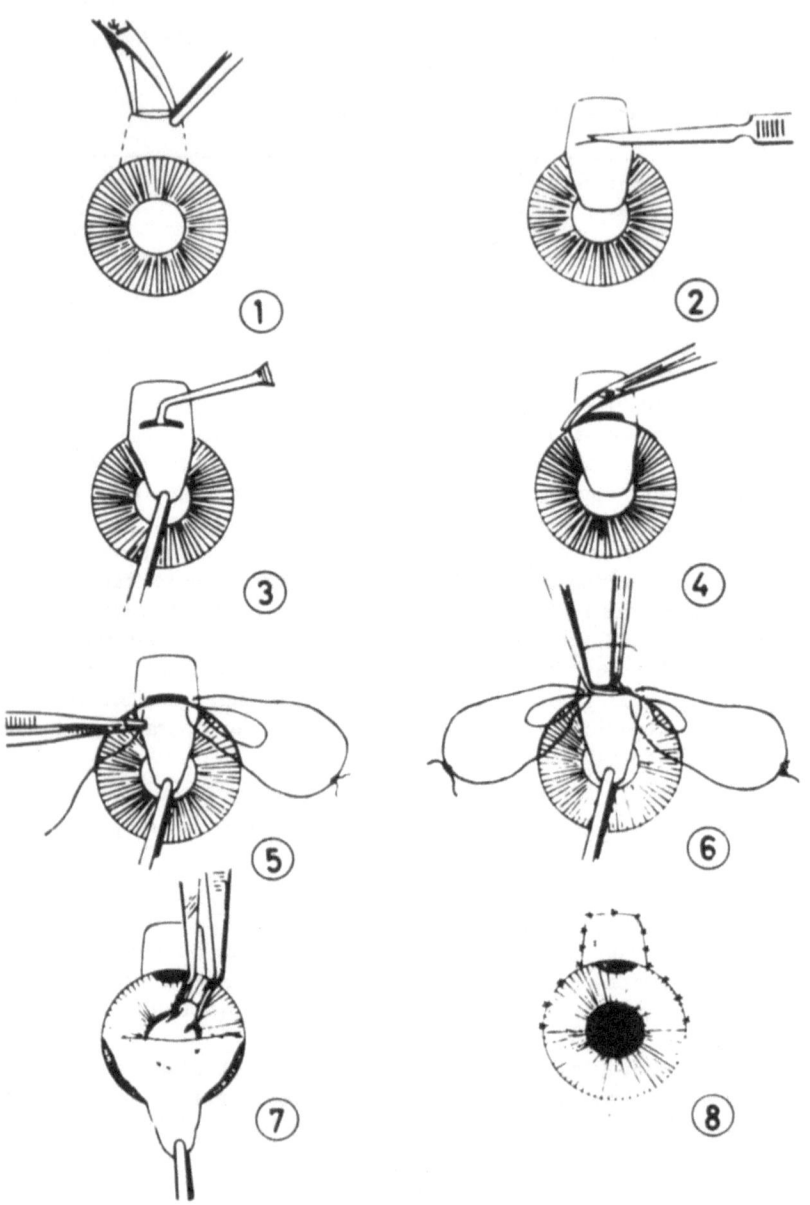

Fig. 1

Through the opening, a scissors blade is introduced into the anterior chamber to make a corneal section from 9 o'clock to 3 o'clock cutting exactly at the level of the limbus, first on the temporal, then on the nasal side.

A suture of virgin silk is placed corneosclerally at each end of the original scleral incision; this corneoscleral suture, which remains under the conjunctive, is ready to be tied as soon as the cataract has been extracted.

Only now do we make a basal iridotomy which must have more or less the same length as the primary incision through the sclera, viz. 5 mm.

All that now remains to be done is to extract the cataract. The lower portion of the lens capsule is tucked and gripped with Green's forceps, which is the best one in our opinion and has given us a total intracapsular extraction in more then 95% of the cases. Actually, this forceps is only used to hold the lens, which is freed by pressing movements and to-and-fro movement of an Arruga hook. This is first placed at the level of the lower limbus, but follows up the lens as it becomes freed and extraction progresses; in this way, the lens expressor not only facilitates the removal of the cataract, but also keeps back the vitreous that might otherwise follow the lens.

We have used alphachymotrypsin only in young patients, below the age of 45—50 years, and the cryoextractor only for intumescent cataract, the capsule of which cannot be tucked.

As soon as the lens is out, we irrigate the iris with 1% acetylcholine to bring about miosis of the pupil. Subsequently, the two sutures previously put into place are tied and the conjunctival flap turned back. This flap is then sutured very carefully, with stitches very close together; virgin silk must be used for all the sutures. Finally, at 11 o'clock and 1 o'clock, i.e. at the extreme limits of the conjunctival flap, we place a corneoscleral suture, which at the same time keeps the conjunctiva in place. Two other corneoscleral sutures are placed between 9 and 11 o'clock, and two between 1 and 3 o clock. Finally, we restore the anterior chamber by an injection of physiological saline.

From the first postoperative day good fistulization can be seen, and this has persisted in 88% of our cases (Fig. 2, Table 2). It should be mentioned that the permanent regulation of the intraocular pressure often occurs only three months postoperatively.

As a rule, the anterior chamber is not flat during the days that follow the operation. Only rarely is it shallow, but usually it reforms in two or three days, if the patient is given Diamox®(2 or 3 tablets per day). We have seen only three cases of choroidal detachment, that persisted for two weeks or longer.

In no patient have we encountered any serious complication (e.g. uveitis). Only two hyphaemas occurred.

The final visual result does not depend on the operation, but on the severity of the glaucoma, which may, of course, have produced a definite decrease of the visual acuity as well as definite defects of the visual field.

II. CATARACT EXTRACTION COMBINED WITH LAGRANGE SCLERECTOMY (FIG. 2)

With a von Graefe's knife we make a corneal incision just at the level of the limbus from 3 to 9 o'clock for the left eye (or from 9 to 3 o'clock for the

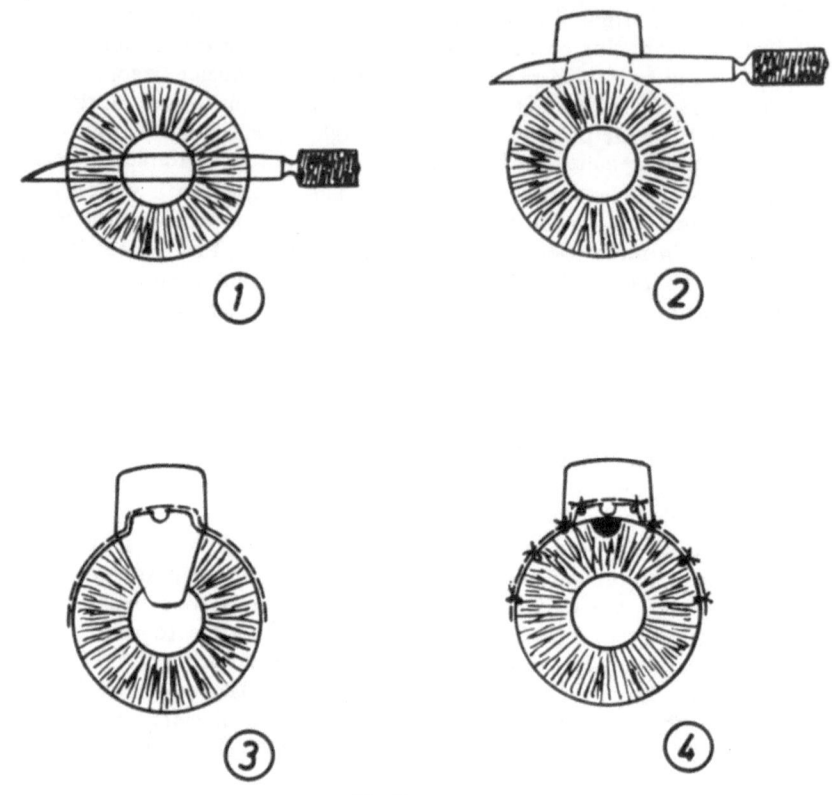

Fig. 2

right eye). When arrived at the superior limbus, instead of leaving the anterior chamber immediately by an incision perpendicular to the eye surface, we slant the knife in order to make an oblique incision, 2 or 3 mm long, in the sclera itself, and to realize at the same time a large conjunctival flap. Thereafter we remove with the aid of Vannas' scissors a semicircular piece, large of 4 mm, at the level of the juxtalimbar part of the scleral wound. An excision of the posterior margin of the scleral wound could also be made, realizing so in fact a trap door sclerectomy just as in trabeculectomy, the anterior scleral strip covering and protecting the filtering fistula. The cataract extraction is performed and the sutures are placed exactly as it has been described for the preceding operation.

After having performed a small basal iridotomy, the lower portion of the lens capsule is gripped with a Green's forceps. This is only used to hold the lens, which is freed by pressing movements and to-and-fro movements of an Arruga hook. This is first placed at the level of the lower limbus, but follows up the lens as it becomes freed and extraction progresses. In this way, the lens expressor not only facilitates the removel of the cataract, but also keeps back the vitreous that might otherwise follow the lens. As soon as the lens is out, a to-and-fro movement of the corneal flap replaces the iris. We then irrigate the iris with 1% acetylcholine to bring about miosis. Subsequently, the 2 sutures previously put into place are tied, the conjunctive being kept in place. Four other corneoscleral sutures are placed between 9 and 11 o'clock and 1 and 3 o'clock. Finally, we restore the anterior chamber by an injection of physiological saline.

A bandage is put into place after instillation of pilocarpine and eserine and an application of Aureomycin.

III. CATARACT EXTRACTION COMBINED WITH TRABECULECTOMY (FIG. 3)

Firstly we dissect a conjunctival flap, starting from the insertion of the superior rectus muscle and continuing right up to the limbus from 11 to 1 o'clock. Thereafter a square scleral flap at limbal hinge, 5 x 5 mm, is cutted, comprising at least half of the sclera. The section of the scleral flap must penetrate into the cornea. An incision of 4 mm is then made in the anterior part of the limbus and with the aid of Vannas' scissors a piece of the trabeculum with a part of the sclera (4 x 3 mm) is excised. Through this opening a scissors blade is introduced into the anterior chamber to make a keratotomy from 9 o'clock to 3 o'clock. The cataract extraction is performed and the sutures placed exactly as it has been described for the preceding operation. At the end of the latter 4 sutures are placed in the scleral flap, 2 laterally and 2 at the extremity.

Our results are summarized in table II.

Table 2. Comparative study of the intraocular pressure normalization after various combined operations for cataract and glaucoma.

Ocular pressure	Miotics	Lagrange No.	%	Scheie No.	%	Trabeculectomy No.	%
normalized	without	5	100	74	91,4	10	71,5
	with	–	–	3	3,7	1	7,1
not normalized		–	–	4	4,9	3	21,4

We had only a few complications in these 100 cases (table III)

Table 3.

Complications in 100 combined operations for cataract and glaucoma	No.	%
Choroidal detachment	11	11
Postoperative iridocyclitis	1	1
Panophthalmia	1	1
Hyphaema	2	2
Vitreous loss	1	1
Vitreous haemorrhage	1	1

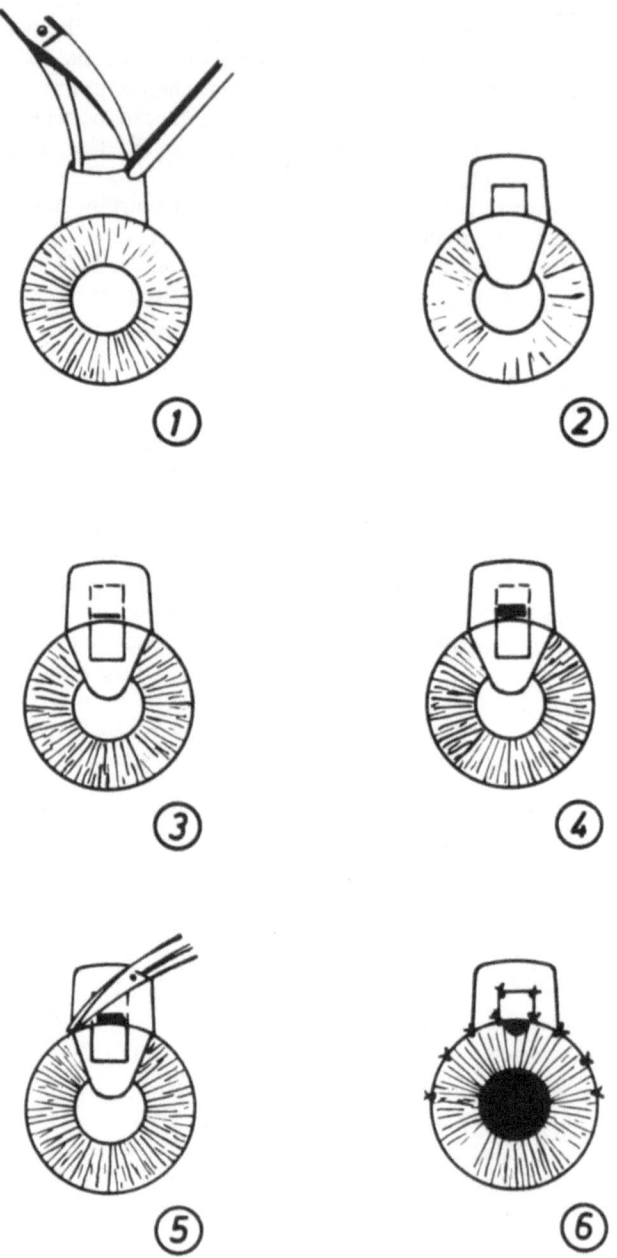

Fig. 3

The choroidal detachment never lasted more than 8 to 15 days and the hyphaema always disappeared in a few days. Serious complications were in fact only seen in 4% of cases.

Although the number of cataract extraction combined with Lagrange's sclerectomy or with trabeculectomy are too few, it seems that, at least in our hands, the cataract extraction combined with Scheie's cauterization gives the best results. The only restriction I have to make that the follow up is not long enough for some cases. On the other hand, the advantage of the trabeculectomy is the fact that big filtering blebs are avoided, although in the 81 cases of cataract extraction with Scheie's cauterizatin we never had a voluminous filtering bleb.

SUMMARY

In cases of cataract and glaucoma, we performed a cataract extraction combined either with a Lagrange sclerectomy, or a trabeculectomy or a Scheie's cauterization. We obtained the best results with Scheie's cauterization.

REFERENCES

Bangerter A. Kombinierte Katarakt-Glaukomoperation. *Ber. Dtsche Ophthal. Ges., Heidelberg*, 65, 84–91, 1963.

Barreau R.K. & Perez R.D.G. A combined operation for the association of glaucoma and cataract. *Arch. Chil. Oftal.*, 28,227-233, 1971.

Bell L.G. Cataract and Glaucoma. *Trans. Ophth. Soc. N.Z.*, 17, 35–43, 1965.

Benedikt O. Einseitige, kombinierte Glaukom.-Katarakt-Operation. *Klin. Mbl. Augenheilk..*, 154, 72–77, 1969.

Bessière E., Le Rebeller M.J. & Gervais C. Aspects actuels des opérations combinées glaucome-cataracte. *Arch. Ophtal., Paris*, 32, 609–614, 1972.

Bessière E. & Pellegris (Mme). Opérations simultanées dans l'association glaucome chronique cataracte sénile (statistique). *Bull. Soc. Ophtal. France*, 62, 369-573, 1962.

Bessière E., Verin P. & Le Rebeller M.J. Opérations combinées de la cataracte et du glaucoma. I. Techniques et résultats. *Arch. Ophtal. Paris*, 29, 7–22, 1969.

Bietti G.B. The possible association of goniotrabeculotomy and cataract extraction in glaucomatous patients. *Boll. Oculista*, 50,389-396, 1971.

Birge M.L. The treatment of cataract with glaucoma. *Amer. J. Ophthal.*, 36, 925–929, 1953.

Boberg-Ans J. Simultaneous operation for cataract and glaucoma. Report on thirty cases. *Trans. Ophthal. Soc. U.K.*, 84, 113–125, 1964.

Borellini S. & Bellomio S. Combined operation in cataract and primary glaucoma. *Ann. Ottalm.*, 97, 621–633, 1971.

Boudet C., Arnaud B. & Miller P. Opérations combinées trabéculectomie phakoexérèse. A propos de quinze cas. *Bull. Soc. Ophtal. France*, 74, 739–745, 1974.

Boyd B.F. Cataract extraction in eyes with open-angle glaucoma. *Highlights Ophthal.*, 12, 259–302, 1969.

Boyd B.F. & Fink A. Cataract surgery in glaucomatous eyes. *Highlights Ophthal.*, 11, 38–86, 1968.

Brancato R. & Campana G. L'intervento combinato nell associazione glaucoma-cataratta. *Ann. Ottal. Clin. Oculistica*, 93, 1326–1340, 1967.

Brégeat P. Trabekulektomie und intrakapsuläre Kataraktextraktion in einer Sitzung. *Klin. Mbl. Augenheilk.*, 167, 505–515, 1975.

Brégeat P. Kombinierte Operation der Katarakt und des chronischen Glaucoms beim Erwachsenen in besonderen Fällen. *Klin. Mbl. Augenheilk.*, 171, 836–841, 1977.

Brégeat P., Hamard H. & Couderc J.L. *Bull. Soc. Ophtal. France*, 74, 13–18, 1974.

Brégeat P., Hamard H., Couderc J.L., Lebuisson D.A. & Lefrançois A. Cataracte et trabéculectomie Indications. Résultats à court terme *Bull. Soc. Franç.Ophtal.*, 87, 137–142, 1975.

Castelli A. Deep anti-glaucoma fistulisation combined with cataract extraction. *Atti Soc. Oftal. Lombarda*, Special no. 125–145, 1971.

Colombi C. Cataratta e glaucoma. *Minerva Med.*, 60, 1362–1368, 1969.

Corbel M., Leser C. & Gibault R. La stabilisation tonométrique dans les interventions combinées cataracte-glaucome. *Bull. Soc. Ophtal. France*, 68, 85–89, 1968.

Cordero-Moreno R. Surgery of the cystalline in cases, complicated by glaucoma. *Ophth. Ibero-Amer.* 23, 43–57, 1962.

Corrado M. L'operazione simultanea del glaucoma e della cataratta. *Ann. Ottal.*, 95, 187–199, 1969.

Couderc J.L. Les interventions chirurgicales associées à l'extraction de la cataracte. *Bull. Soc. Ophtal. France*, 75, 865–873, 1975.

David M., Popescu M. & Antal I. Extraction of cataractous lens in a glaucomatous eye according to the Jules François method. *Ophtalmologia*, 15, 251–256, 1971.

Dellaporta A. Combined trepano-trabeculectomy and cataract-extraction. *Trans. Amer. Ophthal.. Soc.*, 69, 113–123, 1971.

Dellaporta A. Combined trepano-trabeculectomy and cataract extraction. *Klin. Mbl. Augenheilk.*, 160, 49–56, 1972.

Demailly P., Bunt J., Clay C. & Rousselie F. Opérations combinées de la cataracte et du glaucoma. II. Extraction du cristallin combinée à un iridencleisis. *Arch. Ophtal., Paris*, 29, 23–32, 1969.

Diotallevi M., Defranco C. & Cocca P. Results of the combined operation for cataract and glaucoma. *Ann. Ottalm.*, 100, 549, 1974.

Eggers C. Trabeculotomy. Technique of the simple ab externo trabeculotomy and of the combination of trabeculotomy and lens extraction. *Arch. Chil. Oftal.*, 28, 158–161, 1971.

Elie G. Le traitement chirurgical en un seul temps de l'association cataracte-glaucome. *Bull. Soc. Ophtal. France*, 67, 848–855, 1967.

Emarah M.H.M. A new combined operation for the manegement of cases of glaucoma and cataract. *Bull. Ophthal. Soc. Egypt*, 66, 231–239, 1973.

Ershkovich I.G. & Redkina E.I. Cataract extraction in glaucoma. *Oftal. Zh.*, 26, 104–107, 1971.

Eustace P. & Harun A.Q.S.M. Trabeculectomy combined with cataract extraction. *Trans. Ophthal. Soc. U.K.*, 94, 1058–1063, 1974.

Ferreira L.E. Cataract and glaucoma. *Rev. Bras. Oftal.*, 30, 147–152, 1971.

Ferreira L.E. Combined surgery of cataract and of glaucoma. *Arch. Soc. Esp. Oftal.*, 32, 1041–1048, 1972.

Fougeres-D'Esperey. Results of combined operations for glaucoma and cataract. *Bull. Soc. Ophtal. France*, 73, 551–558, 1973.

François J. Kombinierte Glaukom und Kataraktoperation. *Klin. Mbl. Augenheilk.*, 155, 608–615, 1969.

François J. A combined operation for glaucoma and cataract. *Ophthalmic Surgery*, 1, 9–13, 1970.

Frankelson E.N. & Shaffer R.N. The management of coexisting cataract and glaucoma. *Canad. J. Ophthal.*, 9, 298–301, 1974.

Galeazzi C. & Vozza R. Cataratta e Glaucoma. Convegno sul Glaucoma primario, Firenze, 459–500, 1967.

Gill E.G. Trend in the surgical treatment of cataract. With special reference to cataract associated with chronic glaucoma. J. Int. Coll. Surg., 32, 661–667, 1959.

Golovine S. A propos de 37 cas d'intervention combinée glaucome-cataracte.. *Arch. Ophtal. Paris*, 31, 355–356, 1971.

Grom E., Maza S., Lobo L., Perez E.Y. & Bermudez A. Simultaneous (combined) operation for glaucoma with cataract. *Ann. Ophthal., Chicago*, 7, 991–994, 1975, and *Bol. I.D.D.I.O.* (Venezuela), 2, 431–437, 1975.

Guyton J.S. Choice of operation for primary glaucoma combined with cataract. *Arch. Ophthal.*, 33, 265–268, 1945.

Harrington D.O. Cataract and glaucoma. *Amer. J. Ophthal.*, 61, 1134–1140, 1966.

Hauer I. A simultaneous cataract-glaucoma operation. *Israel Med. J.*, 19, 254–256, 1960.

Hilsdorf C. Combined trabeculectomy and lens extraction. *Klin. Mbl. Augenheilk.*, 164, 298–303, 1974.

Hommer K. Goniotrephining with scleral flap and mitred incision as combined glaucoma-cataract operation. *Klin. Mbl. Augenheilk.*, 160, 327–329, 1972.

Hughes W.L. Report on a combination operation for cataract with glaucoma. *Amer. J. Ophthal.*, 48, 1–14, 1959.

Hughes W.L., Kazdan M.S., Brackup A.H. & Marinakos C.H. Combination operation for cataract and glaucoma. *Amer. J. Ophthal.*, 56, 391–394, 1963.

Ismail A.M.A.R. A combined operation for glaucoma and cataract. *Bull. Ophthal. Soc., Egypt*, 63, 315–322, 1970.

Jaffe N.S. The lens. *Arch. Ophthal.*, 85, 485–500, 1971.

Jebejian R. L'opération combinée cataracte-glaucome sous anesthésie locale et akinésie potentialisée. *Ann. Oculistique*, 199, 497–508, 1966.

Johnson S.B. Combined cataract extraction and scleral cautery (includes 8-year follow-up in 9 cases). *Ann. Ophthal., Chicago*, 3, 1163–1166, 1971.

Khasanova N.K. & Fedorova N.V. Combined cataract extraction and sinuso-trabeculectomy. *Vestn. Oftal.*, 92, 3–4, 1975.

King J.H. Jr. Cataract complicated by glaucoma or by corneal disease. *Trans. Pacif. Cst Oto-Ophthal. Soc.*, 51, 175–184, 1971.

Kliachko L.I. Auxiliary operations in the regional treatment of glaucoma and cataract. *Oftal. Zh.*, 28, 142–151, 1973.

Klouman O.F. Combined glaucoma and cataract operation. *Acta Ophthal., Kbh.*, 47, 30–32, 1969.

Küchle H.J. Katarakt und Glaukom. *Klin. Mbl. Augenheilk.*, 140, 645–656, 769–779, 1962.

Kudoyarov G.K. & Chemodanova L.E. Cataract extraction in a glaucomatous eye (in Russian) *Vestn. Oftalm.*, 4, 24–29, 1961.

Labib M.A.M., Emarah M.H.M. & Abdalla S.I. The combined operation for cataract and glaucoma. Evaluation of the results of 135 cases. *Bull. Ophthal. Soc. Egypt*, 66, 195–229, 1973.

Lee O.S. & Weilh J.E. Results of operation for cataract with primary glaucoma. *Arch. Ophthal.*, 44, 275–284, 1950.

Legrand J. Les problèmes thérapeutiques posés par l'association cataracte-glaucome. *Bull. Soc. Ophtal., France*, 68, 67–84, 1968.

Leydhecker W. & Knapp E. Gleichzeitige Operationen von Katarakt und Glaukom. Vergleich verschiedener Verfahren. *Klin. Mbl. Augenheilk.*, 155, 328–333, 1969.

Loh R.C.K. Cataract and glaucoma. A combined operation. *Orient. Arch. Ophthal.*, 7, 190–201, 1969.

Lugossy G. Cataract surgery combined with iridencleisis in glaucoma. *Szemeszet*, 114, 4–9, 1977.

MacMillan J.A. Discussion of Ramsey's paper on glaucoma and cataract. *Arch. Ophthal.*, 43, 195, 1950.

Mandras G., Protonotarios P. & Chilaris G. Combined glaucoma and cataract surgery by a modified Stallard operation. *Bull. Soc. Hellén. Ophtal.*, 37, 264–278, 1969.

Marchi V. Descrizione di una technica associante nello stesso intervento l'estrazione della cataratta e la ciclodiastasi di Strampelli con filo di supramid. *Ann. Ottalm. Clin. Oculistica*, 93, 137–150, 1967.

Maumenee A.E. & Wilkinson C.P. A combined operation for glaucoma and cataract. *Amer. J. Ophthal.*, 69, 360–367, 1970.

Mawas E., Chabat H. & Parizot H. Bilan de quatre années d'opérations combinées de la cataracte et du glaucome en un temps. *Bull. Soc. Ophtal. France*, 67, 842–848, 1967.

McDonald P.R. Glaucoma complicated by cataract. *Trans. Penn. Acad. Ophth. Oto-laryng.*, 20, 15–18, 1967.

Menezo J.L. Nusstro proceder quirurgico en la extraccion de la catarata en pacientes glaucomatosos. *Arch. Soc. Oftal. Hisp. Amer.*, 25, 225–252, 1965.

Mukhina E.A. Experience with one stage cataract extraction and trabeculectomy. *Vestn. Oftal.*, 91, 35–37, 1975.

Nagpaul P.N., Charan H. & Sarda R.P. Cataract and iridencleisis. One stage operation. *J. All-India Ophthal. Soc.*, 14, 31–35, 1966.

Nath K. & Shukla B.R. Two pillar iridencleisodialysis with cataract-extraction in cataract glaucoma. *J. All-India Ophthal. Soc.*, 14, 21–25, 1966.

Naval C.I. & Dizon J. Combined cataract cryo-extraction and glaucoma filtering operations. *Philipp. J. Ophthal.*, 2, 91–101, 1970.

Nectoux R., Chabat H., Mawas F. & Parizot M. L'opération en un temps de la cataracte associée au glaucoma. *Bull. Soc. Ophtal. France*, 64, 377–384, 1964.

Neetens A. Combined glaucoma-cataract surgery. *Ophthalmologica*, 171, 288–295, 1975.

O'Brien C.S. Ocular surgery. *Arch. Ophthal.*, 37, 1–7, 1947.

O'Donoghue H.N. A combined glaucoma-cataract operation. *Trans. Ophthal Soc. U.K.*, 92, 359–369, 1972.

Offret G. & Pouliquen Y. Opération mixte de la cataracte et du glaucome dans un seul temps. *Bull. Soc. Ophtal. France*, 64, 890–892, 1964.

Palimeros G., Chimonidou E., Magouritsas N. & Velissaropoulos P. Cataract extraction in chronic simple glaucoma. *Ophthal. Surg.*, 5, 62–66, 1974.

Pittar C.A. Combined operation for cataract and glaucoma. *Trans. Ophthal. Soc. Australia*, 25, 59–64, 1966.

Preste E. Estrazione di Cataratta con contemporanea sclerectomia antiglaucomatosa di Arruga. *Ann. Ottalm. Clin. Oculistica*, 92, 289–298, 1966.

Protonotarios P. A combination of cyclodialysis and sclerotomy with inclusion of a silicone sheet in a simultaneous glaucoma and cataract operation. *Bull. Soc. Hellén. Ophtal.*, 38, 252–253, 1970.

Rich W. Cataract extraction with trabeculectomy. *Trans. Ophthal. Soc. U.K.*, 94, 458–467, 1974.

Rodriguez Gonzalez A. Combined cataract and glaucoma surgery. *Rev. Soc. Colomb. Oftal.*, 6, 33–37, 1975.

Roveda J.M. Opération combinée de la cataracte et du glaucoma. *Ann. Oculistique*, 205, 193–197, 1972.

Sambursky J.S., Teixeira J.B. & Ferreira G.P. Ciclodialise e facectomia concomitantes. *Rev. Bras. Oftal.*, 26, 405–408, 1967.

Sakic D. Beitrag zu Staroperationen im glaukomatosen Auge. *Dtsche Ophthal. Ges., Heidelberg*, 63, 350–354, 1960.

Sarda, R.P., Jain M.R. & Ahluwalia C.J.S. Iridostasis and double sphinctero-iridotomy with cataract extraction. *Brit. J. Ophthal.*, 52, 486–488, 1968.

Sautter H., Demeler U. & Naumann G. Simultaneous trabeculotomy and intracapsular cataract extraction. *Klin. Mbl. Augenheilk.*, 164, 65–71, 1974.

Sbordone G., Nastri G. & Romano A. Personal technique of combined glaucoma and cataract surgery. *Atti LIII Cong. Soc. Oftal. Ital.*, 27, 342–345, 1971.

Scuderi G. On the surgical therapy of the association: chronic glaucoma and cataract. *Ann. Inst. Barraquer*, 7, 557–570, 1967.

Scuderi G. & Cardia L. Novita'nelle terapia chirurgica della associazione morbosa cataratta-glaucoma. *Int. Surg. Chicago, Section I*, 49, 478–483, 1968.

Scuderi & Schillaci C. Sulla scelta dell'intervento chirurgico nella associazione morbosa glaucoma cronico semplice-cataratta. *Riv. Ital. Tracoma*, 16, 39–57, 1964.

Shmeleva V.V. One-stage cataract extraction and trabeculectomy. *Vestn. Oftal.*, 85, 44–47, 1972.

Shmeleva V.V. & Mukhina E.A. Combined cataract extraction and cyclodialysis. *Vestn. Oftal.*, 85, 30–33, 1972.

Simon J.M. Sobre el tratamiento del glaucoma con catarata. *Arch. Soc. Oftal. Hisp.-Amer..*, 25, 348–354, 1965.

Spaeth P.G. Combined cataract and glaucoma surgery. *Trans. Austr. Coll. Ophthal.*, 2, 60–66, 1970.

Stelzer R. Indications for the combined operation for glaucoma and cataract. *Klin. Mbl. Augenheilk.*, 165, 475–477, 1974.

Stocker F.W. Cataract extraction combined with scleral cauterisation. Results and revised technique. *Eye, Ear, Nose, Thr., Monthly*, 48, 322–324, 1969.

Stocker F.W. & Young J.A. Symposium: Recent advances in cataract surgery. Cataract extraction combined with scleral cauterisation. *South Med. J.*, 58, 1423–1425, 1965.

Streiff E.B. Terapia chirurgica della associazione morbosa cataratta-glaucoma. Simp. Chirurgia Ocular, Bari, 1967.

Suga K. & Nagata M. Surgery of cataract with simple glaucoma. *Rinsho Ganka*, 25, 1479–1484, 1971.

Takats I. & Pinter E. Combination of iridencleisis and cataract extraction. *Acta Chir. Acad. Sci. Hung.*, 12, 281–285, 1971.

Thyer H.W. & Wilson M. Trabeculectomy. *Brit. J. Ophthal.*, 56, 37–40, 1972.

Tizio (Di) A. & Leonardi A. Cataratta e glaucoma. Intervento combinato. *Atti XLVII Cong. Soc. Oftal. Ital.*, 21, 227–239, 1963.

Vancea P.P. & Schwartzenberg T. La trabéculectomie combinée avec l'extraction du cristallin cataracté. Technique et résultats cliniques immédiats et tardifs. *Ann. Oculistique*, 207, 337–351, 1974.

Vasilev V. Cryo-Extraction of the lens and filtering iridectomy as a combined operation in senile cataract with glaucoma. *Ophthalmologia, Sofia*, 20, 10-16, 1972.

Veirs E.R. & Tate C.B. Jr. Adjunctive surgical techniques for glaucoma. A preliminary report. *Ann. Ophthal., Chic.*, 3, 196–200, 1971.

Verin P., Yacoubi M., Berbich A. & Morax S. Opération combinée pour cataracte et glaucome chez les malades trachomateux. Bull. *Soc. Ophtal., France*, 71, 502–504, 1971.

Verzella M. Estrazione di cataratta con contemporanea irido-encleisis. *Atti XLV Cong. Soc. Oftal. Ital.*, 19, 318–321, 1961.

Verzella M. Opération combinée cataracte et iridencleisis. *Ann. Oculistique*, 196, 688–708, 1963.

Vorosmarthy D. & Ballschuh G. Linsenextraktion an glaukomatösen *Augen. Klin. Mbl. Augenheilk.*, 153, 382–386, 1968.

Wenaas E.J. & Stertzbach C.W. Cataract extraction with iris inclusion. *Amer. J. Ophthal.*, 39, 71–75, 1955.

Wolfe O.D. Glaucoma and cataract. *J. Iowa Med. Soc.*, 42, 522–524, 1952.

Wright R.E. Lectures on cataract. *Amer. J. Ophthal.*, 20, 376–387, 1937.

Yigitsubay V. Concomitant peripheral iridencleisis and lens extraction in the surgical treatment of glaucoma associated with cataract. *Cerrahpasa Tip Bult.*, 6, 195–202, 1973.

Zuccoli A. L'iridettomia basale filtrante nell'operazione della cataratta associata a glaucoma. *Atti Soc. Oftal Lombarda*, 20, 175–183, 1965.

Zuccoli A. Résultats d'une expérience de 9 ans de l'iridectomie filtrante dans l'intervention simultannée pour le glaucome associé à la cataracte. *Ann. Oculistique*, 201, 516–526, 1968.

Author's address:
Graef de Smet de Naeyerplein 15
B–9000 Gent
Belgie

INTRODUCTION TO OPTICAL AND FUNCTIONAL TREATMENT OF APHAKIA

DAVID PATON, M.D.

(Houston, Texas, U.S.A.)

In the 17th century a Florentine physician, scholar, scientist and poet – Francesco Redi – wrote what is probably the first reference to the use of spectacles (Figure 1). In searching through old monastery manuscripts, Redi found one dated 1299 in which a monk had written: 'I am so weighted with years that without the glasses (occhiali) I could neither read nor write. These have lately been invented to the convenience of poor old people whose sight is enfeebled.'

It was also Francesco Redi who was the first to demonstrate the falsity of the doctrine of spontaneous generation. His ductum 'omne vivum ex viva' was the first major biological generalization that was based upon biological research. Using Galileo's experimental method for the study of the physical sciences, Redi showed for the first time that experimental methods are the most effective means of arriving at the truth concerning biological phenomena.

It is appropriate that a congress of ophtalmology be held in Florence where Redi did most of his important work, for never before has there been a greater need for scientists and physicians to appreciate the importance of objective conclusions derived from sound scientific studies. Huxley said, 'Nature, like a witness, reveals her secrets when put to torture.' Let me rephrase Huxley's confirmation of Redi's discovery by the following extrapolation to the realities of our own work: It is the task of ophthalmologists today to search further for the truth about the nature of the eye and its surgery, while at the same time avoiding the tortures of any ill-conceived clinical investigations.

As mentioned, Redi gave us the first significant essay on the topic of spectacle correction. Glasses have endured rather well. Today, the majority of the world's aphakic patients still have glasses rather than contact lenses or intraocular implants. However, we now have extraordinary new techniques and remarkable new technology to provide us with a multiplicity of options for the management of our patients with cataracts. The basic theme of the papers that I will be giving at this meeting – and I suspect this is true of many others as well – is that the management decisions of the individual doctor for a specific patient are as vital as surgical skills themselves. No ophthalmologist can translate his own repertoire into exactly the same operation as done by his colleague. There are personal, national and even

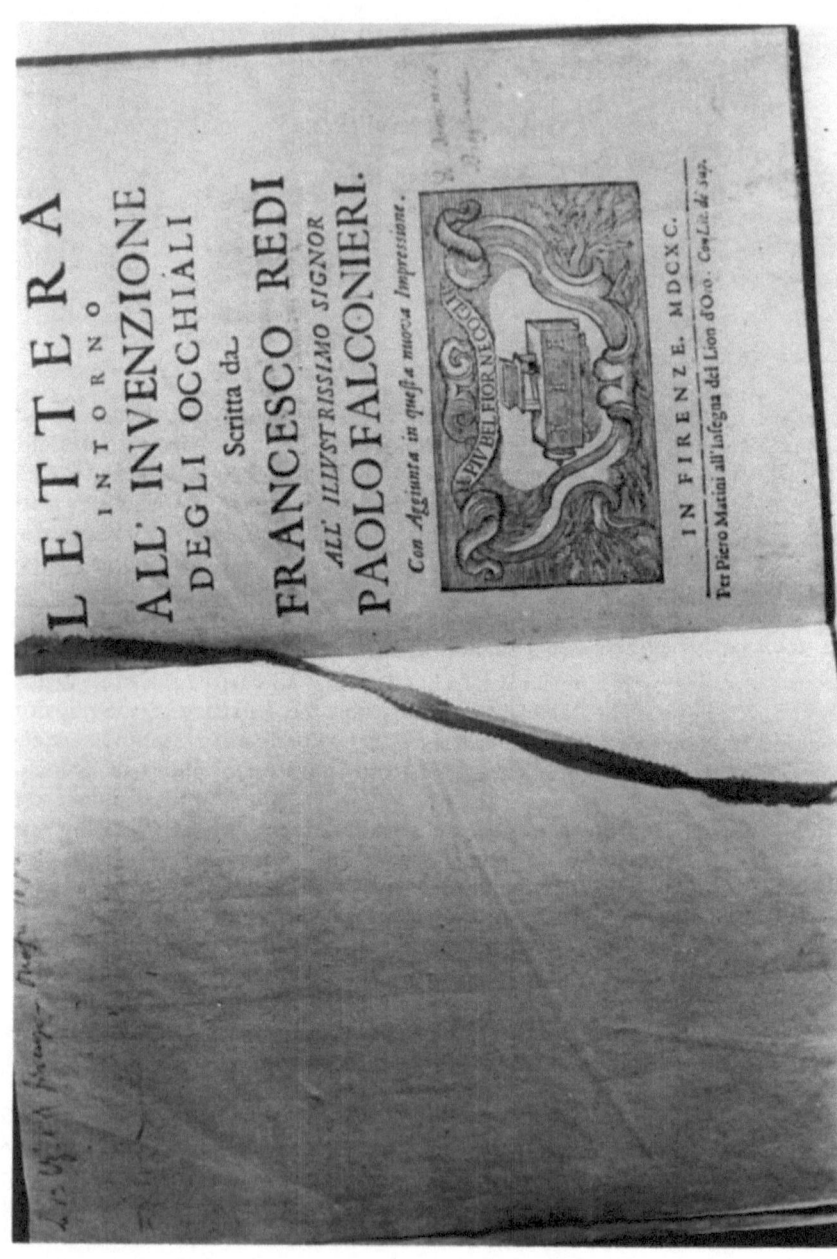

Fig. 1.   Francesco Redi: *Lettera Intorno All' Invenzione Degli Occhiali.*

international factors that make for separate identities in our professional performances. Thank goodness that there is variety and a flux of ideas! In the opera of life, Joe Green is not Giuseppe Verdi.

No personal insecurities or disguised self-interests should prevent each of us from acknowledging that there are 'super-surgeons' for cataracts. Such colleagues, whether in the eye camps of Asia or the operating rooms of industrialized nations, are extracting scores of cataracts every week. Other doctors, more versatile in the practice of ophthalmology, must be cautious in undertaking complex methods that require unfamiliar skills. What is good technique for one surgeon is bad for another. In this meeting we will hear and see the modern magic of some super-specialists. Whereas we may each decide that we should not try to master some of these complete systems of cataract surgery, we can learn a great many fine points that are very much applicable to the surgery that each of us performs. Our changes should be gradual and considered.

One of the most fascinating topics of the meeting is that of intraocular lenses, primarily espoused in Europe and North America. They are truly amazing devices that can give a more nearly perfct restoration of vision than the less convenient and more cumbersome contact lenses and spectacles. Let us not rush to finalize judgment of these implants but, cognizant of the lessons of their history, let us look for sound experimental evidence — clean clinical data. To that I am sure Francesco Redi would give strong approval.

In closing, one last bit of metaphysics from the lessons of this great country: What we see is not necessarily the truth, for the mind makes assumptions that can play tricks on the prejudiced observer. Since I believe

A

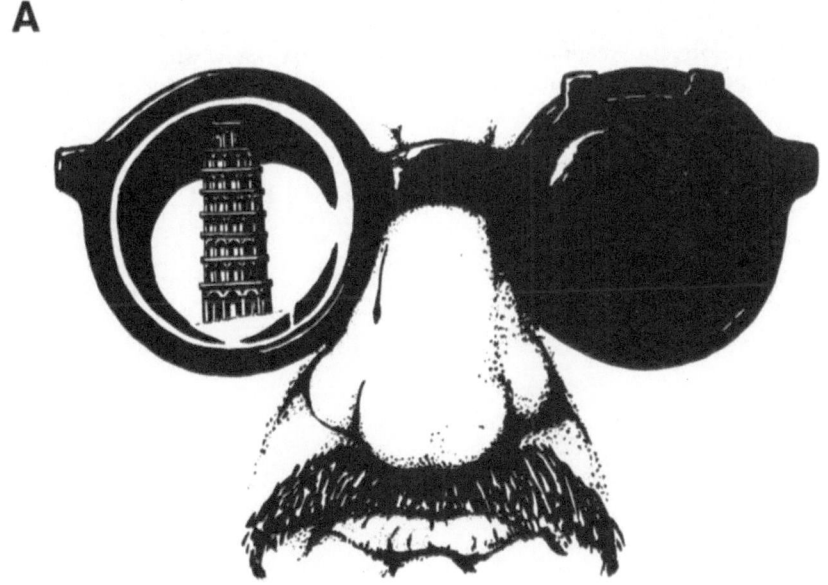

B

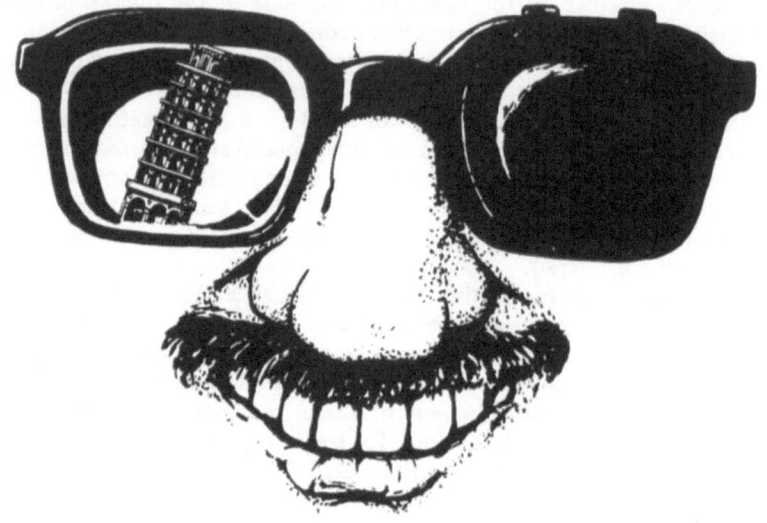

that astigmatism remains the most neglected preventable complication of cataract surgery, I have asked my friend and associate, Dr. John Craig, to illustrate that point by showing a monocular aphake (Figure 2). He is observing a familiar tower, not far from the homes of Redi and Galileo, with a bad lens that is then changed to provide the proper cylindrical correction and the correct perception. The patient, of course, knew what he should see — for he is Italian. Not all of us would have recognized the deception.

PSYCHO-OPTICAL ASPECTS OF THE APHAKIC CONDITION

A. ALAJMO

(Venice, Italy)

If we consider the anatomical-physiological variations induced by surgery in general, we can immediately assert that the very attainment of the final end that surgery sets itself is, in many cases, the first complication of the operation.

The first complication in cataract surgery is therefore the aphakic condition itself that is to be achieved. Such complications that, due to pre-existing visual conditions may not be significant from the subjective point of view, in consideration of the great functional advantage that the operation restores, can in certain cases represent the partial or total failure of the aim of the patient's general well-being, which is the goal of both patient and surgeon.

A concise and drastic enunciation of the operative indication for cataract can display similar contingencies. A mere few minutes of pre-operative explanation can spare the prolonging of the post-operative crisis of adaption which is at times even very long.

This can occur in subjects who are still young in age for basically optical reasons, and in patients of very advanced age, for fundamentally psychological reasons. Dubois-Poulsen has illustrated these aspects in which everyday practice offers us different examples.

Due simply to the different anatomical conditions that develop, a post-operative aphakic condition, even in order, represents above all a possible source of complications, wich, however, by being noted generally only by the surgeon, have no importance from the psychological point of view for the patient.

Without going into the critical evaluation of the operations for the 'prosthetophakia' with their differing methods, I think that the intra-ocular fitting of an acrylic lens can create problems of a psychological nature, more or less accentuated, and analogous to those of a user of an artificial cardiac valve, a pacemaker, a femoral pin, etc. . . . . The psychological motivations, with which, however, I have not had direct experience, can be due to the fear which is always produced by the presence of a foreign body in our own organism, and in the consciousness of being dependent on an instrument.

Again, psychological problems arise in a person with the aphakic condition in relation to sensorial factors which are linked with his new visual condition. These factors are mainly in connection with the variations of the retina's image, the alterations of the visual field and certain distortions of the peripheral vision associated with spherical and chromatic aberration caused by the use of the optical correction.

With the traditional optical correction, the distortion of the peripheral vision is added to the concentric shrinking of the visual field, and the so-called 'Jack in the box' phenomenon and alternations in the apparent speed of displacement of objects is so situated in the peripheral zone that their different angular relationships to the direction of sight determine either an increase or a decrease in the apparent velocity of movement, thus creating noticeable hindrances, particularly while driving automobiles; these phenomena have already been clearly illustrated by Welsh and Dubois-Poulsen.

The alteration of spatial relations, which represents the first impact with his surroundings for a patient recovering from a cataract operation, is even better known.

All of these alterations create noticeable psychological and adaptation problems and can even influence other aspects of the subject's life, once he has become aphakic.

Certainly, correcting the aphakic condition with corneal lenses remedies such eventualities by improving the quality of the retina's image and eliminating the various causes of visual alteration. An analogous defense can be put forth, even if more cautiously, in favour of intraocular lenses.

Soft corneal lenses, the opportune intra-operative prevention of post-operative astigmatism, its eventual correction by means of 'equivalent spherical' lenses, in particular the attainment of 'continuous wearing' of the corneal lenses by means of technical perfection, already in use, all allow for the obtaining of an improved visual comfort' with better adaptation to certain circumstances of vision.

The use of dioptric lenses which are progressively variable do not seem to have given satisfactory practical results in the field of strong ametropia of a person with the aphakic condition while, on the other hand, better prospects are opening up with the introduction of the 'four drop' lenses.

In addition, 'confusional' problems must be observed in aphakic patients without correction, as summarized by Gernet (1977): 1. Binocular vision is troubled by the aphakic image, in spite of less than 1/20 visual acuity; 2. The patient perceives a dim image especially in the far vision; 3. The patient presents diplopia without strabismus; 4. The patient is troubled by an alteration of the stereoscopic sense; 5. The patient, finally, perceives at night clear rings around luminous sources.

All these symptoms may be suppressed by means of a 'contact lens plus conventional lens' correcting system both in the far and near vision.

In Jaffe's opinion, the conventional lens usually produces in an aphakic eye, a 25% enlargement of the image. The enlargement with contact lens and intraocular lens is respectively 7% and 2%.

Besides, stereoscopic vision is reestablished in 45% of contact lenses users and in 82% of patients receiving an intraocular lens.

Also, it must be remembered that the hard or soft contact lenses are always difficult to apply for aged patients who, after many trials, return to the conventional correction.

486

To reach the goal of a complete functional recovery, the introduction of an intraocular lens seems to be preferable, and so the different percentages, from 10-20% to 80%, of a similar operative indication must be explained.

In contrast with the negative psycho-optical aspects, to which I have briefly alluded, fortunately there is a positive side which balances the clinical and at times operative delicacy necessary for the extraction of a cataract from an extremely myopic eye. The most delicate problem remains, in my opinion, that of foreseeing possible difficulties pertaining to his near vision which must be evaluated, and explained to the patient.

In conclusion, I hold that the evaluation of the psycho-optical aspects created by the aphakic condition must not be disregarded in any single case, but must be explained in full honesty to the patient without being overrated and above all which must be evaluated according to the following considerations: 1. a refractive and psychological pre-operative evaluation of the clinical situation; 2. information for the patient in cautious and appropriate terms; 3. instruction about type of available optical correction for use after the operation; 4. the appropriate surgical technique used to obtain the optical correction; 5. the earliest post-operative correction possible should be worn by means of suitable glasses, even during the first days of the post-operative period for a faster and better re-insertion of the patient; 6. the correct psychological treatment of a patient that shows signs of a sequel of a psycho-optical nature; 7. the eventual modification of the type of optical correction being used; 8. a strict attitude with 'difficult' patients, asking the same also of his immediate household; 9. the suggestion of the advisable visual norm, encouraging the patient to renounce certain activities and to take up others; 10. in the cases of unilaterial aphakia, in which the restoration of the binocular vision is not possible, the functional sacrifice of the the operated eye, perhaps with a brilliant success, for the advantage of temporarily more comfortable vision out of the un-operated or not yet operated eye.

This 'decalogue', which I have chosen to present to you below the stern look of Michelangelo's Moses, concludes this short exposition that has fundamentally, I believe, one main moral:

'A cataract operation must, above all, be useful to the patient'.

Author's address:
Primario Oculista Osp. Civile
Venezia 33100 Italia

Note: But as it happens for 'The ten Commandments' not all of us are wont to trust, and the Believers also do not always succeed in respecting them.

Docum. Ophthal. Proc. Series, Vol. 21

OPTICAL CORRECTION OF APHAKIA

M. MAIONE & F. CARTA

(Parma, Italy)

The choice of the type of optical correction of the aphakic not fitted with intraocular lenses must be made taking into account a series of parameters which reflect the optical characteristics of the operated eye, the physical and mental condition of the patient and the mono- or bilateral nature of the aphakia. This last aspect of the problem will not be treated here, since it has already been widely discussed by others with great competence.

The aphakic eye is, from the optical point of view, substantially an optical instrument delimited by the corneal surface and diaphragmed by the pupil. As the cornea is not a surface of revolution and the operation not infrequently provokes a more or less accentuated displacement of the pupil, the correction of the ametropia is often conditioned by these two phenomena, and the search for the most efficacious retinal section of the caustic, which is not necessarily the sharpest but rather which has better light distribution, becomes empirical.

It is not unusual that the trial correction performed in the ophthalmologist's or optometrist's office, and regularly prescribed, differs substantially in dioptric value and visual efficacy from that which would be necessary for the final, definitive lens, to the patient's dissatisfaction. This is even more evident when dealing with contact lenses rather than a traditional correction; often a supplementary correction, usually cylindrical, must be added. Even when the aphakic eye has a pupil which is round and well-centered, an analogous discrepancy between trial conditions and definitive conditions may be present for the following reasons:

1. The possibility that the trial lenses and those of the definitive spectacle of correction do not have the same alignment in respect to the patient's visual axis (variations of spherical power and of astigmatism).

2. The possibility that the trial lens and the definitive lens do not have the same inclination in respect to the visual axis (variations of astigmatism).

3. The possibility that the trial lenses and the definitive ones have a different distance from the vertex of the cornea (variations in spherical power).

4. The possibility that the two lenses have a different form factor (variations in magnification).

To obviate these difficulties, Welsch has created an 'Aphakic Refracting Kit' consisting of six pairs of aspheric lenses of +11 diopters mounted on permanent frames having the most common interpupillary distances; there is a special bracket for the insertion of any necessary supplementary corrective device. This permits the ophthalmologist to give the technician all the necessary information for making the glasses without too many tiring sittings, and gives the patient the opportunity of choosing proper frames.

The correction of aphakia with contact lenses is always experimental in the aphakic, especially if the patient is a child or an old person, not infrequently affected with senile enophthalmos. Such correction may become impossible when the aphakic eye has a strong astigmatism or a marked updrawing of the pupil or when the contact lens adheres badly. The adherence of a contact lens depends not only on correspondence between cornea and lens, but also on pressure exerted by the eyelid, on the amplitude of the fornices, on the quantity of lacrimal secretion, on the weight of the lens, etc. This makes it essential that the trials are made with contact lenses having adequate power, and that the ophtalmologist, carefully evaluating the advantages, is sure that they abundantly outweigh the disadvantages, enough to create a psychological motivation. This evaluation must take into account visual acuity, which may be conditioned by sensorial deprivation or by ocular malformations in the case of congenital cataract or by macular degenerations in senile cataract. Remaining in the area of Gaussian approximation, it must be remenbered that the retinal image in the conventionally corrected aphakic eye, even with the variations due to differences in the form factor, is about 30% larger than that which would be found in the same eye after correction with a contact lens. Consequently, visual acuity is better with conventional correction and can be maximized with the proper choice of lens form. Often moreover the patient, either spontaneously or because instructed to do so, by holding the glasses at a certain distance from his eyes can improve magnification even further when necessary, for example, to read a price-tag or the number of a bus.

It follows, therefore, that in all of those conditions in which the patient's visual acuity is low, correction with conventional glasses is to be preferred, and sometimes even a modest degree of undercorrection, which permits better utilization of the spy-glass effect, should be considered. Of course in correction for close vision, greater magnification may be obtained with overcorrection which permits objects to be brought closer.

The ophthalmologist may thus be faced with having to choose whether it is better to achieve a problematical binocularity through the use of a contact lens, or a better acuity trough a conventional correction. In the case of binocular cataract, it seems obvious that the choice should be in favour of a better acuity. In the case of monocular cataract, a suggestion of Enoch's, which seems rational, should be mentioned. A negative contact lens of sufficient power, placed on the phakic eye, permits simultaneous binocular correction of both eyes, (facilitates the various systems of penalization used in treatment of amblyopia) and allows the patient to resort to the spy-glass effect in an emergency.

The optical aberrations of traditional lenses provoke astigmatism for oblique incidence, curvature of the field and a reduction of the field of vision which are very annoying for the patient. These distortions may be minimized by using lenses with an aspheric anterior surface and a concave or

490

toric posterior surface (curvature between 3 and 4 diopters).

There is no doubt that contact lenses give a field of vision which is greater than that which can be obtained by conventional correction. Less evident is their effect on the other two aberrations: the spherical form of the anterior surface of the contact lenses reduces the spherical aberration and consequent curvature of field and neutralises the astigmatism for oblique incidence provoked by decentral displacement of the pupil. These phenomena are exacerbated by a bad choice of contact lens, where the pupil is not centered on its vertex. From this can be seen the utility of aspheric contact lenses for aphakics.

It can be said that for correction of aphakia not complicated by diseases influencing the acuity or by distortions of the ocular objective consequent to operative complications, the choice between correction with glasses or with contact lenses may be left to the patient, who should evaluate his motivations, degree of manual dexterity, etc. In all other cases the choice must be made by the physician, who will take into account whether it is opportune to favour attainment of the best possible acuity to the detriment of the best possible field of vision, what are the possibilities that supplementary traditional correction over the contact lenses may allow greater exploitation of residual visual capacity, and within what limits he can count on the collaboration of the technician in achieving the best possible results.

As regards cataract in children, we must distinguish between congenital, total cataracts and incomplete cataracts developing later. If the cataract is monocular, total, and already present at birth or shortly thereafter, post-operative visual results are almost non-existent and the problem of correction of aphakia does not present itself, even when the operation is performed very early. When the monocular cataract is incomplete, an attentive case-by-case evaluation of the residual visual capacity will serve to decide the best moment for the operation, which should be postponed the longer, the more useful is the residual vision. However, if the mono-or binocular operation has been performed on a child under the age of two, many physicians prefer a modest degree of over-correction of the defect (1.5 diopters) since the child's interests are limited to a relatively small area around him. In this way the necessity for bifocal glasses is avoided. The correction will utilize a contact lens which is direct or inverse, i.e., applied to the other eye if the aphakia is monocular.

The greatest practical problem to be dealt with in the choice of optical correction of non-complicated aphakia is the difficulty presented by stairways and sidewalks. Looking downwards with a well-centered lens introduces an annoying astigmatism for oblique incidence and an increase in the focal power of the lens which renders the image blurred and out of focus. Moreover the prismatic effect causes variance between the actual rotation of the eyes and the rotation of the direction of viewing, and between the actual and the apparent size of the object, all of which create real difficulty for the patient, who ends up moving in a very awkward manner.

A good aspheric lens with the proper curvature of base and the proper framing can reduce these phenomena to tolerable limits. The best type of lens for aphakics is considered to be the aspheric lens of lenticular form,

491

with a 40 mm. diameter of the lens. It permits good centering when the frames are properly chosen, an acceptable aesthetic effect as the zone of support of the lens is covered by the glasses' frames, a sufficiently wide field of vision, and considerably lighter-weight glasses.

The existence of these aberrations is the prime motivation for using contact lenses. The correction of aphakia with well-fitted contact lenses, with the consequent immediate disappearance of awkwardness of movement, creates great enthusiasm in a large percentage of highly-motivated patients. This enthusiasm, however, cannot be uncritically shared. In reality, more than 50% of aphakic contact lens wearers return, after a period of time which varies according to the patient's age, to the conventional, easier-to-wear, type of correction. In these cases, the learning of a new vision-capability correlation has only been postponed, with obvious psychological harm to the patient.

One other advantage of correction by means of contact lenses is the facility of providing adequate correction for short-focus vision with ordinary bifocal glasses. The contact lens wearer may use these without much difficulty. Bifocal glasses for the aphakic non-contact lens wearer are much more complex, for various reasons. Due to the power of the correcting lenses for short-focus vision, a strong externally-bases prismatic effect is introduced, which must be corrected by an adequate decentralization of the lens towards the inside. Such a decentralization, for 16-diopter lenses may be more than 5 mm. for each lens and is in any case always much greater than would be thought on the basis of technical considerations taking into account interpupillary distance and distance from working surface.

There are two great categories of contact lenses, soft and hard. Different types of soft contact lenses differ according to the amount of water they can absorb. Their main advantage in aphakia is their greater diameter, which makes the lens less mobile and more adaptable even in the presence of total iridectomy. Moreover they are usually better tolerated even for long periods of time. Their defects are a lesser capacity for correcting astigmatism, a greater deformability, which may in itself cause astigmatism due to the effect of eyelid pressure, a greater sensibility to the temperature and humidity of the environment which causes variability of their optical effect, and a greater difficulty in handling them. Hard contact lenses require more careful fitting, made difficult by the weight and form of the lens, but are more easily handled and in general are more satisfactory from the optical point of view. Silicon lenses too may be utilized; these share the advantages of the other two types, but deteriorate more rapidly.

Author's address:
Direttore Clinica Oculistica Università
Parma 43100
Italy

EXTENDED WEARING OF CONTACT LENSES:
AN OVERVIEW

G. PETER HALBERG*

(New York, N.Y., U.S.A.)

Under the pressure of the ever expanding intraocular lens surgical field there is a steadily increasing demand for contact lenses that can be worn by patients longer than one day. This type of lenses in the United States are called extended wear contact lenses. World wide efforts are being made to find the proper material that would be universally accepted by the patients, especially aphakic patients, who because of their age, and often due to their lack of manual skill, have difficulty in handling the contact lenses on a daily basis. Many intraocular lens surgeons use this as their major argument: with intraocular lens surgery the visual rehabilitation after cataract surgery is instanteneous, with contact lenses in patients who are unable to handle the lens it is not possible.

There are many studies under way in Europe, the United States and Japan, with the aim of finding the best possible combination for the contact lens material, and the best possible geometry of the contact lens that would permit extended wearing with minimal limitations.

Up to the present time we have found that independent of what kind of material is being used the patient population to be fitted with an extended wearing contact lens break down statisically into two groups. A group, approximately 60% of the patients, that can wear extended wear contact lenses under optimum fitting conditions. Another group, about 40% of the patients, that cannot wear extended wear contact lenses even under optimum fitting conditions. This would not be an unfavorable distribution if we would have safe predictors that would tell us in advance with which group we are faced at the time. Unfortunately, in spite of very intensive investigational work, up to this time we do not have any safe predictors that would assure us about individual patients. Therefore even under optimal circumstances, the patients have to be monitored with greatest of care, for a long period of time.

The first week in our service, independently of the material we are working with, we have the patient seen daily, the second week, three times a week, from the third week on twice a week and weekly for eight to ten

---

* President International Contact Lens Council of Ophthalmology Chief Contact Lens Service, St. Vincent's Hospital and Medical Center of N.Y.

weeks thereafter. This is an enormous burden, both for the patient and for the ancillary personnel, another real factor is cost.

We are investigating high water content, hydrophilic polymers, Poly-2-Hydroxy-Methylmetacrylate and its modifications. We are also investigating contact lenses fabricated of silicone rubber that is made optically clear and is molded into the shape of a contact lens. Usually 11 mm in diamter with smooth transition zones of the periphery, a fair edge design, with a good optical zone and clear optics.

Silicone rubber is originally hydrophobic but the manufacturer of silicone contact lenses in the United States, the Dow-Corning Corporation, Danker and Wohlk succeeded in modifying the silicone rubber lenses so that they are wettable on the surface. Unfortunately we do not have long enough experience to know how long the surface treatment of the lens does last. We have to believe that some of the failures that we have seen recently are due to the fact that in certain cases the surface treatment is wearing off in a matter of several months, after which the lens becomes intolerable for the patient.

Other problems with the silicone rubber lenses are the soiling of the surface by protein and debris from the tear film which varies from individual patient to individual patient. Some patients show absolutely no tendency toward such depositions, on the other hand, other soil the lens in a matter of hours or days. We had some very fortunate cases in the 60% group that can wear the lens on an extended basis and we have also some near disaster cases in the 40% group that cannot wear the lenses.

Another one of the serious problems is the frequent inability of the patient to recognize early danger signals, some patients will disregard the early reddness and discomfort in the eye with the extended wearing silicone lens and will be returning to the office or the clinic only when mild or destructive ulceration of the cornea is already present.

The problem with extended wearing is that we are cutting down in almost all cases on the oxygen available for the corneal epithelium. Some eyes are capable of adapting to the reduced amount of oxygen better than others. Studies show that a minimum of 7 to 9% oxygen in the tear film has to reach the corneal epithelium for it to maintain its integrity.

If the geometry and/or the material characteristics of the contact lens are such that the proper level of oxygen supply cannot be maintained, then there is only very little hope that the patient can wear successfully in an extended fashion the contact lens.

High water content lenses are being tested, especially in the HEMA group, as high as 85% water content is being tried. One must not lose perspective by indiscriminately increasing the water content of the extended wearing lenses without taking into account meticulously the status of the available water in the anterior segment of the eye. Correct assessment of the available water should be performed by careful observation of the marginal tear strip by slit lamp microscope, the Schirmer Tear Test, the tear film breake up time.

If there is not enough water present to maintain the polymer saturated at the level for which it was designed (cross linked), the following profound changes will take place in the polymer and the lens which is fabricated of it:

1. The consistency of the material will change, making the material sticky
2. The refractive index will change
3. The radius of curvature of the contact lens will shorten, making the lens steeper
4. The refractive power will change
5. Ultimately the contact lens will deform and will become a harsh irritant in the eye, not infrequently, completely rejected by the eye and the patient might find it difficult to keep the lens in place.

In summary, we must state that the patient has to be evaluated whether or not he or she is capable of tolerating extended wearing lenses. It must be kept in mind that the high water content hydrophilic lenses are dependent on the available water in the anterior segment and it should be emphasized that besides the characteristics of the polymers, such as silicone rubber or high water content hydrophilic lenses, the geometry of the lens is of utmost importance. Great emphasis must be placed on honest evaluation of the situation otherwise serious disappointment may ensue both for the patient and the physician.

Author's address:
40 West 77th Street
New York, New York 10024,
U.S.A.

Docum. Ophthal. Proc. Series, Vol. 21

SILICONE LENSES IN APHAKIA EVALUATION AFTER ONE YEAR

A. TRAYKOVSKI & C.F. TRAYKOVSKI

(New York, U.S.A.)

This is a study of Silicone Lenses manufactured by Danker-Wohlk under F.D.A. status, N.D.A. The silicone rubber lens is a corneal type lens which can be fitted like a hard lens and tolerated as well as a soft lens. It is gas permeable with rubber-like softness, inert, thermally stable and durable.

The silicone material is hydrophobic and becomes hydrophilic with irradiation of Cobalt $_{60}$ in the presence of oxygen.

The size of the lens is 11 mms and has a transparency of 94% with a refractive index of 1.42. The lenses should remain in a constant wet state in order to maintain the hydrophilic properties.

The lenses can be checked with conventional instruments as with hard lenses. Lensometer, radioscope and keratometers can be used.

The aphakic lenses are .5 mms to .7 mms thickness depending on the plus power. They are molded with an aspheric posterior surface and lenticular cut. The edges are thin and rounded.

Patient selection: The general indication for both hard and soft lenses are applicable for Silicone Lenses as well. Patients with mild dry eye may be fitted with supplemental use of tear substitutes on a regular basis.

Aphakics: with neovascularization at the limbus and old inactive keratitis can be fitted. The patients should be able to handle the lenses independently or have assistance from a cooperative relative or friend for weekly cleaning and removal.

Astigmatism: Patients with astigmatism up to two diopters can achieve satisfactory visual acuity. Surprisingly the patients with high astigmatism of 3 to 5 diopters have a greater reduction of their astigmatism when fitted on an intermediate meridian.

Complete ophthalmological examination as for hard lenses should be done.

Criteria for fitting: Select a lens from a trial set closest to the flatter meridian and insert like a hard lens. The patient can be evaluated in 5 to 10 minutes.

1. **Centration:** The lens centers well and rests on the peripheral 3 mms of the cornea. When fitted flatter than the flattest K, the lens slips down 2 mms from the lower limbus. Depending on the corneal contour, the lens may overlap the limbus for 1 to 2 mms. This occurs more frequently with highly astigmatic corneas, irregular corneas and post keratoplasty.

2. **Movement:** With each blink or ocular rotation the lens should move approximately 1 mm. When fitted for extended wear it is imperative that the lens moves and that adequate tear exchange occurs. A small percentage of patients with mild dry eyes exhibit a non-moving lens or a 'gripper'. These patients must remove the lens daily and use substitute tear products.

3. **Flourescein:** Testing reveals freely flowing flourescein underneath the lens with minimal central pooling and even peripheral touch. The lens does not discolour after flourescein application.

4. Clear retinoscopic reflex should be visualized in all meridians.

5. Vision is stable and as good as with spectacle correction provided there is no excessive astigmatism.

6. **Removal:** Remove the lenses at the end of the day, week, or month and evaluate the cornea. The epithelium shows minimal punctate staining which disappears after one hour. The Keratometry reading and the corneal thickness should remain unchanged. The patients with a 'gripper' and 'dry eyes' show more staining which persists for several hours. These are daily wear candidates and their corneas should return to a normal state each morning.

Mode of Wear: The adaptation is rapid. Most patients exhibit minimal foreigh body sensation of the upper eyelid. After determination of patient tolerance over a period of 1½ hours, the patient is advised to wear the lenses 6 to 8 hours the first day and all day long the following day. Check up is made after 24 hours and a decision is made for appropriate length of wear.

Trial Set: A limited trial set of the following base curves is indicated: 7.50, 7.70, 7.80, 7.90, 8.00, 8.10 and 8.20 in various powers form +12.00 to +15.00. Patients and relatives are taught insertion and removal with the DMV suction cup, which is wetted with Soaclens.

ADVERSE REACTIONS

Minor Problems

1. Slip off: may occur rather commonly and patients or relatives must be taught repositioning.

2. 'Gripper' – The lens doesn't move and the patient is predisposed to developing corneal abrasions and iritis.

3. Loss of hydrophilic surface results in dry spots with decrease in vision. This occurs after approximately one year but may happen earlier in patients with exposure, poor blink reflex and dry eyes. These lenses may be returned to the laboratory for recoating. A spare lens is advisable in these cases.

4. Papillary conjunctivitis with congestion of the conjunctiva of the upper eyelid may occur rarely. Lens loss from the eye is extremely infrequent.

Major Problems

Corneal abrasions and iritis occurred in patients with high plus lenses +16.00 to +20.00 who were unable to remove the lenses. These difficulties developed after one to two weeks extended wear. If possible, they should be converted to daily wear; if not, discontinue the lenses.

Clinical Study

This particular study of 23 aphakics, 13 unilateral and 5 bilateral was done on patients in this practice. The bilateral aphakics require assistance from a relative or friend with insertion and removal. Those patients who had support of a spouse or nearby friend managed well. The clinic population in this study, generally did not make good candidates as the followup isn't always reliable, and they may have difficulties following instructions.

Eleven patients out of nineteen accepted the lenses, eight were returned to us for various reasons. (fig. 2 & 3). Many of these rejections had anxieties about insertion and removal and in spite of repeated attempts of teaching by a trained contact lens technician were unable to manage or alleviate their fears.

75% of these patients were 65 or over, 20% were between 45–60, and 5% an adolescent high myope. The eldest aphakics managed well if they had good eye hand coordination or support of an alert relative. The younger

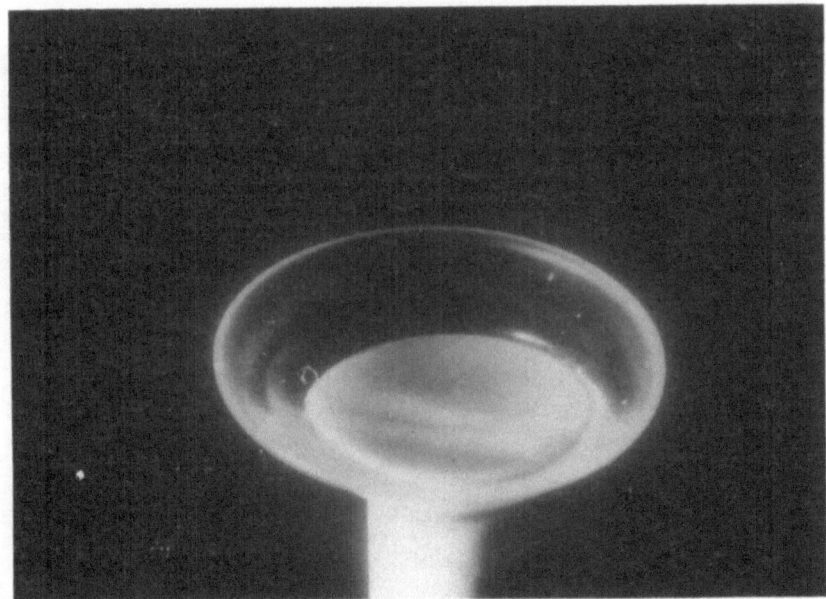

Fig. 1. **Wearing time of all patients studied**

Presently worn: (patient number)	Wearing time:
12	14 months, OU
17	12 months
6	11 months
15	7 months, OU, intermittant
2, 19	6 months
8, 18	1–3 months

group managed independently other than the high myope who was assisted by a sister.

The longest trial is 14 months (No. 12, fig. 1). The lenses are in excellent condition and stable acuity is maintained. Two patients experienced severe 'clouding' of vision after six months of wear. The central portion of the lens became hydrophobic. These were with removal every three days. Replacements were made. On the whole longevity is equal or superior to soft lenses. Further evalution should be carried out in this area, as we do not have a high enough percentage of patients with lenses over 12 months duration in this study.

Four patients fitted developed complications. All of these were fitted on an extended wear basis. A maintenance worker whose environment was dusty developed uveitis and a corneal abrasion. His correction was +19.00. Perhaps the thickness of the lens contributed to his difficulties. Two other aphakics developed similar complications, both were +15.50 or higher. These lenses were discontinued.

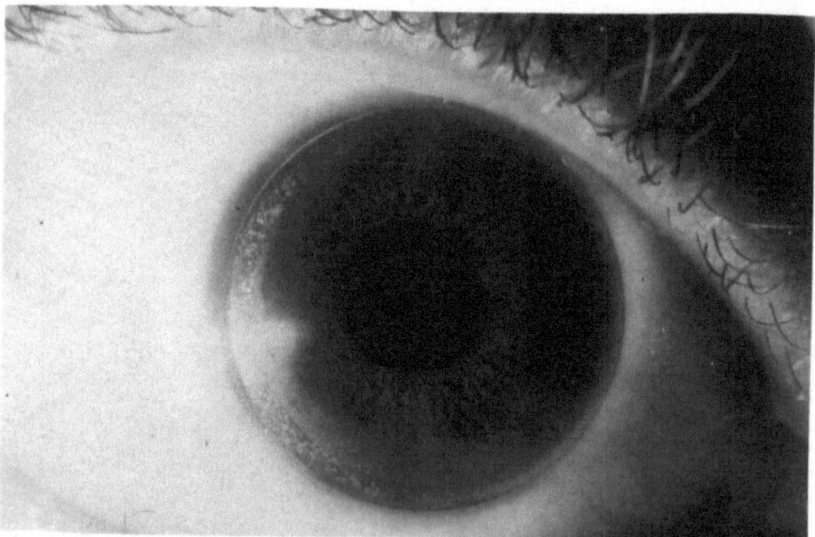

Fig. 2. Terminated cases

Terminated wear: (patient number)	Reason:
3	slipping and anxiety
5	unreliable followup
7	unreliable followup
9	unable to handle, dusty environment, high, plus
10	refused
11	unable to handle
12	refused, multiple problems due to systematic disease

Fig. 3. Total statistics

Diagnosis:	Number of cases:	Accepted:	Rejected:
Aphakia	6 patients 8 eyes	8	4
Aphakia and Post Keratoplasty	6 patients 6 eyes	4	2
High myopia	1 patient 2 eyes	1	

Best results in visual acuity, longevity and a 'quiet eye' are obtained by removal every three days or daily. Good results can be obtained for patients with adequate tear production for extended wear up to a week. Lenses are removed on retiring and reinserted the next morning. Bilateral aphakics alternate, so they have use of one eye for insertion and removal.

Alle extended wear patients are checked with lenses in their eyes. Satisfactory criteria are good lens centering, good mobility with flourescein freely flowing underneath the lens. The lenses are removed and the cornea shows fine punctate staining which disappears after 30 minutes. The keratometry readings and the refraction before starting the lenses was usually unchanged. The corneal thickness remained unchanged pre and post wearing. The patients who had complications due to extended lens wearing such as, corneal abrasions and iritis recovered their original corrected vision after treatment.

In conclusion Danker-Wohlk Silicone Lenses are suitable for aphakic patients for extended wear provided they are fitted in accordance with summarized criteria. Patient selection should include only those able and willing to follow the routine and have minimal assistance. Failures occur with poor followup or if assistance at home was unavailable.

SUMMARY

The Silicone Lenses are safe and effective for correction of aphakia. They may be worn daily or as an extended wear lens.

The practictioner will find the fitting procedure simple with the usual ophthalmic instruments in his office. A small trial set is necessary.

These corneal lenses are gas permeable, durable elastic and flexible.

The optics are of high quality due to molding and the thin edge. The advantages over hard lenses are easy adaption and tolerance, better centering and a greatly decreased loss rate.

Advantages over soft lenses are durability and better optical performance especially in astigmatism.

They are easier to insert and remove by patients and relatives. The Silicone Lenses are more suitable for mild dry states where the soft lenses have failed. They do not cause neovascularization.

The major disadvantage is loss of hydrophilic surface after one year.

Docum. Ophthal. Proc. Series, Vol. 21

KERATOPHAKIA TODAY

BRUCE MATHALONE

(London, England)

The operation of keratophakia involves changing the refraction of the eye by carving a convex lens from the substantia propra of a donor cornea to build up the host cornea. It was thought of and developed by Jose Barraquer following his original work on keratomileusis. (Barraquer, 1964) The usual indication is after cataract extraction and most usually in unilateral cases.

This paper will try and put the operation in perspective with the recent developments in intraocular and contact lenses.

THE OPERATION

The technique involves the use of a lathe with a freezing device using CO_2 or N_2O gas to freeze the lap and cutting edge. After a retrobulbar injection of 4 mm of saline, a reference mark is placed on the patient's cornea. The eye is fixed by a pneumatic ring, through which passes an electromicrokeratome. This operates like a carpenter's plane and shaves a parallel faced corneal disc from the patient's own cornea. A 10.0 continuous perlon suture is inserted and left loose.

A keratoctomy is then made on the donor eye to obtain a thick corneal disc and this is carved on the epithelial side after freezing. The tissue lens is thawed in glycerol 10% and then placed in the centre of the keratectomy. The interfaces are carefully washed and the corneal disc centred. The continuous suture is now adjusted and tied.

The change in corneal curvature is immediately apparent and a monocular bandage applied. The refraction is changed according to the power of the carved tissue lens. This is a more satisfactory way of getting a hypermetropic correction than using the technique of keratomileusis in which the lens is carved from the original lamellar cut. The patient is kept on local steroids and mydriatics and the continuous suture is removed in 21 days.

The dimensions and detailed descriptions of the special tools designed by Barraquer for this technique and the basis for the calculations have been fully described elsewhere. (Barraquer 1967, 1969)

As there are two interfaces it is rare to obtain a visual acuity of 6/6 and in our hands 6/12 — 6/9 was the usual result after a succesful case; however the change was constant without the use of any visual aids.

It is important to take care to prevent amblyopia in children.

INDICATIONS FOR THE OPERATION

Keratophakia can be used in any cases of hypermetropic anisometropia of over 5D. In our hands it was not very successful in the treatment of aniso-metropic amblyopia probably because of the period of occlusion and rela-tively poor vision after surgery. It was most successful in cases of traumatic aphakia in children and adults and also in cases of unilateral aphakia. We did one case in which a posterior chamber Ridley implant had to be removed because of glaucoma after many years of good vision and the patient would not tolerate a contact lens. There is also a case for doing the operation in elderly cataractous patients who find aphakic glasses difficult to use and contact lenses often impractical.

Complication of the operation are few. Amorphous opacities, usually not central, can occur in the interface. Foreign bodies in the interfaces can result unless care is taken when inserting the lenticule. Correction of over 15D can result in such a thick lenticule that substantial optical aberrations can occur. Poor centering can similarly reduce the visual acuity.

RESULTS

By far the majority of cases of keratophakia have been performed by Bar-raquer and have been fully reported. I will just desribe in detail two selected cases to show the type of results than can be expected.

1. **Child age 6 years following injury to the cornea and traumatic cata-ract.**

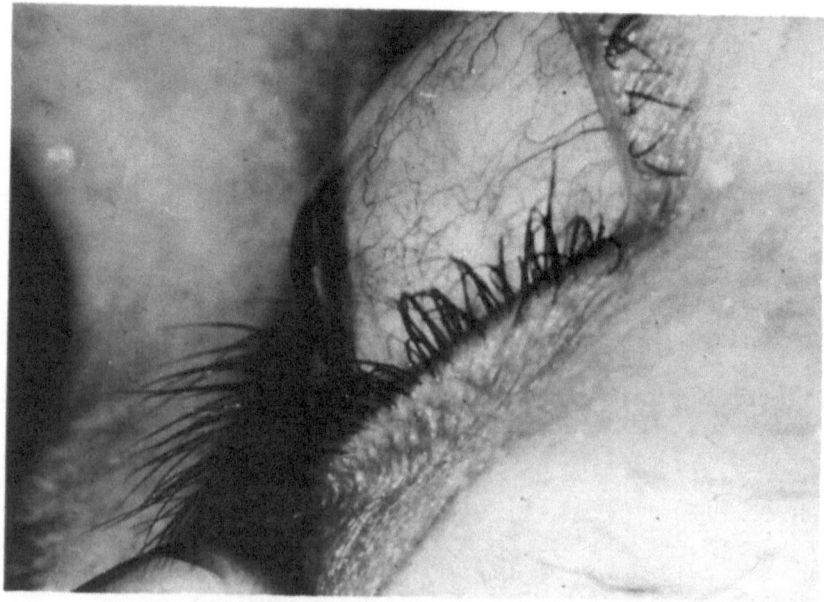

Fig. 1. Change in corneal curvature after Keratophakia.

Visual Acuity 6/36 with + 11.50 Sph.

Post operation 6/24 unaided   6/12 + 2 with + 1.0 Sph.

2. Man aged 23 years who wished to do a job requiring a minimal 6/12 unaided vision in the worse eye.

Visual acuity: 6/24 unaided
 6/18 part with $\dfrac{+\ 4.0\ \text{Sph}}{+\ 2.0\ \text{Cyl}}$

Post operation 6/9 −2 unaided   6/9 with $\begin{array}{l}+\ 0.5\ \text{Sph}\\ -\ 1.0\ \text{Cyl.}\end{array}$

These two unselected cases are typical of two different types of problem. In (1) a young child with unilateral traumatic aphakia benefitted with good unaided vision without any aids, and preserved good binocularity.

In (2) such a good result was not predicted, and in general this is probably not a good indication for the operation, but in this case was worthwhile.

Unlike some of the keratomileuses cases the keratophakias did not lose correction in the post-operative period.

DISCUSSION

Since Barraquer's original work and our earlier cases, many improvements have been made in intraocular and contact lenses and these have been given much publicity. Their main advantage over keratophakia is that adaptations of the routine cataract operation are relatively much less complicated than in keratophakia. However there is little doubt that the complication rate in the long term follow-up of intraocular lenses is much higher and when there has been iris damage in traumatic cases, it is more difficult to apply a lens satisfactorily.

With contact lens wear, it is known that the aphakic cornea is less sensitive than the phakic one, and hard lens wear is often successful especially in younger people. However, older patients find them very difficult to manage and frequently give up trying. The continuous wear lens has problems after cataracts. I have some patients with deep corneal vascularisation − a complication much less likely in unoperated eyes. Also they are prone to infections and the lens will not correct any appreciable residual astigmatism.

SUMMARY

Keratophakia is a difficult and complicated operation which in a few specialised centres has a small but definite place in cataract surgery. In the future the most suitable cases will probably be in traumatic aphakia and possibly in the elderly.

This paper is dedicated to the enormous amount of work done by Jose Barraquer in thinking of and developing the technique and to Derek Ainslie whose painstaking work has largely been the basis of this paper.

REFERENCES

Barraquer, J. I (1964). *Arch. Soc. Am. Oftal. Optom.* 5, 27

Barraquer, J. I (1967). *Arch. Soc. Am. Oftal. Optom.* 6, 21.

Barraquer, J. I (1969). Corneo-Plastic Surgery, Pergamon Press.
Proceedings of the Second International Corneo-Plastic Surgery Conference, London 1967. 409–433.

Author's address:
St. Stephens Hospital
Fulham Road
Chelsea SW10 9TH
England

THE CHOYCE ANTERIOR CHAMBER IMPLANTS

D.P. CHOYCE

(London, England)

The anterior chamber implant was invented by Benedetto Strampelli of Rome in 1953 and was next in the time sequence after the Ridley posterior chamber lens. Also made of polymethylmethacrylate, this was placed in front of the iris and pupil, the central portion containing a bi-convex optic to correct the aphakia and with a blunt point at one end and a dovetail at the other. Thus 3-point, sutureless fixation within the anterior chamber was achieved. Primarily designed for secondary implantation and technically a simpler procedure than the Ridley operation, it was widely used initially. Unfortunately the earlier models were of doubtful purity, as well as being too thick and too steeply curved, thus bringing them dangerously close to the cornea which was therefore exposed to both chemical and mechanical trauma. The ensuing high incidence of corneal dystrophy led many surgeons to abandon intraocular lens implantation altogether, or to experiment with the pupillary lenses of Epstein, 1955 or Binkhorst, 1957.

One who did not, however, was myself. I persevered with the anterior chamber implant and introduced many modifications designed to increase its safety and extend its range of usefulness. The Choyce Mark VIII anterior chamber implant introduced in 1963 is only 0.25 mm. thick except for the central 6 mm. diameter optic whic is 0.9 mm. thick. A dovetail at each end provides 4-point sutureless fixation. Flattening the feet and using an implant 1 mm. longer than the horizontal corneal diameter carries the whole implant well away from the cornea, thus reducing the incidence of corneal damage to acceptable proportions. According to an independent survey by Pearce (1975) of my secondary implants, it is 1½% after an average follow-up period of 5½ years. I have also been responsible for the production by Imperial Chemical Industries of sheets of polymethylmethacrylate, coloured and opaque and inert, which can be fused with a clear plastic to provide anterior chamber implants with coloured opaque haptics. These are available in blue, brown and grey-green so that surrounding a 4 mm. diameter optic, colour matching of the individual iris is available. These coloured haptic implants are advised on optical and cosmetic grounds when the iris is deficient and/or discoloured as a result of previous injury, surgery or disease.

The final addition to the sophisticated range of Choyce anterior chamber implants is the external fixation Mark VIII implant, used when nearly all the iris is missing. In these, the coloured haptic implant is provided with nylon monofilament loops at either end so that it can be anchored inside the anterior chamber by trans-limbal subconjunctival suturing. The Mark VIII range of implants has been in use for almost 15 years. As of now, I have inserted a total of approximately 1,500 anterior chamber implants to correct aphakia and 75 for other uses, for instance as a form of internal scaffolding prior to perforating keratoplasty, in occasional patients with very high myopia, for cosmetic reasons, etc. They are usually used as a secondary procedure to correct pre-existing aphakia, but only slight modification to conventional cataract surgery is required for them to be used as a primary implant. Indeed my indications for primary implantation are basically second eyes, i.e. where one eye has been successfully treated in two stages and the second eye develops a cataract, or on the grounds of age and infirmity. The end result then after using a clear haptic Choyce anterior chamber implant is an anterior chamber with physiological depth about 3.0 mm., with a non-dislocatable pseudophakos with its optical centre at or very close to the nodal point of the eye, immediately in front of an untrammelled pupil, that is one free to react naturally to light and accommodation. Drugs affecting the pupil, particularly mydriatics may be used when indicated, for diagnostic purposes or in the management of retinal pathology, e.g. detachment surgery, photocoagulation procedures, etc.

I admit to a powerful bias in favour of secondary implantation, particularly for patients who are already aphakic in one or both eyes when first seen by the ophthalmologist. These patients have a serious problem in obtaining full visual rehabilitation. They have tried and found wanting cataract spectacles and contact lenses. It is my experience that longstanding, uncomplicated cases of aphakia are very favourable for secondary Mark VIII implantation. In addition, secondary implantation makes it easier to choose a pseudophakos of correct power by means of retinoscopy and subjective testing in the usual way without recourse to complicated and expensive apparatus like A-scans, ultrasonography, etc. Another advantage is that one has a visual acuity target at which one can aim. All too often in primary implantation if one does not know the eye at all well, what it should see after surgery is a matter of guess work. Then one can eliminate additional pathology which may be present and finally, it is always possible to go through the motions of a contact lens trial. All of these are not possible with primary implantation.

For the decade 1965-75, little interest was taken in the anterior chamber implant technique apart from myself and one or two others but then a great change came over the picture, mainly because of the enthusiastic way in which Tennant of Dallas, Texas took up the Choyce Mark VIII implant. This created within 6-12 months a demand for their product which Rayners, the makers of Rayner/Choyce Mark VIII implants, were unable to satisfy. In an effort to meet this demand certain American implant manufacturers entered the field, in the belief that it was possible to make safe anterior chamber implants to what they called the 'Choyce design' using a different plastic, in this case Röhm & Haas polymethylmethacrylate, which has a lower melting point than the Perspex CQ from which Rayner/Choyce lenses are made and which can therefore be subjected to injection moulding, i.e. a mass-produced lens as opposed to a craft-made or custom-made lens.

The use of injection moulded AC implants over the past 18 months to 2 years has led to an epidemic of serious complications, mainly in North America where they have been used in large numbers, consisting of attacks of increasing severity of uveitis, heamorrhage, glaucoma, vitritis and macular oedema connected with the name of Ellingson of Bismarck, North Dakota. The reason we attach the name of Ellingson to this UGH syndrome is because he was the first to point out correctly that this syndrome does not occur with Rayner lenses, and therefore it must be an implant-induced complication. Why should injection moulded AC implants cause these problems? The following factors seem to be involved:-

a. *Chemical.* The PMMA may be altered by injection moulding so that irritant monomers are released within the eye, initiating a chronic uveitis.

b. *Mechanical.* Imparting a really smooth finish all the way round the perimeter of the implant is more difficult and sharp posterior edges undoubtedly traumatise the delicate anterior iris stroma and initiate neovascularisation in the angle.

c. Warping of one or more feet has occurred after implantation, causing torsion of the implant and pressure on the trabecular meshwork.

The treatment is to remove the injection moulded lens and replace it with a Rayner lens, after the eye has settled down. Unfortunately, however, once the UGH syndrome is well established, implant removal may not suffice to bring the situation under proper control. The American Intra-Ocular Implant Society was so concerned over this situation that on 1st February, 1978 it ussued a Warning Notice to all its members regarding the dangers of injection moulded AC implants.

From the surgical point of view, the key to Mark VIII implant surgery, whether it be primary or secondary, is to pick a lens of the right length. Most of my lenses centre round the 12.5 mm. length in the proportion of 1 x 12.0 mm.: 2 x 12.5 mm.: 1 x 13.0 mm. It is necessary to make a somewhat corneal section so as to create a corneal shelf or ledge behind which the proximal feet may be tucked at the time of implant insertion. Therefore the surgeon must guard against making an incision too far back which in turn makes it easier to put in an implant which is really too long. Adequate openings in the iris are essential; I think two iridotomies or iridectomies are necessary. The incision, of course, should be securely sutured − I favour interrupted sutures, and the anterior chamber re-inflated with balanced salt solution.

CONCLUSIONS

1. The Choyce Mark VIII AC implant has been very successful in the hands of those who have used the recommended implants and have studied the correct technique for their insertion. It is equally satisfactory as a primary or a secondary procedure, following intra-capsular or extra-capsular surgery or phacoemulsification.

2. The surgeon should take care not to make his incision too far back or to insert an implant which is too long.

3. Unfortunately because Rayner-made implants are in short supply, injec-

tion moulded imitations have been used in large numbers, giving rise to an epidemic of complications (the UGH syndrome of Ellingson), very reminiscent of the complications encountered by Strampelli and Barraquer 25 years ago, probably for the same non-surgical reasons.

4. Once this supply problem has been solved, the AC implant will take its rightful place, as envisaged by Strampelli and Barraquer many years ago, as the most catholic and versatile of all pseudophakoi.

REFERENCE

Pearce, J.L., (1975). Long-term results of the Choyce anterior chamber lens implants Marke V, VII, VIII. *Brit. J. Ophthal.* 57, 99.

Author's address:
9 Drake Road
Westcliff-on-Sea
Essex 550 8LR
England

Docum. Ophthal. Proc. Series, Vol. 21

SPECULAR MICROSCOPY OF THE CORNEAL ENDOTHELIUM AND LENS IMPLANT SURGERY

C.D. BINKHORST, PER NYGAARD & L.H. LOONES

(Terneuzen, The Netherlands)

INTRODUCTION

Adequate function of the endothelial cells is necessary for a perfectly clear cornea.

Endothelial function is endangered in all intraocular surgery, but especially in cataract surgery. The latter, in most instances, gives rise to a transient insufficiency of endothelial function (striate keratitis) and in rare instances, causes permanent functional disorder, either immediately after surgery (surgical corneal dystrophy) of in a later phase (late corneal dystrophy).

The addition of further endothelial trauma caused by the act of lens implantation, is likely to compromise the endothelium even more. Lens implantation techniques of the past suffered from an unacceptably high incidence of corneal dystrophy. But also the latter techniques of iris and/or capsule fixated intraoculair lenses (Binkhorst 1959, 1961, 1967) have given unnecessary high incidences of corneal dystrophy in the hands of some surgeons. Most surgeons, however, practicing these techniques within acceptable limits. (Binkhorst 1972, 1973, 1977). It would have been interesting, however, to know how much damage had been done to the corneal endothelium in cases without manifest corneal dystrophy.

Specular microscopy of the corneal endothelium has contributed to our knowledge of the latter to a great extent.

Altred Vogt (1930) described the principle of 'Spiegelmikroskopie with the slitlamp in great detail.

The slitlamp, however, offers only limited possibilities for magnification (Fig. 1).

David Maurice (1968) developped a 'specular microscope' for laboratory use that allowed magnifications up to 400 X. This instrument was adapted for clinical use by Laing, Sandstrom, and Leibowitz (1975), and by Laing, Sandström, Berrospi, and Leibowitz (1976) (Fig. 2). The specular microscope visualizes differences and defects of light reflection.

The intercellular boundaries do not reflect light and become visible as dark lines (Fig. 3). So specular microscopy enables the study of gross cell morphology and the determination of cell size, the latter usually expressed as cell density (number of cells per mm^2). Also other defects of reflection show very nicely, for example excrescences of Descemet's membrane (cornea guttata) (Fig. 4).

It is generally accepted that human endothelial cells do not possess the

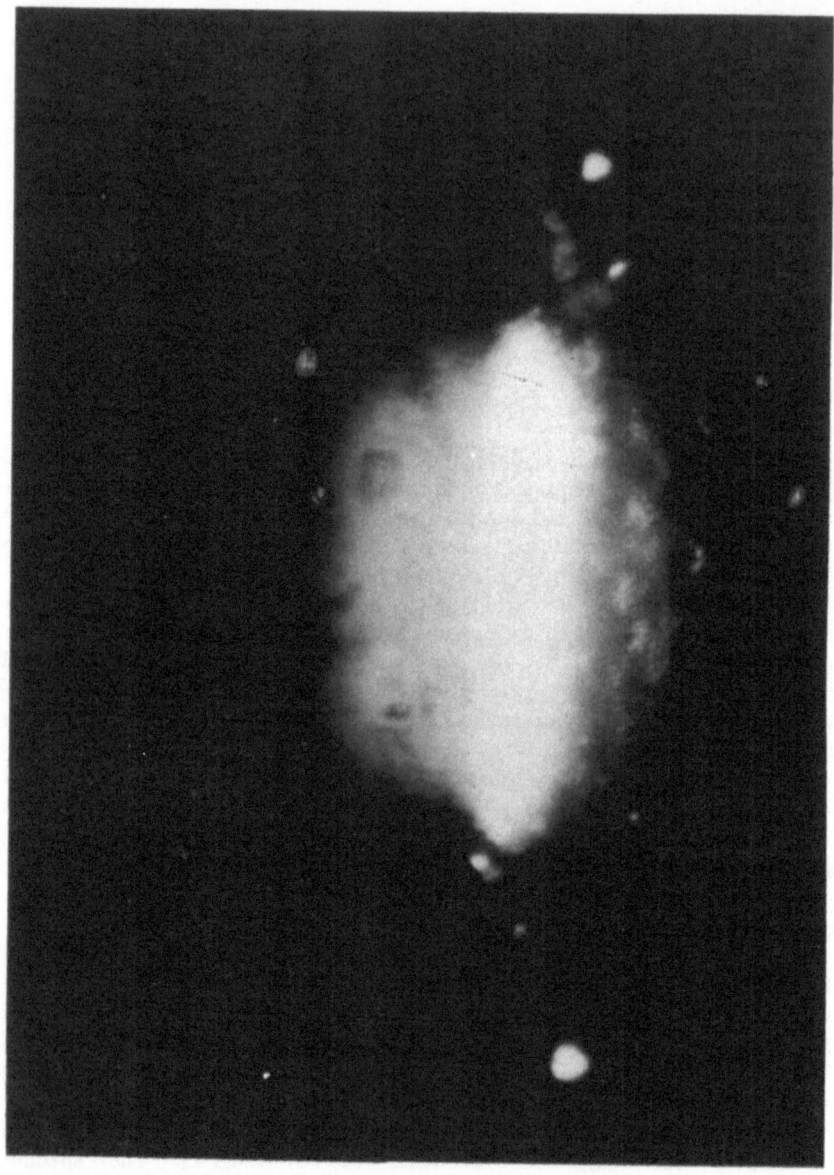

Fig. 1. Corneal endothelium of a 58 year old woman. The hexagonal cell pattern can just be distinguished in the guttated cornea (Zeiss photo-slitlamp 40 X).

ability of regeneration through mitosis. The area of lost cells is covered by citoplasmic extensions from the surrounding cells, which accounts for enlargment of cells and decrease of cell density. Through this process it is thought that the function of the endothelium as a whole is compromised. The 'healing reserve' (Bourne & Kaufman 1976) may become insufficient

512

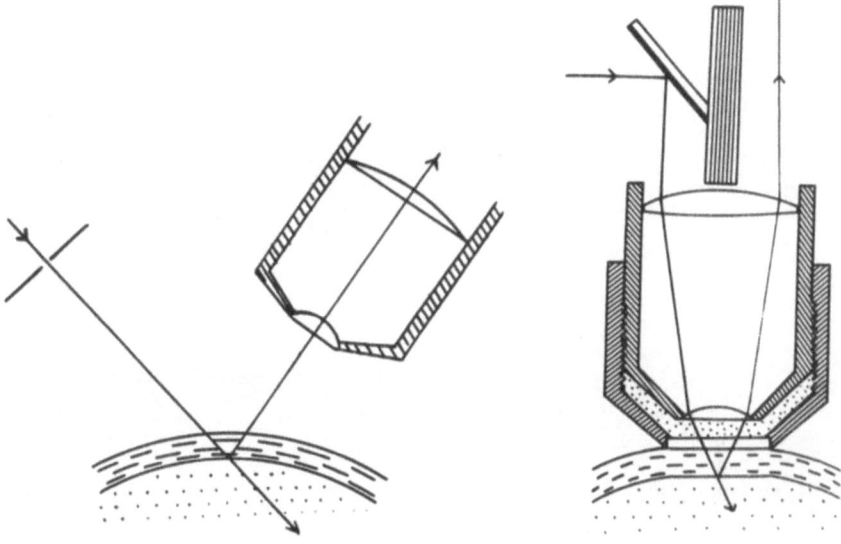

Fig. 2. The principle of specular microscopy.
a. with the slitlamp.
b. with Maurice's specular microscope.

Fig. 3. Normal corneal endothelium. The intercellular boundaries do not reflect the light and show as dark lines (Maurice's specular microscope 100 X). Top: endothelium of an 11 year old boy (3650 cells per mm^2). Bottom: endothelium of a 72 year old man (2124 cells per mm^2). Pleomorphia of cells.

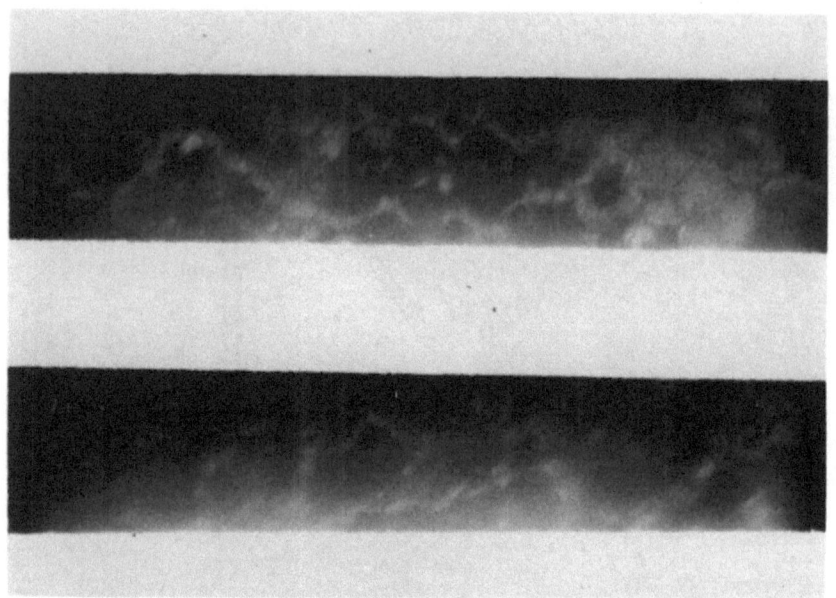

Fig. 4. Multiple, rather sharply-defined areas without reflection of light, probably caused by excrescences of Descemet's membrane (cornea guttata) in a 46 year old woman. (Maurice's specular microscope 100 X).

with the consequence of breakdown when further endothelial desintegration occurs.

It is well know that endothelial cell density decreases with ongoing age (Kaufman, Robbins & Capella 1965; Capella 1971; Stocker 1971). It suffers through eye disease, and through injury of the eye, including eye surgery. This contribution mainly deals with the determination of endothelial cell density in the field of cataract surgery, without, but mainly with lens implantation.

MATERIAL AND METHODS

The specular microscope was used for the examination of the corneal endothelium in six series.

Series A: 41 eyes to be subjected to extracapsular cataract extraction and lens implantation for senile cataract.

Series B: 13 eyes carriers of an intraocular lens after intracapsular cataract extraction and 13 eyes carriers of an intraocular lens after extracapsular cataract extraction for senile cataract.

Series C: 23 patients carriers of an intraocular lens in one eye after intracapsular cataract extraction and in the other eye after extracapsular cataract extraction for senile cataract.

Series D: 26 children and young adults wearing lens implants after surgery for traumatic cataract.

Series E: 14 pseudophakic eyes carrying lens implants with supramid loops and 22 pseudophakic eyes carrying lens implants with platium-irridium loops.

Series F: 9 eyes to be subjected to extracapsular cataract extraction with implantation of a four-loup lens, and 45 eyes to be subjected to extracapsular cataract extraction with implantation of a two-loop lens.

RESULTS AND DISCUSSION

In our study of the endothelium of clear corneas we have used endothelial cell density of the central area of the cornea as a parameter for endothelial damage and for endothelial function. However, we also detected many instances of supposed endothelial or subendothelial edema, reminding the 'leaking points' described in donor eyes by Bigar, Schimmelpfennig & Gieseler (1976) and indicating instances of subclinical endothelial microdecompensation (Fig. 5).

Fig. 5. **Ill-defined areas without reflection of light, probably patches of edema.** (Maurice's specular microscope 100 X).

Up to now only a few surgeons have reported about cell loss due to cataract surgery. Bourne & Kaufman (1976) examined 16 patients. They found statistically significant cell loss only in 4 cases, in 2 of which cell loss continued after surgery in the presence of complications (vitreous prolaps, iridocyclitis).

Forstat, Blackwell, Jaffe & Kaufman (1977) calculated 8 per cent cell loss after uncomplicated intracapsular surgery (5 patients). Troutman & Kaye (Pers. comm.) determined a cell difference of 9,9 per cent when intracapsular aphakic eyes were compared with the normal fellow eye (45 patients) and in another series 16 per cent cell loss through intracapsular surgery (25 patients).

Increased endothelial damage can be expected when cataract surgery is combined with lens implantation. Several authors had this experience, although figures of cell loss diverge largely. Bourne & Kaufman (1976) mention 34 to 70 per cent cell loss after extracapsular cataract surgery and lens implantation in 5 patients, 2 of which presented vitreous loss. Forstat, Balckwell, Jaffe & Kaufman (1977) report 28,6 per cent cell loss in a series of eyes after intracapsular surgery without complications and 43,5 per cent difference with the other eye in another series of eye after intracapsular surgery without complications and 43,5 per cent difference with the other eye in another series of eyes after intracapsular surgery. In patients with extracapsular surgery this difference was about the same (47,5 per cent). Between aphakic and pseudophakic eyes they found an average difference of about 40 per cent. Troutman & Kaye (Pers. comm.) report 26 per cent cell loss after intracapsular surgery with lens implantation.

A series of 41 eyes was examined by the authors before and after extra-capsular cataract extraction and lens implantation (Series A). Nearly all surgery had been performed by one of us (C.D.B.). We found an average cell loss of 6,7 per cent (Binkhorst, Loones & Nygaard 1977) (Fig. 6). Generally the cornea was almost completely clear on the first postoperative day. In 4 out of these 41 eyes during surgery the anterior chamber was much flatter than usual and it was striking that in these cases an average cell loss of 31,6 per cent was found versus 4 per cent in the other 37 cases. This fact may well indicate the importance of a soft eye and of a deep anterior chamber during surgery. We even consider a flat anterior chamber a contraindication for lens implantation. Although implantation under difficult conditions like a flat chamber may seem succesfull and although consequences for the cornea may seem to be absent, the chances for late corneal dystrophy are certainly not to be neglected. Several surgeons have faced this situation many times without understanding why.

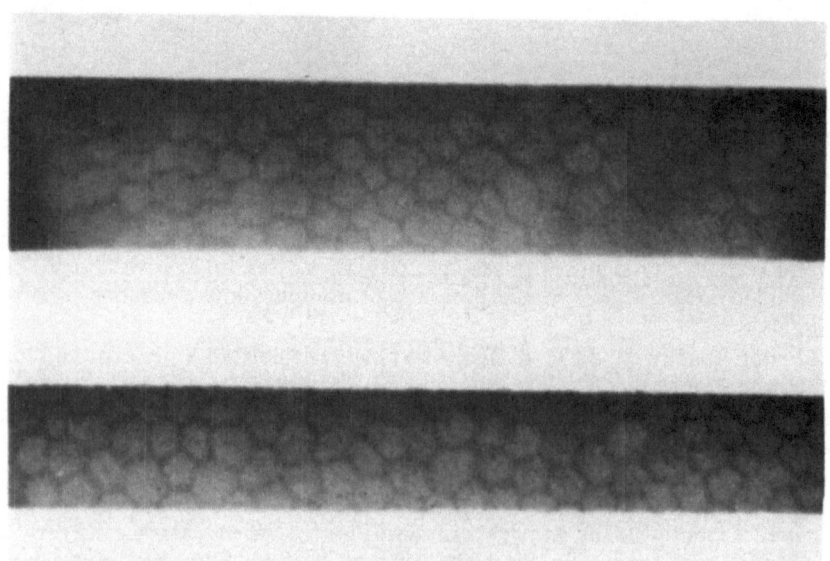

Fig. 6. Corneal endothelium of the right eye of a 71 year old man. Top: prior to surgery (2650 cells per mm²). (Maurice's specular microscope 100 X). Bottom: after extracapsular cataract extraction and implantation of lens implant with two poly-propylene loops. (2635 cells per mm²). Deep chamber technique.

Several authors have proposed techniques of lens implantation to avoid endothelial contact. Sheets (1976) uses a 'lens glide' or 'lens carpet' in combination with a large air bubble in the anterior chamber. Kaufman (1977) advised 'coating' of the lens implant with polyvinylpyrolidone. Our personal development in this respect is a so-called 'deep chamber technique' (Binkhorst, Loones & Nygaard 1977). In this technique the anterior chamber is kept deep during most of the procedure of cataract extraction and lens implantation bij means of air and/or fluid. This technique is illustrated and described in detail in Fig. 7. Specular microscopy of the corneal endothelium surely had contributed already much to the art of lens implantation.

Of great concern to-day is the place of lens implant surgery in the resident's training program (Keates 1975; Worthen 1976; Reinhart & Annable 1977). Also here specular endothelial microscopy could be of help to select the future lens implant surgeon. And why should this means of determining surgical trauma not be used for the same purpose by the established profession? Corneal dystrophy in pseudophakic eyes surely can be avoided to a large extent.

Intracapsular and extracapsular pseudophakic eyes were as closely as possible matched as to the age of the patients and as to the wearing time of the lens implant. All patients had suffered from senile cataract and were successfully treated. All cornes were perfectly clear (Fig. 9 and 10). We compared 13 intracapsular pseudophakic eyes with 13 extracapsular pseudo-

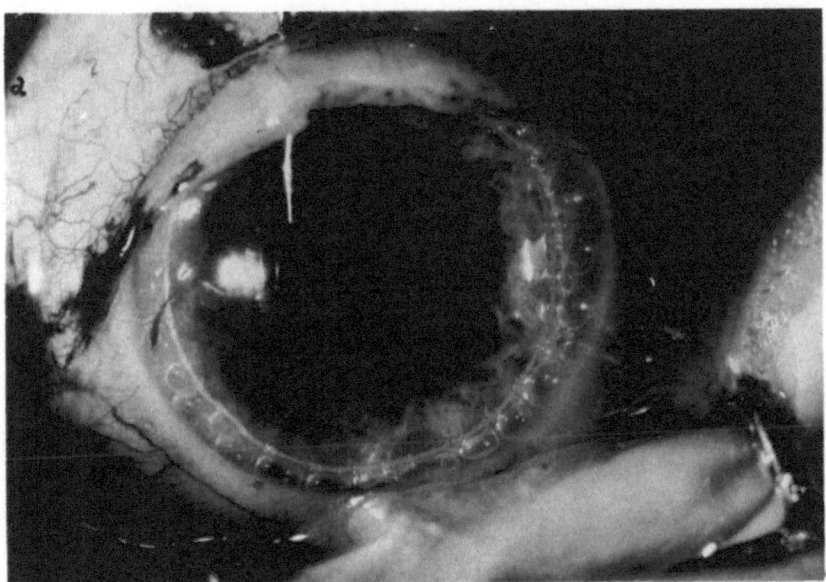

Fig. 7. The main surgical steps of extracapsular cataract extraction and implantation of a lens implant with two polypropylene loops. Deep chamber technique.
a. 3 mm wide keratome incision under a small limbus-based conjunctival flap. The anterior chamber then is completely filled with air with a fine canula.

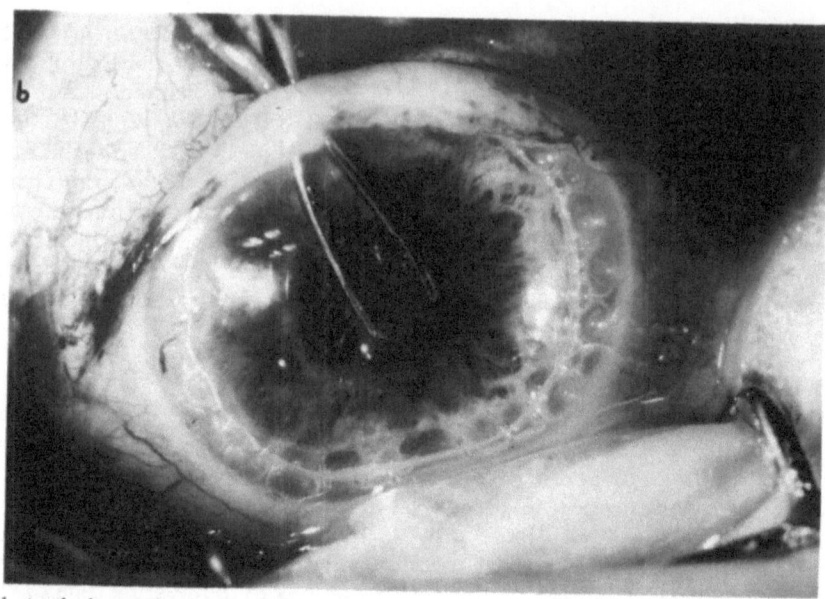

b. teethed capsular forceps of Vogt (Grieshaber, length of arms 6 mm) is introduced to grasp and to extract the middle third part of the anterior capsula without endothelial contact.

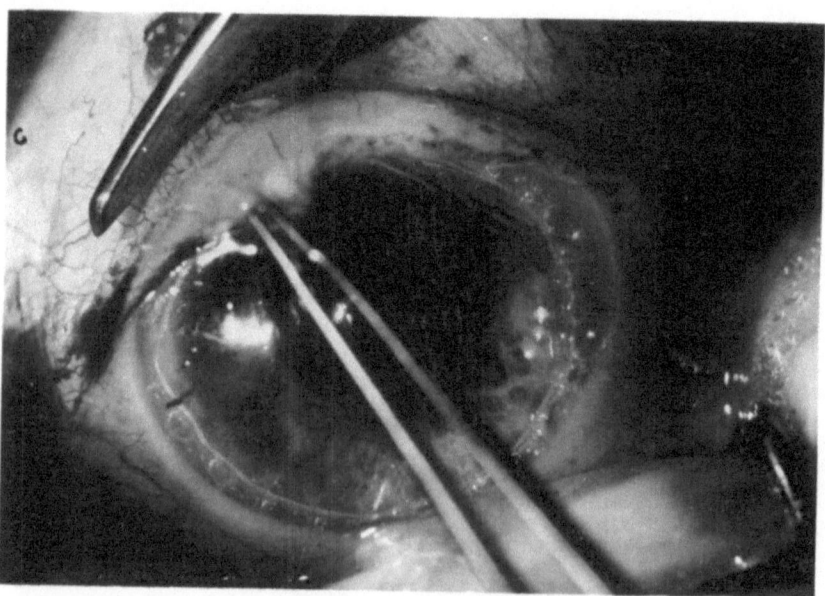

c. One leg of Castroviejo corneo-scleral scissors is introduced first to one side and then to the other side into the anterior chamber filled with air to widen the keratome incision to about 110 degrees. The air bubble prevents endothelial contact and also lesion of the iris.

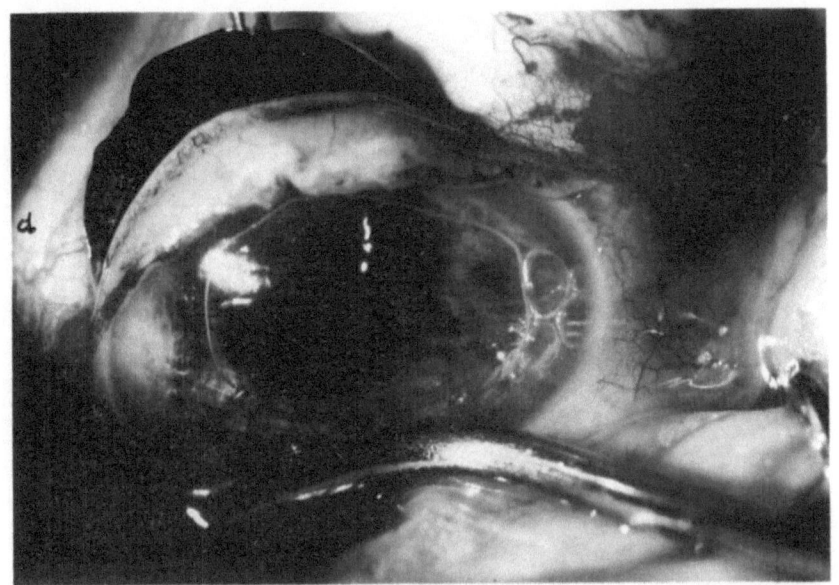

d. Delivery of the nucleus takes place the anterior chamber being partly filled with air. The air bubble acts as protection against rubbing of the endothelium with the nucleus. Delivery is obtained through pressure at 12 o'clock and at 6 o'clock without any movement of the muscle hook over the cornea. Delivery of cataract without endothelial contact is a unique procedure, only possible in extracapsular surgery.

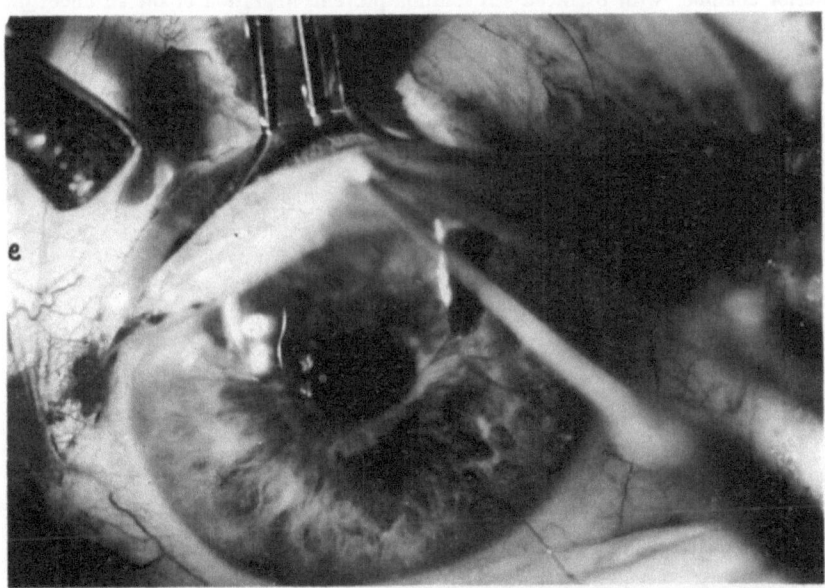

e. After irrigation and occasional aspiration of cortex remnants two peripheral iridectomies are performed at the ends of the incision. Both iris colobomas are then fully opened and all iris adhesions loosened with a fine repositor. The incision can be reduced just to fit the lens implant by corneo-scleral sutures at both ends. The principle of insertion of the lens implant into a deep chamber is to keep the anterior chamber filled with balanced salt solution during the act of inserting the lens ("aqueous push"). For this purpose a wide canula is used. The inferior loop is placed into the capsular bag at 6 o'clock, whereas the superior loop still rests on the iris.

519

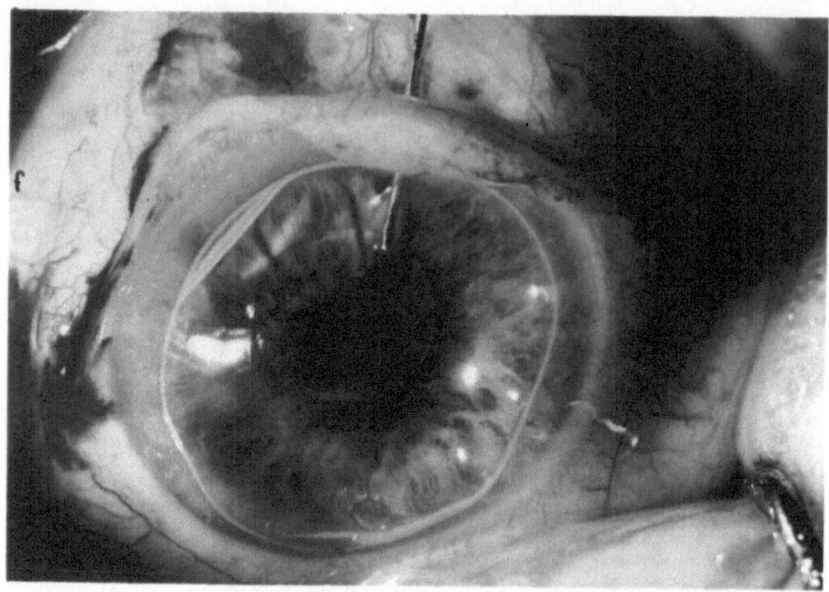

f. The anterior chamber is now partially filled with air. Simultaneous deepening of the anterior chamber with balanced salt solution prevents migration of the air under the lens.

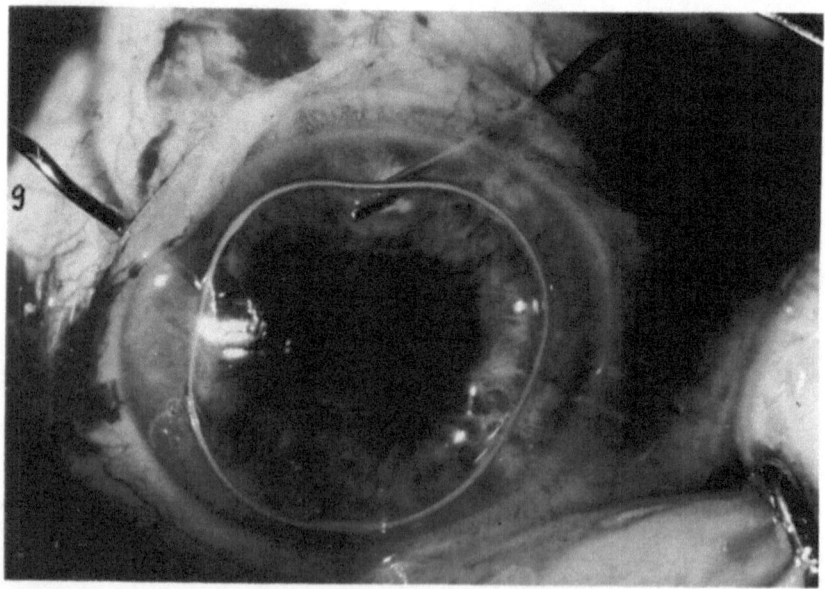

g. The iris is placed over the upper loops with a blunt iris hook, a wire repositor holding the lens steady. More air is injected now into the anterior chamber and the incision is completely sutured up.

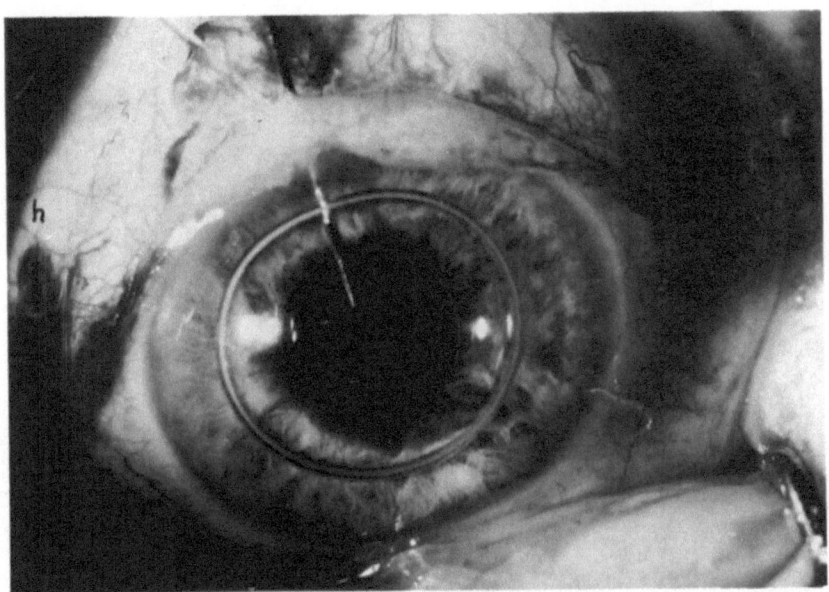

h. At the end of the operation the air is removed and balanced salt solution is allowed to replace it, again in a simultaneous procedure of aspiration and external application of a fine fluid stream.

phakic eyes of different patients (series B). The average age of the intracapsular pseudophakic eyes was 71 years and of the extracapsular pseudophakic eyes 65 years. The average post-operative period was 63 months and 61 months respectively. There was a marked difference in cell density between the intracapsular and the extracapsular eyes, being 975 to 1950 (average 1495) cells per mm^2 and 1300 to 2750 (average 2408) cells per mm^2 respectively. The intercapsular eyes had an average cell deficit of 38 per cent when compared with the extracapsular eyes.

An even more interesting comparison between intra- and extracapsular pseudophakic eyes could be obtained on 23 bilateral pseudophakic patients, wearing a lens implant after intracapsular extraction in one eye and after extracapsular extraction in the fellow eye (series C).

The average age of the patients was 71 years. The average wearing time was 86,8 months for the intracapsular eyes and 65,7 months for the extracapsular eyes. Here cell density difference between the intracapsular and the extracapsular eyes was even higher, being for the intracapsular eyes 442 to 2275 (average 1064) cells per mm^2 and for the extracapsular eyes 692 to 3058 (average 2166) cells per mm^2. Average cell deficit here even amounted to 50,8 per cent (Binkhorst, Loones & Nygaard 1977). After having ruled out a possible influence of lens implant material, of lens design, of minor events that took place during and after intracapsular surgery, and of the use of chymotrypsine, two possibilities remain to explain this significant difference between intracapsular and extracapsular pseudophakic eyes. The first possibility is that our intracapsular surgery had been much more traumatic

Fig. 8. Corneal endothelium of a 16 year old boy (Maurice's specular microscope 100 X). Top: normal right eye (3182 cells per mm²). Bottom: aphakic left eye after perforating injury (1167 cells per mm²). Because of low cell density the eye was not subjected to secondary implantation.

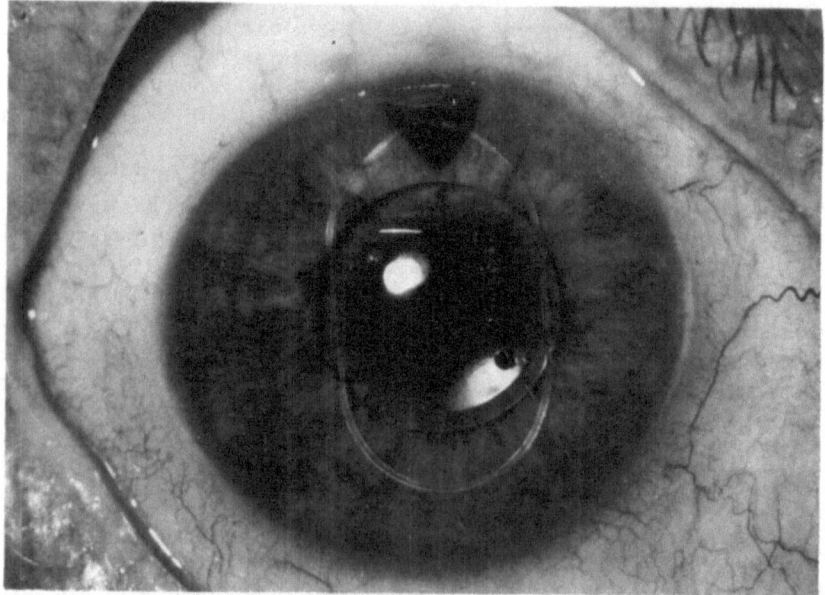

Fig. 9. Intracapsular pseudophakic eye (four-loop iris clip lens).

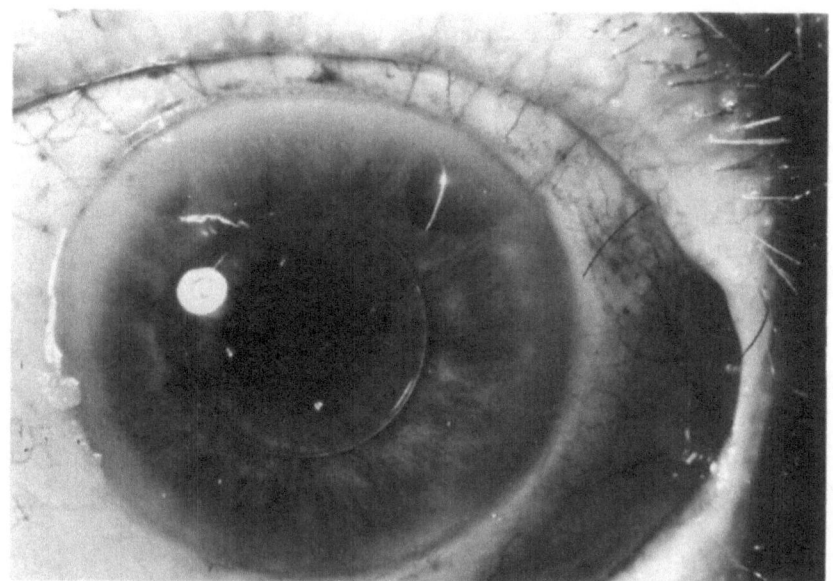

Fig. 10. Extracapsular pseudophakic eye (two-loop iridocapsular lens).

then our extracapsular surgery. A prospective comparative study of endothelial surgical damage has recently been started and thus far can not confirm this. The second possibility is that the fixation of the lens implant is responsible for this different behaviour of the corneal endothelium. Extracapsular extraction provides the eye with a stable capsular membrane and capsular fixation is stable fixation of the lens implant.

Intracapsular extraction causes instability in all corners of the eye, a situation which is best described as 'endophthalmodonesis'.

Iridodonesis is the sign through which "endophthalmodonesis" betrays itself. The iris-fixated lens implant moves with the iris ("pseudophakodonesis") and perhaps reinforces the movements of the iris. We feel that unphysiological hydrodynamics in the anterior chamber may cause progressive endothelial cell disintegration, the essence of which could be named "turbulance endotheliopathy". This more or less mechanical theory does not exclude the existence of other endothelium-destroying factors that may be present in the intracapsular aphakic eye. A prospective long-term study of intracapsular aphakic eyes without lens implant is under way.

Determination of endothelial cell density can help to evaluate eyes with complicated cataract, such as after uveitis, in glaucoma, after injury, cataract in the presence of endothelial corneal dystrophy, and possibly also cataract associated with systemic disease.

A series of 26 young patients wearing lens implants for prolonged periods of time for the correction of unilateral posttraumatic aphakia have recently been examined retrospectively (Binkhorst, Loones and Nygaard 1977), (Series D). An average cell deficit of 38.7 per cent was registered in the injured eyes when compared to the normal eye. In two eyes cell density was even less than 1000 cells per mm^2 which must be regarded as an ominous sign for the future transparency of the cornea. Recent prospective cell counts in similar cases have told us when and when not to undertake lens implantation.

The decision whether to perform secondary lens implantation in an aphakic eye rather than to insist on contact lens correction, can very much be influenced by endothelial cell density (Fig. 8).

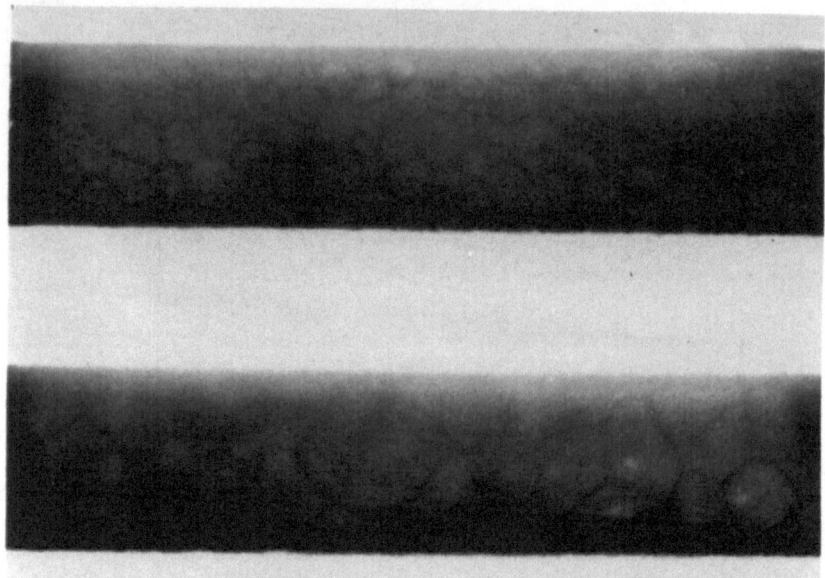

Fig. 11. Corneal endothelium of a 79 year old man (Maurice's specular microscope 100 X). Top: right eye 9 years after extracapsular cataract extraction and implantation of irido-capsular lens with two platine-iridium wire loops (2718 cells per mm^2). Bottom: left eye 11 years after intracapsular cataract extraction and implantation of iris clip lens with four supramid wire loops (558 cells per mm^2). Leaking points (micro-decompensation).

Endothelial cell counts may be of help to decide if cataract surgery, without or with lens implantation, should be performed with simultaneous corneal grafting.

There likely is a place for specular microscopy of the endothelium to decide if and when, after implantation into the first eye, the second eye should be treated in the same way.

Finally, the decision whether to do lens implantation in case of presenile cataract, can, apart from other factors involved also be made depending on the findings with the specular microscope.

In all the above mentioned instances the specular microscope is a useful tool to help estimate how much damage the endothelium is likely to stand, in other words to help estimate the "endothelial trauma allowance" (Binkhorst 1973).

If our findings in intracapsular pseudophakic eyes as compared with extracapsular pseudophakic eyes indeed originate from the fact that the cataract has been extracted intracapsularly then the intracapsular aphakic and pseudophakic eye must be considered a diseased eye (Barrier Deprivation Disease).

Endothelial studies, further more, could be helpful to evaluate the situation in the presence of chronic inflammation, in case of suspicion upon endothelial contact of the lens implant or of toxicity of the implant, and in case of repeated dislocations. The decision whether to remove a lens implant or not could be influenced by the detection of real low cell density.

We found an indication for a possible toxicity of supramid used as loop material (Binkhorst, Loones and Nygaard 1977). In 14 extracapsular pseudophakic eyes with supramid-looped lens implants an average cell density of 1867 cells per mm^2 was found versus 2499 cells per mm^2 in 22 extracapsular pseudophakic eyes with lens implants fitted with platina-iridium loops (Series E). The finding reminds tissue culture studies of Galin, Chowchuvech, and Galin 1975 from which also to toxicity of supramid was concluded. Not only for this reason, but also for reasons of weight reduction several manufacturers now provide lens implants fitted with polypropylene loops.

The usefulness of endothelial studies for the evaluation of lens implant design, of method of sterilisation, and of lens implants from different manufacturers can only be accepted when all other parameters, including the surgeon are equal.

In 9 extracapsular pseudophakic eyes with four-loop lens implants we determined an average postoperative cell density of 2446 cells per mm^2 and in 45 extracapsular pseudophakic eyes with two-loop lens implants of 2472 cells per mm^2 (Series F). No difference in the use of these two designs, thus, was found. Other reports are not available.

Finally corneal endothelial studies may contribute to answer still disputed questions in the field of lens implant surgery.

Anterior chamber angle fixation of lens implants as introduced by Strampelli and later practiced by many others has in the past given rise to very high incidences of late complications, such as glaucoma, iritis, but above all corneal dystrophy. One refined lens implant design for angle support, the Choyce Mark VIII implant, has survived and today is even gaining popularity especially in the United States of America (Choyce 1977; Tennant 1977). It would be interesting to know not only the surgical effect on the cornea that, because implantation is easy indeed, could be very mild, but specifically the long-term behaviour of the corneal endothelium that is so close to the haptics of the lens implant. Up to now, no such endothelial studies have been published.

There is a difference of opinion as to the desirability of lens implantation in a two-stage rather than in a one-stage operation. We allude to the case in which the decision to cataract extraction and lens implantation has been made and not to the aphakic eye in which lens implantation for whatever reason has been missed at the time of cataract surgery. The pros and cons of both procedures are still amply being discussed. Our personal experience with corneal distrophy has always been in disfavour of secondary implantation and endothelial cell studies in our opinion will no doubt confirm the higher demand on the corneal endothelium, also in cases with a clear cornea, in a two-stage procedure.

No reports are available on the corneal endothelium of eyes that underwent successful phakoemulsification and lens implantation for senile cataract. The only patient that we personally had the opportunity to examine had bilateral surgery and cell counts in the right eye and in the left eye of respectively only 1065 and 1105 cells per mm^2, some months after surgery. The patient had suffered from presenile cataracts at the age of 37 years.

Prospective and retrospective endothelial studies on patients treated with phakoemulsification without and with lens implantation are urgently required.

SUMMARY

The specular microscope is a relatively new instrument for the examination of the corneal endothelium. Its value in the field of intraocular surgery is discussed.

The specular microscope helps to estimate the endothelial viability long before clinical signs of decompensation occur. Therefore specular microscopy is useful for the selection of eyes for lens implantation in general, for the prognosis of the eye with a lens implant, for the evaluation of the method of cataract surgery, of lens implantation techniques, and possibly of lens design, material and manufacturing.

A long-term study of intracapsular and extracapsular pseudophakic eyes revelaed that the intracapsular pseudophakic eyes had significantly less endothelial cells, which could partly be explained by toxicity of the supramid used as loop material, but mostly by assuming continuing endothelial desintegration in the intracapsular eyes.

The extracapsular technique of the authors in 41 patients was found to have caused an average cell loss of only 6,7 per cent and is described in detail.

REFERENCES

1 Binkhorst, C.D.: Iris supported artificial Pseudophakia. A new development in intra-ocular artificial lens surgery. *Trans. Ophthalm' Soc. U.K.* 79, 569-584, 1959.

2 Binkhorst, C.D.: Uber die endgültige Verträglichkeit künstlicher Augenlineen bei der Aphakie und deren Verbesserung mittels Fixation der Linse in der Pupille. *Klin. Mbl. Augenhk.* 134, 536, 1959.

3 Binkhorst, C.D.: Aktive und rationelle Behandlung der Altersstar mit der "iseikonischen" Pupillarlinse (Iris-Klipp-Linse). Ber. 64 Zusammenkunft Dtsch. Ophthalm. Ges. Heidelberg, 1961.

4 Binkhorst, C.D.: Eigene Verfahren der Pseudophakia. *Klin. Mbl. Augenhk.* 151, 21, 1967.

5 Binkhorst, C.D.: Praxis und Theoris der "Iris-Klipp-Linse" und der "Irido-Kapsular Linse". Sitzungsbericht 125 Versammlung des Ver. Rhein-West-fal. Augenärzte 33-50, 1972.

6 Binkhorst, C.D.: The iridocapsular (two-loop) lens and the iris-clip (four-loop) lens in pseudophakia. *Trans. Amer. Acad. Ophthalm. Otolaryng.* Sept.-Okt. 589-617, 1973.

7 Binkhorst, C.D.: Five hundred planned extracapsular extractions with irido-capsular and iris clip lens implantation in senile cataract. *Ophthalmic Surgery*, 8, 37-44, 1977

8 Vogt, A.: Lehrbuch und Atlas der Spaltiampen Mikroskopie des lebenden Auges. Julius Springer Verlag, Berlin, 1930.

9 Maurice, D.M.: Cellular membrane activity in the corneal endothelium of the intact eye. *Experientia* 24, 1094, 1968 (Basel).

10 Laing, R.A., Sandström, M.M. & Leibowitz, H.M.: In vivo photomicrography of the corneal endothelium. *Arch. Ophthalm.* 93, 143-145, 1975.

11 Laing, R.A., Sandström, M.M., Berrospi, A.R. & Leibowitz, H.M.: Changes in the corneal endothelium as a function of age. *Exp. Eye Res.* 22, 587-594, 1976.

12 Bourne, W.M. & Kaufman, H.E.: Specular microscopy of human corneal endothelium in vivo. *Am. J. Ophthalm'* 81, 319-323, 1976.

13 Bourne, W.M. & Kaufman, H.E.: Endothelium damage associated with intraocular lenses. *Am. J. Ophthal.* 81, 482-485, 1976.

14 Bourne, W.M. & Kaufman, H.E.: Cataract extraction and the corneal endothelium. *Am. J. Ophthalm.* 82, 44-47, 1976.

15 Bigar, F., Schimmelpfennig, B. & Gisseler, R.: Routine evaluation of endothelium in human donor corneas. Graefe's Archiv. *Klin. Exp. Ophthalm.* 20, 195-200, 1976.

16 Kaufman, H.E., Robbins, J.E. & Capella, J.A.: The endothelium in normal and abnormal corneas. *Trans. Amer. Acad. Ophthalm. Otolaryng.* 69, 931-942, 1965.

17 Capella, J.A.: The pathology of corneal endothelium. *Ann. Ophthalm.* 3, 397-400, 1971.

18 Stocker, F.W.: The endothelium of the cornea and its clinical implications. Ed 2, Springfield, III. Charles C. Thomas Publisher, p 13, 1971.

19 Forstat, S.L., Blackwell, W.L., Jaffe, N.S. & Kaufman, H.E.: The effect of intraocular lens implantation on the corneal endothelium. *Trans. Amer. Acad. Ophthalm. Otolaryng.* 83, 195-203, 1977.

20 Troutman, R.C. & Kays, D.S.: Personal communication.

21 Binkhorst, C.D., Loones, L.H. & Nygaard, P.: The clinical specular microscope. Documents ophthalmologica. Proceedings series. Junk Publishers, the Hague, Netherlands, 1977. In press.

22 Binkhorst, C.D., Loones, L.H. & Nygaard, P.: Biomicroscopic observations on the human corneal endothelium. *Trans. Ophthalm. Soc. U.K.* 1977. In press.

23 Sheets, J.: Personal communication. 1976.

24 Kaufman, H.E.: Corneal endothelial damage due to intraocular lenses. *Trans. Am. Acad. Ophthalm. Otolaryng.* 1977. In press.

25 Keates, R.H.: The place of intraocular lenses in ophthalmic training program. *Contact and Intraocular Lens Med. J.* 4-6, 1975.

26 Worthen, D.M.: The role of the university in teaching the correction of aphakia. *Contact and Intraocular Lens Med. J.* 2, 41-47, 1976.

27 Reinhart, W.J. & Annable, W.L.: Intraocular Lens Surgery on a Resident's Service. Ophthalmic Surgery 8, 156-161, 1977.

28 Galin, M.A., Chowchuvech, E. & Galin A.: Tissue culture methods for testing the toxicity of ocular plastic materials. *Am. J. Ophthalm.* 79, 665, 1975.

29 Choyce, D.P.: The Choyce Mark VIII anterior chamber implant. Primary and secondary implantation compared. *Ophthalmic Surgery*, 8, 49-53, 1977.

30 Tennant, J.L.: Results of primary and secondary implants using Choyce Mark VIII lenses. *Ophthalmic Surgery* 8, 54-56, 1977.

Docum. Ophthal. Proc. Series, Vol. 21

BARRAQUER SHEARING INTRAOCULAR LENS

R.P. KRATZ

(Los Angeles, California, U.S.A.)

The Barraquer intraocular lens has been modified by Shearing for use in extra capsular cataract extraction. The overall length of the prolene loops is 13 mm and the optic is 6 mm. It has the advantage of being easy to insert with minimal intraocular manipulation and excellent centration. Subluxation is rare and the lens is single plane and single size for each power. Since it is a posterior chamber intraocular lens there is no corneal touch, trabecular touch, Choyce type ocular tenderness and no pain on scleral depression. The iris is free of hooks, sutures and cutting from loops or haptics. The pupil may be widely dilated or miotics may be used. There are no pupillary synechiae. There are no oval pupils associated with iris tucking or lacerated or displaced pupils. There is no pseudo phaco-denesis. Optically the problems of glitter, dazzle, flutter, edge glare and image magnification are minimzed.

The Barraquer-Shearing intraocular lens may be used in a shallow anterior chamber. Filtering surgery or Keratoplasty may be performed at a later date with little risk to the corneal endothelium. Cosmetically the eyes are normal in appearance Aniscoria is minimized. Visual results have been good.

The disadvantages are primarily short follow up (one year) and the small number of cases. It is for use in extracapsular cataract extraction but not for intracapsular cataract extraction. The long term results of gentle pressure on the ciliary body are not known but probably are little different than the support used by the more rigid Choyce intraocular lenses. Post operative capsulotomies are a little more difficult than with other intraocular lenses.

Author's address:
15225 Vanowen Street
Van Nuys, Calif. 91405
U.S.A.

UNILATERAL TRAUMATIC AND COMPLICATED CATARACT IN CHILDREN AND YOUNG ADULTS AS A SPECIAL INDICATION FOR INTRAOCULAR LENS IMPLANTS.

R. KERN

(Lucerne, Switzerland)

SUMMARY

The occlusion of one eye by an acquired cataract or by an aphakia causes amblyopia and loss of binocularity in children, loss of binocular vision and depth perception in young adults. The deterioration of binocularity is manifested by an increasing strabismus, at the beginning of the intermittent, then of the concomitant type with horizontal deviation only (grade 1 - 4). A rotatory component is finally added at grade 5 (= "malign stabismus"). To restore full binocular vision and depth perception in children or in young adults, the implantation of an intraocular lens is strictly indicated before the formation of a "malign strabismus".

To restore good visual acuity, surgery is necessary in the case of an advanced traumatic or complicated cataract. The extracapsular or intracapsular mode of extraction may be chosen according to the age of the patient as well as to the habits of the eye-surgeon. The ophthalmic practitioner generally decides about the "when" of the operation, and afterwards about the "how" of the correction. To obtain optimal results both, the eye-surgeon and the ophthalmic practitioner, have to keep in mind the answer to the following question: What is the goal of our treatment in the case of an unilateral traumatic or complicated cataract? It is two fold:
- to prevent amblyopia and/or squint
- to restore full binocular vision and depth perception for far and near distance.

Five possibilities to correct aphakia are available today: none, the 'classical' aphakic spectacles, the hard or soft contact-lens, the keratophakia or the intraocular lens. To correct monocular aphakia a patient with a normal second eye will not accept an unilateral aphakic glass. Resignation by both the ophthalmic practitioner, and especially by the patient is the result in all those cases, where other modes of corrections are impossible.

If binocular vision is desired or necessary, a contact-lens, a keratophakia or an intraocular lens are potential possibilities to restore binocularity with depth perception.

Keratophakia, proposed by Jose Barraquer (1976), is still in an experimental stage and not further discussed. The contact-lens or the intraocular lens (Binkhorst, Gobin & Leonard; Choyce 1977; Hiles 1977; Kern 1978; Percival & Yousef 1976; Ridgway 1977) therefore remain as practically advisable corrections in uniocular aphakia. The question, which now arises, is: are there cases, where the implantation of an intraocular lens is highly indicated?

The problem will be indirectly solved by answering the two following questions: 1.) Are there patients with unilateral aphakia, corrected by contact-lenses, who exhibit a **high incidence** of failure to wear contact-lenses? 2.) Is an **irreversable** deterioration of the monocular or binocular function the consequence of such a failure? If the answer is twice "yes", then the implantation of an intraocular lens is strongly indicated.

The danger of amblyopia or squint is minimal in middle-aged or old people in the case of unilateral cataract or aphakia. Full monocular and binocular functions are reestablished, whenever - even years later - clear media and an adequate correction are achieved. Children and young patients behave differently: the continous occlusion of one eye by either a traumatic or complicated cataract, or by an absent optical correction is followed by a convergent or - more often - a divergent strabismus. Five stages of dispersing binocularity are observed:

— **Stage one:** normal motility despite interrupted binocular vision.
— **Stage two:** an intermittent strabismus is then noted.
— **Stage three:** it later turns into a main concomitant squint with horizontal deviation only and a spontaneous reversibility as soon as clear media and adequate correction are achieved. Orthoptic exercises and a decreasing prismatic correction are indicated in some of those cases.
— **Stage four:** there is still a pure horizontal deviation, however of a larger angle. Binocular vision can be obtained by an additional operation on the extraocular muscles only.
— **Stage five:** As soon as a rotatory component, mostly combined with a vertical deviation, is observed, a normal binocular vision between the two eyes is definitely impossible, even under optimal optical conditions. Diplopia due to a horror fusionis is the consequence of restoring clear media, combined with the implantation of an intraocular lens or with the wearing of a contact-lens. That stage five of strabismus is called "malign strabismus".

The operation on an unilateral traumatic or complicated cataract followed by the implantation of an intraocular lens or by prescribing a contact-lens is indicated from stage one to stage three; it is allowed at stage four, but it is strictly contraindicated at stage five of a squint.

The interval between the onset of occlusion and the beginning of strabismus id highly individual: no prediction of time is therefore possible.

Consequence number 1: an unilateral acquired cataract in children and young patients should be operated on and optimally corrected as soon as possible, at least before the onset of a "malign strabismus".

Now back to the two questions: 1.) Are there patients with a high incidence of failure to wear contact-lenses? There are indeed: children from age 3 to 8 to 10 years and patients, who live or work in dry, windy or dusty areas. 2.) Is an irreversible deterioration of the monocular and/or binocular function the consequence of such a failure? Yes, it is in children and young patients, who are unable to wear contact-lenses, due to age or to socio-economic reasons.

Consequence number 2: The implantation of an intraocular lens is strongly

532

indicated in all those cases to save the monocular and/or binocular function. The interval between the onset of a rather dense cataract and the implantation of an intraocular lens should be minimal, at least not later than stage three to four of strabismus. The knowledge of the visual acuity of the non-fixing eye and binocular functions in children as well as of the unstable binocular vision and depth perception in young adults is essential to planning an early optimal rehabilitation in the case of an unilateral acquired cataract: intraocular lens plus glasses for far and near distance (bifocal).

REFERENCES

Barraquer, Jose: Keratomileusis and keratophakia. Proc. Second World Corneal Congress, Washington, D.C., 1976.

Binkhorst, C.D., M.H. Gobin & P.A.M. Lenoard: Post-traumatic artificial lens implants (Pseudophakoi) in children. *Brit. J. Ophthal. 53, 518–529* (1969).

Choyce, D.P.: Restoration of binocular vision. *Ophthal. Surg. 8, 102–104,* (1977).

Hiles, D.A.: The need for intraocular lens implantation in children. *Ophthal. Surg.* 8, *162–169* (1977).

Kern, R.: Einseitige Aphakie und Pseudophakos. *Acta Ophthal. 36, 74–79,* (1978).

Percival, S.P.P. & K.M. Yousef: Treatment of uniocular aphakia. A comparison of iris-clip lenses with hard corneal contact lenses. *Brit. J. Ophthal. 60, 642–644* (1976).

Ridgway, A.E.A.: Orthoptic consequences of Binkhorst lens implantation for unilateral cataract. *Ophthal. Surg. 8, 170–173* (1977).

Author's address:
Eye Clinic, Kantonsspital
Spitalstr. 4
6004 Lucerne
Switzerland.

INTRA- OR EXTRACAPSULAR LENS IMPLANTATION

G. BAÏKOFF

(Nantes, France)

At the present we reserve implants to senile aphakia and to unilateral traumatic aphakia in young adults.

Functional recovery after unilateral traumatic cataract in the very young child has, as of yet, not been resolved (and the same goes for the unilateral congenital cataract). In our experience, the traumatized eye is nearly always condemned to amblyopia. Contact lenses for permanent wear are regularly lost. Children, parents and doctors grow weary. The few implantations which we have effected have been well tolerated, yet have always required the discission of a secondary membrane often of a very dense nature.

At this age, the placing of an implant is fraught with difficulties due to a (fibrinous aqueous humour and to a tendency to anterior synechiae in the incision. In the child aged under five, surgery of the crystalline lens by means of small corneal incisions is well regulated, while large corneal incisions complicate the operation (limbic keratotomy, or transfixing keratoplasty).

SENILE APHAKIA

In France the implant technique has spread most cautiously due to the recollection of the implants of Ridley. At present the indication is essentially accepted in the case of a unilateral cateract after having informed the patient as to the specific character of the operation.

A first series of intra-capsular implantations with the Worst medallion lens was made. A number of serious accidents led to stopping this practice. But, above all, the frequency of macular edema accompanied by a significant decrease of visual acuity was striking. This was observed in 27% of patients, yet it must be emphasized that more than 80% of these have recovered, without consequences, in more or less long delay periods (photograph 1).

This abnormal frequency has often been attributed to the type of lens used, but had the patients not been very closely watched, certain maculopathies could have gone unnoticed. Use of the extra-capsular would seem to make these disappear, but the macula is in this case not always easily observed.

We reserve the extra-capsular (photographs 2-3) with 'Irido-capsular lens

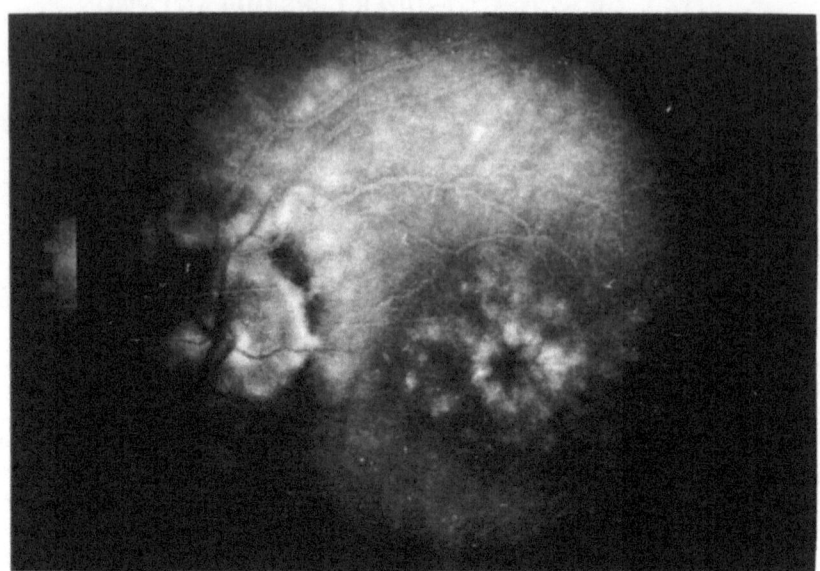

Fig. 1. Cystoid macular edema with decrease of visual acuity which has come about after placing a medallion lens in the intracapsular.

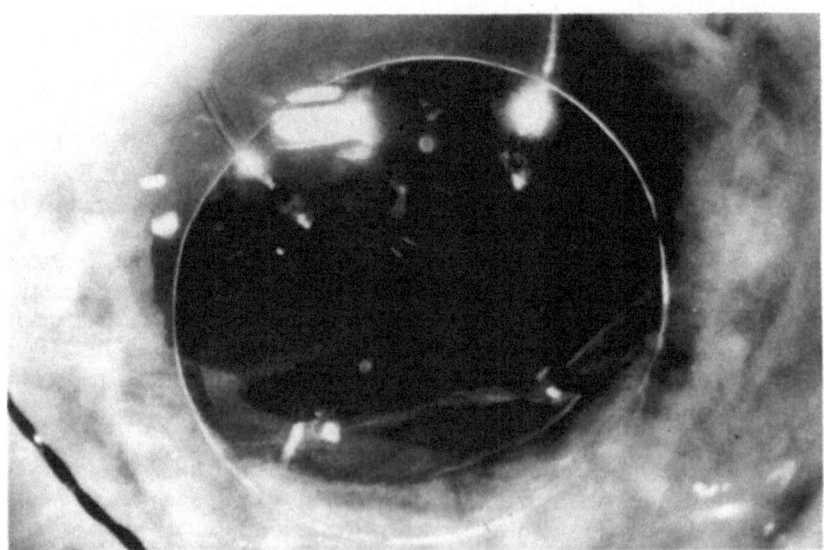

Fig. 2. During the operation, strong microscopic magnification is indispensable for making sure that the posterior ansae of the implant are well placed between the anterior and the posterior capsules.

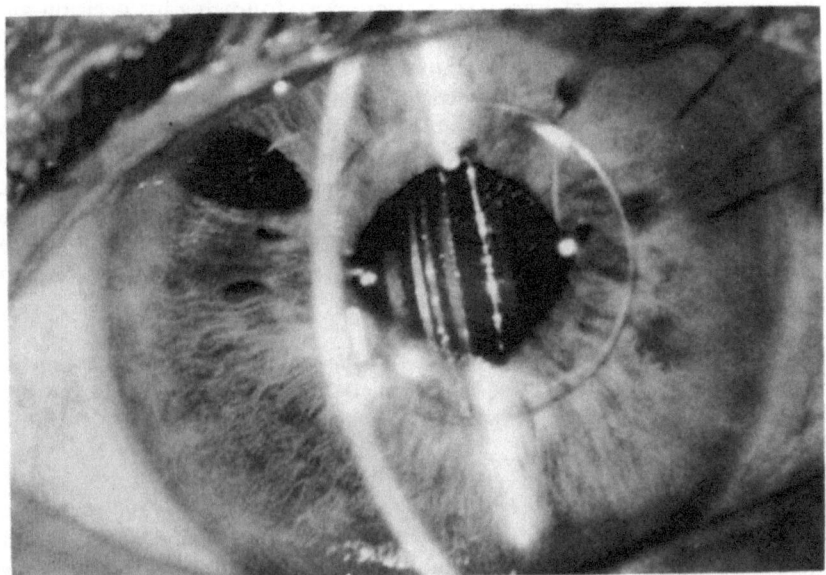

Fig. 3. An optical cut showing the cornea, the anterior and posterior faces of the implant, the posterior capsule and the anterior hyaloid.

of Binkhorst to the youngest of our patients, as in their case the endothelium would seem to be at its least fragile. On the other hand, the intracapsular would seem to be more suitable to patients of an advanced age, as in their case the cornea is certainly more fragile. Hence intraocular manoeuvres are reduced to a minimum, the time for the surgery being hardly longer than for a mere cataract.

UNILATERAL TRAUMATIC APHAKIA IN THE YOUNG PATIENT

In this case the traumatology is at the origin of a complex pathology. In effect, apart from lens damage, hypertonicity, corneal opacity, and accidents of the retina can be encountered. In these cases, contact lenses are far from solving all the problems of the aphakic patient. The period of amblyopia is long, professional re-insertion can only be considered once the adaptation period is over and additional correction has been prescribed. Tolerance is mediocre; in effect, our casualties come from the steel industry and from the building industry. Following the accident, the poor tolerance of the lens and the disturbance of binocular sight become the original reason for a professional demotion for 30% of manual labourers: changing of jobs, protected employment, changing of profession or calling, even unemployment.

All of these arguments can justify the introduction of an artificial cyrstalline lens. This practice does not resolve all the problems, but at least eases a number of them. The implant can only be proposed to the patient (there is no question of imposing it upon him); following his decision and the state of the cornea, a number of different approaches are possible:

— given the absence of a wound of the cornea, and if the patient refuses the implantation, then an extra-capsular is performed; hence if the contact lenses are a failure, it remains possible to consider a secondary implantation.

— if there does exist a wound of the cornea, it is not always so easy to predict, before extraction of the crystalline lens, its harmful on the optical result: a. the patient refuses the implant: the surgeon therefore performs an extra-capsular, dealing very gently with the posterior capsule. If a kerato-plasty is necessary, it will then accordingly be simple to consider also an implant at the same time (photograph 4).

b. the patient accepts the implant, but the wound of the cornea seems to be negligible: the implantation is then made in a first phase. If the corneal wound is bothersome, a keratoplasty is made in a second phase (photograph 5).

c. the implant is accepted by the patient and the graft is indispensable: the restoration of the anterior segment is carried out in one sitting. This is the solution which makes it possible to obtain a funtional result most rapidly. (photograph 6).

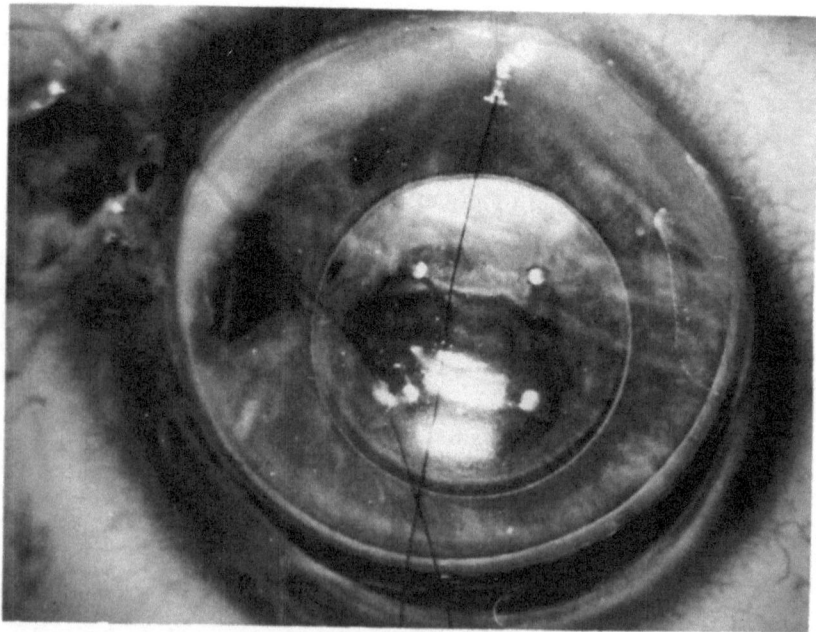

Fig. 4. Implantation and perforating keratoplasty at the same time.

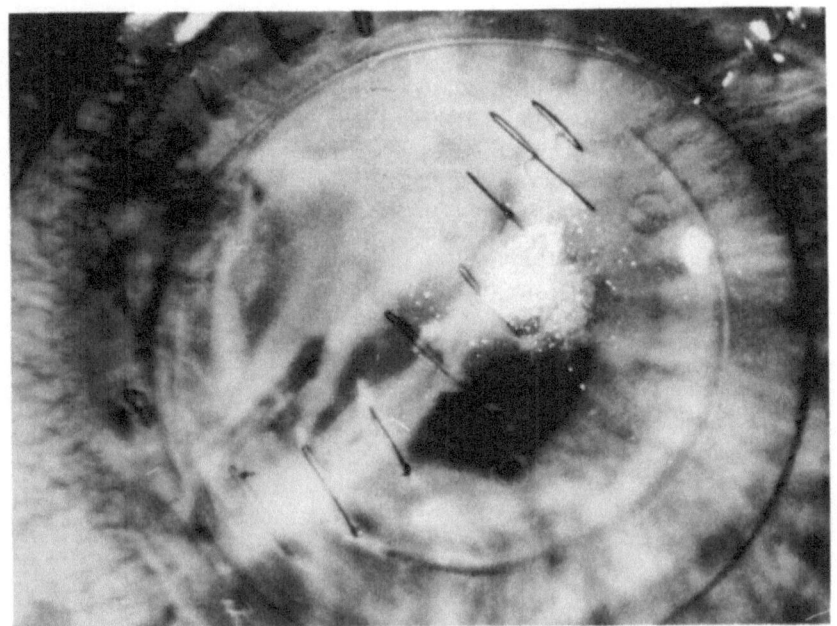

Fig. 5. Indication of perforating graft following an implantation; the corneal cicatrix hinders visual acuity.

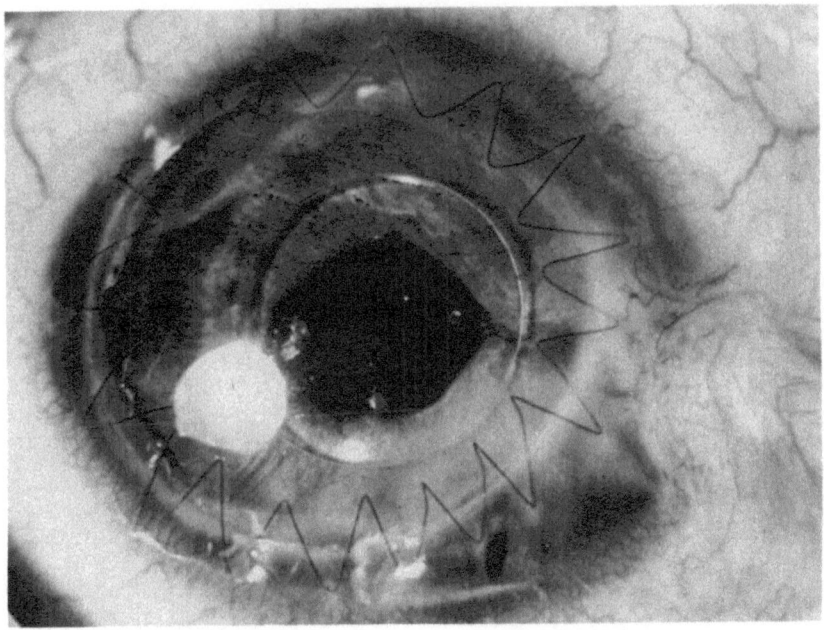

Fig. 6. Perforating graft and implant.

Three conditions seem to be indispensable: a. the surgeon must avoid having to carry out the implantation after perforating keratoplasty: he would very much risk endangering the transparency. b. if the surgeon wishes to retain the possibility of a secondary implantation, it is essential that he respect the posterior capsule of the crystalline lens. c. risk to the retina is a formal contraindication, nad this is why we refuse to make implantations in the following cases:

— intraocular retro-crystalline foreign body;
— after anterior vitrectomy;
— after hemorrhage of the vitreous humour;
— when there is a laceration or a detachment of the opposite eye.

Author's address:
Centre Hospitalier Regional de Nantes
Nantes 44035
France

Docum. Ophthal. Proc. Series, Vol. 21

COMPLICATIONS WITH INTRAOCULAR LENSES

DAVID PATON, M.D.

(Houston, Texas, U.S.A.)

A most significant honor of my life was to be among the hosts to Dr. C.D. Binkhorst when he recently gave a major lecture on intraocular lenses at a meeting in Houston. It was a commensurate honor during that same meeting period to have my picture in the paper with Dr. Joaquin Barraquer, who had summoned me to join him in an interview with a newspaper reporter. Unfortunately, the reporter wanted only to discuss intraocular lenses. Dr. Barraquer, no longer using intraocular lenses, was in a difficult position but was very mild in his statements; it was I who tried to explain to the reporter my own complex feelings in regard to lens implants. You can imagine how embarrassing the published article was to me as a host at the same time to Dr. Binkhorst, and I apologized to him then as I apologize to him again now. He is among the great masters of intraocular lenses — and his work deserves great acclaim.

I think the intraocular lens is the most satisfying way of restoring vision that has ever been available to the cataract surgeon. I also believe it is one of the most hazardous devices that the ophtalmologist can use if his patients are not properly selected, if his technique is less than excellent, or if he and his patient just plain have bad luck, for which there is a multiplicity of causes. Admittedly, we still can not say with certainty whether present day lenses will be tolerated by a large percentage of eyes harboring them for many years. Indications are that most of the recipient eyes will do well indefinitely. There is a term from American history which may be applicable to my own position regarding these devices: Mugwump. This is defined as a person on a fence with his mug on one side and his rump on the other. I do have a middle-of-the-road attitude: excitement and also concern regarding the future of intraocular lenses. I use them, not in large numbers.

My exposure is skewed. I receive referrals of the cases that get into trouble and I see far more of these than of the patients whose post-operative course remains uneventful. In presenting this paper I will illustrate a variety of problems that can occur from a variety of intraocular lenses: endothelial trauma at the time of surgery; the pendulum effect causing corneal damage from a loose iris-clip lens; hyphema with an anterior chamber lens, etc.

In the United States, the Food and Drug Administration now requires surgeons who use devices to report their experience with each case. If the study is properly conducted (and I am uncertain that it will be), the data derived

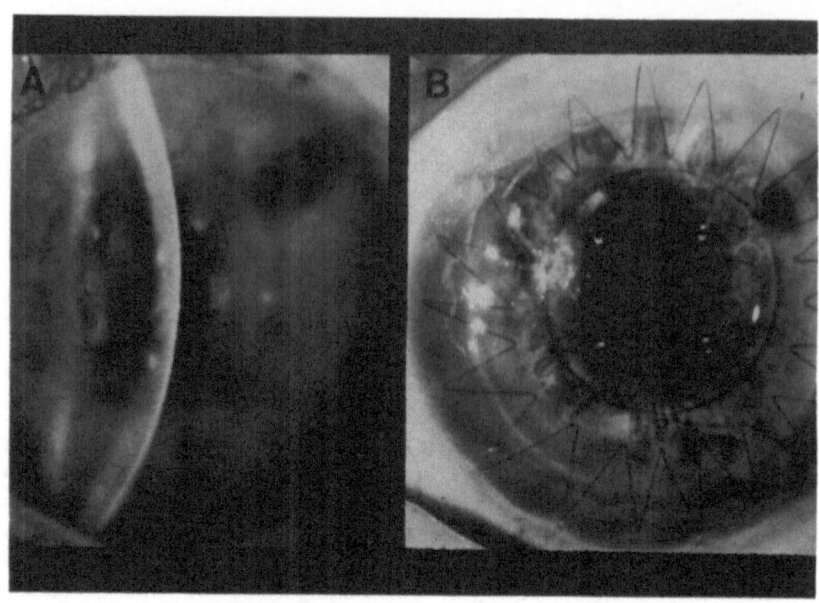

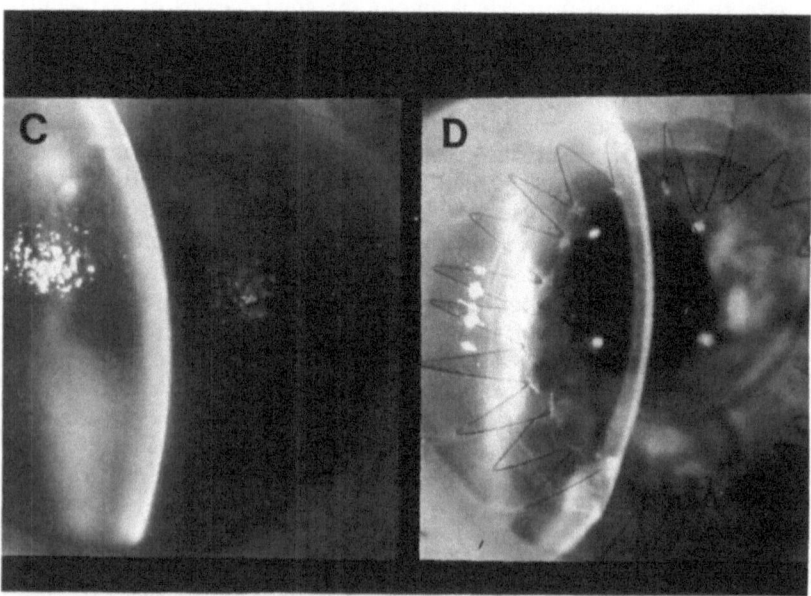

Fig. 1. Representative examples of eyes with bullous keratopathy following placement of intraocular lenses are demonstrated in A and C. The same eyes following penetrating keratoplasty with the implants remaining in position are shown in B and D.

542

should be helpful to the profession. In the meanwhile, there is a healthy hesitancy admixed with much enthusiasm that permeates the majority of implant surgeons in the States.

When bullous keratopathy occurs – and in my observations this is the most common of the major complications – penetrating keratoplasty has an excellent chance of restoring corneal transparency. In most circumstances, at the time of keratoplasty a lens in proper position should not be removed, for it prevents the otherwise inevitable necessity of performing an anterior vitrectomy. Representative examples are shown in Figure 1.

The ideal secure intraocular lens probably remains to be developed. For a presentation at the Fifth Cataract Congress in Miami, Dr. John Craig prepared this illustration of what the perfectly secure lens should look like (Figure 2).

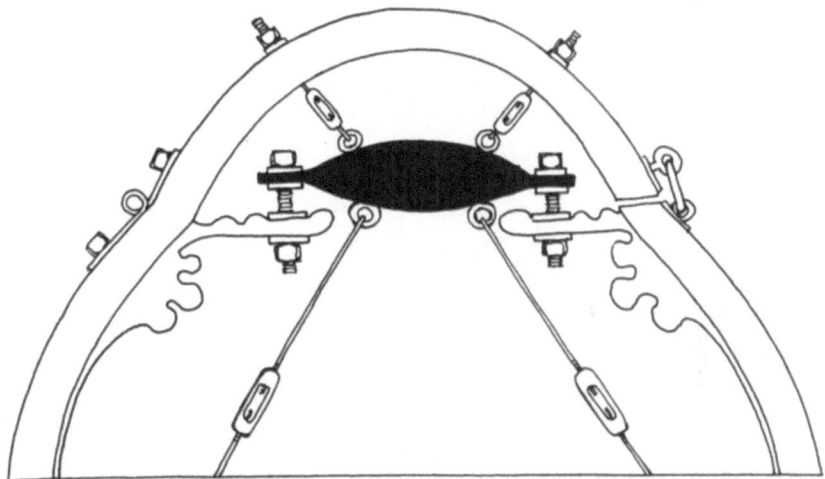

Fig. 2.

Docum. Ophthal. Proc. Series, Vol. 21

COMPLICATIONS WITH INTRAOCULAR LENSES

J. BARRAQUER

(Barcelona, Spain)

Early complications may be caused by technical defects; we encountered such complications in the first years of our experience, from 1954 to 1961.

Late complications, extremely serious, have appeared in many cases after 8, 10 or 15 years of perfect tolerance. The most serious complication is secondary endothelial dystrophy, both from the mechanical effect of contact with the lens and from the degradation of the Supramid of the suspension axis.

The speaker discusses other complications such as atrophy of the iris, secondary glaucoma, dispersion of pigment, etc.

There are also cases where lenses have been well tolerated for 20 years and more; in these cases, we advise prophylactic extraction. If the patient does not agree to this, we advise strict medical control, since once the complications have begun, their consequences can be disastrous.

Docum. Ophthal. Proc. Series, Vol. 21

INTRAOCULAR IMPLANTS IN EXTRA AND INTRACAPSULAR EXTRACTION INCIDENTS AND COMPLICATIONS

B. STRAMPELLI

(Rome, Italy)

From the scientific point of view, the remarkable technical progress made in artiphakia (or pseudophakia as it is sometimes called) by the various authors who have dealt with this subject during the last thirty years, expecially the more recent Worst and Binkhorst, is most praise-worthy. But from the practical point of view the aphorism 'primum non nocere' must never be forgotten.

At present, notwithstanding the notable improvements made in the technique of artiphakia or psuedophakia (including keratophakia), until there is a 100% assurance that no complications will ensue, such an operation should be done only in special cases, i.e., in cases of unilateral aphakia where it is impossible to obtain, with the use of the most highly perfected corneal contact lenses, binocular vision good enough to allow the patient continue his professional activity.

A look at the history of intraocular implants in aphakia shows that such an assurance has never been achieved; thus several different techniques have been tried: from implant in the posterior chamber (generally, introduced into the capsular sac), pioneered by Ridly in 1949, we have gone on to the introduction of the artificial lens in the anterior chamber (Baron, Strampelli, Bietti, Schreck, Barraquer, Charf, Salleras, Dannheim, Boberg, Coyce, Ridley himself, and at present Kermann).

We have then gone on to iris-pupillary fixation, proposed by Sourdille and performed by Vortham, Schillinger, Schearer-Levige, Epstein, Bink-horst, Worst, Baikoff, Feodorov, and Krasnow; finally, the trend has been toward Ridly's first idea, intracapsular fixation in the posterior chamber (Worst, Tearce).

Another method devised in 1956 (Madrid Congress) makes use of an acrylic lens placed in the anterior chamber and anchored to the corneal-scleral covering by means of supramid threads. (An analogous fixation was tried by Apollonio in 1956 and by Parri in 1958).

This technique, which has been in use for more thans 22 years, is shown in the following illustrations (Fig. 1-15). Such a lens can be used even in cases of aniridia and of large coloboma iridis. If necessary, the lens can very easily be removed. Results have been most encouraging in hundreds of cases; however, the supramid threads may become thinner and break even after 15 or 20 years, with luxation and sublixation of the lens and with

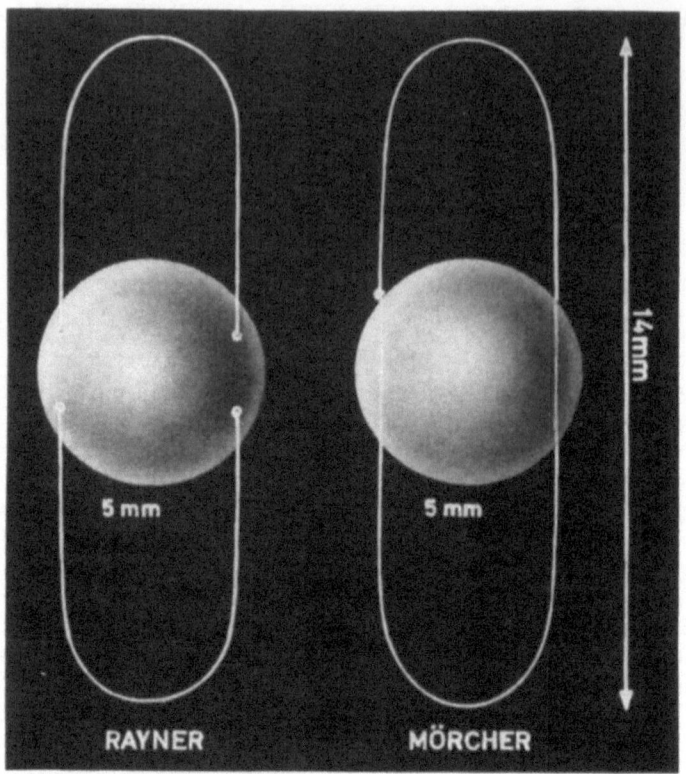

Fig. 1. Acrylic lens for anterior chamber. Rayner Model - Mörcher Model.

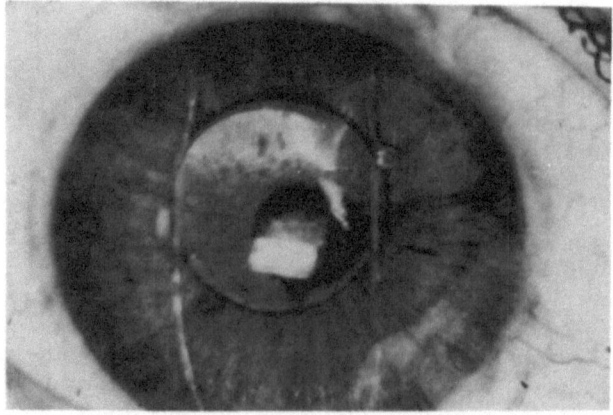

Fig. 2. See text.

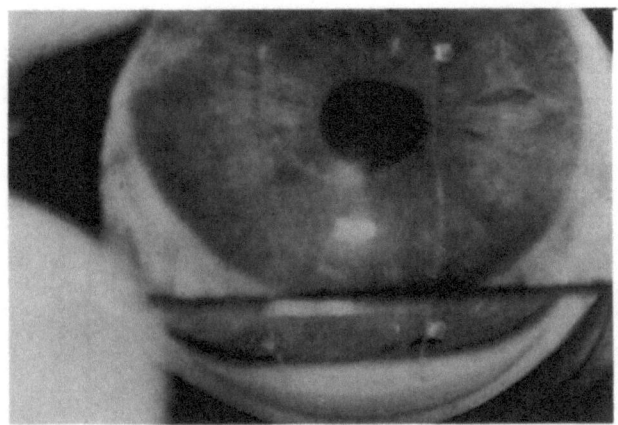

Fig. 3. Same as Fig. 2 upon examination with Goldman's gonioscope. In the mirror, near the bottom, the upper threads which perforate the corneal-scleral membrane are visible.

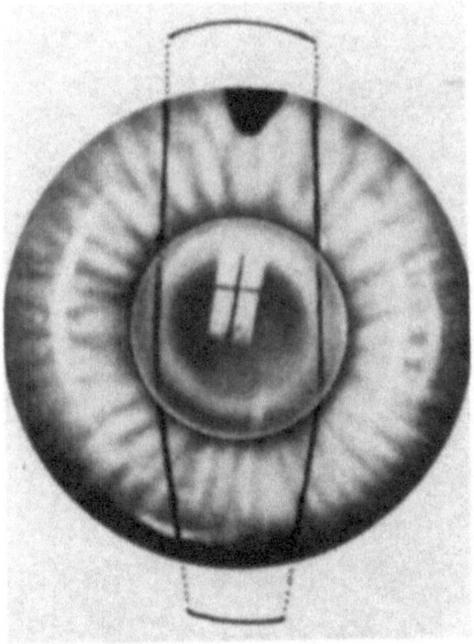

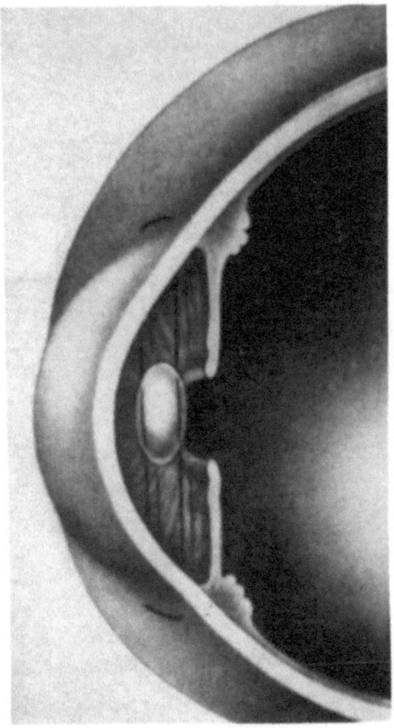

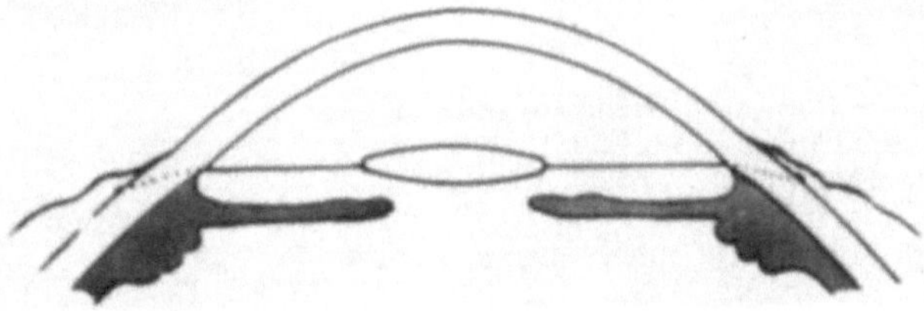

Figs. 4, 5 and 6. See text.

549

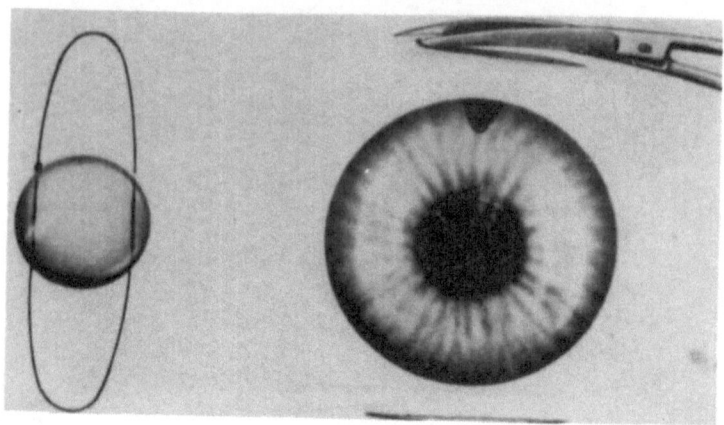

Fig. 7. Incision of the conjunctiva above and below near to the insertion of the rectus muscles.

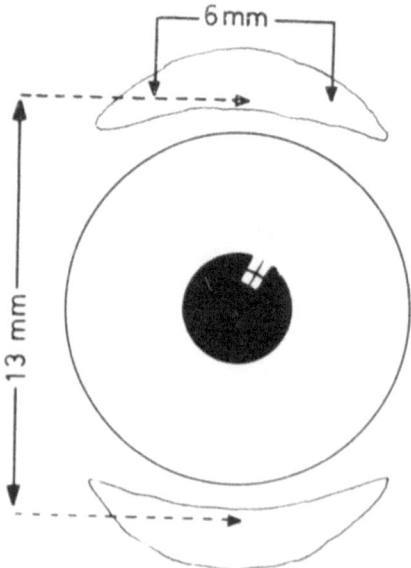

Fig. 8. The points where the lens threads will emerge is indicated above and below, 1 mm. less than the length of the lens itself. Above, the width of 6 mm. is indicated, 1 mm. more than the width of the lens, which is 5 mm.

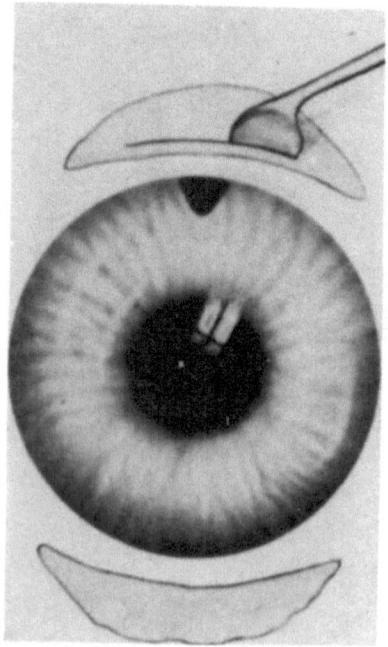

Fig. 9. Incision 'ab externo' of the sclera above.

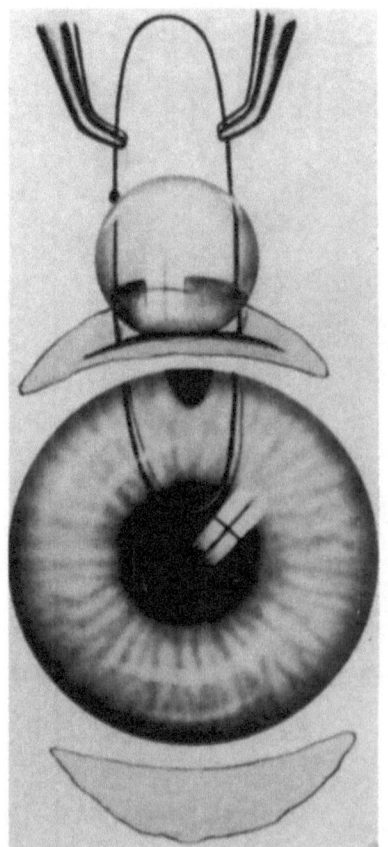

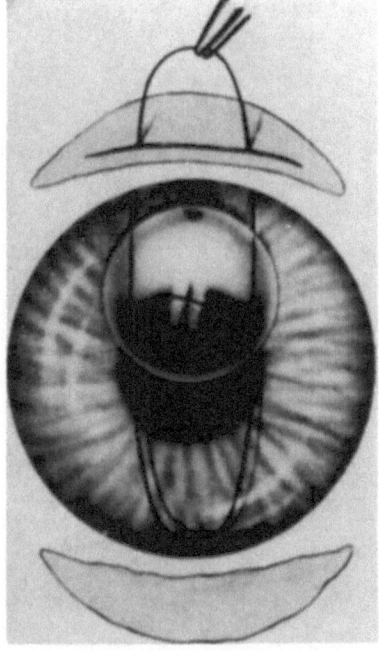

Figs. 10-11. Having opened the anterior chamber and performed an irisdectomy (if not already done previoysly), the lens is introduced into the anterior chamber, leaving the upper loop on the exterior.

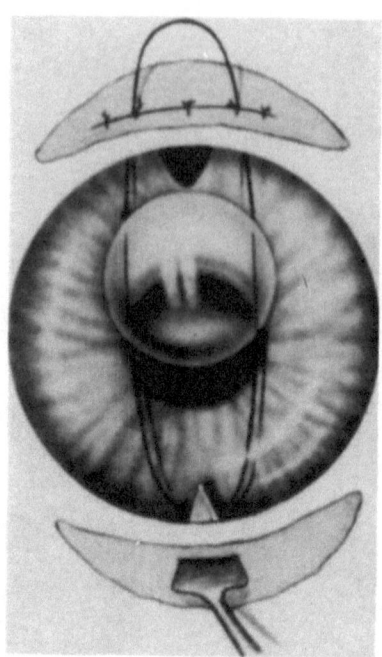

Fig. 12. After having sutured the upper wound with virgin silk, the sclera is opened below with a lancet.

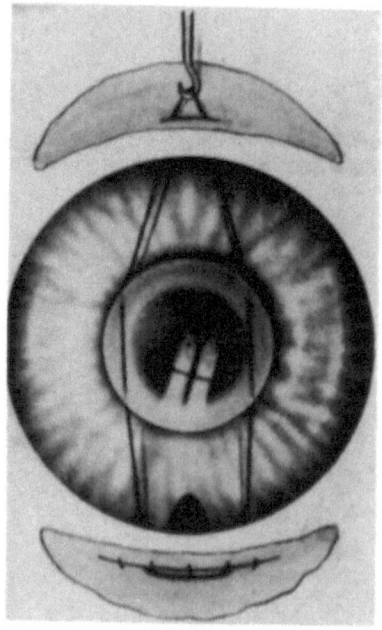

Fig. 13. The lower loop of supramid is pulled out with a small hook.

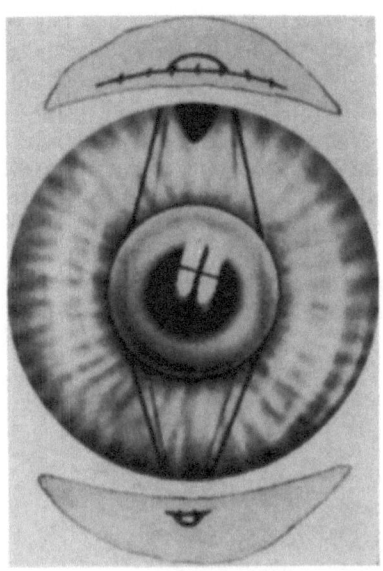

Fig. 14. The lower opening too is sutured, leaving outiside a small loop of supramid thread.

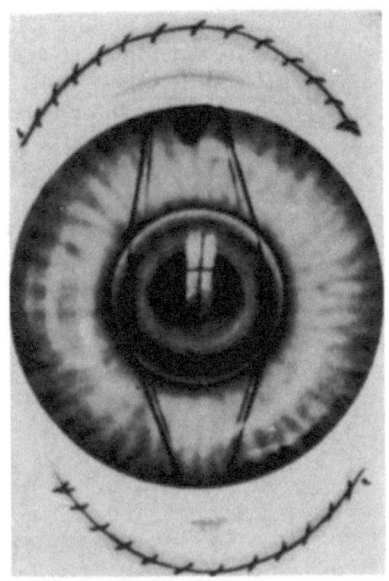

Fig. 15. Finally the upper and lower limbus are sutured in catgut.

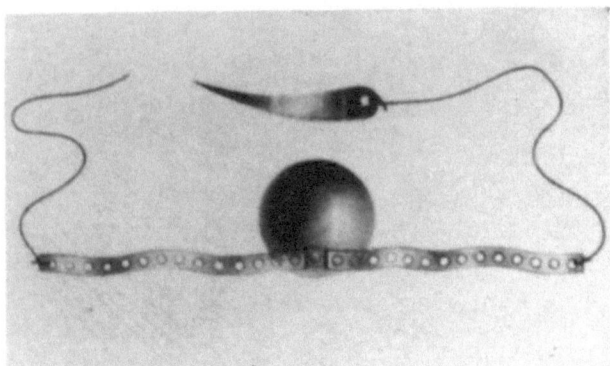

Fig. 16. See text.

unpleasant complications; thus it is better to use propylene or platiniridium threads. For this reason, (see illustrations, Fig. 16-21), fixing the lens with silastic blades or with a pediculate autograft of tenonian tissue (see photo 22) has been tried.

Further improvements have been made in the method of anchoring the attic supports of the lens intrasclerally.

Two successfull cases, operated more thans 21 years ago, can be used as illustration. In the fist case (M.L.), an all-acrylic lens was implanted in the anterior chamber (1953). The patient was a station-master who had had a traumatic cataract in the rigt eye, intracapsularly ɩemoved with excellent results (10/10). In spite of this result, he was prohibited by law from continuing to work as station-master, even using glasses or contact lenses. As he would lose his job otherwise I have then implanted an acrylic lens in the anterior chamber. Five years after the implant, it was necessary to effect a discission due to secondary cataract, and two years later detached retina occured, which was fortunately replaced by operation successfully. The patient is still working as station-master, with excellent binocular vision. In the illustrations (Fig. 23, 24), the final result after 21 years can be seen. This is clearly a case in which artiphakia was necessary.

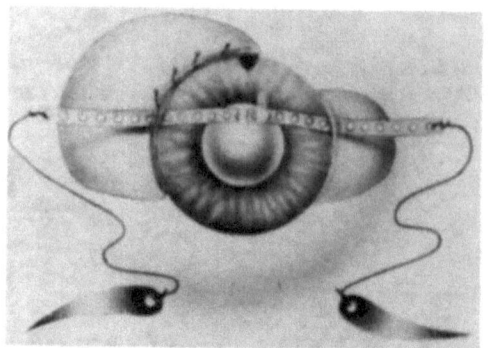

Fig. 17.

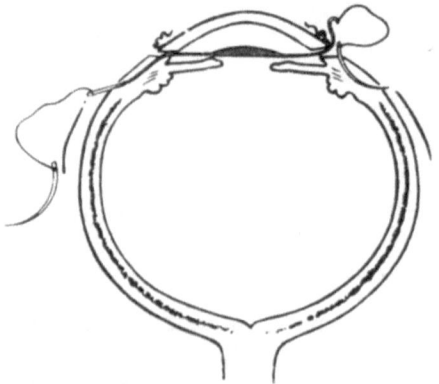

Fig. 18.

554

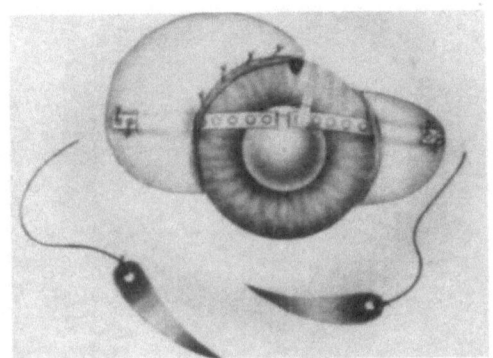

Fig. 19.

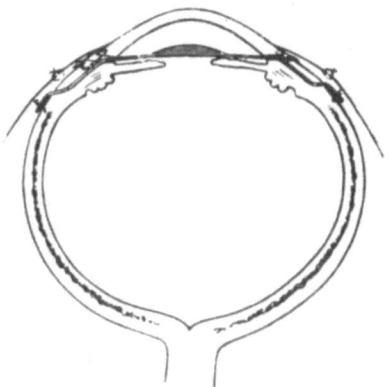

Fig. 20.

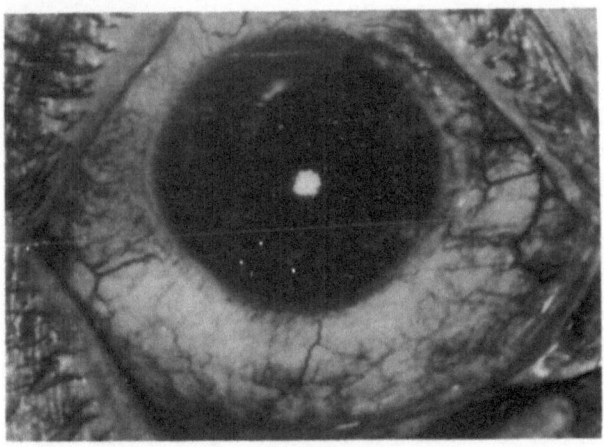

Fig. 21. Lens anchored with tiny silicone straps.

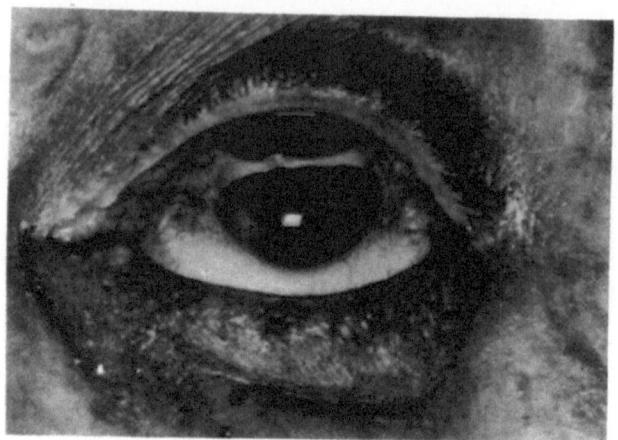

Fig. 22. Lens anchored with tenonian capsule with pediculate flap.

I also operated on another case (C.G.) 21 years ago. In the right eye, a completely acrylic lens was implanted, while in the left eye, an acrylic lens with supramid anchoring to the sclera was implanted. In the photographs (Fig. 25, 26, 27, 28, 29, 30, 31) the results can be seen. The patient has excellent binocular vision without glasses. However, despite the excellent results, such an operation today would not be necessary, since it is now possible to obtain the same results with corneal contact lenses.

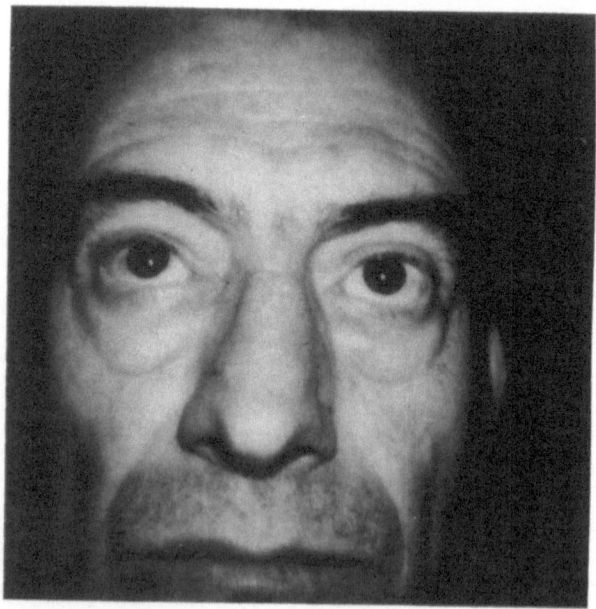

Fig. 23. See text.

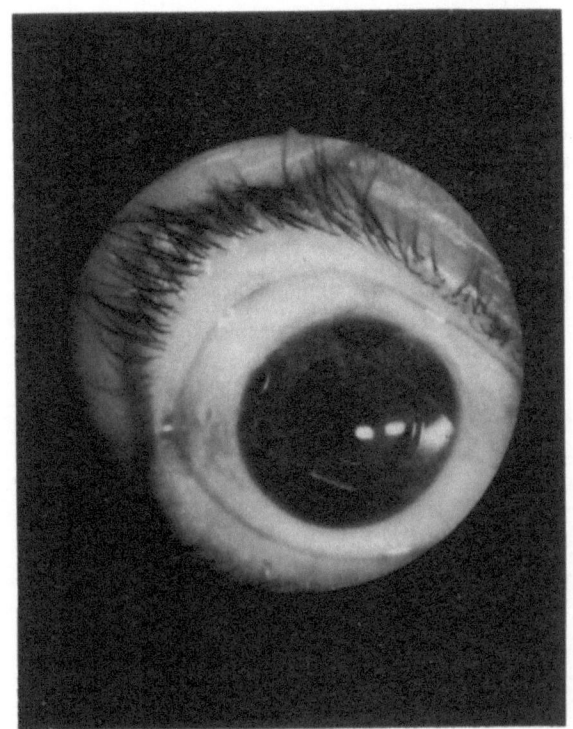

Fig. 24. See text.

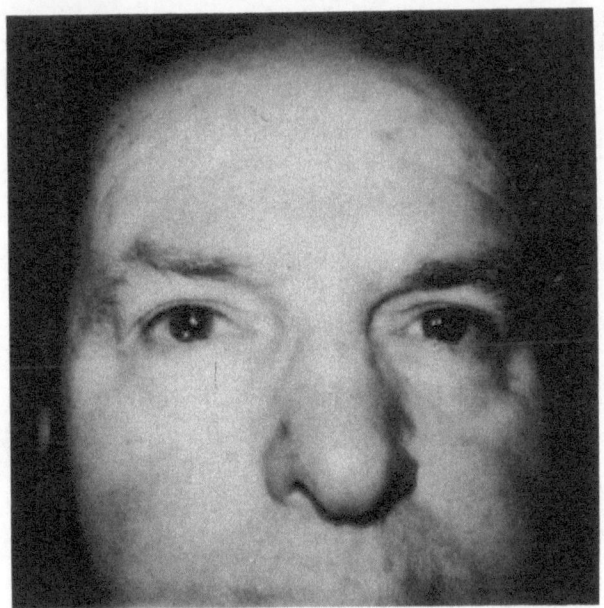

Fig. 25. See text.

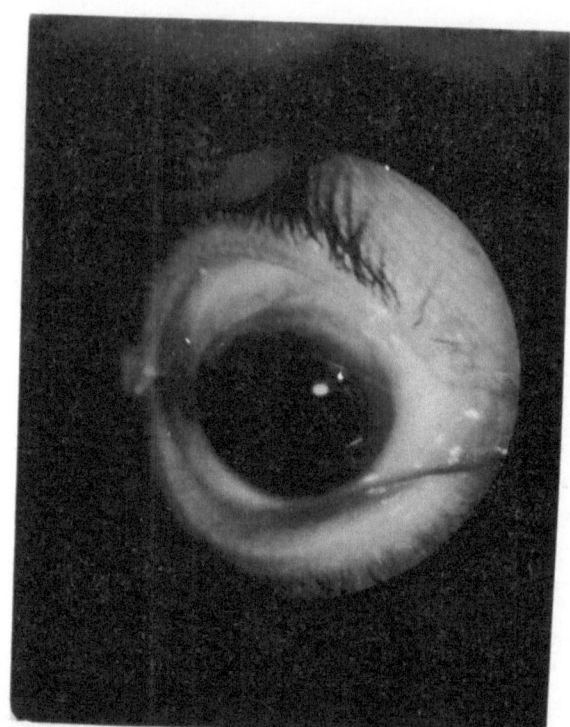

Fig. 26. See text.

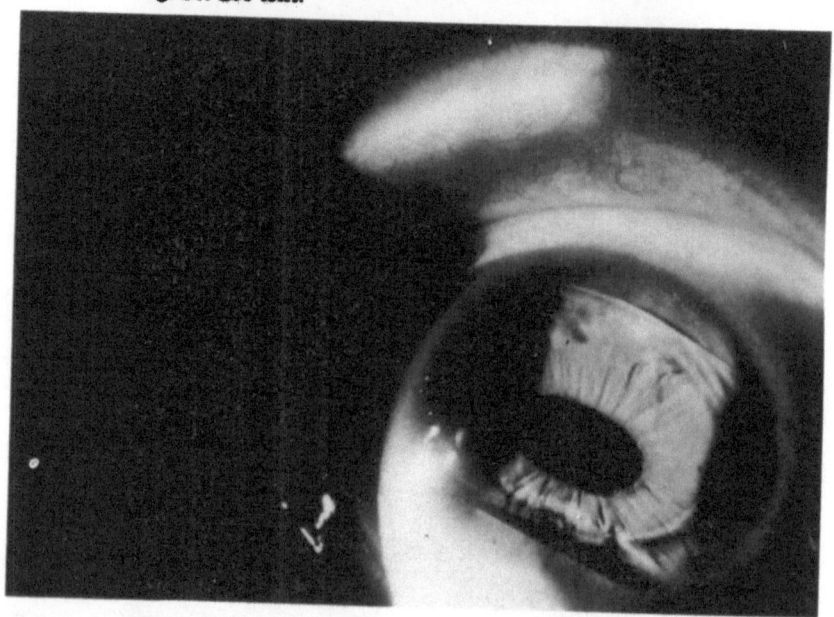

Fig. 27. See text.

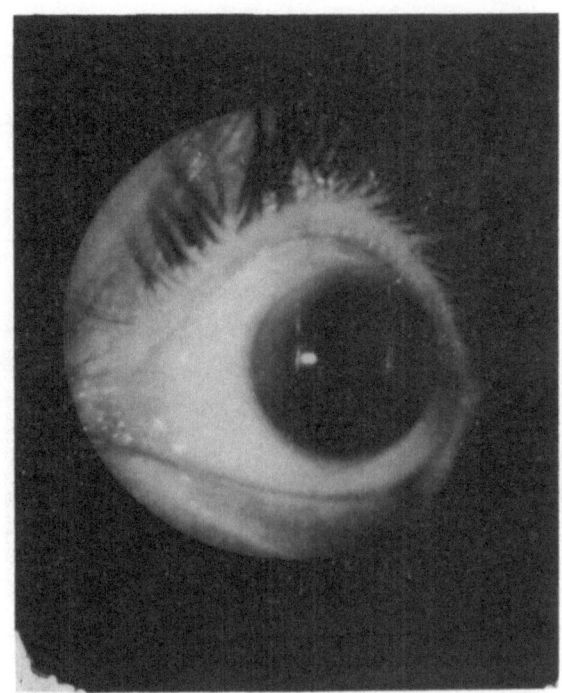

Fig. 28. See text.

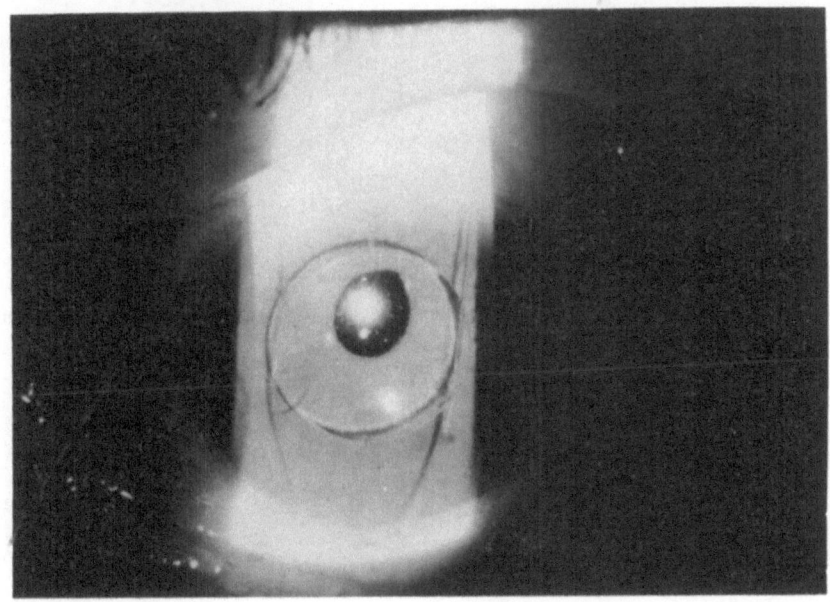

Fig. 29. See text.

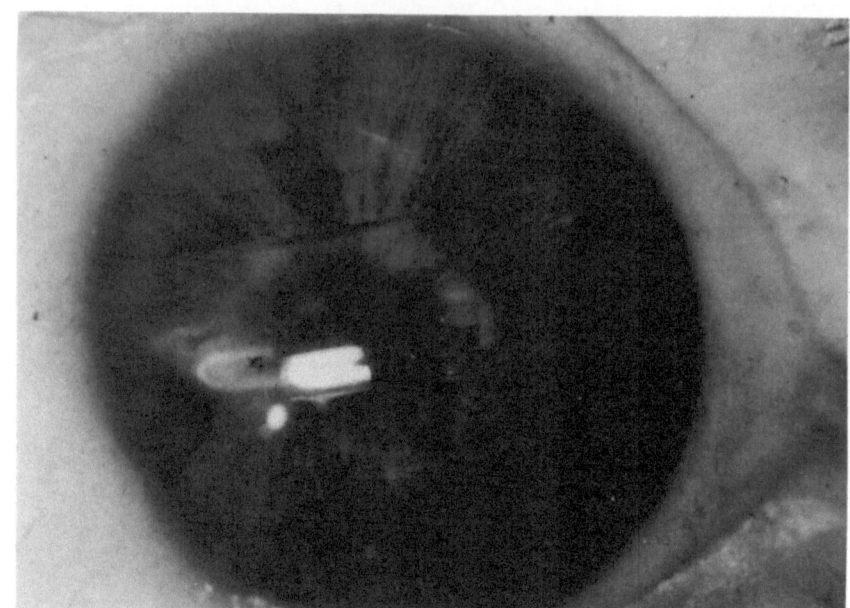

Fig. 30. See text.

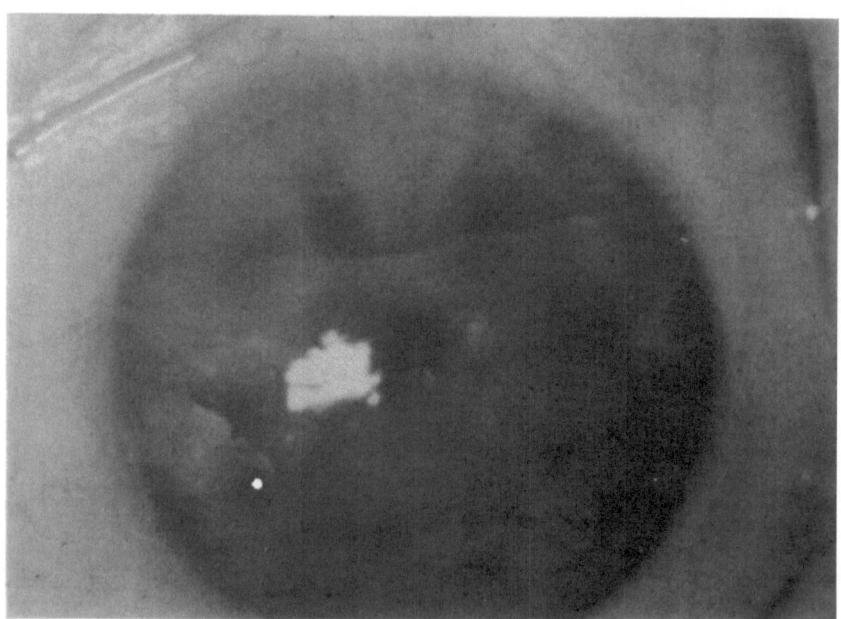

Fig. 31. See text.

560

These two cases show no complications after 21 years, but there are other cases in which, even after 10-15 years, following a period of excellent tolerance, and in the absence of technical errors or displacement of the lens, bullous keratitis had occurred, requiring removal of the lens and keratoplasty.

Thus it must be repeated that artificial lens implant is not to be done without serious forethought, and only in cases of extreme necessity.

Author's address:
65 Cir ne Cornelia
Rome
Italy